D1710154

Invertebrate Medicine

Invertebrate Medicine

Gregory A. Lewbart

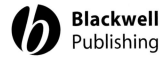

Blackwell Publishing

Gregory A. Lewbart, M.S., V.M.D., Diplomate ACZM, is Professor of Aquatic Animal Medicine, North Carolina State University, College of Veterinary Medicine, Department of Clinical Sciences, Raleigh, North Carolina.

©2006 Blackwell Publishing
All rights reserved

Blackwell Publishing Professional
2121 State Avenue, Ames, Iowa 50014, USA

Orders: 1-800-862-6657
Office: 1-515-292-0140
Fax: 1-515-292-3348
Web site: www.blackwellprofessional.com

Blackwell Publishing Ltd
9600 Garsington Road, Oxford OX4 2DQ, UK
Tel.: +44 (0)1865 776868

Blackwell Publishing Asia
550 Swanston Street, Carlton, Victoria 3053, Australia
Tel.: +61 (0)3 8359 1011

Authorization to photocopy items for internal or personal use, or the internal or personal use of specific clients, is granted by Blackwell Publishing, provided that the base fee of $.10 per copy is paid directly to the Copyright Clearance Center, 222 Rosewood Drive, Danvers, MA 01923. For those organizations that have been granted a photocopy license by CCC, a separate system of payments has been arranged. The fee codes for users of the Transactional Reporting Service are ISBN-13: 978-0-8138-1844-3; ISBN-10: 0-8138-1844-3/2006 $.10.

First edition, 2006

Library of Congress Cataloging-in-Publication Data

Lewbart, Gregory A.
    Invertebrate medicine/Gregory A. Lewbart.—1st ed.
        p. cm.
    Includes bibliographical references and index.
    ISBN-13: 978-0-8138-1844-3 (alk. paper)
    ISBN-10: 0-8138-1844-3 (alk. paper)
    1. Invertebrates—Diseases. 2. Veterinary medicine. I. Title.

    SF997.5.I5L49 2006
    639.7—dc22

                                2005017249

The last digit is the print number: 9 8 7 6 5 4 3 2 1

DEDICATION

To my parents, Marvin and Virginia, for their constant love and support and for introducing me to the wonders of the natural world.

CONTENTS

CONTRIBUTORS

Robert S. Bakal, DVM, MS
US Fish and Wildlife Service
Warm Springs Regional Fish Health Center
Warm Springs, GA 31830, USA
e-mail: Robert_Bakal@FWS.gov

Ilze K. Berzins, PhD, DVM
The Florida Aquarium
Tampa, FL 33602, USA
e-mail: IBerzins@flaquarium.org

Michael S. Bodri, MS, VMD, PhD
North Georgia College and State University
School of Natural and Health Sciences
Health and Natural Sciences Bulding
Dahlonega, GA 30597
e-mail: MSBodri@ngcsu.edu

Robert A. Bullis, DVM, MS
Advanced BioNutrition Corporation
Columbia, MD 21045, USA
e-mail: rbullis@advancedbionutrition.com

John R. Chitty, BVetMed, CertZooMed, CBiol, MIBiol,
    MRCVS
Strathmore Veterinary Clinic
Andover, Hants SP10 2PH, UK
e-mail: xmo32@dial.pipex.com

John E. Cooper, DTVM, FRCPath, FIBiol, FRCVS
Wildlife Health Services (UK)
Comparative Pathology and Forensic Services
Present address:
School of Veterinary Medicine (Mount Hope)
University of the West Indies (UWI)
St Augustine, Trinidad, West Indies
e-mail: NGAGI@vetaid.net

Flavio Corsin, MS, PhD
Network of Aquaculture Centres in Asia-Pacific (NACA)
Department of Fisheries
Kasetsart University Campus
Bangkok 10900, Thailand
e-mail: flavio.corsin@enaca.org

Daniel S. Dombrowski, MS
North Carolina State University
College of Veterinary Medicine
Raleigh, NC 27606, USA
and
North Carolina Museum of Natural Sciences
Raleigh, NC 27601, USA
e-mail: dan.dombrowski@ncmail.net

Laura Foster
North Carolina State University
College of Veterinary Medicine
Raleigh, NC 27606, USA
e-mail: lfoster74@aol.com

Murray E. Fowler, DVM, Dipl ACZM, Dipl ABVT, Dipl
    ACVIM
University of California
School of Veterinary Medicine
Davis, CA 95616, USA
e-mail: mefowler@ucdavis.edu

Fredric L. Frye, DVM, MS, CBiol, FIBiol
La Primavera Farm
Cloverdale, CA 95425-9428, USA
e-mail: FredFrye@aol.com

Amy L. Hancock, VMD
The Philadelphia Zoo
Philadelphia, PA 19104, USA
e-mail: hancock.amy@phillyzoo.org

Craig A. Harms, DVM, PhD, Dipl ACZM
North Carolina State University
Department of Clinical Sciences
College of Veterinary Medicine
Center for Marine Sciences and Technology
Morehead City, NC 28557, USA
e-mail: craig_harms@ncsu.edu

Mac Law, DVM, PhD, Dipl ACVP
North Carolina State University
Department of Population Health and Pathobiology
College of Veterinary Medicine
Raleigh, NC 27606, USA
e-mail: mac_law@ncsu.edu

Jay F. Levine, DVM, MPH
North Carolina State University
College of Veterinary Medicine
Department of Population Health and Pathobiology
Aquatic Animal Epidemiology and Conservation Genomics
    Laboratory
Raleigh, NC 27606, USA
e-mail: jay_levine@ncsu.edu

Gregory A. Lewbart, MS, VMD, Dipl ACZM
North Carolina State University
Department of Clinical Sciences
College of Veterinary Medicine
Raleigh, NC 27606, USA
e-mail: greg_lewbart@ncsu.edu

Michael J. Murray, DVM
Monterey Bay Aquarium
Monterey, CA 93940, USA
e-mail: mmurray@mbayaq.org

Edward J. Noga, MS, DVM
North Carolina State University
Department of Clinical Sciences
College of Veterinary Medicine
Raleigh, NC 27606, USA
e-mail: ed_noga@ncsu.edu

Esther C. Peters, PhD
Registry of Tumors in Lower Animals
Experimental Pathology Laboratories, Inc.
Sterling, VA 20166-4311, USA
e-mail: administrator@pathology-registry.org

Romain Pizzi, BVSc, MS, CertZooMed, FRES, MRCVS,
    MACVSc(Surg)
Edinburgh University
Royal (Dick) School of Veterinary Studies
Department of Veterinary Clinical Studies
Midlothian EH25 9RG, UK
e-mail: romain.pizzi@ed.ac.uk

Joseph M. Scimeca, DVM, PhD
Southern Illinois University
Research Development and Administration—SIUC
Carbondale, IL 62901, USA
e-mail: jscimeca@siv.edu

Stephen A. Smith, DVM, PhD
Department of Biomedical Sciences and Pathobiology
Virginia/Maryland Regional College of Veterinary Medicine
Virginia Polytechnic Institute and State University
Blacksburg, VA 24061-0442, USA
e-mail: Stsmith7@vt.edu

Roxanna Smolowitz, DVM
Marine Biological Laboratory
Woods Hole, MA 02543, USA
e-mail: rsmol@mbl.edu

Michael K. Stoskopf, DVM, PhD, Dipl ACZM
Department of Clinical Sciences
North Carolina State University
College of Veterinary Medicine
Raleigh, NC 27606, USA
e-mail: michael_stoskopf@ncsu.edu

FOREWORD

It has been interesting to witness the evolution of modern veterinary care for nontraditional animal species. The year 1950 heralded the founding of the American Association of Zoo Veterinarians and attracted veterinarians interested in all types of captive wild animals. A year later, in 1951, the Wildlife Disease Association was founded. Both of these organizations had as their founding goal the sharing and dissemination of information.

With an increased interest in birds in many veterinary practices, a new group, the Association of Avian Veterinarians, was formed and with it came a plethora of literature on the subject. A number of books on reptile and amphibian medicine stimulated an intense interest in these animals, and the Association of Reptilian and Amphibian Veterinarians came into being.

If history repeats itself, the publication of this comprehensive book on the medicine of invertebrates will stimulate greater interest in the innumerable species of animals without backbones (and rightfully so, as 80% of the animal biomass of this planet consists of invertebrates, not elephants and blue whales). Insects alone account for more than three quarters of the world's animal species.

When I began working with nontraditional animals, I would kid my colleagues that they dealt with only 2–8 species of domestic animals while I was concerned with nearly 50,000 vertebrates and millions of species of invertebrates. Early in my career, a neighbor's little girl came to my door with a shoebox containing a crayfish that she had acquired as a pet. "Dr. Fowler, is this crayfish a boy or a girl?"—a pretty basic question that I couldn't answer; however, I learned and answered the girl's question.

Insectariums have become important attractions in many zoos, with some exhibits traveling from one zoo to another on contract. A zoo in Japan designed a building with the roof in the form of a butterfly. International tourists are permitted to visit a butterfly farm on the Island of Aruba on the north coast of Venezuela.

The interest in the medical care of invertebrates is not limited to the United States. A recent conference in Brazil spotlighted a veterinarian who provides intensive care, including fluid therapy, for spiders, scorpions, and praying mantises.

Interest in invertebrate medicine is not limited to captive species. A catchword in the 21st century is *biodiversity*. Invertebrates are important contributors to the food chain for vertebrates, including humans. Invertebrates may be involved in the transmission of epidemic diseases and may cause disease themselves.

Invertebrates are subject to many toxic substances and may become locally or regionally extinct from pollution. The Mexican red-kneed spider is currently listed in Appendix 2 of the Convention on International Trade in Endangered Species of Wild Fauna and Flora (CITES), one of many CITES-listed invertebrate species throughout the world. Should captive breeding be contemplated to reestablish a population of endangered spiders or other invertebrates, knowledge of their diseases and medical management could be critically important.

For veterinarians to provide optimal veterinary care, they must have a basic understanding of the biology of the species they are attempting to help. Although this book is not meant to be a definitive natural history of invertebrates, it does provide basic biology.

The editor has brought together a varied group of authors who have a specialized interest in each topic, many of whom have research or clinical experience with invertebrates. The result is a comprehensive volume on the veterinary care of invertebrates that are harvested or reared for human food, are kept in captivity as pets or for exhibition, or are being used as research models. The editor and authors are fully aware that there are significant gaps in the scientific information available on some taxa. Nevertheless, this foundation work will spur others to take steps to observe, conduct research, and provide clinical care for these special animals that are the ultimate beneficiary of the dedication and efforts of the editor and authors.

Murray E. Fowler, DVM, Dipl ACZM, Dipl ABVT, Dipl ACVIM
Professor Emeritus, Zoological Medicine
School of Veterinary Medicine
University of California
Davis, California

PREFACE

For many decades, invertebrates have been kept as pets, displayed in aquariums and zoos, used for research, and consumed. Maintaining live invertebrates in captivity is becoming more sophisticated and popular as time passes. Arthropod zoos and insectariums, jellyfish exhibits, and captive living coral reefs are relatively commonplace today but were rare or nonexistent 20 years ago. Despite this popularity, diversity, and economic importance, though, veterinary medicine has traditionally paid little attention to this huge chunk (over 95% of the earth's animal species) of the animal kingdom.

My own interest in invertebrates started on a family trip to Campobello Island in New Brunswick, Canada, nearly 4 decades ago. Finding a sand dollar test on the beach was an exciting moment for a young boy, as was the subsequent quest to identify it. Years later, I found myself studying invertebrate zoology at Gettysburg College; my professor was Dr. Robert D. Barnes. After exciting field trips with Dr. Barnes to the Duke University Marine Laboratory in Beaufort, North Carolina, and the Bermuda Biological Station, I was definitely hooked! These educational experiences were a pivotal point in my life and I hold a special place in my heart and mind for Dr. Barnes and his inspirational teaching.

I began thinking about working on a veterinary text for invertebrates in the early 1990s and was very happy (and just a little apprehensive) when I signed a contract to edit this text with Blackwell Publishing Professional (at the time Iowa State University Press) in 2001.

This book is the product of a concerted effort by a group of dedicated authors on the topic of invertebrate animal medicine. This is not an invertebrate zoology text and is by no means comprehensive with regard to the anatomy, physiology, natural history, and taxonomy of the myriad of invertebrate taxa. This is a veterinary text about invertebrate animals that includes pertinent biological data as well as state-of-the-science information pertaining to medicine and the clinical condition. It is my hope that this book will be a valuable guide to those charged with the medical care and well-being of both captive and wild invertebrate animals.

At the North Carolina State University College of Veterinary Medicine (NCSU-CVM), my students and colleagues continually inspire me. Several years ago, the veterinary students started the Invertebrate Medicine Club, and we now offer an intensive 1-week elective course on invertebrate medicine. The NCSU-CVM administration has been extremely encouraging of these efforts, and I am grateful and fortunate to be working in such a rich, supportive environment.

I am very excited about invertebrate animal medicine and hope you will join me in this excitement. There is much work to be done in this realm in which the opportunities are truly endless.

Gregory A. Lewbart, MS, VMD, Dipl ACZM
Professor of Aquatic Animal Medicine
Department of Clinical Sciences
North Carolina State University
College of Veterinary Medicine

ACKNOWLEDGMENTS

A project like this could not come to fruition without the help, support, and assistance of many individuals.

For their instruction, inspiration, guidance, support, and mentoring during my student years, I thank all of my mentors and professors, but, in particular, Donald Abt, Robert Barnes, Philip Bookman, Dale Dickey, John Gratzek, Louis Leibovitz, William Medway, Trish Morse, Nathan "Doc" Riser, Ralph Sorensen, and Richard Wolke. Doc was my master's thesis advisor and I am especially grateful for his knowledge, wisdom, and patience. I am fortunate to be associated with the North Carolina State University College of Veterinary Medicine (NCSU-CVM), a fine, progressive institution of higher learning. I am grateful to all of my NCSU-CVM friends and colleagues. Oscar Fletcher, Craig Harms, Edward Noga, Elizabeth Stone, and Michael Stoskopf have been especially supportive. Craig Harms reviewed many of the chapters, and I am indebted to him for his keen eye, advice, patience, and friendship.

I also collectively thank the veterinary students I have worked with, both at the NCSU-CVM and those from other colleges of veterinary medicine. They are the bright future of our profession, and I know some days they teach me more than I teach them. Dan Dombrowski, one of this book's authors, deserves special mention as an inspiration to all those interested in keeping and caring for the earth's invertebrates.

The following individuals were generous in providing case material, images, suggestions, and other assistance: Genevieve Anderson, Rich Aronson, Herman Berkhoff, Charles Bland, Shane Boylan, James Brock, Mike Buchal, Rick Cawthorn, James Clark, Angelo Colorni, David Engel, Carlton Goldthwaite, Stacey Gore, Malcolm Hill, Sarah Joyner, Kelly Krell, Wade Lehmann, Douglas Mader, Stuart May, Jim Moore, Alf Nilsen, Hendrik Nollens, David Rotstein, Clay Rouse, Melanie Rembert, Johanna Sherrill, Jerry Stevens, Cinamon Vann, and Nicole Webster. Richard Fox and Eric Borneman were especially generous in providing images, and Esther Peters's input on neoplasia and other aspects of the book were invaluable.

I am grateful to Alison Schroeer and Brenda Bunch, both outstanding biological illustrators, who provided high-quality images and were tolerant of my numerous requests and deadlines. I also thank the helpful personnel of the NCSU-CVM Biomedical Communications Department.

I am very grateful to the talented group of authors that constructed this diverse collection of chapters; there would be no *Invertebrate Medicine* without their hard work, dedication, and commitment to the project. As the book's editor, I take full responsibility for any errors or omissions.

The folks at Blackwell Publishing have been exceptional through this entire process. They are true professionals and a pleasure to work with. I specifically acknowledge David Rosenbaum, the person who "signed me up"; Cheryl Garton, who helped in the early stages; Antonia Seymour, the editorial director supervising this project; Jamie Johnson, who patiently waited for appropriately formatted figures; Judi Brown, who made certain everything was in order for the presses; and, finally, Dede Pederson, my managing editor, who was always there for this book and me. Thanks Dede!

John Flukas did a tremendous job of copyediting the manuscript and deserves special mention. His meticulous proofreading and editorial skills have greatly improved the book. He's also one of the most calm and easygoing people I've ever worked with.

I really don't think I could have completed this book without the dedicated and selfless help of Shane Christian during the past 3 years. He is simply the most reliable and competent person I know, and his efforts allowed me the time to focus on this project. Thanks Shane!

Finally, I am so very grateful for the love and support I consistently receive from my wonderful wife, Diane Deresienski. Her advice is always sound. Her ideas always good. Her hugs always warm. And she's a top-notch veterinarian who I deeply admire and respect.

Gregory A. Lewbart

Invertebrate Medicine

Chapter 1

INTRODUCTION

Gregory A. Lewbart

The book before you is the product of a concerted effort by a group of dedicated authors on the topic of invertebrate animal medicine. This is not an invertebrate zoology text and is by no means comprehensive with regard to the anatomy, physiology, natural history, and taxonomy of the myriad of invertebrate taxa. This is a veterinary text about invertebrate animals. It includes pertinent biological information as well as state of the science information pertaining to medicine and the clinical condition.

What sort of topic is invertebrate medicine? And what exactly are invertebrates? Ruppert and Barnes (1994) have said that the invertebrates are a group of unrelated taxa that share no universal "positive" traits. Undergraduate and graduate courses are dedicated to invertebrate zoology or even to specific parts of this topic, such as entomology, malacology, or protozoology. Simply put, the invertebrates are a collection of animals, comprising more than 95% of the earth's species, unified by the lack of a vertebral column. Depending on the text or investigator, there are currently over 30 recognized phyla of invertebrates (not including the protozoans). Many of these might be considered obscure, but for no better reason than they may contain few species, microscopic representatives, or have no obvious economic value to humans. In reality, each phylum and its members are important to the diversity and survival of the planet, even if the group is only studied by a small number of investigators. Unfortunately, very little is known about the veterinary aspects of many of these taxa, and writing a comprehensive text for all invertebrate phyla would currently be a daunting and somewhat inefficient task. Consequently, I have elected to include, at least in this volume, the most economically important and "visible" metazoan taxonomic groups. Exclusively parasitic taxa (e.g., trematodes, cestodes, and acanthocephalans) are only touched upon. Table 1.1, which lists the major taxonomic groups (along with brief descriptions) that do not have their own chapter, has been included in an effort to remind readers of the diversity of the invertebrate animal kingdom. Table 1.2 provides a snapshot of animal diversity with regard to number of described species and habitat. I encourage interested readers to obtain one or more of the general invertebrate zoology texts listed under General Invertebrate Zoology References, where detailed descriptions of the various groups in Table 1.1 and throughout this book can be found.

Table 1.1. Invertebrate phyla and major classes not reviewed in this book

Placozoa: A monotypic phylum containing only the species *Trichoplax adhaerens.* This primitive amoeboid metazoan is flattened, less than 3 mm in diameter, and exhibits extracellular digestion of detritus and algae.

Orthonectida: A very small phylum (about 20 species) of very small (no larger than 1 mm) internal parasites of other invertebrates such as bivalves, polychaetes, tunicates, turbellarians, and nemerteans.

Dicyemida: This phylum contains about 75 species of very thin renal parasites of cephalopods.

Nemertea: This diverse phylum contains approximately 1150 species of *ribbon worms,* which tend to be much larger and longer than flatworms. Unlike flatworms, nemerteans have a true coelomic circulatory system. Most are marine, but there are a few freshwater and terrestrial forms. Nemerteans are predators and use a long, eversible proboscis to capture and retain prey.

Mollusk groups

  Aplacophora: This class consists of about 300 species of small, vermiform, marine animals that live at depths of between 200 and 7000 m.

  Polyplacophora: Commonly known as the *chitons,* these interesting mollusks are mobile but spend most of their time tightly adhered to rocky substrates. There are approximately 800 exclusively marine species described. All have eight valves or plates (hence the name of the class) that overlap and are connected by soft tissue and surrounded by a muscular "girdle." Most species could rest in your palm, but one, *Cryptochiton* sp., the stocky gumshoe chiton, can reach a length of about 40 cm.

  Scaphopoda: Known as the tusk or tooth mollusks because of their shell shape. The approximately 500 species are all marine, and most are burrowers with the head facing down within the substrate.

Echiura: Commonly known as the *spoon worms,* most of the 150 species either live in U-shaped burrows or between rocks closely associated with the marine environment. Most are deposit feeders, and some are an important food source for fishes. The name comes from the large and flared prostomium that resembles a spoon or small scoop.

(continued)

Table 1.1. *(continued)*

Sipuncula: The sipunculids, or *peanut worms*, are a group of about 150 marine burrowing species. Most are smaller than 10 cm, but some can reach 70 cm in length. They possess an interesting feeding structure termed the *introvert* that can be expelled from or retracted into the main body or trunk.

Onychophora: This group of tropical, terrestrial animals (110 known species) are commonly referred to as *velvet worms* or *walking worms*. They are segmented and aligned with arthropods. In fact, some workers include the phyla Onychophora, Tardigrada, and Arthropoda in the superphylum Panarthropoda. Velvet worms prey on smaller arthropods by capturing them with slime ejected from paired glands near the mouth.

Tardigrada: If the *water bears*, as they are commonly known, grew larger (most are less than 1 mm long), they would surely be common and popular pets and display animals. There are marine, freshwater, and terrestrial representatives among the 800-plus species in this group of taxonomically mysterious animals. They have features in common with the arthropods but are different enough to warrant their own phylum. Perhaps their most interesting attribute is their ability to undergo cryptobiosis and form desiccated *tuns*, which can withstand adverse environmental conditions. In fact, some tardigrades may live as long as 100 years with the aid of cryptobiosis.

Gastrotricha: Many of the 500 species belonging to this microscopic phylum are interstitial. Most appear like miniature bowling pins atop two small pegs. There are freshwater and marine forms.

Nematomorpha: The *horsehair worms* superficially resemble nematodes but are very long and free-living as adults. The larvae usually parasitize either crustaceans or insects. Approximately 325 species have been described.

Priapulida: This small phylum containing just 18 species is all marine and benthic. They are cylindrical and resemble a small cactus.

Loricifera: This interesting and microscopic marine phylum (all appear to be interstitial) was not known to science until 1983. Many of the 100 or so known species have not yet been described due to the difficulty in examining fresh, living specimens. These little creatures are so dogged in their attachment to sand grains that only freshwater will dislodge them, causing osmotic damage and distortion of their anatomy.

Kinorhyncha: The *mud dragons* somewhat resemble the Gastrotricha in general shape but have an oral feeding structure called the *oral styles* at the end of a movable introvert. Most are microscopic and are either interstitial or benthic on mud and sand. There are approximately 150 species and all are marine.

Gnathostomulida: Virtually all 80 known species are marine, interstitial, and less than 1 mm long. They are vermiform and were not known to science until 1956.

Rotifera: Most occur in freshwater, but there are marine and terrestrial (primarily in water films) species. They are defined and frequently identified by the ciliated corona or *wheel organ* near the head. Some rotifers are extremely important in freshwater and marine food chains (in some cases, hundreds may be found in a liter of water) and are also commonly reared to support invertebrate and finfish aquaculture. There are approximately 2000 described species.

Acanthocephala: A totally parasitic group containing 1150 species. They are commonly known as thorny-headed worms, and some are important parasites of wild and domestic vertebrates. Most use other invertebrates as intermediate hosts.

Kamptozoa: Also known as Entoprocta, the 150 species are nearly all marine. Most are stalked, and some people refer to them as *nodders* because of the zooid's tendency to nod or rock at the end of the stalk. Although some zoologists still classify them as bryozoans, these animals differ in their complete lack of a coelomic cavity. Some zoologists feel the morphological similarities between the groups are convergent.

Cycliophora: This small (in size and species number) phylum was not introduced to science until 1995. The single described species, *Symbion pandora*, exhibits a commensal lifestyle with a lobster (*Nephrops* sp.). Other as yet undescribed species are commensal with other crustaceans, including the American lobster, *Homarus americanus*. They are suspension feeders and have a complex reproductive cycle with both asexual and sexual life stages. None of the life stages are over 0.5 mm long.

Phoronida: There are just 14 species in two genera of these sessile marine creatures. These vermiform animals live in chitinous tubes that they secrete. Although externally they are bilaterally symmetrical, internally the left side is dominant. They feed by means of a lophophore and are grouped into the superphylum Lophophorata along with the bryozoans and brachiopods.

Brachiopoda: The brachiopods, or *lamp shells*, are an interesting group of 350 extant marine species that grossly resemble bivalve mollusks. Thousands of species are known from the fossil record, in part due to their mineralized valves that are preserved well. They are not related to mollusks, and the hard valves that protect the soft body are oriented opposite that of the bivalve's. They feed with the aid of a lophophore, placing them in the superphylum Lophophorata. Most are the size of small *cherrystone* clams and frequently turn up in shops specializing in fossils. Most species occur in colder waters.

Bryozoa: Known as the *moss animals*, these are common animals that can be found on many marine substrates (there are a few freshwater species), including rocks, algae, pilings, and even living animals such as sea turtles. With nearly 5000 species, this phylum is the best known of the Lophophorata and is usually studied as part of nearly all basic invertebrate zoology courses. The vast majority are colonial, although there is one solitary genus. From a distance, they may look more like plants than animals to casual observers. Some colonies are polymorphic, whereas other species are monomorphic. They are filter feeders, using the lophophore to trap and retain small food items.

Arthropoda

Pycnogonida: Known commonly as the *sea spiders*, this class of arthropods contains about 1000 known species. They are all marine and widely distributed, with most occurring in benthic habitats. Very few species are larger than 1 cm, and although they resemble a true spider, they are not close relatives.

Taxonomy and descriptions are from Ruppert et al. (2004).

Table 1.2. Habitats and approximate metazoan species numbers

Phylum	Benthic Marine	Pelagic Marine	Benthic Freshwater	Pelagic Freshwater	Terrestrial	Ectosymbiotic	Endosymbiotic
Porifera	###	—	#	—	—	#	—
Placozoa	#	—	—	—	—	—	—
Orthonectida	—	—	—	—	—	—	#
Dicyemida	—	—	—	—	—	—	#
Cnidaria	###	##	#	#	—	#	—
Ctenophora	#	#	—	—	—	—	—
Platyhelminthes	###	#	###	—	##	#	####
Nemertea	##	#	#	—	#	#	—
Mollusca	#####	#	###	—	###	#	#
Annelida	####	#	##	—	###	##	—
Echiura	##	—	—	—	—	—	—
Sipuncula	##	—	—	—	#	—	—
Onychophora	—	—	—	—	##	—	—
Tardigrada	#	—	##	—	#	—	—
Arthropoda	####	###	####	###	#####	###	###
Gastrotricha	##	—	##	—	—	—	—
Nematoda	###	#	###	#	###	###	###
Nematomorpha	—	—	—	—	—	—	##
Priapulida	#	—	—	—	—	—	—
Loricifera	#	—	—	—	—	—	—
Kinorhyncha	##	—	—	—	—	—	—
Gnathostomulida	#	—	—	—	—	—	—
Rotifera	#	#	##	##	#	#	#
Acanthocephala	—	—	—	—	—	—	###
Kamptozoa	##	—	#	—	—	#	—
Cycliophora	—	—	—	—	—	#	—
Phoronida	#	—	—	—	—	—	—
Brachiopoda	##	—	—	—	—	—	—
Bryozoa	###	—	#	—	—	—	—
Chaetognatha	#	#	—	—	—	—	—
Hemichordata	#	—	—	—	—	—	—
Echinodermata	###	#	—	—	—	—	—
Chordata (Cephahochordata and Urochordata)	###	#	—	—	—	—	—
Chordata (Vertebrata)	###	###	##	###	####	#	#

#, 1–100; ##, 100–1000; ###, 1000–10,000; ####, 10,000–100,000; and #####, over 100,000.
Modified from Pearse et al. (1987), p. 7; with taxonomic and number updates from Ruppert et al. (2004).

References

Pearse V, Pearse J, Buchsbaum M, and Buchsbaum R. 1987. Living Invertebrates. Blackwell Scientific, Palo Alto, CA, 848 pp.

Ruppert EE and Barnes RD. 1994. Invertebrate Zoology, 6th edition. Saunders College, Philadelphia, pp 499–595.

Ruppert EE, Fox RS, and Barnes RD. 2004. Invertebrate Zoology: A Functional Evolutionary Approach, 7th edition. Brooks/Cole—Thomson Learning, Belmont, CA, 963 pp.

General Invertebrate Zoology References

Barnes, RSK, Calow P, Olive PJW, Golding DW, and JI Spicer. 2001. The Invertebrates; A Synthesis, 3rd ed. Blackwell Science Ltd., 497 pp.

Barrington EJW. 1979. Invertebrate Structure and Function, 2nd ed. John Wiley & Sons Inc., New York, 765 pp.

Brusca RC and GJ Brusca. 2003. Invertebrates, 2nd ed. Sinauer Associates, Inc., Sunderland, Massachusetts, 936 pp.

Cohen WD (ed.). 1985. Blood Cells of Marine Invertebrates: Experimental Systems in Cell Biology and Comparative Physiology. Alan R. Liss, Inc., New York, 295 pp.

Conn DB. 1991. Atlas of Invertebrate Reproduction and Development. John Wiley & Sons, Inc., New York, 252 pp.

Fretter V and A Graham. 1976. A Functional Anatomy of Invertebrates. Academic Press, London, 600 pp.

Harrison FW. 1991-1999. Microscopic Anatomy of Invertebrates (fifteen volumes). Wiley-Liss, New York.

Hyman, LH. 1940-1967. The Invertebrates (Vol. 1-6). McGraw-Hill, New York.

Kozloff EN. 1990. Invertebrates. Saunders, Philadelphia, 866 pp.

Meglitsch PA and FR Schram. 1991. Invertebrate Zoology, 3rd ed. Oxford University Press, New York, 623 pp.

New TR. 1995. Introduction to Invertebrate Conservation Biology. Oxford University Press, Oxford, 194 pp.

Pearse V, Pearse J, Buchsbaum M, and R Buchsbaum. 1987. Living Invertebrates. Blackwell Scientific, Palo Alto, CA, 848 pp.

Ruppert EE, Fox RS, and RD Barnes. 2004. Invertebrate Zoology: A Functional Evolutionary Approach, 7th ed. Brooks/Cole—Thomson Learning, Belmont, CA, 963 pp.

Sherman IW and VG Sherman. 1976. The Invertebrates: Function and Form, 2nd ed. Macmillan, New York, 334 pp.

Stachowitsch M. 1992. The Invertebrates: An Illustrated Glossary. Wiley-Liss, New York, 676 pp.

Young CM, Sewell MA, and ME Rice. 2002. Atlas of Marine Invertebrate Larvae. Academic Press, London, 626 pp.

General References for Invertebrate Medicine, Husbandry, Culture, and Pathology

Frye FL. 1992. Captive Invertebrates: A Guide to Their Biology and Husbandry. Krieger Publishing, Malabar, Florida.

Kinne O. (ed). Diseases of Marine Animals (vols. 1-4), John Wiley & Sons.

Mitsuhashi J. 2002. Invertebrate Tissue Culture Methods. Springer-Verlag, Tokyo, 446 pp.

Mothersill C and B Austin. 2000. Aquatic Invertebrate Cell Culture. Springer Praxis Publishing, Chichester, UK, 409 pp.

Stolen JS, Fletcher TC, Smith, SA, Zelikoff JT, Kaattari SL, Anderson RS, Soderhall K, and BA Weeks-Perkins. 1995. Techniques in Fish Immunology, Fish Immunlogy Communications 4 (FITC 4), SOS Publications, Fair Haven, NJ, 258 pp. plus appendices.

Chapter 2

SPONGES

Gregory A. Lewbart

Natural History and Taxonomy

The phylum Porifera is a diverse group of primitive animals commonly referred to as the sponges. Until the middle of the 18th century, sponges were actually classified as plants (Ruppert and Barnes, 1994). Sponges occur in the fossil record back to the Precambrian (over 600 million years ago) and were the most important contributors to reefs during the Paleozoic and Mesozoic Eras (Hooper and Van Soest, 2002). All members lack defined organs; differentiated cells within connective tissue perform necessary biological functions. A unique system of water canals facilitates transport of food, waste products, and gametes. Nearly all are sessile and most species are marine. Of the approximately 8,000 species belonging to over 680 genera, only about 3% occur in freshwater (Ruppert and Barnes, 1994; Hooper and Van Soest, 2002). Sponges are normally found on firm substrates in shallow water, although some occur on soft bottoms.

Taxonomy*

Phylum: Porifera (Sponges). Approximately 8000 species (Ruppert et al., 2004).

Class: Calcarea. Members of this group have calcium carbonate spicules. No spongin. Most are small (less than 10 cm). The class contains asconoid, syconoid, and leuconoid members. Important genera include *Leucosolenia* and *Sycon.*

Class: Hexactinellida. Members of this group have hexagonal, siliceous (glass) spicules and are commonly referred to as glass sponges. Most are symmetrical, and some display a lattice-like morphology. These sponges are medium sized (10–30 cm) and are generally found at depths between 200 and 1000 m (Barnes, 1987). A good example from this class is Venus's flower-basket (*Euplectella* sp.)

Class: Demospongiae. The largest class of sponges with over 90% of the species (Barnes, 1987). The skeleton may be composed of spongin, siliceous spicules, or a combination of the two. All are of the leuconoid morphotype, and most are irregularly shaped. The economically important bath sponges belong to the family Spongiidae and possess only spongin fibers. *Spongia* and *Hippospongia* are the most commonly harvested genera (Barnes, 1987).

Class: Sclerospongiae. Members of this small class are associated with cryptic areas of coral reefs (Jackson et al., 1971; Barnes, 1987). They have a skeleton composed of calcium carbonate, siliceous spicules, and spongin fibers.

Anatomy and Physiology

There is a wide size variability among sponges, and very few are regularly or consistently shaped. Many are brilliantly colored, especially the marine forms.

Porifera means "pore bearing." In the basic body plan, numerous external pores, known as *ostia,* open into a large central cavity called the *atrium* or *spongocoel.* The atrium terminates in a single large opening termed the *osculum.* Water enters the sponge through the ostia, percolates into the atrium, and then exits via the osculum (Figure 2.1).

The body wall, known as the *pinacoderm,* is composed of epithelial cells called *pinacocytes.* Some pinacocytes can produce an adhesive that fixes the sponge to the substrate. Circular porocytes form the ostia and extend from the surface of the sponge to the atrium. A connective tissue-like matrix lies beneath the pinacoderm. This layer, which frequently contains skeletal elements and amoeboid cells, is termed the *mesohyl.* The skeletal elements may be spongin, silicium, calcareous, or some combination of these. *Spongin* is a protein that is comparable to collagen. Skeletal elements are the primary means of determining sponge taxonomy. In some cases, skeletal elements may extend through the pinacoderm to the sponge's surface (Figure 2.2).

There are a number of amoeboid cells in the mesohyl. These cells carry out the basic body functions. Archeocytes are large, phagocytic, and totipotent. Collencytes secrete collagen, sclerocytes secrete skeletal spicules, and spongocytes produce spongin. Choanocytes move water through the sponge to obtain food. All sponges lack a gut.

There are three basic sponge body plans: asconoid, syconoid,

---

*For a detailed account of sponge classification, see Hooper and Van Soest (2002). Some workers divide the phylum into two subphyla: Symplasma and Cellularia. Symplasma is synonymous with Hexactinellida, and Cellularia contains the major sponge groups (Ruppert et al., 2004).

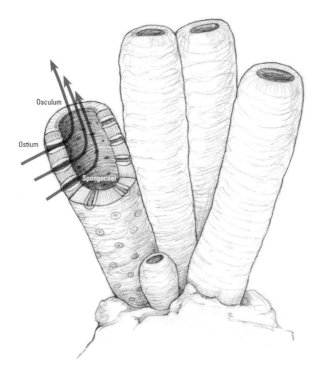

Figure 2.1. Basic sponge body plan illustrating water flow patterns. Drawing by Brenda Bunch.

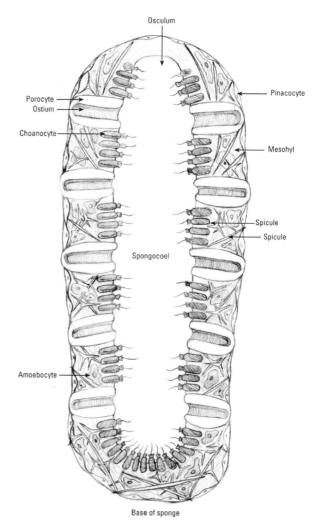

Figure 2.2. Microscopic diagrammatic view of the sponge. Drawing by Brenda Bunch.

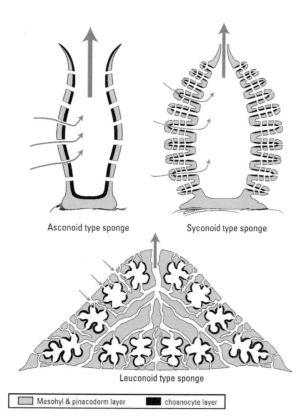

Figure 2.3. Three different types of body plans. Drawing by Brenda Bunch from several sources.

and leuconoid (Figure 2.3). Most sponges, and certainly the larger, more typical sponges, follow the leuconoid plan. The simple and primitive asconoid plan, with its radial symmetry and single atrium, has a limited surface area and hence a small maximum size. Evolving sponges solved this problem by increasing surface area by folding of body surfaces: the more folds, the more choanocytes, and the more choanocytes, the more water flow. In the intermediate syconoid body plan, the choanocytes do not line the spongocoel but are located along open channels called *radial canals*. The leuconoid sponge is the most evolved and has the most body folding and surface area. In this type of sponge, the choanocytes are in flagellated chambers and the spongocoel is frequently reduced to numerous canals connected to the osculum. Leuconoid sponges can grow large because mass increase leads to an increase in the number of flagellated chambers. Many forms possess more than one osculum. De Vos et al. (1991) have provided a detailed atlas of gross and microscopic sponge morphology.

Water flow sustains the life of a sponge, delivering food and removing waste products. Sponges are remarkably efficient animals with regard to water flow. *Leuconia*, a small leuconoid sponge (approx. 10 × 1 cm) has 2,250,000 flagellated chambers and may pump 22.5 L/day (Ruppert and Barnes, 1994). These water currents are produced by asynchronous beating of the choanocyte flagella. In some cases (environment and species dependent), there is a passive component to water flow.

Sponges are filter feeders and subsist primarily on microscopic organisms, organic matter, and minute plankton (Reiswig, 1971). The food elements are phagocytosed by all types of sponge cells. Larger particles (5–50 μm) are consumed by pinacocytes and archeocytes while tiny pieces (<1 μm) are absorbed by choanocytes. Most digestion occurs in the archeocytes and choanocytes; archeocytes then transport nutrients to different cells. Some marine sponges use photosynthesis via symbiotic organisms—normally, blue-green algae (*cyanobacteria*). Some sponge species harbor *zooxanthellae* (nonmotile dinoflagellates). The zooxanthellae frequently impart a color to the sponge (Figure 2.4, Color Plate 2.4).

Sponges accomplish gas exchange by simple diffusion and secrete ammonia as their primary nitrogenous waste product. Ammonia is removed by water coursing through the sponge.

Sponges lack a nervous system; message substances travel from cell to cell via diffusion.

Sponges reproduce in a variety of ways: regeneration, asexual reproduction, and sexual reproduction. Most sponges are sequential hermaphrodites. Choanocytes produce sperm, and either archeocytes or choanocytes produce eggs. Environmental changes may trigger the production of gametes. Sperm are expelled through the ostia and enter other sponges via the inhalant channels. Gametes fuse, and a parenchymella larva develops. Larvae leave via the ostia and may swim freely for a period before settling and attachment. In some species, given time and the proper environment, pieces from a mature sponge will grow into a new large sponge. Some freshwater sponges (and a few marine forms) display an interesting strategy of surviving a harsh winter. Clusters of nutrient-rich archeocytes are surrounded by amoebocytes that secrete a firm coating around the cluster. These cellular survival pods, known as *gemmules*, can survive freezing and desiccation, developing into an adult sponge during the spring and summer months. The temperate marine sponge *Microciona prolifera* undergoes marked morphological changes (Figure 2.5, Color Plate 2.5), including *apoptosis* (programmed cell death), during the winter (Kuhns et al., 1997). The surviving archeocytes become encased in a protective tissue matrix, likely waiting for warmer temperatures, when differentiation can occur (Kuhns et al., 1997).

Sponges secrete metabolites that are toxic to fish and other potential predators. Not all predators are deterred, and some sea turtles eat a diet primarily composed of sponges and excrete the undigestable spicules in their feces. Although not thoroughly understood, the sponge immune system is simple compared with higher invertebrate and vertebrate phyla and relies on cell-

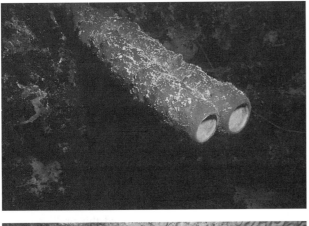
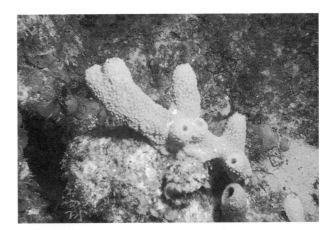
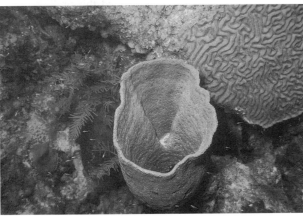
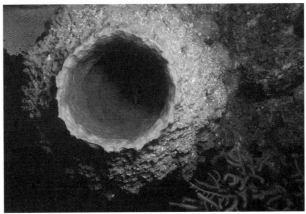

Figure 2.4. Four different sponges from the Turks and Caicos Islands. Symbiotic zooxanthellae can impart striking colors upon the sponge.

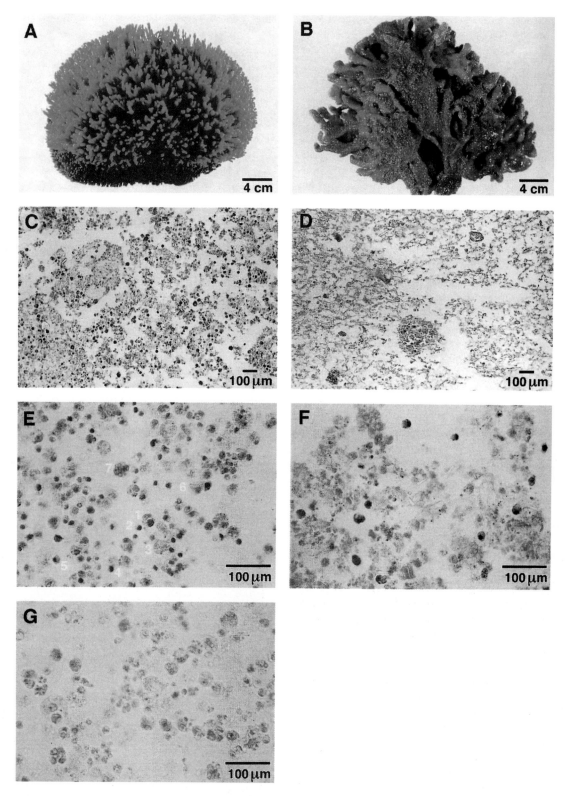

Figure 2.5. Gross and histological comparison of summer and winter *Microciona prolifera*: summer sponge **(A)** and winter sponge **(B)**. The winter sponge displays less color and integrity. Microscopic view of summer sponge **(C)** shows more cellularity than that of the winter sponge **(D)**. A TUNEL (terminal deoxyribonucleotidyl transferase-mediated dUTP nick end label) assay shows fragmenting nuclear DNA as brownish red **(E)**, whereas **G** is the counterstained control (no TUNEL). *Yellow numbers* are as follows: *1* and *7*, phagocytosed apoptotic cells; *2* and *5*, small apoptotic cells; and *3*, *4*, and *6*, macrophage-type (apparently healthy) and small apoptotic cells. In the winter sponge TUNEL assay **(F)**, a small number of healthy stem cells (blue nuclei) are mixed with clumps of apoptotic debris. From Kuhns et al. (1997), Figure 1 (pp. 239–240). Reprinted by permission of the Marine Biological Laboratory, Woods Hole, MA.

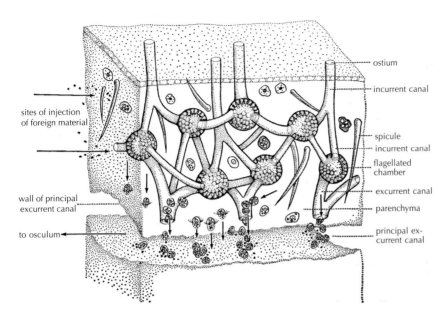

Figure 2.6. Serial section reconstruction of *Terpios zeteki* body wall with ink-laden archeocytes (*arrows*). Note that the cells are expelled through the excurrent canals. From Cheng et al. (1968a), Figure 1 (p. 303). Reprinted by permission of Academic Press, New York.

mediated immunity (Van de Vyver and Buscema, 1990). Phagocytosis, primarily by archeocytes, appears to be the primary mode of defense against invading pathogens (Cheng et al., 1968a, 1968b; Rützler, 1988). These foreign body-laden phagocytic cells migrate to the excurrent canals and are expelled (Figure 2.6). In a study examining a variety of heterografts in the sponge *Terpios zeteki*, it was noted that human erythrocytes were completely phagocytosed by slightly smaller archeocytes, indicating the sponge cell's hypertrophic capability (Cheng et al., 1968b).

Some sponges harbor antimicrobially active bacteria and can produce antibacterial and antifouling compounds (Nigrelli et al., 1959; Jakowska and Nigrilli, 1960; Burkholder and Ruetzler, 1969; Bakus et al., 1990; Thakur-Narsinh et al., 2003). Thakur-Narsinh et al. (2003) used the marine sponge *Suberites domuncula* and found antimicrobial *Proteobacteria* and a perforin-like protein with antibacterial activity associated with this species. Ectyonin, an extract of *Microciona prolifera* (the red beard sponge), showed in vitro antimicrobial activity against Gram-negative, Gram-positive, and acid-fast bacteria, as well as against *Candida albicans* (Nigrelli et al., 1959). Preliminary tests in this study indicated that ectyonin (parenterally injected) is not toxic to killifish (*Fundulus heteroclitus*) and mice. Sorbicillatone A, a bioactive alkaloid produced by *Penicillium chrysogenum* (a fungus that lives on the Mediterranean sponge *Ircinia fasciculata*), is cytotoxic to murine leukemic lymphoblasts and warrants further study (Bringmann et al., 2003).

Faulkner (1999, 2000) and Müller (2003) provide detailed accounts of natural products produced by sponges and their symbionts. This is an active research area involving the disciplines of molecular biology, organic chemistry, and biotechnology. For obvious reasons, successful maintenance and cultivation of sponges can contribute to ongoing research efforts in these areas. Brümmer and Nickel (2003) review the topic of captive sponge propagation, and Table 2.1 contains a list of pertinent data.

Sponges frequently serve as home for many other animals, including echinoderms, worms, and crustaceans.

Environmental Disorders

As aquatic, sessile animals, sponges rely on a constant flow of life-sustaining water. Adverse water-quality parameters can have an immediate and detrimental effect on sponges because they cannot escape or avoid environmental challenges. Although there are some freshwater sponges, most are marine, and tolerance for sudden changes in salinity varies between species (De Laubenfels, 1947). *Iotrochota birotulata*, a marine sponge, was found to tolerate salinities between 23 and 38 ppt but die in water below 20 ppt and higher than 40 ppt (De Laubenfels, 1932). One study (De Laubenfels, 1947) found that the sponge *Hymeniacidon* sp. could maintain a core temperature higher than the surrounding air and water (33°C for the sponge and 29°C for the environment). No explanation was given for this temperature differential.

A number of references address the topic of sponges as models for assessing impact of pollutants on aquatic animals (Zahn et al., 1983; Francis and Harrison, 1988; Hansen et al., 1995). Laboratory experiments (Hill et al., 2002) on developing freshwater sponges (*Heteromyenia* sp. and *Eunapius fragilis*) showed that ethylbenzene, nonylphenol, and bisphenol (all endocrine disrupters) produced developmental anomalies and retarded growth rate in these animals (Figures 2.7 and 2.8). The mechanisms for these effects are not well understood, but collagen synthesis disruption has been proposed for the freshwater sponge *Ephydatia fluviatilis* when exposed to azetidine 2-carboxylic acid (Mizoguchi and Watanabe, 1990).

It was determined that both copper and zinc are toxic to the freshwater sponge *Ephydatia fluviatilis* at concentrations of 1×10^{-7} in water with a total hardness of 60 mg/L (Francis and Harrison, 1988). The two metals exhibited different toxic ef-

Table 2.1. Mediterranean Sea sponges in captivity that were collected from a variety of localities

Species	Interim Storage	Recovery After Transport	Long-term Maintenance	Growth
Acanthella acuta	Excellent	Excellent	Months/year	Not observed
Agelas oroides	Excellent	Excellent	Months/year	Not observed
Aplysina aerophoba	Excellent	Excellent	Months/year	Good
Aplysina cavernicola	Excellent	Excellent	Months	Not observed
Axinella polypoides	Excellent	Excellent	Months	Not observed
Axinella verrucosa	Excellent	Excellent	Months	Not observed
Cacospongia sp.	Possible	Impossible	Impossible	Not determined
Chondrilla nucula	Excellent	Excellent	Years	Good
Chondrosia sp.	Excellent	Excellent	Years	Excellent
Clathrina clathrus	Excellent	Good	Months/year	Not observed
Clathrina coriacea	Good	Good	Weeks	Not observed
Cliona vermifera	Excellent	Excellent	Months	Not observed but possible
Cliothosa hancocki	Excellent	Excellent	Months	Not observed but possible
Crambe crambe	Good	Good	Weeks/months	Not observed
Dysidea avara	Excellent	Good	Months/year	Good/possible
Haliclona sp.	Not determined	Good	Weeks	Not observed
Hexadella racovitzai	Excellent	Excellent	Months	Not observed
Ircinia sp.	Impossible	Impossible	Impossible	Not determined
Petrosia ficiformis	Excellent	Excellent	Months/year	Not observed
Spirastrella sp.	Good	Good	Weeks/months	Not observed
Suberites domuncula	Excellent	Excellent	Years	Good
Sycon raphanus	Excellent	Excellent	Months/year	Good
Tethya aurantium	Excellent	Excellent	Weeks/months	Not observed but possible

Modified from Brümmer and Nickel (2003).

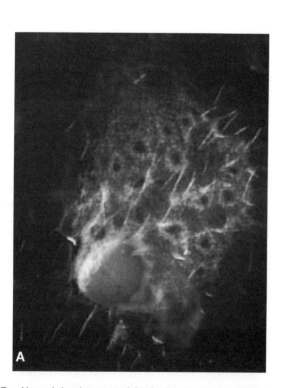
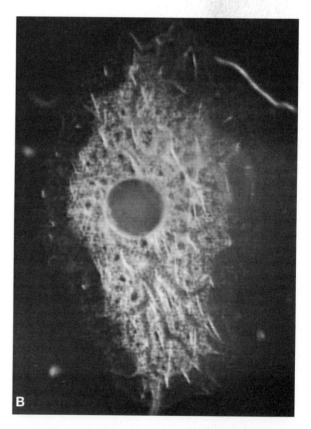

Figure 2.7. Normal development of the freshwater sponge *Heteromyenia* sp. **A:** The solid gemmule is at *lower left* with developing spicules and multiple ostia clearly visible within the parenchyma. **B:** Another example with a more centrally located gemmule and a visible canal system. From Hill et al. (2002), Figures 1 and 3 (pp. 297–298). Reprinted by permission of Elsevier.

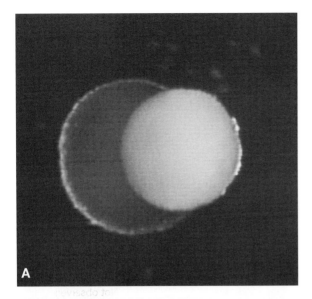

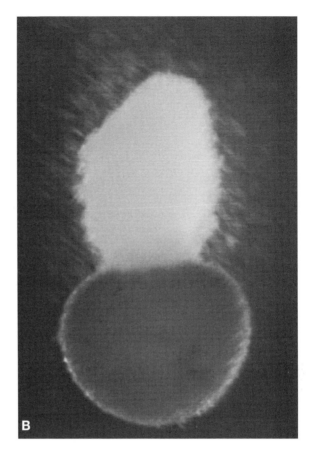

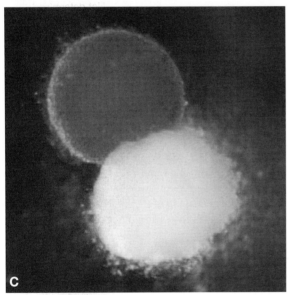

Figure 2.8. Abnormal development of the freshwater sponge *Heteromyenia* sp. after in vitro exposure of developing sponges to 11 ppm nonylphenol **(A)**, 22 ppm nonylphenol **(B)**, and 16 ppm bisphenol **(C)**. Note the lack of organization and tissue differentiation evident in Figure 2.7. The white, consolidated, and undifferentiated tissue is arising from the darker gemmules.

From Hill et al. (2002), Figures 1 and 2 (pp. 297–298). Reprinted by permission of Elsevier.

fects. Cultured sponges exposed to 4×10^{-7} copper displayed a generalized deterioration, whereas in sponges exposed to 4×10^{-7} zinc the archeocytes were most affected. The authors concluded that the dermal tissues were more resistant to zinc than were the other tissues. In the same study, the authors found that *E. fluviatilis* required 1×10^{-8} copper and zinc for normal growth. The authors noted that toxic levels might be lower in softer water.

It is well documented that suspended sediments can reduce or even eliminate populations of marine filter-feeding invertebrates (Bakus, 1968; Rhoads and Young, 1970; Dodge et al., 1974). A laboratory study on the tropical marine sponge *Verongia lacunose* determined that pumping rates decreased with an increase in suspended sediments (Gerrodette and Flechsig, 1979).

Living organisms can overgrow and outcompete wild sponge populations. Such a case was documented in New South Wales,

Australia (Davis et al., 1997). *Caulerpa scalpelliformis*, a green alga invader, spread rapidly in Botany Bay during the mid-1990s while populations of sessile marine invertebrates (primarily sponges) declined dramatically. Sponges are known to adapt to these types of biological challenges, but the result may mean less diversity or smaller sponges (Rützler, 1970; Sara, 1970; Carballo et al., 1996).

Infectious Diseases

Lauckner (1980) provides a comprehensive review of poriferan infectious diseases.

Infectious diseases of sponges in the wild have not been well characterized. A major complicating factor is differentiating between a primary and secondary/opportunistic pathogen.

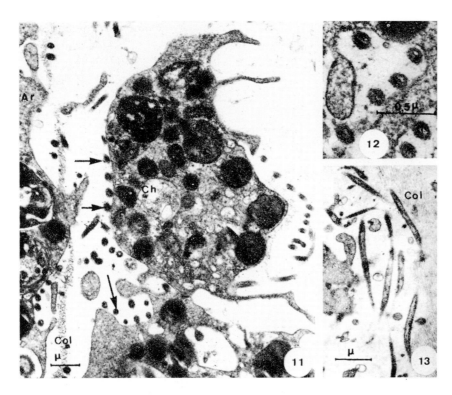

Figure 2.9. Transmission electron microscopy shows bacteria associated with the cells of *Pleraplysilla spinifera*. *Arrows* **(11)** indicate bacteria closely associated with a choanocyte (*Ch*). An archeocyte (*Ar*) and collagen (*Col*) are also visible in **11**. Transverse view of bacteria **(12)**. Longitudinal view of bacteria **(13)**. From Vacelet and Donadey (1977), Figures 11–13 (p. 308). Reprinted by permission of Elsevier/North-Holland Biomedical.

Diseased sponges in the wild are soon infested with a wealth of bacteria and other microorganisms (Rützler, 1988). It has been demonstrated that many sponges harbor symbiotic bacteria belonging to a wide range of genera (Colwell and Liston, 1962; Madri et al., 1967, 1971; Vacelet and Donadey, 1977; Reiswig, 1981; Rützler, 1988). It appears that in general the bacteria isolated from sponges are representative of the local aquatic bacteria (Lauckner, 1980). There is likely a mutualism between the bacteria and the sponge host. The bacteria consume metabolic waste from the sponge, and the sponge phagocytoses excess symbiotic microorganisms (Lauckner, 1980). In some cases, the bacteria can overwhelm the host and cause disease. This was reported in the marine bacteriosponge *Geodia papyracea* by Rützler (1988). Bacteriosponges may contain so much bacterial mass that the bacteria exceed the weight of the primary sponge tissues (Reiswig, 1981). It seems transfer of symbiotic bacteria can be vertical in some sponges (Bertrand and Vacelet, 1971). Hentschel et al. (2003) provide a detailed review of marine sponge microbial diversity.

Widespread cyanobacterial blooms have been associated with massive sponge mortality in the Florida Bay (Butler et al., 1995). This loss of sponge habitat had a negative impact on spiny lobsters (*Panulirus argus*), as juveniles of this species use sponges for shelter.

During the mid-1980s, massive mortalities decimated the Mediterranean commercial sponge industry. This mortality event was well studied, and several articles linked the sponge mortality to a bacterium (Gaino and Pronzato, 1989; Vacelet, 1994; Vacelet et al., 1994) that could cause tissue necrosis. Although the link between the unidentified bacterium and the sponge mortality appeared strong (including electron microscopy evidence), a bacte-rial organism was never cultured from the affected sponges. In 1998, a diseased wild Great Barrier Reef sponge (*Rhopaloeides odorabile*) was confirmed to have an α-proteobacterium infection (Webster et al., 2002). The authors named this organism *NW4327* and were able to fulfill Koch's postulates and establish this as the first confirmed case (with bacterial isolation) of a primary bacterial disease of sponges (Figure 2.10).

In the late 1930s, mass mortalities among commercially valuable sponges (*Hippospongiae lachne, H. gossypina, Spongia barbara, S. dura,* and *S. graminea*) of the Bahamas and British Honduras (now Belize) were attributed to fungal disease (Galtsoff et al., 1939; Smith 1939, 1941). The majority of the affected British Honduras sponges were cultivated from cuttings of naturally occurring species. The sequence of areas affected were correlated with water currents (Galtsoff et al., 1939). Funguslike filaments were found in most diseased tissue examined and not in healthy sponges. Infections appeared to begin internally and spread peripherally. This epizootic had a significant impact on the Gulf of Mexico commercial sponge industry, reducing populations to about 5% of preepizootic numbers (De Laubenfels, 1953) and completely eliminating the harvest in some areas (Dawson and Smith, 1953; De Laubenfels, 1953).

Protozoal diseases of sponges have been uncommonly reported. One flagellate, *Syncrypta spongiarum*, parasitizes the radial channels of *Grantia compressa* and *Sycon ciliatum* (Tuzet, 1973; Lauckner, 1980). A number of ciliated protozoans have been associated with sponges, but defining clinical etiology and pathogenicity has proved difficult (Wenzel, 1961a, 1961b; Lauckner, 1980).

A large variety of metazoan animals, mostly invertebrates, are known to be closely associated with sponges (Lauckner, 1980).

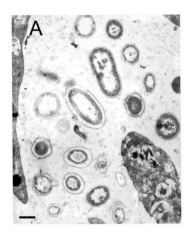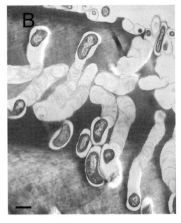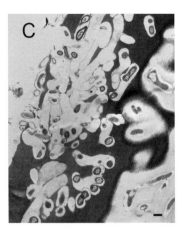

Figure 2.10.   Transmission electron micrographs of the Great Barrier Reef sponge (*Rhopaloeides odorabile*) affected by the bacterium NW4327. **A:** The bacterial organisms are normal (control sponge) and display varied morphology. **B and C:** From sponges inoculated with 10^6 CFU/mL of the bacteria. **C:** Note the necrosis and displacement of normal sponge tissue. Scale bars = 500 nm. From Webster et al. (2002), Figure 2 (p. 307). Reprinted by permission of Inter-Research (www.int-res.com).

In most cases, these relationships are not parasitic and have little, if any, negative impact on the sponge. Taxonomic groups with documented sponge relationships include coelenterates, mollusks, crustaceans, echinoderms, polychaetes, and fishes (Lauckner, 1980). De Laubenfels (1947) conducted an interesting experiment in which he allowed three *Hymeniacidon* sp. totaling about 800 mL in volume to lie stagnant. Within a couple hours, the dish holding the sponges contained the following: 50 macroscopic nematodes, 1000 microscopic nematodes, 100 macroscopic annelids, 200 microscopic annelids, 500 macroscopic amphipods, and 800 microscopic amphipods. The author felt that some of these animals (at least some of the nematodes) were parasitic but could not prove this.

Rotifers have been described as both parasites and commensals of freshwater sponges (Berzins, 1950). In this report, the rotifers *Lecane clara* and *Lepadella triba* were described as "gnawing" shallow notches (less than 50 μm) in the outer layers of the sponge *Spongilla lacustris*. The author noted that these two parasitic rotifers were not specialized and did not differ morphologically from free-living rotifers.

In some cases, polychaete worms can initiate fibrogenesis and tissue proliferation in sponges (Connes et al., 1971). The sponge *Geodia cydonium* had a marked histological reaction to the polychaete *Eunice siciliensis* (Connes et al., 1971).

There are numerous instances where crustaceans, including barnacles, amphipods, and decapods, have close associations with sponges (De Laubenfels, 1947; Connes et al., 1971; Lauckner, 1980). There is good evidence that some of these crustaceans consume sponge tissue, but the clinical impact on the sponge is hard to quantify (Arndt, 1933).

Mites belonging to the genus *Unionicola* frequently use freshwater sponges (as well as mollusks) during their development (Smith and Oliver, 1986; Proctor and Pritchard, 1989). Mite eggs, prelarvae, protonymphs, and tritonymphs (resting stage) can all be found in sponge tissues. These mite life stages appear to have little or no detrimental affect on the sponge host.

Analgesia, Anesthesia, and Surgery

No reports were located on either anesthesia or analgesia for sponges. People have been performing surgery on sponges for many decades, as cuttings and grafting are techniques used in the commercial culture of sponges (Ruppert and Barnes, 1994). Sterile techniques are not employed, and at least some species of sponges handle these manipulations well. Although autografts are successful in the Mediterranean sponge *Axinella polypoides*, allografts and xenografts are not (Van de Vyver and Buscema, 1990). The authors of this study also determined that sponges have a cellular immune response to a variety of nonsponge materials, including cork, glass, granite, and polyvinyl chloride (PVC) foam. The most marked rejection reaction was in response to the granite.

References

Arndt W. 1933. Die biologischen Beziehungen zwischen Schwämmen und Krebsen. Mitt Zool Mus Berl 19:221–305.

Bakus GJ. 1968. Sedimentation and benthic invertebrates of Fanning Island, Central Pacific. Mar Geol 6:45–51.

Bakus GJ, Schulte B, Jhu S, Wright M, Green G, and Gomez P. 1990. Antibiosis and antifouling in marine sponges: Laboratory versus field studies. In: Rützler K, ed. New Perspectives in Sponge Biology. Smithsonian Institution Press, Washington, DC, pp 102–108.

Barnes RD. 1987. Invertebrate Zoology, 5th edition. Saunders College, Philadelphia, pp 71–91.

Bertrand JC and Vacelet J. 1971. l'Association entre éponges cornées et bactéries. C R Hebd Seances Acad Sci Paris 273:638–641.

Berzins B. 1950. Observations on rotifers on sponges. Trans Am Microsc Soc 69:189–193.

Bringmann G, Lang G, Mühlbacker J, Schaumann K, Steffens S, Rytik PG, Hentschel U, Morschhauser J, and Müller WEG. 2003. Sorbicillactone A: A structurally unprecedented bioactive novel-type alkaloid from a sponge-derived fungus. Prog Mol Subcell Biol 37:231–253.

Brümmer F and Nickel M. 2003. Sustainable use of marine resources: Cultivation of sponges. In: Müller WEG, ed. Sponges (Porifera): Progress in Molecular and Subcellular Biology. Springer, Berlin, pp 141–162.

Burkholder PR and Ruetzler K. 1969. Antimicrobial activity of some marine sponges. Nature 222:938–984.

Carballo JL, Naranjo SA, and Garcia-Gomez JC. 1996. Use of marine sponges as stress indicators in marine ecosystems at Algeciras Bay (southern Iberian Peninsula). Mar Ecol Prog Ser 135:109–122.

Cheng TC, Rifkin E, and Yee HWF. 1968a. Studies on the internal defense mechanisms of sponges. II. Phagocytosis and elimination of india ink and carmine particles by certain parenchymal cells of *Terpios zeteki*. J Invertebr Pathol 11:302–309.

Cheng TC, Yee, HWF, Rifkin E, and Kramer MD. 1968b. Studies on the internal defense mechanisms of sponges. III. Cellular reactions in *Terpios zeteki* to implanted heterologous biological materials. J Invertebr Pathol 11:29–35.

Colwell RR and Liston J. 1962. The natural bacterial flora of certain marine invertebrates. J Insect Pathol 4:23–33.

Connes R, Paris J, and Sube J. 1971. Reactions tissulaires de quelques demosponges vis-à-vis de leurs commensaux et parasites. Nat Can 98:923–935.

Davis AR, Roberts DE, and Cummins SP. 1997. Rapid invasion of a sponge-dominated deep-reef by *Caulerpa scalpelliformis* (Chlorophyta) in Botany Bay, New South Wales. Aust J Ecol 22:146–150.

Dawson CE and Smith FGW. 1953. The Gulf of Mexico sponge investigation. Fla State Board Conserv Mar Lab Tech Ser 1:1–27.

De Laubenfels MW. 1932. Physiology and morphology of Porifera, exemplified by *Iotrochota birotulata* Higgin. Carnegie Inst Washington Publ 435:37–66.

De Laubenfels MW. 1947. Ecology of the sponges of a brackish water environment, at Beaufort, N.C. Ecol Monogr 17:31–46.

De Laubenfels MW. 1953. Sponges from the Gulf of Mexico. Bull Mar Sci Gulf Caribb 2:511–557.

De Vos L, Rützler K, Boury-Esnault N, Donadey C, and Vacelet J. 1991. Atlas of sponge morphology. Smithsonian Institution Press, Washington, DC, 117 pp.

Dodge RE, Aller RC, and Thomson J. 1974. Coral growth related to resuspension of bottom sediments. Nature 247:574–577.

Faulkner DJ. 1999. Marine natural products. Nat Prod Rep 16:155–198.

Faulkner DJ. 2000. Marine natural products. Nat Prod Rep 17:7–55.

Francis JC and Harrison FW. 1988. Copper and zinc toxicity in *Ephydatia fluviatilis* (Porifera: Spongillidae). Trans Am Microsc Soc 107:67–78.

Gaino E and Pronzato R. 1989. Ultrastructural evidence of bacterial damage to *Spongia officinalis* fibres (Porifera, Demospongiae). Dis Aquat Org 6:67–74.

Gaino E, Pronzato R, Corriero G, and Buffa P. 1992. Mortality of commercial sponges: Incidence in two Mediterranean areas. Boll Zool 59:79–85.

Galtsoff PS, Brown HH, Smith CL, and Smith FWG. 1939. Sponge mortality in the Bahamas. Nature (Lond) 143:807–808.

Gerrodette T and Flechsig AO. 1979. Sediment-induced reduction in the pumping rate of the tropical sponge *Verongia lacunosa*. Mar Biol 55:103–110.

Hansen IV, Weeks JW, and Depledge MH. 1995. Accumulation of copper, zinc, cadmium and chromium by the marine sponge *Halichondra panicea* Pallas and the implications for biomonitoring. Mar Pollut Bull 31:133–138.

Hentschel U, Fieseler L, Wehrl M, Gernert C, Steinert M, Hacker J, and Horn M. 2003. Microbial diversity of marine sponges. In: Müller WEG, ed. Sponges (Porifera): Progress in Molecular and Subcellular Biology. Springer, Berlin, pp 59–88.

Hill M, Stabile C, Steffen LK, and Hill A. 2002. Toxic effects of endocrine disrupters on freshwater sponges: Common developmental abnormalities. Environ Pollut 117:295–300.

Hooper JNA and Van Soest RWM. 2002. Systema Porifera: A Guide to the Classification of Sponges, volumes 1 and 2. Kluwer Academic/Plenum, New York.

Jackson JBC, Goreau TF, and Hartman WD. 1971. Recent brachiopod–coralline sponge communities and their paleoecological significance. Science 173:623–625.

Jakowska S and Nigrilli RF. 1960. Antimicrobial substances from sponges. Ann NY Acad Sci 90:913–916.

Kuhns WJ, Ho M, Burger MM, and Smolowitz R. 1997. Apoptosis and tissue regression in the marine sponge *Microciona prolifera*. Biol Bull 193:239–241.

Lauckner G. 1980. Diseases of Porifera. In: Kinne O, ed. Diseases of Marine Animals, volume 1. John Wiley, New York, pp 139–165.

Madri PP, Claus G, Kunen SM, and Moss EE. 1967. Preliminary studies on the *Escherichia coli* uptake of the redbeard sponge (*Microciona prolifera* Verill). Life Sci 6:889–894.

Madri PP, Hermel M, and Claus G. 1971. The microbial flora of the sponge *Microciona porifera* Verrill and its ecological implications. Bot Mar 14:1–5.

Mizoguchi H and Watanabe Y. 1990. Collagen synthesis in *Ephydatia fluviatilis*. In: Rützler K, ed. New Perspectives in Sponge Biology. Smithsonian Institution Press, Washington, DC, pp 188–192.

Müller WEG, ed. 2003. Sponges (Porifera): Progress in Molecular and Subcellular Biology. Springer, Berlin, 258 pp.

Nigrelli RF, Jakowska S, and Calventi J. 1959. Ectyonin, an antimicrobial agent from the sponge *Microciona prolifera* Verrill. Zoologica (NY) 44:173–176.

Proctor HC and Pritchard G. 1989. Variability in the life history of *Unionicola crassipes*, sponge-associated water mite (Acari: Unionicolidae). Can J Zool 68:1227–1232.

Reiswig HM. 1971. Particle feeding in natural populations of three marine demosponges. Biol Bull Mar Biol Lab Woods Hole, 141:568–591.

Reiswig HM. 1981. Partial carbon and energy budgets of the bacteriosponge *Verongia fistularis* (Porifera: Demospongiae) in Barbados. Mar Ecol 2:273–293.

Rhoads DC and Young DK. 1970. The influence of deposit-feeding organisms on sediment stability and community trophic structure. J Mar Res 28:150–178.

Ruppert EE and Barnes RD. 1994. Invertebrate Zoology, 6th edition. Saunders College, Philadelphia, pp 499–595.

Ruppert EE, Fox RS, and Barnes RD. 2004. Invertebrate Zoology: A Functional Evolutionary Approach, 7th edition. Brooks/Cole—Thomson Learning, Belmont, CA, 963 pp.

Rützler K. 1970. Spatial competition among Porifera: Solution by epizoism. Oecologia (Berl) 5:85–95.

Rützler K. 1988. Mangrove sponge disease induced by cyanobacterial symbionts: Failure of a primitive immune system? Diseases of Aquatic Organisms 5:143–149.

Rützler K, ed. 1990. New Perspectives in Sponge Biology. Smithsonian Institution Press, Washington, DC, 533 pp.

Sara M. 1970. Competition and co-operation in sponge populations. Symp Zool Soc Lond 25:273–284.

Smith FGW. 1939. Sponge mortality at British Honduras. Nature (Lond) 144:785.

Smith FGW. 1941. Sponge disease in British Honduras, and its transmission by water currents. Ecology 22:415–421.

Smith IM and Oliver DR. 1986. Review of parasitic associations of larval water mites (Acari: Parasitengona: Hydrachnida) with insect hosts. Can Entomol 118:407–472.

Thakur-Narsinh L, Hentschel-Ute, Krasko-Anatoli, Pabel-Christian T, Anil-Arga C, and Mueller-Werner EG. 2003. Antibacterial activity of the sponge *Suberites domuncula* and its primmorphs: Potential basis for epibacterial chemical defense. Aquat Microb Ecol 31:77–83.

Tuzet O. 1973. Eponges calcaires. In: Grassé P-P, ed. Traité de Zoologie, volume 3. Masson, Paris, pp 633–690.

Vacelet J. 1994. Control of the severe sponge epidemic—Near East and Europe: Algeria, Cyprus, Egypt, Lebanon, Malta, Morocco, Syria, Tunisia, Turkey, Yugoslavia. Technical Report: The Struggle Against the Epidemic Which Is Decimating Mediterranean Sponges. FI:TCP/RAB/8853. FAO, Rome, pp 1–39.

Vacelet J and Donadey C. 1977. Electron microscope study of the association between some sponges and bacteria. J Exp Mar Biol Ecol 30:301–314.

Vacelet J, Vacelet E, Gaino E, and Gallissian MF. 1994. Bacterial attack of spongin skeleton during the 1986–1990 Mediterranean sponge disease. In: Van Soest RWM, van Kempen ThMG, and Braekman JC, eds. Sponges in Time and Space. AA Balkema, Rotterdam, pp 355–362.

Van de Vyver G and Buscema M. 1990. Diversity of immune reactions in the sponge *Axinella polypoides*. In: Rützler K, ed. New Perspectives in Sponge Biology. Smithsonian Institution Press, Washington, DC, pp 96–101.

Webster NS, Negri AP, Webb RI, and Hill RT. 2002. A spongin-boring proteobacterium is the etiological agent of disease in the Great Barrier Reef sponge *Rhopaloeides odorabile*. Mar Ecol Prog Ser 232:305–309.

Wenzel F. 1961a. Ciliaten aus marinen Schwammen. Pubbl Stn Zool Napoli Mar Ecol 32:272–277.

Wenzel F. 1961b. Notisen über *Ophryodendron multiramosum* n. sp. und seine Konjugation. Arch Protistenkd 105:269–272.

Zahn RK, Zahn G, Müller WEG, Michaelis ML, Kurelec B, Rijavec M, Batel R, and Bihari N. 1983. DNA damage by PAH and repair in a marine sponge. Sci Total Environ 26:137–142.

Chapter 3

COELENTERATES

Michael K. Stoskopf

Introduction

Much of the concern about health of coelenterates is focused on their important ecological role in the wild. Considerable information and speculation have been published on factors causing declines in coral reef ecosystems and much of the concern about these declines centers on loss of the reef-forming corals. The dynamics of these alterations are complex. Anthropogenic causes, including overfishing and nutrient loading, affect the balance of community structure. This in turn can have major impacts on individual species abundances. However, other non-infectious factors, including physical disturbances from major storms, can have important impacts on key reef communities, some of which may be drivers of normal succession in these communities (Ostrander et al., 2000). Infectious diseases of coelenterates have received careful attention only relatively recently, and our progress in identifying disease agents greatly outstrips the progress in identifying useful diagnostic and therapeutic approaches to the diseases. At the same time, maintenance of many coelenterate species in private and display aquaria has grown geometrically, and this experience has resulted in important knowledge of basic requirements and improved understanding of health management approaches. Captive coelenterates have even helped us better understand our own health through their use as models of human disease, such as in the study of hydra basement membrane changes in response to D-glucose that mimic those seen in diabetic patients (Zhang et al., 1990). However, there remains an important need to improve our understanding of the health management of coelenterates, both at the population level in the wild and at the individual and colony level in captivity.

Natural History and Taxonomy

This chapter focuses on the group of animals historically classified together under the phylum Coelenterata (Greek *Koilos*, meaning "hollow," plus *enteron*, meaning "intestine") because of their shared radial symmetry and other structural similarities. Modern taxonomists, however, now describe two distinct phyla—Ctenophora and Cnidaria—that contain the species that once comprised the Coelenterata. For convenience sake, the term *coelenterate* will be used throughout the chapter to refer to the two phyla in combination.

Comb Jellies

The phylum Ctenophora (Greek *Cten*, meaning "comb," plus *phora*, meaning "bearer"), or the comb jellies, is relatively poorly studied. Estimates of species numbers range from 90 to 150, with speculation that many species remain to be described. Common names include the sea gooseberry, the sea walnut, and Venus's girdles. Comb jellies are found in all ocean habitats from tropical to Arctic waters and from deep ocean to coastal shallows. They live in all ranges of the water column and include deep benthic species as well as surface floaters. Most are free-swimming organisms, though benthic species may creep on the bottom or more commonly on the other animals they live upon (sponges, etc.). They are taxonomically unified by the presence of eight rows of fused cilia that form stacked combs or comb plates (ctenes) used in locomotion (Figure 3.1). These combs have interesting light refraction properties that can give comb jellies an elegant appearance. Some, but not all, will also have long tentacles that assist in the prey capture (copepods, planktonic fish, and mollusk larvae). Most comb jellies are also luminescent, a property that should not be confused with the iridescence of the combs. Pigmentation in deep benthic species is thought perhaps to mask or alter their luminescence to reduce risk of predation. The predator comb jellies are preyed upon by jellyfish, sea turtles, and some fishes. Though the further classification of comb jellies remains controversial, taxonomists seem to have agreed on dividing the phylum into six classes: Cydippida, Platyctenida, Beroida, Thalassocalycida, Cestida, and Lobata (Mills, 1998–present; Podar et al., 2001).

The taxonomic separation of the comb jellies from the Cnidaria is based on several lines of evidence. Once thought to have stinging cells, it is now known that nematocysts found in comb jellies are remnants of stinging cells from prey they have ingested. An exception to this rule is the genus *Haeckelia*, a group still classified as comb jellies but having nematocysts (Mills and Miller, 1984). Rather than nematocysts, most comb jellies rely on sticky cells called *colloblasts* to gather and hold prey. Comb jellies are essentially radially symmetrical but have several features reminiscent of structures in bilaterally symmet-

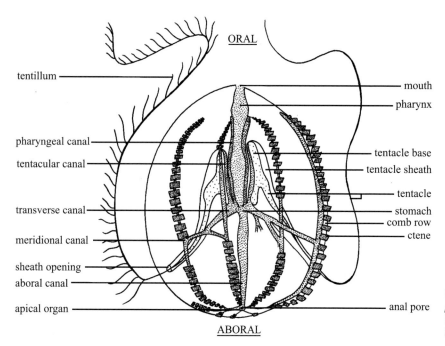

ORAL

tentillum

mouth
pharynx

pharyngeal canal
tentacular canal

tentacle base
tentacle sheath

tentacle

transverse canal

stomach
comb row
ctene

meridional canal

sheath opening
aboral canal

apical organ

anal pore

ABORAL

Figure 3.1. The comb jelly *Pleurobrachia pileus*. Schematic drawing reproduced from Richard Fox, Lander University, by Alison Schroeer.

rical animals. These include the presence of a pair of anal pores, and a third tissue layer between the endoderm and the ectoderm. Molecular studies have not supported hypotheses suggesting the comb jellies are closely related to the bilaterally symmetrical phyla, but these structural differences are strong evidence for separating them from the Cnidaria. The natural history of the comb jellies is also quite different than for most Cnidaria because the former have a simple life cycle without metamorphosis. Many comb jelly species spend their entire life as a planktonic form (holoplanktonic). Most comb jellies are self-fertilizing hermaphrodites that spawn free-floating eggs and sperm into the sea. Once fertilized, eggs develop to a larval stage that hatches and grows to adult size. These species can reproduce when they are very small and have very short generation times. Full-sized animals spawn more frequently and prolifically than smaller ones, and can spawn daily if there is enough food. When no food is present, spawning ceases and the animals shrink. Not all comb jelly species follow this pattern. Some species, such as the sea walnut (*Mnemiopsis leidy*) hold their fertilized eggs internally until larvae develop.

Cnidarians

The animals classified together in the phylum Cnidaria [Greek *Knide* for "nettle"] share a radial symmetry, hydrostatic skeleton, diploblastic composition, dimorphic development, and the ability of many species to inflict a sting by using *nematocysts*, specialized organelles produced by cnidocytes. The approximately 9000 species in this phylum are among the simplest of metazoa. Within the phylum Cnidaria, taxonomists generally agree on three classes: Hydrozoa, Scyphozoa, and Anthozoa. Recently, however, a fourth class has begun to emerge—the Cubozoa, which are now recognized as a separate class by many taxonomists.

Hydrozoa (Hydra and Fire Corals)

The class Hydrozoa is comprised of animals with distinct tissues, distinguishing them from the Porifera. They are commonly classified into five orders. The Trachylinida have a small medusa stage that develops directly from a crawling larva called an *actinula*. They have no polyp stage. The largest order of the class, the Hydroida are for the most part colonial species that have alternating medusa (Figure 3.2A) and polyp stages, though some genera (*Hydra*) consist of solitary polyps (Figure 3.2B). This order has a chitinous exoskeleton (Figure 3.2C). The two orders Milleporina and Stylasterina are sometimes combined as a single order called the Hydrocorallina or *fire corals*. These hydrozoa are colonial and create an aragonite (calcium carbonate based) skeleton. Their common name comes from the potency of their nematocysts. The fifth order of hydrozoans is known as the Siphonophorida. The best known of these complex colonial organisms with specialized polyps for feeding, swimming, prey capture, and reproduction is the Portuguese man-of-war (*Physalia physalis*).

Scyphozoa (Jellyfishes)

The class Scyphozoa is generally characterized by having a much larger medusa stage than polyp stage (with the exception of the Stauromedusae) (Figure 3.3). They lack the shelf of tissue projecting in from the margin of the bell of the medusa found in the box jellies (Cubozoa). Most taxonomists recognize four orders of Scyphozoa. The order Stauromedusae includes small sessile organisms usually living in cold water that adhere to hard substrates by a peduncle. They do not have a free-swimming medusa stage but instead cycle between a polyp, like an adult, and a creeping benthic larval stage. The members of the order

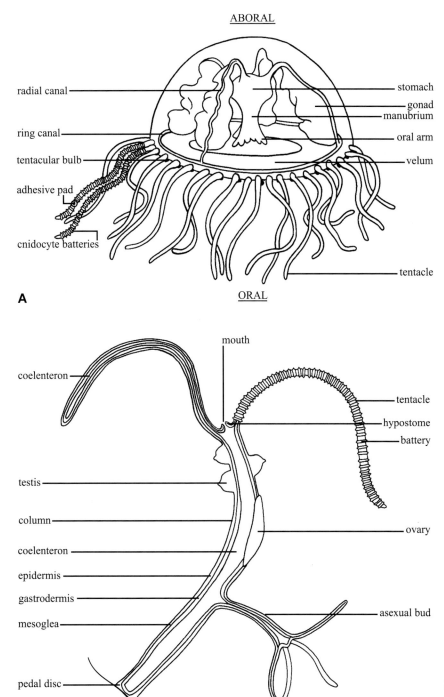

ABORAL

radial canal

ring canal

tentacular bulb

adhesive pad

cnidocyte batteries

A

ORAL

stomach

gonad
manubrium

oral arm

velum

tentacle

mouth

coelenteron

testis

column

coelenteron

epidermis

gastrodermis

mesoglea

pedal disc

B

tentacle

hypostome

battery

ovary

asexual bud

Figure 3.2.   A: The medusa of the hydrozoan *Gonionemus*. **B:** The simple hydrozoan, *Hydra* sp. Schematic drawings A and B reproduced from Richard Fox, Lander University, by Alison Schroeer.

Coronatae are distinguished by a groove around the bell of the medusa. Many Coronatae are heavily pigmented deep-water species. Their polyp forms resemble hydroids and are similarly protected by a chitinous tube. The medusa stages of members of the order Semaeostomeae have tentacles along or beneath the margin of the bell or umbrella, and long oral arms hanging down from the mouth, but no coronal groove. The medusae of the order Rhizostomeae have no marginal tentacles, and their oral arms are fused and bear numerous small mouth openings.

Jellyfishes have complex life cycles. Medusae of most species are dioecious, with the fertilized egg developing into a very small, ciliated, free-swimming larva (*planula*). The planktonic larvae settle to the bottom and develop into tentacle-bearing polyps (*scyphistomae*). The sessile scyphistoma can then repro-

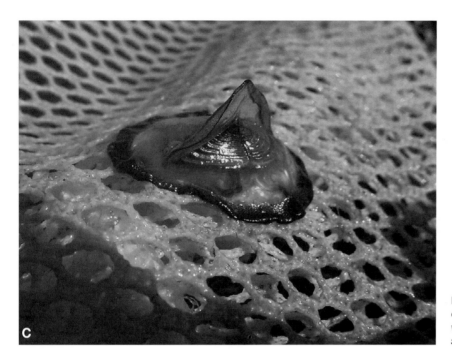

Figure 3.2.   C: The small (approx. 5-cm diameter) colonial, pelagic hydrozoan (*Velella velella*), known commonly as the *by-the-wind sailor.*

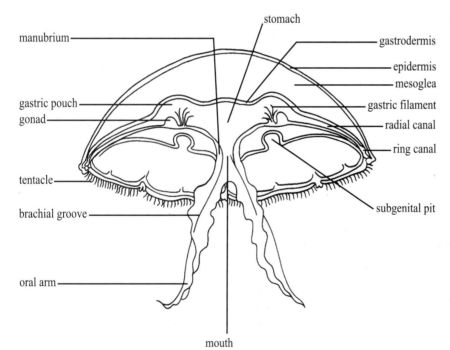

Figure 3.3.   The moon jellyfish, *Aurelia aurita*. Schematic drawing reproduced from Richard Fox, Lander University, by Alison Schroeer.

duce asexually, usually by budding or podocyst formation. If environmental conditions are correct, scyphistomae can undergo *strobilation*, which is transverse segmentation, and segment metamorphosis, where the segmented parts of the polyp become incipient medusae that eventually break loose to become free-swimming ephyrae. The ephyra completes the life cycle by growing into an adult medusa. Meanwhile, the basal part of the strobila reverts to a scyphistoma that after growth can reproduce asexually or strobilate again.

Anthozoa (Sea Anemones and Corals)

The taxonomy of the class Anthozoa is controversial, to say the least. The variety of classification schemes is somewhat daunting. In general, the class is comprised of the vast majority of species commonly referred to as sea anemones and corals. They are distinguished by their life history, existing exclusively as polyps, completely without a medusa life stage (Figures 3.4 and 3.5). The Anthozoa are routinely divided into various subclasses, though the number of subclasses and spelling are highly

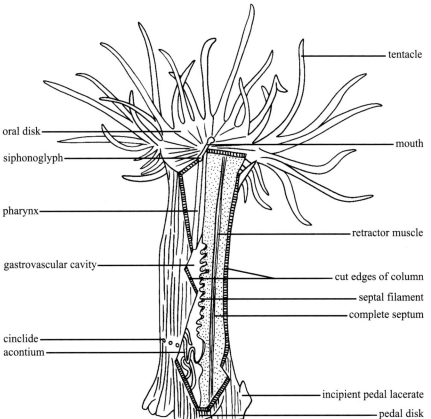

tentacle

oral disk

mouth

siphonoglyph

pharynx

retractor muscle

gastrovascular cavity

cut edges of column

septal filament

complete septum

cinclide

acontium

incipient pedal lacerate

pedal disk

Figure 3.4. *Aiptasia pallida*, a common Atlantic sea anemone of the southeastern United States. Schematic drawing reproduced from Richard Fox, Lander University, by Alison Schroeer.

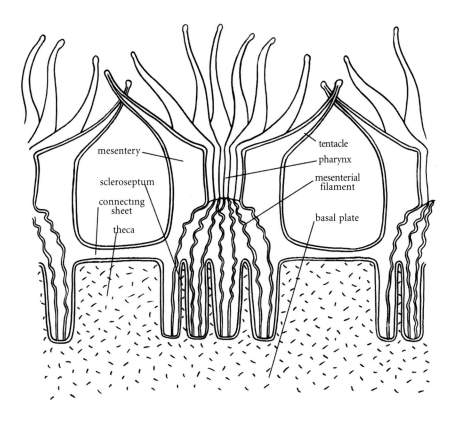

mesentery

tentacle

pharynx

scleroseptum

mesenterial filament

connecting sheet

theca

basal plate

Figure 3.5. The basic scleractinian coral anatomy of three polyps. The major anatomical features are identified. Schematic illustration by Allison Schroeer, after Barnes, 1980.

variable. The elegant three-volume *Corals of the World* (Veron, 2000) provides some valuable keys for the reef-forming corals and divides the Anthozoa into three subclasses: Octocorallia, Hexacorallia, and Ceriantipatharia.

Octocorallia

The subclass Octocorallia, commonly known as *soft corals*, is a diverse group of species, not very closely related to the true corals (Scleractinia). The polyps of octocoralliarians have eight tentacles. The octocorals are traditionally divided into five or six orders (Telestacea, Alcyonacea, Gorgonacea, Pennatulacea, Helioporacea, and sometimes Stolonifera). Most do not develop skeletons. Exceptions to this rule include the monotypic order Helioporacea, which is comprised of the single Indian and Pacific Ocean species *Heliopora coerulea* (blue coral) and the pipe organ corals of the genus *Tubipora* usually placed in the order Alcyonacea or their own order Stolonifera. Most octocorals form spicules within their tissues, and some produce calcified holdfast structures or long, rodlike internal supports. All octocorals have pennate tentacles where small branches come off of the main tentacle, giving it a featherlike appearance. All of the octocorals are colonial, including the sea fans and sea whips (Gorgonacea). In some, the sea pens and sea pansies, for example (Pennatulacea), the polyps are specialized for specific functions. In the sea pens, the base or primary polyp grows large and loses its tentacles. It forms the central axis of the colony and has a contractile bulb at its base that is used to attach the colony to substrate. Branching off the primary polyp are various secondary polyps. Typical feeding polyps are called *autozooids*; larger *siphonozooids* take in water and circulate it through the colony to keep it upright. The secondary polyps can be arranged in clusters that resemble leaves. This is seen in the Subselliflorae, but most sea pens are less ornate.

Hexacorallia

The subclass Hexacorallia is comprised of six orders, two of which are extinct, the order Rugosa and the order Tabulata. These organisms were major reef builders in the Paleozoic Era, but no members survived the Permian extinctions. The orders Actinaria and Zoanthidia contain the simple sea anemones and the colonial anemones, respectively. The order Scleractinia contains the true stony or reef-building corals. The order Corallimorpharia or mushroom corals are sometimes referred to as *false corals*.

Actinaria and Zoanthidia (Anemones)

Most of the soft-bodied anthozoans known as *sea anemones* are classified in the Actinaria. There are over 1000 species of sea anemone. Actinarians generally have column-shaped bodies with the mouth at one end and a muscular pedal disk for attachment to substrates at the other. The mouth is ringed with rows of tentacles. Though actinarians have soft bodies and do not form hard parts, some coat themselves with sand grains and/or mucuslike secretions. Most actinarians are relatively sessile, either not moving or moving very slowly by contractions of the pedal disk. Some anemones burrow into sand, and a few can swim short distances. Actinarian anemones can reproduce ei-

ther sexually or asexually, but they do not form true colonies with permanent tissue connections between members, as seen in the superficially similar zoanthiniarian anemones.

The Zoanthiniaria are a small group of polypoid anthozoans that differ from most sea anemones (Actinaria) in details of internal anatomy. Also, unlike most sea anemones, zoanthiniarians can form true colonies in which all members are connected by common tissue. Zoanthiniarians make no hard parts and leave no fossil record. However, they are more closely related to extinct coral taxa (Tabulata and Rugosa) than they are to other soft-bodied anthozoans.

Scleractinia (True Stony Corals)

The scleractinians are the largest group of anthozoans, with approximately 3600 extant species (Ruppert et al., 2004). This prominent taxon provides the calcium carbonate building blocks for the world's coral reefs. The aragonite (calcium carbonate) skeleton is secreted by the epidermis and is present in all members of this order (Ruppert et al., 2004). The order Scleractinia is usually divided into 18 families: Acroporidae, Astrocoeniidae, Pocilloporidae, Euphylliidae, Oculiidae, Meandrinidae, Siderastreidae, Agariciidae, Fungiidae, Rhizangiidae, Pectiniidae, Merulinidae, Dendrohylliidae, Caryophylliidae, Mussidae, Faviidae, Trachyphylliidae, and Poritidae. Each is classified by morphological features of colony growth and various soft-tissue features. The Pocilloporidae are comprised of relatively few species but are heavy contributors to reef formation, second only to the Acroporidae in reef contribution worldwide. The Acroporidae are mostly in two genera, *Acropora* and *Montipora*. These are fast-growing forms with both asexual and sexual reproduction.

Some scleractinians, like members of the genus *Fungia*, are solitary and can be relatively large: up to 50 cm in diameter (Ruppert et al., 2004). Most, however, are colonial, with polyp size generally 3 mm or less in diameter. Individual scleractinian colonies, some composed of thousands of polyps, may be several meters in diameter and weigh hundreds of kilograms.

Corallimorpharia (False Corals)

The Corallimorpharia are largely unstudied, and their taxonomy has shifted greatly over time. Recent use of molecular taxonomy probes has provided evidence for dividing the order into four families: Discosomatidae, Ricordeidae, Corallimorphidae, and Sideractidae. The Discosomatidae (formerly Actinodiscidae) are individual polyps that often can be colonial. Their taxonomy beyond genus is very problematic. Species range in size from 2.5 to 30 cm across. The Ricordeidae are often polystomatous and have oval rather than round mouths. They are not very motile, if at all, and deeper-living species are more solitary. The Corallimorphidae are mostly temperate species from deep water. They are rarely kept in captivity. The Sideractidae are relatively poorly known.

Ceriantipatharia

The subclass Ceriantipatharia is comprised of two orders: the Antipatharia or black corals and the Ceriantharia or tube anemones. The taxonomy of these animals is not very well agreed upon, and efforts to establish any relevance of the taxonomic classifications to health issues would be somewhat premature. There are approximately 24 genera of Antipatharia and 125–150 species. They are sometimes called *little thorn corals* because of their small polyps. They occur in all oceans but are most commonly confined to deep water, although a couple of unusual antipatharian species can be found in water as shallow as 1 m. Normally, they prefer low light conditions even when found in shallows, and they lack any symbiotic zooxanthellae. The ceriantharians are classified into approximately 59 genera and about 150 species. They are often mistaken for anemones, but these ceriantharians live only in soft sediments and have distinctive anatomical features.

Cubozoa (Box Jellies)

The box jellies are the topic of considerable taxonomic discussion. Commonly placed in the class Scyphozoa or true jellyfishes, they have a different life cycle and a distinct structure that many taxonomists believe warrants a separate classification into the class Cubozoa, with the single order Cubomedusae. The approximately 20 species considered in the Cubozoa are thought by some to be more closely related to the Hydrozoa than to the Scyphozoa. They all have a square appearance when viewed from above and four tentacles or sets of tentacles attaching to each corner of their boxlike bell. Two families are proposed: the Carybdeidae, with a singe tentacle connected to each of the four pedalia (a fleshy pad attached to the bell); and the Chirodropidae, which have multiple tentacles attached to each pedalium. Perhaps the most widely known of the Cubozoa is the chirodropidid *Chironex fleckeri*, also known as the sea wasp, marine stinger, or the Australian stinger. This potentially deadly, large, fast-swimming cnidarian predator reaches 30 cm in diameter and has up to 60 tentacles that reach 5 m in length when extended for feeding. A person can die within minutes of injection of the multicomponent toxin by the nematocysts. Estimates of human mortality range between 15% and 20% of stung victims, with lethal outcomes more common when 10% or more of the skin surface area is stung. Immediate first aid consists of application of ammonia to inactivate embedded nematocysts, and administration of an antivenin of sheep IgG (3 vials intramuscularly) as soon as possible when there is evidence of potentially lethal envenomation (collapse and cardiovascular abnormalities).

Anatomy and Physiology

As might be expected from such a broad group of organisms, there is considerable variation in their natural history, anatomy, and physiological adaptations to survival. Figures 3.1–3.5 illustrate the basic cnidarian body plan. Most jellyfishes and comb jellies are predators, but the size and type of food they use vary significantly by species and by life-cycle stage. Corals and sea anemones can harbor unicellular algae (zooxanthellae) that supplement the nutrition of their host, but most capture animal prey as their main nutrition source. Some species feed on planktonic food borne by currents, and some species can absorb

significant portions of required nutrients directly from seawater. Nutrition of these species in captivity remains a challenge. A variety of approaches are employed, and theories of how much and what to feed are outlined in many of the better books on the husbandry of these species (Sprung and Delbeek, 1994; Borneman, 2001).

There are records of temperate anemones surviving for many decades in commercial aquaria, and one small sea anemone in New Zealand has been calculated to live over 300 years. Colonial organisms are potentially immortal, but most estimates for corals and anemones conservatively place the normal life span of a colony at around 20 years. Studies on the Great Barrier Reef of Australia have calculated the average age of an *Acropora* colony at between 4 and 7 years and for massive corals (*Porites* spp.) at between 7 and 11 years (Borneman, 2001). Jellies and comb jellies are considered more ephemeral, but with improvements in husbandry and captive care, we are learning that many species live longer than previously thought.

All cnidarians reproduce sexually. Some species are hermaphroditic, and others have separate sexes. Typically, sperm and eggs are released into the sea, where fertilization occurs. A free-swimming larva develops and then settles into an appropriate habitat to metamorphose and develop. In some species, eggs are not released but are fertilized internally by sperm entering with the water being pumped in and out of the female. Environmental cues (e.g., a full moon and a low tide) can be important to the timing of spawning and have been used in captivity to propagate various species of commercial or conservation interest. Some cnidarians can also undergo asexual reproduction. They may divide longitudinally into two smaller individuals, which usually takes a couple of days. This results in genetically identical organisms—essentially clones. Cloning can also occur through fragmentation and regeneration. Larger specimens are less likely to clone than smaller animals.

Coelenterates have an array of defenses against injury and disease. Mucus production is a primary defense of corals and anemones. Some species are better at this than others. Stressed or injured animals secrete large amounts of mucus, which can be physically protective and may contain bioactive defense molecules. Corals do possess a functional cellular immune system, with many cell types and molecules analogous to vertebrate immune systems. Phagocytes that are capable of mounting a directed or a general response to potential invaders are present, and many corals, particularly soft corals, secrete bioactive compounds with antibiotic efficacy. No humoral immunity has been identified in the corals.

Environmental Diseases and Preventive Medicine

In captive management of these species, health care focuses nearly entirely on environmental management. This is particularly appropriate with this group of organisms because basic issues of water composition and quality, nutrient supply, and trauma appear to be the largest contributors to morbidity and mortality. In the wild, the complex interaction between reef communities and their environment has been the focus of considerable study and speculation, and is clearly a major concern in maintaining healthy reefs.

Water Quality

As a general rule, coelenterates thrive best with excellent water quality. Ammonia levels should effectively be undetectable at all times, though there have been reports of levels up to about 20 μM stimulating zooxanthellae growth (Borneman, 2001). Nitrate can be directly absorbed by corals, and there is some evidence of coral growth enhancement with supplementation of low levels of nitrate. However, successful propagators of captive corals recommend that nitrate levels always be well below 10 ppm. Though nitrogen can be a limiting nutrient to coral growth, when zooxanthellae experience high environmental nitrogen levels, they reduce translocation of nutrients and oxygen to their host animal. This can result in excessive growth of the zooxanthellae population, which in turn creates a high demand for carbon dioxide, possibly exceeding supply. When this happens, photosynthesis is blocked due to interference with photon absorption (Borneman, 2001). Excess nitrogen can also reduce calcification and skeletal density in stony corals in addition to reducing photosynthesis and respiration. Similarly, most corals can use dissolved organic matter for nutrition, but high levels reduce coral growth and stimulate algal growth. Dissolved organic matter should be held in the range of 0.5–3.0 ppm in captive reef systems.

Phosphate is also a limiting nutrient for most coelenterates. In captivity, additions from food and makeup water can result in excess water phosphate content. This will depress calcification in skeleton-forming species and at the same time help to induce algal proliferation. Most corals are adapted to very low phosphate levels and, when water phosphate content exceeds 0.3 ppm, problems occur (Borneman, 2001). Ideally, water phosphate levels should be below detection limits with routine testing equipment.

Water calcium levels are of particular concern in captive propagation or management of skeleton-forming coelenterates. Coral polyps constantly absorb calcium from seawater, requiring active management to maintain the necessary levels of at least 400 ppm or preferably 450 ppm calcium ion. This can be accomplished through the careful addition of saturated lime water, often referred to as *Kalkwasser*. Preparation of the Kalkwasser is time consuming, and very careful attention to dosing is required. For these reasons, many aquarists are shifting to safer and less labor intensive 2-part calcium additives that consist of a carbonate buffer solution and a concentrated calcium-ion solution. Calcium reactors can also be used but require significant capital outlay. The use of calcium chloride for acute manipulations of calcium-depleted water work, but over time there is concern about the accumulation of excessive chloride ions, especially in small systems (Borneman, 2001). A syndrome of decalcification occurs spontaneously in many stony corals despite good polyp expansion and outward appearances of health. In this condition, the skeleton becomes unable to support itself and fractures or collapses spontaneously without obvious trauma. This is thought to be due to lack of bioavailable calcium and other minerals in aquaria, but also is seen in the wild, and more likely represents a complex pathogenesis. Boring sponges and worms as well as algae are thought to be associated with the condition in the wild, but there is no good description or study of the condition. It should be mentioned that decalcification of skeleton is thought to be normal in some fungiid corals as part of their asexual reproduction.

More volatile in freshwater systems, pH remains an important water parameter to monitor in captive management of coelenterates. Diurnal shifts as wide as 0.2 pH points are not uncommon, with lower pH occurring at night. Ideally, pH should be maintained between 8.2 and 8.4 and, if it is necessary to err, it is better to be slightly more alkaline. Alkalinity in natural reefs is generally about 2.5 mEq/L, but most aquarists maintain higher levels, between 3.2 and 4.5 mEq/L. This increased buffer capacity seems to be beneficial, stabilizing and reducing pH shifts.

Salinity varies considerably with ocean habitat and can flux significantly, even on a diurnal basis, in some reef environments. Aquarists generally measure specific gravity as a surrogate for salinity and try to hold a specific gravity of 1.027 for maintaining anemones and stony corals in captivity.

There is considerable controversy over the exact trace-element requirements of corals and other coelenterates. It certainly makes sense from analysis of coral skeletons that there would be optimal levels to maintain strong skeletal construction. Nevertheless, there is no consensus on how important strontium, iodine, magnesium, iron, molybdenum, bromide, fluoride, vanadium, and other trace elements are to coral growth, and certainly no consensus on proper supplementation rates.

Temperature

As a group, the coelenterates are found in an extremely wide range of temperatures, but for individual species, the temperature ranges they tolerate are much narrower. Corals and anemones are rapidly killed if temperatures range outside of their tolerance limits. Water temperature affects the function of critical enzymatic processes required for digestion, tissue maintenance, and detoxification of free radicals generated during photosynthesis by zooxanthellae. High temperatures outside of the tolerance range are particularly damaging because elevated metabolic rates demand more oxygen at the same time that oxygen saturation of water decreases. This is particularly a challenge at night, when zooxanthellae convert to oxygen consumption rather than photosynthetic production, placing further demand on scarce oxygen resources. Affected animals can be seen with persistently open mouths and everted bodies, or they may be collapsed and shrunken. Tropical species of anemones generally experience problems below 20°C or above 31°C, and the optimum temperature is often around 24°C (Sprung and Delbeek, 1997). Temperate anemone species usually can survive at 24°C but are more robust and healthier when maintained at 20°C (Sprung and Delbeek, 1997) Temperature optima and ranges for corals are generally similar to those of anemones.

Water Motion

For the medusae stage of jellies and comb jellies, water flow patterns can be all important, providing transportation as well as the means for nutrient gathering (Figure 3.6, Color Plate 3.6). A flow that is too high can push captive animals into traumatic collisions with enclosures. Too little flow can also be a significant problem. Anemones and corals need some water motion. The amount of motion varies with species. For example, the anemone fish hosts *Heteractis magnifica*, *H. crispa*, and *Stichodactyla mertensii* all experience strong surges of water frequently, though intermittently, in their natural habitat. In contrast, *Stichodactyla giganta*, a quiet back-reef species, only experiences high flow with strong tidal currents in the wild.

All coelenterates need sufficient water motion for oxygenation of tissues, and, for sessile species, the flushing away of debris. When anemones or corals in captivity are seen holding their mouth open persistently, or everting themselves, it can be a sign of inadequate oxygenation, which may (at least in part) be due to inadequate water flow. This can particularly be a problem in specimens that are experiencing other challenges. One common protective response of corals and anemones is the copious generation of protective mucus. Unfortunately, this mucus can significantly reduce the ability of the organism to absorb oxygen. It can also trap debris, resulting in sedimentation effects that further exacerbate oxygen depletion as well as encourage increased bacterial growth. Corals with branching skeletons are less prone to this problem. Increasing water flow in the face of high mucus production helps to flush excess mucus and sediment and reduces the development of localized anoxic zones that may initiate polyp death and necrosis.

Light and Nutrient Issues

Many coelenterates, particularly anemones and corals, rely on a symbiotic relationship with zooxanthellae to supply their nutrient needs. Without careful attention to light and water-quality management, these species can lose their zooxanthellae after a short time in captivity. This results in a loss of normal color and, more important, the loss of a critical nutrient source. Affected anemones take on odd shapes and postures, begin to shrink, and generally experience a negative nitrogen balance that can be irreversible. Though more easily appreciated in the anemones, similar problems occur with all of the species in these taxa that rely on symbiosis with commensal zooxanthellae.

Interpreting the implications of a shrinking anemone can be challenging. A deflated anemone may simply be following a normal rhythm in its life cycle, including normal asexual reproduction, but prolonged deflation or shrinking is not a good sign. It can be an indication of infection or predation, but often is a sign of malnutrition. Anemones that are not getting sufficient nutrients may begin to digest their own tissues. Another early sign of starvation can be a loss of stickiness as animals are unable to support the synthesis and replacement of spent cnidocytes (Sprung and Delbeek, 1997). Though anemones are routinely fed at least weekly in captivity with appropriate prey, refusal of food is not an indication for force feeding. If the anemone is otherwise normal, it may not be feeding because it is receiving adequate light to enable the zooxanthellae to meet its needs. Adequate light is actually the first concern when signs of starvation appear. Shrinking or deforming anemones should be placed where they will receive appropriate light levels and wavelengths while normal voluntary feeding is maintained at least weekly. With too little light, anemones become pale, may shrink gradually, and climb as close to the light sources as they can. Conversely, when too much light is provided, anemones will retreat from the light source while seeking lower-intensity areas.

Excessive light, particularly in the ultraviolet (UV) wavelengths can cause morbidity and mortality, induce bleaching, or cause algal overgrowth. Anemone bleaching is somewhat analogous to what occurs in coral bleaching though no infectious agent has been tied to the phenomenon in anemones. It is thought that anemones respond to overillumination, particularly in the UV wavelengths, by extruding zooxanthellae as superoxide radicals build up from excessive photosynthetic activity in addition to trying to move away from the light. If caught early enough, the condition is reversible by providing proper lighting. What is considered proper lighting is controversial among experts in the captive husbandry of these species. Most

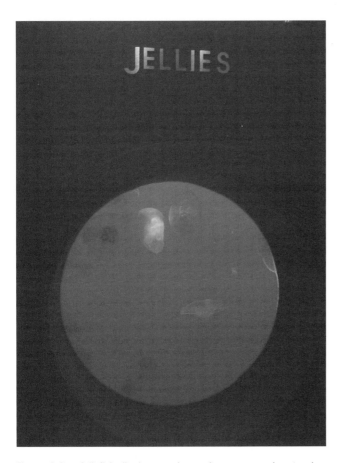

Figure 3.6. Jellyfish displays are becoming very popular at public aquariums and zoological parks, as well as some restaurants. Jellies are typically displayed in cylindrical tanks with carefully controlled water flow and attractive lighting. This public display contains Western Atlantic moon jellyfish (*Aurelia aurita*).

agree that attention must be paid to both spectral quality and quantity (photon flux density per wavelength interval) to achieve proper lighting. For zooxanthellae-harboring animals, photosynthetically active radiation (400–700 nm) is needed, preferably with more flux density between 400 and 550 nm and less between 650 and 700 nm. Obviously, species living at deeper levels may need less light than those of more shallow habitats. In cases of anemone bleaching or photoavoidance, decreasing the light intensity is appropriate. Alteration of the pattern of light intensity (cloud simulation) can also improve the condition. There seems to be a benefit in varying lighting intensity as opposed to constant strong illumination. Photoavoidance and even bleaching can occur when no changes have been made in the lighting of a well-established system. One cause of this phenomenon is any sudden change in water clarity. Aggressive use of ozone or activated carbon can rapidly remove organic compounds in the water and increase light exposure, requiring that the intensity of light delivery at the surface be decreased to maintain appropriate illumination in the tank (Sprung and Delbeek, 1997).

Trauma

Reports of impacts of direct trauma are most common for stony corals and jellies, but all coelenterates are susceptible to trauma. Captive management of jellies first became practical with the design of special tanks with circulation to prevent jellies from sustaining trauma from collisions with tank walls and water flow apparatus (Figure 3.6). Trauma remains the most significant identified cause of specimen loss for species where nutritional needs are reasonably well established. Traumatized jellies benefit from timely sharp debridement of the damaged tissues. Stony coral trauma has best been examined in the wild, where

studies of ship groundings and anchor damage have documented the impact on coral colonies. Appropriate debridement and potentially prophylactic treatment to reduce secondary bacterial or protozoan infections are beneficial in captive situations, though generally considered impractical in large-scale injuries in the wild.

Anemones are susceptible to a similar form of trauma from interaction with tank components to that seen in the jellies, just with a relatively slower time course. Anemones seem drawn to migrate to pump intakes, where they sustain what is usually fatal trauma. Anemones are easily pulled through mesh strainers and, besides their own death, can precipitate problems for the entire tank by blocking critical filtration flow. The elimination of pumps and powerheads inside the aquarium or the judicious use of large foam baffles over intakes can reduce or eliminate the problem. Submersible heaters are also a source of trauma for anemones that may attach while the heating element is off and then be unable to release their hold quickly when the heating element turns on. The result is usually a fatal burn (Sprung and Delbeek, 1997).

Community Balance Shifts

Predator–prey relationships, and interspecific and intraspecific competition for space and optimal water and lighting conditions, make the reef communities that support many species of coelenterates complex and dynamic. Any number of imbalances can occur, setting the community into a cascade of population shifts. These challenges are constant both in wild and in captive communities. Much study has been devoted to both situations, though, appropriately, more aggressive manipulation of community balance and dynamics has been reserved for captivity situations.

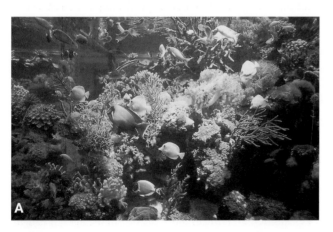
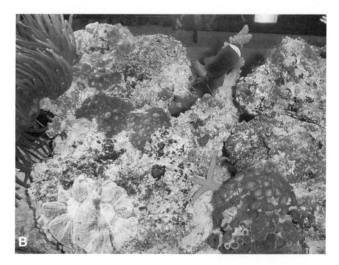

Figure 3.7. Private coral reef aquariums are becoming very popular throughout the world. **A:** An 11,000-L system owned by David Saxby in London. **B:** Many hobbyists are enjoying much smaller systems like the animals in this 600-L aquarium. Photo A courtesy of www.bio-photo.net.

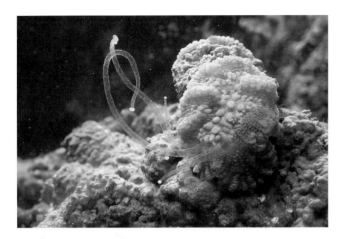

Figure 3.8. *Favia maxima* with many sweeper tentacles extruded. Photo courtesy of E.H. Borneman.

Contact Inhibition and Interspecific Aggression

Interspecific aggression between colonies of scleractinian corals occurs. Corals have been observed to generate mouthless, elongated sweeper tentacles on polyps at the outermost part of colonies (Figure 3.8). These sweeper tentacles attack competing adjacent corals. The toxicity of these tentacles varies with species. Many hard corals (e.g., *Favia, Scolymia,* and *Pavona*) also can possess mesenterial (mesenteric) filaments in their stomach that are capable of killing and digesting polyps of other coral species on contact. This sort of interspecific aggression in stony corals is perhaps best studied for *Stylophora pistillata,* where it is well documented that contacting colonies result in necrosis in one of the colonies. This necrosis initially is restricted to layers interspersed with polyps, but later the nonliving central corallum is destroyed by foreign microorganisms. The necrosis may be mediated by carbonic anhydrase, which has been found to be induced in areas of coral in close contact with nonisogenic tissues. In some cases, the necroses heal with a living septal layer or with a calcareous plug (Muller et al., 1984)

Soft corals can compete with adjacent organisms by releasing terpenoid compounds that injure or kill competitive species, clearing the way for expansion of the soft coral. These competitive mechanisms observed in captive situations probably occur in wild reefs, as well, and are likely balanced by movement of more mobile specimens. These interactions are likely responsible for the geospatial segregations of cnidarian species that are observed in natural reefs. In captivity, this situation can require active management. Generally, corals of the same genus do not damage each other on contact, but there have been exceptions. Some corals are much more aggressive than others and will completely overgrow adjacent colonies of less aggressive corals (Table 3.1). It has been observed that some corals (*Euphyllia, Fungia,* and *Catalaphyllia*) become more aggressive when hungry, so proper planes of nutrition would be expected to reduce the problem. Physical removal of sweeper tentacles from adjoining corals that are touching has been used as a management strategy in small reef tanks. Care needs to be taken to avoid microalgal colonization of the resulting wounds, which will heal rapidly if not infected.

Abrasion-mediated polyp retraction is one of the primary mechanisms of competition used against scleractinian corals (*Porites porites*) by tall macroalgae (*Sargassum hystrix*) (River and Edmunds, 2001).

Algal Competition

The adaptability and resilience of algae make them a key challenge in the maintenance of reef community balance. A well-reported problem in Caribbean reefs developed after an epizootic reduced the abundance of the herbivorous sea urchin (*Diadema antillarum*) in a wide range. The population decline of the urchin was followed by a surge in macroalgae abundance (Ostrander et al., 2000). This overgrowth of macroalgae, in concert with the effects of a massive bleaching event that reduced hard coral abundance, caused reef communities rapidly to become dominated by macroalgae. With the recovery of *Diadema* populations, reefs with macroalgal dominance are beginning to shift back to a dominance by corals and algal turf. In areas where *Diadema* are recovering, macroalgae are rare and the density of juvenile corals is much higher than in zones where *Diadema* are less common (Edmunds and Carpenter, 2001).

Algal overgrowth is also a major problem in captive management of corals and anemones. In addition to imbalances in communities caused by too few algal grazers, accumulation of water nutrients (phosphates, nitrates, and silicic acid) and improper lighting can favor macroalgal and microalgal exuberance that is detrimental to corals and anemones. Nonbiological approaches to combating algal overgrowths in aquaria focus primarily on

Table 3.1. Aggressiveness of corals, listed from most to least aggressive

Catalaphyllia plicata	Most Aggressive
Euphyllia ancora, E. fimbriata,	
E. glabrescens, E. cristala	
Pterogyra sinuosa	
Physosyra lichensteini	
Fungia actiniformis	
Goniopora spp.	
Trachyphyllia seofroyi	
Turbinaria peltata	
Galaxea fascicularis	
Favia spp.	
Clavularia spp.	
Sarcophyton spp.	
Dendronephthva spp.	
Sinularia spp.	
Cladiella spp.	
Gorgonacea	
Anthelia spp.	
Xenia spp.	
Rhodactis spp.	
Actinodiscus spp.	Least aggressive

Adapted from Paletta (1990).

limiting the sources of nutrients for algae (nitrate, phosphate, and silicate). Use of highly purified water (distilled or reverse osmosis) for generating makeup water can be useful in small-scale operations to reduce nitrogenous and organic nutrients. Similarly, extensive use of filtration with activated carbon (bituminous coal and lignite processed with steam to make it highly porous) will reduce nitrogenous and organic nutrient loading. Organic carbon loads can also be reduced by using potassium permanganate (Thiel, 1998), but this approach has a severe effect on the redox potential of the treated water. Chemical filtration with ferric hydroxide has been used to remove phosphates as well as arsenic. Aluminum hydroxide has also been used to remove phosphates, but soft coral species are reported to be sensitive to the process. Additions of calcium hydroxide (Kalkwasser) to boost pH will help precipitate phosphate, making it unavailable to algae. Another approach for reducing available nutrients is to culture algae in a filter outside of the primary enclosure. *Algal scrubbing*, or using macroalgal cultures to reduce available nutrients from system water, have been employed with some success for many years. A twist on this concept is the culture of soft corals (Xenieidae) in a similar manner to the use of algal scrubbers. These are rapid-growing species that can pull nutrients used by algae from system water and possibly generate a commercial product in the process (Sprung, 2002).

Mechanical filters can be used intermittently to reduce large particulate organic matter and reduce detritus buildup, but unless carefully managed can become a source of dissolved inorganic nutrients that promote algal growth. Ultraviolet sterilizers can be used to kill floating spores and algal filaments as they pass the filter. This approach can be effective when combined with other means of control when faced with cyanobacteria or filamentous algal problems. Protein skimmers (foam fractionators) remove phosphates and amino acids needed for algal growth. Ozonation can also reduce the nutrient supply to algae by oxidation of organics and impacts on the redox potential. When filamentous algae are colonizing between polyps or zoanthids, physical removal using old toothbrushes, scrapers, toothpicks, or wooden skewers is about all that is available for control other than the use of appropriate herbivores. Care needs to be taken to avoid breaking up the algae excessively; otherwise, regrowth from algal fragments can rapidly overwhelm the system.

Normally some form of biological control is required in addition to physical and chemical control methods to bring a captive reef community into balance once exuberant algal growth has begun. Many corals are thought to produce antifouling substances to combat algal invasion. *Porites*, *Sarcophyton* (Figure 3.9), *Lobophytum*, *Sinularia*, and many gorgonians produce a waxy film that is periodically shed into water currents to remove attached algae (Sprung, 2002). Other corals produce copious mucus or use shading strategies by expanding their tissues to block out light to algae trying to establish on their base. *Acropora* is reported to kill adjacent algae by using digestive filaments (Sprung, 2002). Most captive coral communities, though, will need additional help to keep algal species in balance. A wide range of herbivores are available—some more specialized than others, and some also more likely than others to graze on coelenterates as well as algae.

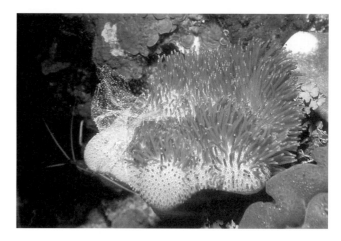

Figure 3.9. Normal shedding of waxy skin by the leather coral *Sarcophyton* sp. Photo courtesy of www.biophoto.net.

Green algae include unicellular microscopic forms and filamentous turf-forming forms, the later being the most aggravating to marine aquarists. Unicellular forms create cloudy green water and must be controlled by reduction of nutrient availability, mechanical filtration, UV sterilization, and protein skimming. *Astrea* snails eat all forms of microalgae, as will some herbivorous copepods, but they are quite small and many are needed for any significant impact. The filamentous endolithic forms such as *Ostreobium* spp. can cause coral tissue to recede from point of attachment. These algae are best controlled by reducing water nitrate and phosphate levels and the use of *Diadema* urchins to graze the algal lawns created by the exposed filaments of the algae. *Alonia macrophysa*, or bubble algae, can rapidly overgrow and smother corals. Rabbitfish (*Siganus punctatus* or *S. puellus*) or Red Sea sailfin tangs (*Zebrasoma desjardinii*) will readily eat these algae, as will emerald crabs (*Mithrax sculptus*), though the crabs are not so fastidious as to eschew a good meal of coral polyps. Most problematic of all are the green hair algae represented by several genera. These algae usually get out of control because of high phosphate levels in the water, making phosphate reduction and water management key. *Derbesia* spp. will be eaten by emerald crabs if the algae are first cropped down by hand. *Enteromorpha* spp. are a bit more palatable. The so-called lawnmower blennies (*Salarias fasciatus*, *Parablennius marmoreus*, *Escenius bicolor*, *E. gravieri*, and *Ophioblennius atlanticus*) and some species of tangs offer hope of control if phosphate levels can be kept low.

Brown algae are members of the Chromista, which includes diatoms and coccolithophorids. They are multicellular photosynthetic protists that contain chlorophyll and undergo complex life cycles. The largest forms are the kelp, which may grow over 30 m in length, and the group includes ecologically important species such as the gas-filled floating Sargassum weed. The brown of the algae is created by the presence of the carotenoid pigment fucoxanthin, but chlorophyll is present. The brown algae are generally considered to have positive effects on water quality from the perspective of coelenterates, but exuberant growth can cause negative impacts on corals through shading. Some species such as *Dictyota* spp. are readily controlled by *Diadema* urchins or mithraculus crabs. Brown hair algae, or *Hincksia* spp., cause problems similar to those posed by green filamentous algae but luckily rarely grow in tropical systems, being a cooler-water species. There is no known herbivore control for this alga. Reduction of available phosphates is thought to be useful in its control (Sprung, 2002).

Red algae (Rhodophyta) are named for their characteristic color caused by their high content of phycobilins, predominately R-phycoerythrin, which reflects red and absorbs blue light. Red algae also contain chlorophyll and carotenes, and come in both unicellular and multicellular forms, including calcifying reef-building species referred to as *coralline algaes*. In captivity, the red hair algaes (*Polysiphonia* and *Asparagopsis*) grow in balls or tufts that spread rapidly and can shade corals or prevent good water flow. Unfortunately, these algae grow in low light conditions as well as bright light and flourish even with low phosphate levels. Quarantine and inspection are the best control strategies because most algae-eating fish and invertebrates do not eat these algae. Efforts to keep nitrate availability down, along with hand removal of algae, can help supplement the use of herbivores. Also, reduction of the amount of red light delivered to the tank may help. The red algae do much better with red light than do most corals. Surgeonfishes may eat *Polysiphonia* but generally refuse to eat *Asparagopsis*. A Pacific snail (*Turbo fluctuosus*) is reported to eat *Asparagopsis*, but the very similar snail *Astrea tectum* from the Caribbean apparently does not eat it at all. *Diadema* urchins, hermit crabs, and perhaps sea slugs (*Aplysia* and *Hermaea*) could be beneficial. Another challenging red algae is wire algae (*Gelidiopsis* spp.), commonly found growing on damaged coral edges. It is controlled with hand removal or the use of surgeon fishes and/or *Diadema* urchins.

Cyanobacteria, or blue-green algae, can smother corals if allowed to get out of balance. A problem genus is *Phormidium* spp. This slime algae can damage coral tissue on contact and is thought by many to be a component of the black band disease complex, since it is found so often in black band lesions. Strong water flow physically prevents colonization. If the algae are established, hand removal or the hermit *Clibanarius tricolor* is used for control.

Predators of Coelenterates

Many reef species are obligate or opportunistic coralivores. Inclusion of these species in captive systems for propagation of coral can lead to failure. Similarly, population shifts in these species can impact wild coral populations. Most marine angelfish, boxfish, butterfly fishes, comb-tooth blennies, filefishes, parrot fishes, porcupine fishes, puffer fishes, spadefish, and triggerfishes predate coral (Borneman, 2001). Predatory gastropods and echinoderms (crown of thorns, *Acanthaster planci*) can be voracious coral predators. Cowries, whelks, cone shells, and some snails predate heavily on coelenterates. *Rapa rapa*, a small snail, feeds on *Sarcophyton*, *Lobophytum*, and *Sinularia* corals by boring into the stalk and eating from the inside. Affected leather corals turn yellow, and polyps may fail to expand properly. Careful examination of the stalk will reveal a small, usually healed, incision. Manual excision of the snail can be successful in restoring the coral. *Heliacus* spp. snails destroy anemone colonies, and *Cyphoma* spp. snails feed on gorgonians. Some nudibranchs feed on corals. Most swimming and box crabs predate corals to some extent, as do several species of shrimp (*Saron* spp., *Lysmata* spp., and members of the Rhynchocinetidae) (Borneman, 2001). It is important to realize that some crabs and shrimp may benefit coral by cleaning debris and removing other deleterious organisms. Some commensal crabs may cause deformations of the coral as gall-like cavities are formed to house them within stony coral colonies, but the net impact on coral growth is positive.

Flatworms, such as the reddish *Convolutriloba retrogemmal*, consume coral tissue and zooxanthellae, creating portals for pathogens to enter the coral. Chemical control of these pests is possible, but caution in this approach is appropriate. Many of these flatworm species accumulate noxious compounds from their prey to help them avoid predation. Killing a large number of these worms suddenly could result in the release of sufficient quantities of noxious or toxic compounds to be of concern. Biological control may be achieved with the mandarin fish (*Synchiropus splendidus*), leopard wrasse (*Macropharyngodon meleagris*), or some types of gobies (Sprung and Delbeek, 1997). Bristle worms and fire worms feed on *Euphyllia* and all soft corals, and polychaetes can wreak havoc on gorgonians and anemones. Generally, these worms are removed manually, though they should be handled with gloves because some species may secrete irritating substances. Many are nocturnal and only do their damage at night. Biological controls are available (wrasses, arrow crabs, and banded shrimp), but unfortunately these usually also destroy the beneficial polychaetes in the system.

Some anemones, particularly *Aiptasia* spp., sting and outcompete corals for space in closed systems. These anemones are serious pests in captive coral systems, and considerable effort has gone into reducing or eliminating their populations, once established. Methods that have been used with at most moderate success include injection of the anemone with boiling water, supersaturated calcium hydroxide, dilute hydrochloric acid, dilute sodium hydroxide, hydrogen peroxide, vinegar, or capsicum. Others have used physical means of removal such as the use of a dental pick to blast *Aiptasia* anemones from substrates. This is only practical if the coral piece being treated can be moved to a separate tank, as regeneration of the fragments of anemones can make the situation worse. The black banded butterfly fish (*Chaetodon striatus*) is a natural predator of *Aiptasia*. A predatory nudibranch, *Berghia verrucicornis*, has been identified that preferentially feeds on *Aiptasia* anemones (Borneman, 2001) but is itself subject to predation, so groups of the nudibranch should be added to the tank at one time. The Majano anemone (*Anemonia* spp.) is a small green anemone that aggressively stings adjacent species. *Centropyge*, *Apolemichthys*, and *Pomacanthus* angels all eat it, but unfortunately they are also quite fond of eating coral.

Toxicities

Heavy Metals

Studies on *Porites lutea* have shown that exposure to copper at relatively low levels (30 ppb or µg/L) greatly reduces primary production of coral endophytes. This effect seems to be dose related. Lower doses (10 ppb or µg/L) did not cause the effect and may even have been protective over the effects of lowered salinity (Alutoin et al., 2001). Coral can be adversely affected by antifouling paint from ships that run aground on reefs. When larvae of the scleractinian coral *Acropora microphthalma* were experimentally exposed to sediment that contained 8 mg/kg tributyltin, 72 mg/kg copper, and 92 mg/kg zinc, larval settlement and metamorphosis were significantly inhibited. Though the exposed larvae survived, they contracted to a spherical shape and ceased swimming and searching. When larvae were exposed to higher contamination levels, 100% mortality was recorded (Negri et al., 2002).

Hydra can be considered more of a pest than a specimen to keep healthy. Though generally hardier than other coelenterates, *Hydra* are susceptible to the same environmental problems that can devastate less hardy species. These conditions include heavy-metal and toxin exposures, extreme temperature, and water condition variations.

Genetic Diseases

Mutant Hydra

Mutant *hydra* are the only mutants identified so far among the coelenterates (Muller, 2002). Greatly enlarged (10-fold normal size) *Chlorohydra viridissima* are considered a mutation from the type species and have no gonad development and do not bud. They exhibit abnormal regeneration patterns, particularly of the basal disc. Laboratory manipulation of these mutants can result in complex multiple branching growth that has been shown to be valuable in the study of autoimmunity (Sugiyama and Fujisawa, 1977; Novak and Lenhoff, 1981).

Diseases of Complex and/or Unknown Etiology

Not unique to coelenterate medicine, it is often difficult to separate noninfectious and infectious contributors to diseases and syndromes. As we learn more about the complex interactions between pathogen, host, and environmental factors in the development of disease in mammals and other terrestrial species, the artificial nature of the distinction between *infectious* and *noninfectious* diseases becomes very apparent. Few, if any, of the diseases of coelenterates can be considered purely infectious, though potential pathogens have been isolated from specimens affected by disease events in the wild and in captivity. In most cases where a potential pathogen has been identified, Koch's postulates are not fulfilled. Nevertheless, most of those diseases have been placed in the section Infectious Diseases. In some cases where considerable work has confirmed a role in disease pathogenesis for an infectious agent, extremely compelling

work also supports roles for environmental factors. I have not been able to place those diseases or syndromes into either Infectious or Noninfectious sections. Therefore, the category of Diseases of Complex Etiology has been created to distinguish these diseases and assuage my prejudice of all infectious disease being the result of a combination of host, environmental, and pathogen factors.

Coral Bleaching

Coral bleaching, though perhaps the most widely and best studied disease of hard corals, is more appropriately considered as a constellation of diseases that cause similar clinical signs. Similar syndromes occur in Cnidaria other than hard corals, but these conditions have received less study. Some of the diseases in this constellation are well documented to be associated with infectious agents, whereas others may be entirely noninfectious. As investigations continue, a combination of environmental factors and the impact of potential pathogens will likely be the more commonly identified pathogenesis for these diseases. The progressive loss of zooxanthellae and resultant loss of color in coral is the cardinal sign that places a disease in the constellation *coral bleaching*. As more work is done, it is likely the discussion of coral bleaching will not be appropriate beyond description of a particularly notable symptom or clinical sign.

Understanding the impact of environmental factors on the pathogenesis of coral-bleaching syndrome is important to comprehend the complexity of the syndrome. The fluorescent pigments of corals help regulate the light exposure to coral tissues. Under low light, they enhance light availability and, in excessive light, they appear to be photoprotective by dissipating excess energy at wavelengths that do not affect photosynthetic activity and by reflecting visible and infrared light. It appears that fluorescent pigments could enhance resistance to mass bleaching of corals during periods of heat stress (Salih et al., 2000). At least some corals (star coral [*Montastraea annularis*] and mountainous star coral [*M. faveolata*]) can act as hosts to many species of *Symbiodinium*, and the composition of these communities is dynamic and seems to depend on the amount of light the corals are exposed to. Some feel that the patterns of bleaching events can be explained by the preferential elimination of a symbiont associated with low irradiance from the brightest parts of a coral's distribution, whereas some corals are protected from bleaching by hosting symbionts that are more tolerant of high irradiance and temperature (Rowan et al., 1997). Other investigators feel that endolithic symbiotic algae may help coral survive bleaching events (Fine et al., 2002).

Other work with coral-bleaching events has established a correlation with increases in sea surface temperature. Looking at the 1998 Maldives event where approximately 98% of Acroporidae and Pocilloporidae (95% of the reef coral population) died, scientists found the monthly mean sea surface temperature was 1.2°–4.0°C above the 1950–1999 average during the warmest months (March–June). The greatest anomaly (+2.1°C) occurred in May. Bleaching was first reported in mid-

April and was severe from late April to mid-May, with some recovery evident by late May. Massive corals (Poritidae, Faviidae, and Agariciidae) survived the bleaching event (Edwards et al., 2001).

One proposed environmental model of coral bleaching sees the clinical signs as a protective defense. This theory is based on knowledge that various stressors, including heat and light, can destabilize the electron transport chain of photosynthesis, causing increased production of reactive oxygen species like hydrogen peroxide. If peroxides and other reactive oxygen products produced by zooxanthellae diffuse into coral tissues at levels that overwhelm the enzymatic and nonenzymatic processes that neutralize them, oxidative damage to the coral would result. As a defense against this, it is hypothesized that the oxidative damage in coral might trigger responses that expel or kill zooxanthellae or reduce their photosynthetic efficiency. In this model, which has been most extensively studied with star coral (*Montastrea annularis* species complex), coral bleaching is a protective defense against oxidative stress that might be triggered by high temperatures or excessive light exposure (Downs et al., 2002). In those studies, levels of oxidative damage products, antioxidant enzymes, and structural integrity indices correlated with bleaching events and increased sea surface temperatures. That coral bleaching is not invariably fatal to affected colonies supports consideration that the actual bleaching may be a protective mechanism to reduce oxidative damage regardless of the source.

Studies focused on mountainous star coral (*Montastrea faveolata*) and boulder star coral (*Montastrea franksi*) in the Caribbean lend an interesting twist to the hypothesis that bleaching is related to the photosynthetic activity of zooxanthellae (Warner et al., 1999). Those studies provide evidence that irreversible damage to photosystem II in heat-stressed symbiotic dinoflagellates within corals occurs during bleaching events. Zooxanthellae lose the photosynthesis II reaction-center protein D1 more quickly than it can be resynthesized at elevated temperatures. However, the observation of higher levels of damage and greater loss of symbionts in deeper corals compared with shallow corals complicates the picture. One hypothesis is that corals resistant to bleaching have a greater capacity for maintaining the photosynthesis II reaction-center reaction at elevated temperatures, perhaps through maintenance of genotypically distinct symbionts (Warner et al., 1999).

Coral bleaching is not limited to corals. Scientists studying the Palau coral-bleaching event following intrusion of warm waters (92°F for over 1 month) caused by the 1998 El Nino event documented significant loss of *Acropora* corals but noted that large carpet anemones also bleached. Many of the affected anemones recovered with the return of cooler waters. Other investigators have suggested that a symbiosis gene (sym32) identified from the temperate sea anemone *Anthopleura elegantissima* may be useful as an early-warning biomarker to detect coral stress leading to coral bleaching. Real-time quantitative reverse transcriptase–polymerase chain reaction (RT-PCR) suggests that the level of sym32 expression is correlated with the abundance of algae in the host anemone (Mitchelmore et al., 2002).

Vibrio shiloi

Vibrio shiloi has been reasonably well established as an infectious cause of coral bleaching in the Mediterranean Sea coral, *Oculina patagonica*. Temperature and infectious causes can work in tandem. In the case of coral bleaching by *V. shiloi*, the disease occurs when seawater temperatures rise, approaching 30°C, and corals recover as the water temperature drops in the fall and winter. The effects of increased temperatures appear to be primarily on the bacteria rather than on the coral itself. For the disease to occur, *V. shiloi* must adhere to the coral surface and penetrate the coral epidermal layer. The major effect of increasing temperature is the expression of virulence genes that code production of an adhesin, enabling the *Vibrio* organism to bind to a receptor in the coral mucus that contains an L-D-galactopranoside group and penetrate into the coral epidermis (Rosenberg and Ben-Haim, 2002). Zooxanthellae must be actively photosynthesizing for this receptor to be produced and secreted in the coral mucus (Banin et al., 2001). Studies have demonstrated that endosymbiotic zooxanthellae contribute to the production of coral mucus and that *V. shiloi* show a distinct positive chemotaxis toward the mucus of *O. patagonica*. *Vibrio shiloi* infects only mucus-containing, zooxanthellate corals (Banin et al., 2000). Once in the coral, the *Vibrio* differentiates into a viable but as of yet nonculturable form and multiplies intracellularly, producing the extracellular toxins that inhibit photosynthesis and bleach and lyse zooxanthellae (Ben-Haim et al., 1999; Banin et al., 2001). The adhesion of the bacteria, intracellular multiplication, and production of the exotoxins are all temperature dependent (Banin et al., 2001). *V. shiloi* also secretes a material designated as AK1-S, which contains a mixture of substances yet to be completely characterized. AK1-S rapidly inhibits photosynthesis of zooxanthellae isolated from at least four species of coral. Other factors in AK1-S that are heat sensitive and nondialyzable also cause pigment loss and zooxanthellae lysis (Ben-Haim et al., 1999).

Vibrio coralyticus

Vibrio coralyticus has been identified as the etiological agent for bleaching stony coral (*Pocillopora damicornis*) in the Red Sea (Rosenberg and Ben-Haim, 2002).

Rapid Wasting

Rapid-wasting disease was first reported in 1996 from the West Indies. Massive corals in middepth and shallow waters are most commonly affected. The syndrome starts as a white lesion that can spread very rapidly (up to 8 cm per day). The coral skeleton is eroded, as well as the soft tissues. No boundary is observed between diseased polyps and disintegrating skeleton material. Algae encroach rapidly onto areas of denuded tissues. It was postulated that a fungal organism was responsible for the condition (Koch's postulates were never fulfilled), but subsequent research has shown that predatory parrot fish (*Sparisoma* sp.) are the source of the lesions (Bruckner and Bruckner, 1998). The disease has been associated with a filamentous fungus that has been observed on affected corals.

Coral Tumors

Tumors of coral have been reported for over 30 years. Some of these reports may be of true tumors, based on the criteria of change in appearance and function, and the ability to metastasize. Normal polyp tissue is destroyed, and tissues are typically lighter in color or white and have decreased or abnormal zooxanthellae populations. Other reports are better characterized as hyperplasia. In *Madrepora* corals, a crustacean symbiont causes development of lesions that mimic a tumor. Algae and fungi are also incriminated as agents in hyperplasias (tumors) on gorgonians.

Tumors of elkhorn coral (*Acropora palmata*), possessing raised, whitened, irregularly shaped skeletal protuberances, grow rapidly and spread along branches. The term *calicoblastic epithelioma* has been proposed for these tumors. Soft tissues surrounding and extending into the skeletal masses revealed proliferation of gastrovascular canals and associated calicoblastic epidermis, with loss of normal polyp structures and zooxanthellae. The slightly atypical tumor calicoblasts were cuboidal to columnar, resembling those found in the rapidly growing apical tips. Stable carbon-isotope ratios of skeletal samples revealed that the tumor skeleton is isotopically lighter than the skeleton in the normal or apical track regions, indicative of higher tissue metabolic rates and lack of carbon-isotope fractionation by zooxanthellae (Peters et al., 1986).

Dark Spots Disease

This is characterized by small discolorations of affected corals (Figure 3.10, Color Plate 3.10). Tissue loss can occur, but corals recover with regrowth of tissue and skeleton, often with a dimpled appearance on the colony surface where the lesion has resolved (Borneman, 2001). The condition is reported to affect *Siderastrea* spp. corals and may be seasonal. No etiological agent has been identified.

Necrotic Patch Disease

An outbreak of necrotic patches affecting *Acropora palmata* in the Mexican Caribbean in the summer of 1999 was reported.

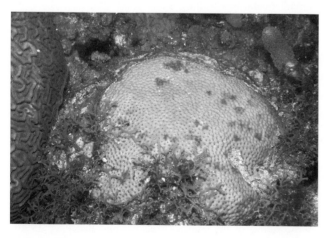

Figure 3.10. Dark spots disease affecting *Siderastrea sideria*. Photo courtesy of E.H. Borneman.

The outbreak was characterized by a rapid increase in the number of new patches, which then leveled off and patches grew in size, sometimes fusing together into very large lesions. The outbreak did not appear to be related to water temperatures (Rodriguez-Martinez et al., 2001). This disease could be synonymous with white pox disease.

Porites *Ulcerative White Spot Disease*

This is thought to be infectious because it can be spread by direct contact between affected and unaffected coral colonies and perhaps by waterborne contact. To date, no specific etiology has been identified. The disease is characterized by discrete, bleached, round to ovoid foci, 3–5 mm in diameter, affecting 3–4 polyps and the coenosteum. These lesions can heal and disappear, which commonly happens. They can also expand and coalesce into larger irregular patches more than 3 cm in diameter, where all coral tissue is lost and colonization with green filamentous algae is common. These lesions do not usually heal, but progress to involve large parts of the coral colony, and can kill the colony. Both branching and massive *Porites* spp. can be affected. Species reported with the disease include *Porites attentuata*, *P. cylindrical*, *P. nigrescens*, *P. horizontallata*, *P. rus*, and *P. annae*. *Porites australiensis*, *P. lobata*, *P. lutea*, and *P. solida* are considered possibly susceptible. The prevalence of *Porites* ulcerative white spot disease appears to correlate with coral density (Raymundo et al., 2003). Some investigators believe bleaching may be the initial event in pathogenesis of *Porites* ulcerative white spot disease, but this is not a uniformly held opinion. In contact transmission studies, lesions develop within a week. Lesions in experimental transmission studies are not discrete and round but are irregular denuded areas, spreading from the point of contact, that progress to tissue loss. Grafting ill colonies onto healthy ones spreads the disease quite effectively.

Purple Ring (Pink Ring) Disease

This condition has been reported affecting *Porites* spp. in the Pacific. The name comes from blotchy areas with algal encroachment that have a distinctive pink/purple ring around them. Fungal hyphae have been described associated with the lesions, but no specific etiological agent has been identified. The purple/pink discoloration is thought to be a response of the coral to stress or injury.

Yellow Band Disease

This is characterized by a broad yellow band that progresses across the coral, leaving behind a denuded skeleton that remains yellow (Figure 3.11). The disease has been reported in finger corals (acroporids) and other corals of the Arabian Gulf. It has also been reported affecting scroll coral (*Turbinaria reniformis*) and the Pacific faviids (*Cyphastrea* spp.). The disease progresses faster in warmer water and is in many ways similar to other coral band diseases. It is sometimes referred to as yellow-line disease but is considered distinct from yellow blotch

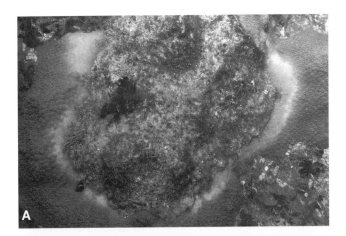

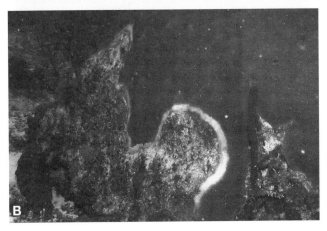

Figure 3.11. Yellow band disease afflicting **(A)** *Montastrea franksi* and **(B)** *M. faveolata*. Photos courtesy of E.H. Borneman.

disease (Korrubel, 1998). The etiology of the condition is unknown.

Yellow Blotch Disease

This is characterized by yellow blotchy patches or rings on the upper surfaces or the sides of coral. These rings spread outward, and filamentous algae accumulate on affected tissues behind the expanding front of the disease. There has been speculation that this disease may be a disease of zooxanthellae rather than of the coral, because of the nature of the discolorations. These appear to be due to pigment changes rather than classic bleaching or necrosis. Atypical zooxanthellae have been observed in diseased tissues of Caribbean corals of the *Montastrea annularis* species complex. These corals host four taxa of symbiotic dinoflagellates (zooxanthellae; genus *Symbiodinium*) in ecologically predictable patterns (Toller et al., 2001). When zooxanthellae depletion from the disease is not extreme, recovering corals generally contain the same types of zooxanthellae as they did prior to the depletion, but, after severe depletion, recovering corals can repopulate with zooxanthellae atypical for their habitat (and in some cases atypical for the coral species) (Toller et al., 2001). In coral colonies where unusual zooxanthellae associ-

ations were established, the original taxa of zooxanthellae were not detected even 9 months after the end of treatment.

Infectious Diseases

Unfortunately, the naming conventions for diseases of coelenterates are based on early terms describing the color, shape, and distribution of lesions. This unfortunate convention is carried forward even when diseases become associated with potential or confirmed pathogens. Coelenterates, as all species, are limited in the ways they can respond to injury and insult. Disease nomenclature based on the limited vocabulary of gross symptomatology generally results in the inappropriate lumping of conditions caused by different agents. This can confound the investigation of control and therapy options. As more careful work is done investigating the etiologies and pathogenesis of these diseases, more appropriate disease names will supplant the confusing and, in many cases, misleading terminology currently in use. An international scientific group called the Coral Disease and Health Consortium is currently working on standardizing coral disease nomenclature and educating coral reef biologists on pathology (E. Peters, personal communication, 2004). In the meantime, I have tried to adhere to the names extant in the peer-reviewed literature.

Viral Diseases

It is not surprising that few viruses have been isolated from coelenterates, much less associated with disease. Considering the breadth of potential pathogen types identified in association with coelenterates in recent years, it is likely that there are many viruses, rickettsia, and other difficult-to-culture and characterize agents yet to be found.

Hydra Adenovirus

This adenovirus causes a disease in *Hydra vulgaris* that is characterized by arrested growth, followed by aggressive budding and regression of the gastric column and tentacles, and then by complete dissolution of the hydra. Histopathology of affected animals shows nuclear hypertrophy in the epithelium of the hydra's stalk. No effective therapeutic approach has been reported. Control measures center on isolation and/or destruction of affected hydra (Van Etten et al., 1982).

Bacterial Diseases
Black Band Disease

This is named for a characteristic black mat that occurs over dying coral tissue (Figure 3.12). The lesion advances at a rate of millimeters per day and leaves behind bare coral skeleton as it progresses. The exposed skeleton is rapidly overgrown by filamentous algae and accumulations of silt. Species of coral considered particularly susceptible to the disease include

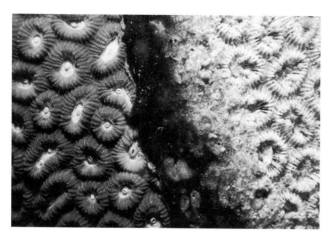

Figure 3.12. Black band disease on a *Favia* sp. specimen. Photo courtesy of E.H. Borneman.

Montastrea annularis, *M. cavernosa*, and *Diploria strigosa*. Very heavy mucus producers like pipe organ coral (*Tubipora musica*) and mushroom corals (fungiids) seem somewhat resistant to the disease, as are those species with large, long-tentacled polyps. Traumatic injury usually predisposes the coral to the disease (E. Peters, personal communication, 2004).

The bacterial community associated with healthy corals is characterized by low bacterial abundance and diversity (Cooney et al., 2002). The microbial mat of black band disease is dominated by large filamentous cyanobacteria originally identified as *Oscillatoria submembranaceae* and later reclassified as *Phormidium corallyticum* (Rützler and Santavy, 1983; Frias-Lopez et al., 2002). Other bacteria identified in the black band disease mat include motile, nonphotosynthetic sulfide-oxidizing *Beggiatoa* spp. (Garrett and Ducklow, 1975; Ducklow and Mitchell, 1979; Rützler and Santavy, 1983) and the sulfate-reducing *Desulfovibrio* spp. (Garrett and Ducklow, 1975; Rützler et al., 1983). Nucleic acid sequences affiliated with the genera *Campylobacter* and *Arcobacter* have been detected in the black band disease mat and on dead coral surface samples (Frias-Lopez et al., 2002). A single cyanobacterial ribotype differing from that identified in *Phormidium corallyticum* black band disease samples, a *Cytophaga* spp., and an α-proteobacterium identified as the etiological agent of juvenile oyster disease have all been found consistently in diseased coral samples (Cooney et al., 2002). In addition, *Clostridium* spp. and *Trichodesmium tenue* have been isolated from the mat of corals affected with black band disease. Microbiological studies of the bacteria communities associated with black band disease of the scleractinian corals *Diploria strigosa*, *Montastrea annularis*, and *Colpophyllia natans* have found no evidence of bacteria from terrestrial, freshwater, or human sources (Cooney et al., 2002). One research group suggests that fish infected with *Cytophaga fermentans* may transmit the disease to healthy corals (Frias-Lopez et al., 2002). Others feel the coral is predisposed to the disease by local injury and exposure to elevated temperatures (Borneman, 2001).

The progression of *Phormidium corallyticum* and *Beggiatoa* spp. across living tissues in black band disease occurs both diur-

nally and nocturnally with the fastest movements by the front of the band during the day and the back of the band at night. The band is very similar to laminated microbial mats found in benthic, sulfide-rich environments. The upper layers in the vertical strata of the band are oxygen rich, whereas the lower layers contain high concentrations of sulfide, which is thought to possibly be a mechanism of coral death as the band progresses. *Phormidium corallyticum* has been shown to occur primarily in the oxygen-rich upper layers of the band. Sulfate reducers like desulfovibrios are found in the lower strata of the band. *Beggiatoa* spp. appear to migrate vertically in the strata of the band, rising toward the band surface at night when these organisms may remain in higher strata nearer the surface of the band than do the *Phormidium* organisms during periods of illumination (Richardson, 1996). Black band disease can halt on its own. This has been observed on rare occasions in aquariums. Removal of affected corals to a treatment tank, and application of a paste of neomycin sulfate brushed onto the band, along with elevation of salinity and 2 or 3 days of darkness, have been reported effective in some cases. Alternatively, debridement approximately 1 cm ahead of the band or siphoning off the band material and applying plasticine modeling clay has been used with modest success (Kuta and Richardson, 1997). It would seem that environmental corrections (low light, reduced water temperature, and increased salinity), combined with aggressive debridement and the use of more efficient antibiotic delivery systems such as drug-impregnated methacrylate, orabase gels, or even plasticine, might improve therapeutic success. Basic antibiotic sensitivity information needs to be developed, and, in captive systems, isolation and careful sanitation protocols will likely contribute to containment.

White Band Disease

This is already subdivided into types I and II. In both types, the disease starts at the shaded base of the coral and progresses toward the branch tips. It can on occasion start in the middle of a branch. There are disagreements about the definition of the disease among researchers, with some holding a very tight definition limiting the disease to acroporid corals and others using a broader definition that is applied to any disease that starts from the base of the coral colony and causes tissue loss (including rapid tissue necrosis). Elkhorn coral (*Acropora palmata*) is the species most commonly reported affected. In type I disease, a clear margin of tissue necrosis advances across the affected coral. The white band expands at a rate of several millimeters per day, leaving bare skeleton exposed. Polyp tissue peels from skeleton in little balls. No consistent accumulation of organisms has been identified in the band, but Gram-negative rod bacteria have been observed on *Acropora* spp. affected with type I disease. Type II disease is more virulent, with a faster progression of necrosis across the coral. The width of the active disease line is variable, and some tissue bleaches before necrosing. *Vibrio charcharia* is associated with type II disease.

Some investigators still do not consider white band disease to be contagious and hypothesize that the disease originates in weakened parts of the coral. Those using the broader definition of the disease associate it with the presence of the corallivorous snail (*Drupella cornus*). However, the disease (particularly type II) appears to be transmissible by direct contact with adjacent coral. Though efforts have been made, no effective treatments have been identified. Antiseptic baths of Lugol's solution or chloramphenicol have been reported occasionally effective, though the key to recovery in captive situations seems to rely on maintaining proper water flow, lighting, and water conditions. Fragmentation and isolated propagation are sometimes employed to avoid total colony loss.

White Plague

This resembles white band disease, and the nomenclature of these related diseases is controversial (Figures 3.13 and 3.14, Color Plate 3.14). White plague has been divided by many workers into two diseases: white plague type I and white plague type II. Type I was first described in the late 1970s from the Florida Keys and is characterized by rapid loss of tissue. The disease is essentially identical to white band disease but is characterized as having a more rapid progression. No causative agent has been identified, and it would not be unreasonable at this point in our understanding of coral diseases to lump the disease with white band disease. Type II is also a fast-progressing disease commonly seen in Caribbean elliptical star coral (*Dichocoenia stokesi*). It was originally split from type I based on spread rates up to 2 cm per day. It has since been demonstrated that the bacterial populations in fragmented remnants of degenerated coral tissues at the lesion boundary in type II are predominantly *Sphingomonas* spp. (Bythell et al., 2002). Infection transmission studies support the small, motile, Gram-negative *Sphingomonas* bacteria as the cause of the disease. A better name for the disease would be *sphingomoniasis*. However, a recent study based on molecular taxonomic techniques has determined that this organism is actually a new species to science and should be in its own genus. The authors have named it *Aurantimonas coralicida* (Denner et al., 2003) and found it to be genetically identical to the *Sphingomonas* organism identified by Richardson et al. (1998) (Figure 3.13). Sphingomoniasis, though first reported to affect *Dichocoenia stokesi*, has since been diagnosed in *Agaricia agaricites*, *A. lamarcki*, *Colpophyllia natans*, *Dendrogyra cylindrus*, *Diploria labyrinthiformis*, *D. strigosa*, *Eusmillia fastigiata*, *Madracis decactis*, *M. mirabilis*, *Manicina areolata*, *Meandrina meandrites*, *Montastrea annularis* species complex, *M. cavernosa*, *Siderastrea siderea*, *Solellnastrea bournoni*, and *Stephanocoenia michelinii* in addition to *Millepora alcicornis* (Richardson et al., 1998). The disease is readily transmitted and can be devastating to reefs or to aquarium collections. No therapeutic or control measures, distinct from those being applied to white band disease, have been developed for white plague I or II.

Red Band Disease

This is also known as coraline lethal orange disease (Littler and Littler, 1995). It primarily affects gorgonians and some stony corals. Current thoughts are that it may have a cyanobacterial etiology, but due to an organism other than *Phormydium coralliticum*. *Schyzothrix* spp. and *Oscillatoria* spp. are also present in a characteristic reddish mat of necrosing tissue and cyanobacteria that advances across affected coral. This disease advances much more rapidly in the day and may become quiescent at night. Another disease of unknown etiology, brown band disease, is lumped with red band disease at this time. No specific therapeutic or control measures have been reported for the disease other than the generalized approaches used with black band disease and white band disease.

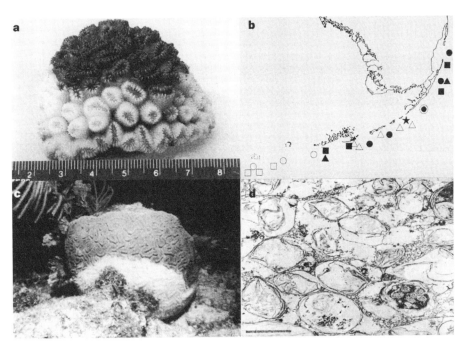

Figure 3.13. *Dichocoenia stokesi* clinically infected by *Sphingomonas* sp. (now more accurately known as *Aurantimonas coralicida*) out of water (centimeter scale) (a) and in the wild (c). (b) Illustrated are the results of a 1995 Florida Reef Tract survey in August (*circles*), September (*squares*), and October (*triangles*). Other symbols and meanings: *black*, active disease; *white*, disease free; *star*, first disease observation; and *double circle*, highest incidence of disease. (d) A transmission electron microsopic image of a diseased gastroderm with collapsed and degenerated zooxanthellae. The *arrow* indicates a periplast membrane (scale bar = 5.0 μm). Reprinted by permission of Nature Publication Group. (from Richardson et al. [1998])

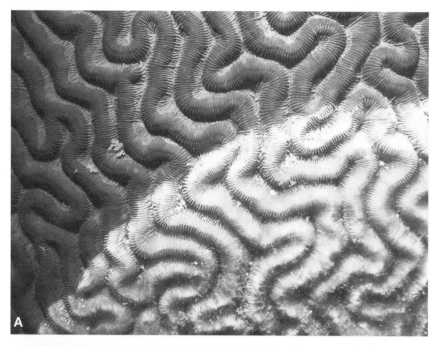

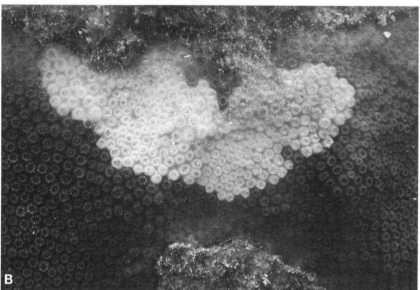

Figure 3.14. White plague disease afflicting **(A)** *Colpophyllia natans* and **(B)** *Montastrea faveolata*. Photos courtesy of E.H. Borneman.

White Pox

This disease (also called white patch disease) affects populations of the shallow-water Caribbean elkhorn coral (*Acropora palmata*) in Florida waters. It is a rapidly progressive disease with tissue loss rates averaging 2.5 cm² per day. Its occurrence is seasonal, with the greatest impact when water temperatures are elevated. The pattern of disease spread fits with a contagion model, with nearest neighbors being most susceptible to infection. A common fecal enterobacterium, *Serratia marcescens*, has been suggested as the causal agent (Patterson et al., 2002). Clinically, the disease appears as scattered blotches of tissue loss. No specific therapeutic or control management of the disease is reported, but basic measures to control other bacterial diseases of coral would be appropriate.

Rapid Tissue Degeneration

This is sometimes referred to as rapid tissue necrosis (Figure 3.15). It is most likely a syndrome rather than a disease, because tissue degeneration or necrosis is a very nonspecific reaction to a wide variety of stressors of coral. The term may be synonymous with the condition referred to by some aquarists as *shut-down reaction*. The condition has been associated with the bacterium *Vibrio vulnificus*, a common potential pathogen that has been isolated from shipping water of affected corals. Koch's postulates have not been fulfilled. The condition is also associated with raised water temperatures and is frequently seen in recently shipped specimens. This argues strongly for the need to apply the key components of preventive health programs, quarantine, acclimation, and routine physical examination to corals

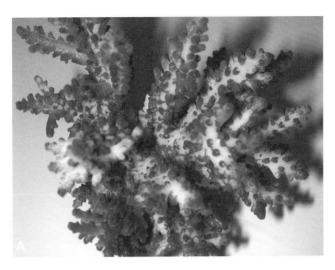
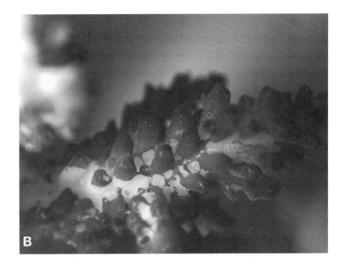

Figure 3.15.   Rapid tissue necrosis (shutdown reaction) afflicting *Acropora* sp. Photos courtesy of E.H. Borneman.

and coelenterates in general. Despite considerable investment in coral stock, which is sometimes irreplaceable, there is a reluctance to accept the value of investing in multiple high-quality holding systems to enable implementation of appropriate quarantine of new colonies, rather than keeping "all eggs in one basket" and risking importation of infectious disease into the collection. Within captive systems, it is recommended that corals be kept well pruned to prevent shading and flow reduction. Management of valuable specimens dispersed in multiple systems is also recommended and can help reduce the dimension of catastrophic losses. In the face of an outbreak, it is recommended that affected corals be removed to treatment systems if at all possible. Affected branches should be debrided and/or pruned. Underwater expoxies have been used to seal the debrided wound edges (Sprung and Delbeek, 1997) with variable success. The technique seems less effective on species with porous skeletons (*Acropora* spp.). This may be because the pathogens can move through the skeleton to infect new tissues. Increasing the water flow on affected corals appears beneficial. Many aquarists facing this disease or syndrome implement any of a variety of antibiotic baths. In particular, chloramphenicol is being touted as a useful treatment, albeit with proper cautioning (Sprung and Delbeek, 1997). The use of antibiotics in the treatment of coelenterate diseases, including this one, requires judicious consideration of the principles of chemotherapeutics. Ideally, some diagnostics should be performed to confirm the involvement of organisms that would be susceptible to the chemical being considered as a therapeutic agent. Culture and sensitivity testing should be more extensively employed in invertebrate medicine. In addition, care should be taken in the selection of antibiotics. Chloramphenicol presents a finite, and small but well-documented, health risk to people genetically susceptible to a dyscrasia of the hematopoietic system known as Grey's syndrome. Though it is an effective broad-spectrum antibiotic, it might be wiser to investigate the use of related compounds, such as florfenicol, that do not pose this risk but have a similar broad-spectrum range of efficacy.

Fungal Diseases

Endolithic Fungi

Endolithic fungi have been identified in corals in a wide variety of states of health. Little work has been reported on the taxonomy of these organisms, and it is difficult to assess their possible role in disease. Researchers looking at *Porites lutea* affected with pink line syndrome found fungi in healthy, partially dead, bleached, and diseased corals (Ravindran et al., 2001). Some investigators believe these fungi may be pathogenic (Bentis et al., 2000).

Sea Fan Aspergillosis

The fungus *Aspergillus sydowii* is considered the causative agent of an epizootic disease affecting sea fan corals (*Gorgonia ventalina* and *G. flabellum*) (Smith et al., 1998; Nagelkerken et al., 1997; Geiser et al., 1998). The disease, which is known throughout most of the Caribbean and the Florida Keys (Nagelkerken et al., 1997), is characterized by galling and purpling of the tissues of the fan corals and can result in death of the colony (Smith et al., 1998). The putative pathogen, *Aspergillus sydowii*, is a mesophilic soil saprobe, which is also known as a food contaminant and occasionally as an opportunistic pathogen of humans (Olutiola and Cole, 1977). It has been postulated that the terrestrial fungus may have infested reef waters via terrestrial runoff (Smith et al., 1998). It has also been hypothesized that *A. sydowii* might be attached to dust particles that settle as aerosols on the sea surface and become suspended in sediment (Shinn et al., 2000). However, strains of *A. sydowii* from terrestrial sources do not appear to be pathogenic to sea fans, whereas strains isolated from sea fans can readily induce disease (Geiser et al., 1998). Sea fans appear to produce antifungal secondary compounds that provide some resistance to disease (Kim et al., 2000), but with elevated water temperatures there is a shift in the coral–fungus interaction favoring the pathogen (Alker et al., 2001). Fungal growth rates increase and the efficacy of the gorgonian-produced antifungal compounds decreases at higher temperatures. Specific therapeutic and control recommendations are not published. The potential for various antifungal drugs to effect cures in captive specimens remains to be explored.

Protozoal Diseases

Hydra Amoebiasis

A seasonal disease of hydra is caused by *Hydramoeba hydroxena*. Numerous amoebic trophozoites can be found in the tentacles of hydra that have stopped feeding. As the disease progresses, the hydra's tentacles will be consumed by the amoebae. The disease is most common in the late summer and early fall, and may be associated with the stress of warmer waters. Green hydra (*Chlorhydra viridissima*) are relatively resistant to the disease. No therapeutic approach has been reported. Control in captive situations involves early diagnosis and removal of severely affected hydra.

Siderastrea Amoebiasis

Large numbers of an unidentified amoeba have been found in calicoblast tissue of starlet corals (*Siderastrea* spp.). No disease condition has been described (Borneman, 2001).

Brown Jelly Infection

A serious acute syndrome of corallimorph anemones may be caused by *Helicostoma nonatum* (Figure 3.16, Table 3.2). Affected anemones melt suddenly in a dark brown jellylike mass that has been compared with a melted chocolate bar (Sprung and Delbeek, 1997). The protozoan spreads by direct contact, so rapid isolation of affected specimens with care not to disperse infected tissues throughout the tank is an important control measure. A similar syndrome is reported in large-polyped corals (e.g., *Cataphyllia* spp. and *Xenia* spp.). It is thought that the disease may be initiated by trauma to the polyp, with secondary invasion by *Helicostoma* sp. Koch's postulates have not been fulfilled. Elevated temperatures and poor water quality have also been associated with initiation of the disease. Reported therapeutic approaches center on careful and complete debridement, freshwater dips, and application of antibiotic pastes. This latter approach would not be expected to be efficacious if *Helicostoma* spp. are indeed the primary pathogens. Prognosis is guarded to poor.

Porites *Hypertrophy*

A condition in finger coral (*Porites porites*) characterized by generalized cellular hypertrophy is thought to be associated with *Nematopsis* spp. infection. The protozoan might have a mollusk or crustacean host, but no studies have been reported. Koch's postulates have not been fulfilled. No therapeutic or tested control measures have been reported (Borneman, 2001).

Gemmocystiasis

The protozoan *Gemmocystis cylindrus* has been isolated from mesenterial filaments of several corals after colonies have displayed patchy necrosis (Upton and Peters, 1986; Borneman, 2001). Koch's postulates have not been fulfilled. No therapeutic or control measures are reported.

Dinoflagellate Diseases

A number of dinoflagellate diseases have been reported in single articles. Little information is provided in the way of patho-

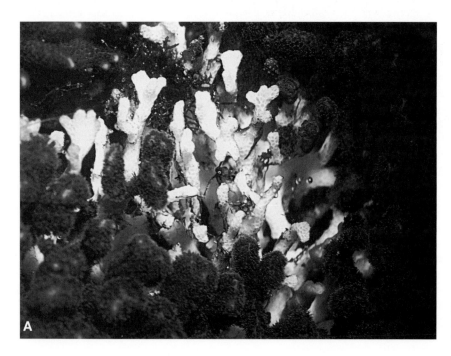

Figure 3.16. A: *Pocillopora damicornis* showing severe damage caused by *Helicostoma* sp.

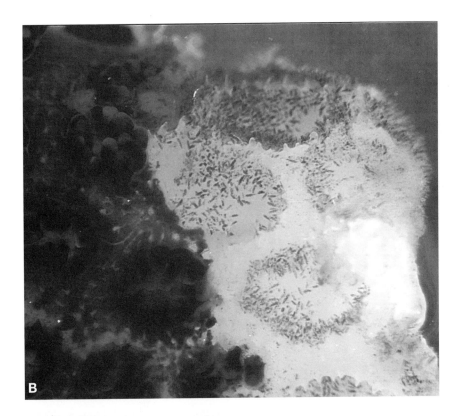

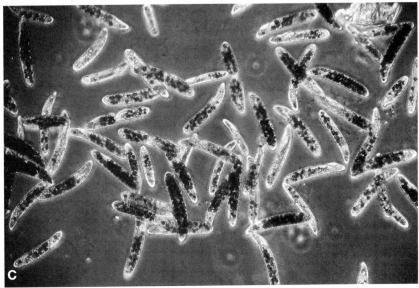

Figure 3.16.   B: Close-up of numerous *Helicostoma* sp. protozoans feeding on the tissues of *Pocillopora damicornis*. **C:** Photomicrograph of a group of *Helicostoma* sp. protozoans with ingested zooxanthellae. Photos courtesy of www.biophoto.net.

genesis or therapeutic response. The taxonomy of the parasites reported is also somewhat confusing. Considerably more work needs to be done with the study of these types of pathogens. Hydromedusae peridinienosis is reported to be caused by the phagotrophic dinoflagellate *Protoodinium chattoni*, also referred to as *Endodinium chattoni* and sometimes considered a symbiotic organism (Goodson et al., 2001). The dinoflagellate parasitizes epithelial cells of gastrozooids and gonozoids of *Velella velella*, *Obelia* spp., *Lizza* spp., and *Podocoryne* spp., among other species. The dinoflagellate *Stylodinium gastrophilum* is reported to parasitize gastrozoids of *Sulculeolaria* spp.

Metazoan Diseases

Corallimorph Flatworm Infestation

A variety of flatworms are commonly seen on *Discosoma* spp. The most common worms are in the genus *Waminoa* and are not considered particularly harmful, but in heavy infestations they can block light from the underlying polyps. These worms also readily transfer from their normal host corallimorphs to stony and soft corals. Other species of flatworm that have been documented to cause problems with large population explosions include *Convolutriloba retrogemma*, a red brown oppor-

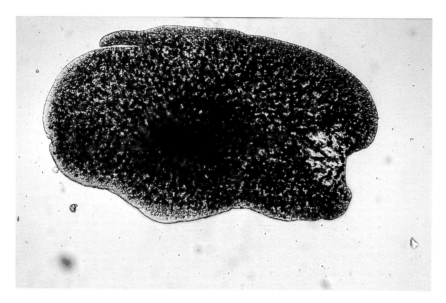

Figure 3.17.   A flatworm found on a soft coral. Photo courtesy of www.biophoto.net.

tunist about 5 mm long with three caudal projections (Figure 3.17). The reddish color of these worms is from incorporation of zooxanthellae into their body wall. Shaking corallimorphs in a saltwater bath prior to placing the specimens in a tank will dislodge a large portion of these worms and retard the buildup of the worm population in the new tank. Corallimorphs will generally tolerate up to a minute in freshwater, and shaking in a freshwater bath rather than saltwater will increase the efficacy of worm removal (Sprung and Delbeek, 1997). There are flatworms that are thought to be parasitic, primarily because they are always found on specific hosts. Mushroom anemones are commonly affected. Large polyp hard corals can also harbor these worms, particularly elegance coral (*Catalaphyllia jardinei*) and bubble coral (*Plerogyra sinuosa*). Soft corals infested include *Sinularia* spp., *Cladiella* spp., *Litophyton* spp., and *Sarcophyton* spp. (Sprung and Delbeek, 1994). The nature of the damage these parasitic flatworms inflict is not well understood, and it may be that their impact, which can cause the decline and even death of a coral specimen, is again primarily from shading and altering water flow to the hosts.

Often the identity of problem flatworms overwhelming tanks is never determined carefully. This leads to some confusion about the efficacy of treatments. Not all flatworms are equally palatable to predators introduced for biological control, nor are all flatworms equally susceptible to chemical or environmental treatments. Whenever possible, collect samples of the worms you are trying to treat and place them in approximately 10 volumes of alcohol to the volume of the worms for fixation and later identification by a trained taxonomist.

Anthelmintic drugs have been used to eliminate flatworm infestations. Levamisole hydrochloric acid delivered at a dose of 8 mg/L in a 24-h bath has eliminated blooms of unidentified (unfortunately) flatworms (A. Tuttle personal communication, 2003). This level of treatment does not cause any apparent harm to a variety of corals, including velvet finger coral (*Montipora digitata*), whorled montipora (*M. capricornis*), *Acropora*

spp., bird's nest coral (*Seriatopora histrix*), and club finger coral (*Stylophora pistillata*). Before conducting treatments of this type on a large scale, it is imperative to test the impact, on a very small scale, of the therapeutant on the organisms you are hoping to help. It is never a good idea to add a therapeutic agent to an entire tank. It is a measure of absolute last resort.

Coelenterate Thynnascariasis

Larval nematodes of the genus *Thynnascaris* have been found associated with *Phialidium* spp., *Polyorchis penicillatus*, and a variety of scyphozoans. The impact of these larval nematodes is not well documented. No successful therapeutic approach has been reported.

Coral Metacercariasis

This disease has been reported in *Porites compressa* and *P. lobata* on Hawaiian reefs. The unspecified metacercariae encyst in a nodule on the edge of polyps. The nodules physically compress adjacent cells and can grow large enough to obscure polyp tentacles. No successful therapeutic approach has been reported.

Analgesia, Anesthesia, and Surgery

Analgesia

The basis for assessing analgesia in coelenterates is not clear. It is arguable that their nervous systems may not be adequate to warrant any significant risk of chemical application on the basis of alleviating pain, but no careful study of this question has been published. Chemical anesthetics have been employed more for control of motion to facilitate imaging, physical examination, or manipulation, than for analgesic purposes. Many procedures are performed with no chemical application. This is

Table 3.2. Clinical signs of disease or normal?

Brown jelly—Brown gelatinous material appears suddenly on the surface of a coral or soft coral. The material is the product of necrosing polyp tissues, and bare skeletal material will become visible as the condition progresses. *Clinical sign.*

Brown oral strings or pellets—These suggest zooxanthellae extrusion, but can be a normal response to rebalance symbiont levels, often responding to shifts in photoperiod or other lighting changes. *Normal.*

Goniopora slow wasting—Lower marginal polyps stop expanding and then die. The condition can progress up the branch until all polyps are gone. *Clinical sign.*

Gorgonian sloughing—This is spontaneous. Starting at the base, the tissue becomes soft and spongy, and separates from core and darkens. *Clinical sign.*

Large polyp recession—Apparently healthy large polyp coral begins to lose tissue at the polyp margins. Algal growth or brown jelly reactions may follow. *Clinical sign.*

Leather coral collapse—Distinct from normal shedding of leather corals (*Sinularia*, *Sarcophyton*, and *Lobophytum*) (Figure 3.9). Polyps stop expanding, turn darker, and after up to several weeks the tissue looses integrity and degenerates rather than renewing. Holes of rotting tissue appear on the capitulum or stalks and grow larger. *Clinical sign.*

Mucus capture webs—These are a normal feeding response of several species. including *Turbinaria* spp. and *Acropora* spp. *Normal.*

Mushroom shrink—Corallimorphs shrink, display mottled and pale tissues, and cannot expand fully. *Clinical sign.*

Nightly collapse—Most soft corals normally collapse when the lights go out. *Normal.*

Polyp coagulative necrosis—Polyp becomes soft, produces a white friable deposit or film on the outer surface, and usually progresses to death. *Clinical sign.*

Polyp extrusion—This appears similar to bleaching, but small round balls (intact polyps) are found floating out from the skeleton of the coral. This occurs often in pocilloprids as part of normal coral expansion. *Normal.*

But it can also occur as a response to disease or stress. *Clinical sign.*

Polyp shutdown—Colonial polyps stop opening for prolonged periods and do not respond to water changes. *Clinical sign.*

Purging—Large polyped corals (*Idiscosoma*, *Cataphyllia*, and *Cynarina*) and large-bodied anemones regurgitate remains of digested food through the oral opening. There is controversy over whether this is normal or a common minor malady.

Soft coral collapse—There is loss of turgor, or collapse or wilt. *Clinical sign.*

Waxy shed—*Porites* and gorgonians as well as *Sarcophyton* spp. and other leather corals normally shed a waxy layer from their surface as a defense against siltation and algae. The process lasts a day to a week, depending on the strength of currents. *Normal.*

White film—Excessive mucus, draped over coral, appears like a white film. It can be a response to irritation or rough handling or a response to chemical irritations from a variety of things, including nearby pockets of anaerobic decay. *Clinical sign.*

White paste—A thick, white, pasty substance that can engulf stony corals is an aggressive response to irritants. *Clinical sign.*

Xeniid melt—Healthy soft corals, particularly in the family Xeniidae, melt to a pile of small fragments and stumps within 24 h. *Clinical sign.*

particularly true for the sessile species. The more mobile jellies can be immobilized with tricaine methane sulfonate (MS-222) or with ethanol to reduce or eliminate pulsing of the bell. Similar techniques, if necessary, would probably be effective for comb jellies.

Surgery

The most common surgical procedures performed on these species is debridement of diseased or damaged tissues and fragmentation for propagation. Debridement should be performed with sharp dissection, taking care to minimize tissue handling and tissue crushing. Debridement of stony corals should extend into the skeleton sufficiently to remove damaged polyps entirely. The appropriate width of margins into apparently healthy tissue has not been well established. It would apparently vary with species and the condition being treated. Further studies in this area are required. Care should be taken to avoid contamination of systems or water with fragments from a debridement. Removed tissue should be treated as infectious and capable of transmitting the disease being treated, even when the infectious nature of the disease is not established.

The issue of whether to fill defects in stony corals after debridement remains controversial. A number of strategies have been used with success measured by the survival of the treated colony. Controlled studies looking at impact on healing time are rare and have had sufficient design flaws to make interpretation difficult. Defects have been filled with antibiotic-impregnated and unimpregnated plasticine clay, plaster of Paris, hydraulic cement (Quick Plug, Ace Hardware), and specialized plastering compounds (Thorite; Standard Dry Wall Products, Cenerville, IN). It would appear that many promising options have not yet been explored. Water-resistant dental compounding bases, methacrylates (superglue), other cyanoacrylate gels, and underwater epoxies deserve further investigation, both with and without drug impregnation.

Fragmentation for propagation needs to be performed correctly or the procedure can put the parent colony or organism at risk for infection and/or deterioration. Many corals are easily propagated, including the soft coral genera *Lobophytum*, *Sarcophyton*, *Sinularia*, *Cladiella*, and *Xenia*, as well as leather corals and *Sinularias*. When fragmenting stony corals, it is important to have a fragment of sufficient size to provide a viable growing colony (Figure 3.18). For branching corals, this is at least 4 cm of branch. Expect healing-over and the initiation of regeneration on the donor site within 2 weeks if the coral is in healthy condition. Some practitioners feel that extending the photoperiod helps improve the culture results and also recommend higher pH (8.2–8.5) to ensure better growth, particularly for soft corals. In general, success will be best with optimal water and lighting conditions combined with proper nutrition.

Several methods have been used successfully to anchor coral fragments to substrate to facilitate handling and provide a base to stabilize the growing colony. An inexpensive and simple method suitable for high production efforts uses sandcast plugs of hydraulic cement (Ace Quick Plug). Up to 10 base plugs are poured at one time and coral fragments placed in the rapidly

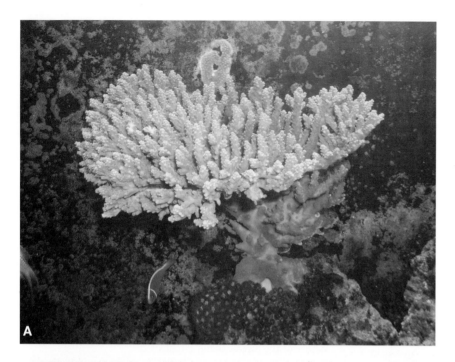

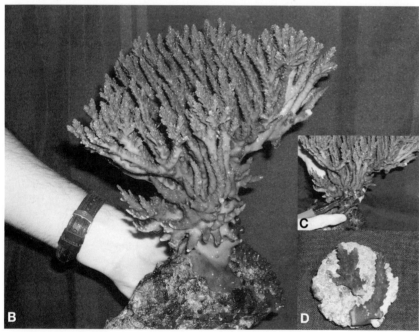

Figure 3.18. Coral fragmentation is a growing and popular aspect of reef-aquarium development and maintenance. Fragmentation of small polyp scleractinian corals occurs by fracturing the underlying corallum (skeleton). Minimizing damage to the epidermis enables fast regrowth of the coral base and reduced likelihood of infection. Fragmentation occurs naturally as physical processes wear on corals in the wild and is mimicked in captivity by use of bone shears or tile snips. Fragments are then adhered to a surface by use of epoxy or cyanoacrylate adhesives. Regrowth and basing begin to occur within a few days. When performed carefully, small cuttings can be safely removed from a larger colony and propagated. **A:** A healthy stony coral colony (*Acropora plana*) in the aquarium. **B:** The same colony removed from the aquarium. **C:** A pair of sharp shears are used to remove 5- to 10-cm pieces of the coral. **D:** The cuttings are cemented to substrate and placed in an aquarium. Photos courtesy of D. Wade Lehmann.

setting cement. By the time the 10th fragment is placed, the first is usually set and ready for removal from the sand. The affixed coral fragments are rinsed to wash off excess mucus, and the plugs are placed in a plastic plant flat to reduce handling trauma and then placed in their grow-out tank. The base of hydraulic cement will be overgrown in as little as 10 days. Two-part underwater epoxies (putty sticks) are used in some less extensive propagation efforts. One should avoid specialized epoxies designed for plumbing applications that may have toxic copper or steel fillers. Underwater epoxies are not very sticky, and care has to be taken in how they are used. They should not be expected

to hold large coral fragments in precarious positions. They can be used effectively as filler to stabilize fragments in a hole or cup. For several days after using underwater epoxies, expect excess skimmer effluent. Cyanoacrylate gels are preferred over underwater epoxies by some propagators because the gels are very innocuous and somewhat more adhesive, but these products rapidly become brittle and also cannot be expected to hold a lot of weight. Neither the epoxies nor the cyanoacrylates bind well to wet items, so careful blotting with a paper or cloth towel is required before the glue is applied (Sprung and Delbeek, 1997).

Diagnostic Techniques

Culture and Sensitivity Testing

Primary Culture

Primary culture of branching scleractinian corals (*Acropora microphthalma* and *Pocillopora damicornis*), *Montipora digitata*, *Stylophora pistillata*, *Seriatopora hystrix*, and *Porites* spp. cells can be accomplished by using supplemented Dulbecco's modified Eagle's media with heat-inactivated fetal bovine serum, antibiotics, and sterile seawater (Kopecky and Ostrander, 1999). This technique can be extremely valuable for in vitro studies examining coral disease processes and should be employed in diagnostic efforts where viral and other unknown agents may be involved in the pathogenesis.

Bacterial and Fungal Culture

Currently a research procedure, the culture of bacteria and fungi associated with lesions in coelenterates needs to become a routine clinical tool. Challenges in this task relate to the need for marine salt-supplemented media to grow many marine organisms and the common need to culture at lower temperatures approximating the environmental temperatures of the coelenterate. Standard automated bacterial identification systems routinely misassign marine organisms, but, with experience, clinical microbiologists can identify those misassignments. In any case, these misassignments may not be as critical to clinical interpretation in coelenterate medicine as they can be in terrestrial species medicine. The evaluation of microbiological features of coelenterate diseases will necessarily involve consideration of assemblages of bacteria and fungi. Researchers have shown that the bacterial communities of healthy corals are characterized by low abundance and diversity (Cooney et al., 2002). Microorganism assemblages in the water above corals can differ significantly from those on the coral surface. Identification of the patterns of change in the complex microorganism assemblages of coelenterates will be an important tool in improving early diagnostic capabilities.

Impression Smears

Direct impression smears of affected polyps, debrided tissues, or even necrotic mats can provide valuable information to guide therapeutic efforts and prognostication. Examination of unstained wet smears is best for identifying motile protozoans and some metazoans. Fixed dried smears can be stained with a variety of standard diagnostic stains to determine preliminary information about bacteria and fungi.

Imaging

Medical imaging brings immediately to mind routine radiographic films commonly associated with diagnosing broken limbs and misplaced organs. Though radiographic techniques can generate elegant images of both soft-bodied and hard-skeletoned coelenterates, their diagnostic usefulness is somewhat limited. Modern diagnostic imaging, however, includes a wide array of sophisticated modalities that have potential for assisting in the early diagnosis, monitoring, and investigation of coelenterate diseases. Magnetic resonance imaging (MRI) is an imaging modality that has been useful in several such applications. Admittedly, access to this equipment is not yet available at local veterinary clinics, and some of the most useful techniques (reverse spectroscopy) are available only on research magnets. Nevertheless, MRI and other imaging techniques capable of evaluating metabolic shifts (positron emission tomography) can be important tools in understanding the pathogenesis and prognostication of the many mystery diseases being identified as biologists, hobbyists, and environmental health professionals begin to examine marine coral reef health closely. Mechanisms to hold marine species successfully for imaging exist, and, where appropriate, these modalities should be employed (Blackband and Stoskopf, 1990).

Histology

Recent advances in histological preparation of biopsies from coral promise to improve our ability to diagnose and characterize lesions. When taking biopsy specimens of hard corals, it is important to take a deep-enough sample to ensure that the structural integrity of the soft tissues is maintained (usually about 0.5–1.0 cm). To improve the ability to visualize the soft structures by fixing them in extended position, some researchers feel that samples should be anesthetized prior to placing them in fixative. This can be accomplished by placing samples in a 1:1 solution of 0.36 mol/L $MgCl_2 \cdot 6H_2O$ and seawater for 30 min before transferring them to fixative (Bythell et al., 2002). Special fixatives may improve the quality of sections. One recently developed for light microscopy consists of 3% gluteraldehyde, 7.5% sucrose, and 0.5% tannic acid in 0.1 mol/L sodium cacodylate buffer (Bythell et al., 2002). When conditions permit, the specimens should be kept at room temperature in this fixative for 1 h and then refrigerated at 4°C for up to 24 h.

To section hard corals, it is necessary to demineralize the sample first. This can alter the architecture of the specimen, particularly with regard to microbial communities in lesions. Encasing the specimen in 1.5% (wt/vol) agarose and then cutting small areas to expose the skeleton to be demineralized helps reduce these artifacts (Bythell et al., 2002). Demineralization is usually accomplished in 10% ascorbic acid in 0.3 mol/L NaCl or 10% (wt/vol) EDTA, which is changed every 12 h. Once the skeleton is demineralized, the specimen can be dehydrated and embedded in resin for sectioning. See Chapter 19 for more information on sample preparation.

Treatment Protocols

Drug Selection and Delivery

The treatment of coelenterate diseases is just entering its infancy. It is exciting to see the efforts that highly trained basic scientists and enthusiastic amateurs are making to identify the causes of and effective treatments for serious conditions of these species, but it is also a time to heed an important caveat for those facing the need to treat a diseased colony or organism. To have an effective treatment, it is highly advantageous to know what you are treating. Aggressively treating diseases caused by agents that will not respond to or be affected by one's therapy will lead to failure, frustration, and possibly the premature abandonment of useful therapeutic approaches. The shotgun application of various drugs in the hopes that one drug or the other will result in a positive outcome for a prize specimen does occasionally work. Unfortunately, without a good diagnosis, we are no wiser as to the benefits of the treatment, even in success. For that reason I urge everyone to invest in the diagnosis of the disease before embarking on treatment.

The first drugs being explored in coelenterate medicine are antibacterial (antibiotics). This makes good sense considering the plethora of bacterial agents being associated with disease states. Tolerance of these drugs is going to vary by taxon, but coelenterates seem to tolerate antibacterial treatments relatively well. Most anemones, for example, tolerate prolonged exposures to 5–10 ppm streptomycin or neomycin without serious damage (Sprung and Delbeek, 1997). This makes sense because some coelenterates (gorgonians, soft corals, and antipatharians) produce their own forms of antibacterial compounds and would be expected to have metabolic methods of detoxification of such compounds (Wilsanand et al., 1999). But the key to therapeutic success will be to select drugs that are effective against the agents actually causing the disease. Antibacterial treatments commonly exacerbate rather than ameliorate fungal infections, for example, and most are relatively ineffective against protozoal or metazoan diseases. Similarly, most antifungal drugs are completely ineffective against most bacterial pathogens and can set the stage for bacterial superinfections. Anthelmintics can be quite specific in the types of organisms they kill. A drug effective against roundworms may have no efficacy against flatworms or trematodes. Much of the needed research to guide drug selection can be conducted in vitro without endangering any coelenterate if cultures of potential pathogens are available. This work needs to be done. In the meantime, coelenterate clinicians will need to rely on the foundation of knowledge that has been amassed on the efficacy of these drugs in treating diseases of other species to select drugs and doses to try on their patients. Having the right diagnosis will be of paramount importance when working with this handicap.

Before conducting treatments of any kind with an agent one has not had experience with, or when one has used the agent but not to treat the coelenterate species one intends to, it is important to test the safety of the treatment on a small scale. Treat one animal, or a single colony first, and then observe it for a prolonged time before proceeding. Some damage by therapeutic agents may not become evident until days after the treatment. Therapeutic agents can be more devastating than the disease on occasion, and sometimes the problem is not the agent itself but rather a toxic metabolite of the original drug. Of course, in emergency situations, where animals are dying rapidly, one may not have the luxury of days to run these tests, but

this judgment needs to be made with the knowledge that proceeding more quickly carries an undefined but real risk of catastrophic outcome when working without prior knowledge.

Treatments should be conducted in separate tanks or containers. It is hard to predict the reactions of the wide variety of organisms that normally inhabit even relatively simple reef tanks, and most anything added will be toxic, even lethal, to at least some organisms (i.e., those one is trying to eradicate). A treatment added to a tank can be very difficult or impossible to remove completely. Never add a therapeutant to a tank unless prepared to lose the animals completely. Be prepared to conduct a major salvage operation should things go awry. Have places to relocate valuable specimens, if necessary. If possible, know and have the appropriate filtration supplements available to try and remove a drug (often activated carbon) and have conditioned makeup water on hand to allow attempts at dilutions through water changes.

Baths and Dips

Freshwater Dips

Large, polyped, stony corals and some soft corals (alcyonarians) can be put in freshwater dips for 1–3 min without undue damage. This procedure is used to reduce or eliminate flatworm infestations and is likely useful against a variety of protozoan and metazoan parasites. The freshwater should be free of chlorines and bromines and the same temperature as the water the coral is acclimated to. It should also be buffered with bicarbonate buffers to a pH of 8.2 or to match the husbandry water of the specimens being treated. This procedure should not be attempted for small polyp corals or xenids. When using the technique on a new species, proceed with caution. Use minimum exposure times and cease the procedure at signs of severe reaction to the treatment.

Lugol's Baths

Lugol's iodine is quite toxic and a very strong oxidant. Tolerance of this treatment is quite variable by coral species. Pulse corals (*Xenia* spp.), including the genus *Anthelia* and star polyps (*Pachyclavularia* spp.), are examples of corals that cannot tolerate this treatment even briefly (Borneman, 2001). It is critical to monitor the bath very carefully and to remove any specimen that shows signs of polyp expulsion or bail out immediately. On removal from the bath, the specimen should be rinsed briefly in fresh, unadulterated seawater to remove residual oxidant. The recommended strength of the bath is 5–10 drops of 5% Lugol's solution per liter of seawater, and baths are routinely conducted for 10–20 min (Borneman, 2001). Lugol's iodine is a good broad-spectrum antiseptic and also cauterizes damaged tissues.

Tetracycline Baths

Tetracycline, which is a broad-spectrum antibiotic that is easily obtainable and comes in water-soluble forms, has been used as a bath treatment for corals suffering from various maladies. The strength of bath reported in the literature to be safe for a wide range of corals is 10 mg/L (Hodgson, 1990). Generally, the efficacy of tetracycline treatments, particularly topical ones, conducted in saltwater is considered suspect. The drug is readily inactivated by binding to calcium ions (Gilman et al., 1990) that are abundant in seawater. Nonetheless, proponents of the practice claim some degree of efficacy. It should be noted that rarely are controlled studies conducted to evaluate whether a coral patient recovers because of the drug, the manipulation, or in spite of the treatment.

Chloramphenicol Baths

Chloramphenicol is a broad-spectrum antibiotic that is uncommonly used in human or veterinary medicine because it can cause a potentially fatal blood dyscrasia known as Grey's syndrome in genetically susceptible individuals. Advanced hobbyists and professional coral propagators have used the drug in a bath treatment for a variety of conditions, not all of which are known to be caused by bacteria. Though their treatment details are not provided here, I would strongly recommend that other antibiotics be explored. Florfenicol, a close relative to chloramphenicol but without the propensity to cause Grey's syndrome, is more readily available and might be more appropriate than chloramphenicol. Authors reporting the treatment technique make a point of the insolubility of chloramphenicol in water, which suggests they are working with the palmitate form of the drug. The succinate form is readily soluble in water. The palmitate form can be dissolved in a small amount of ethanol and then dissolved in water. This bath treatment should never be conducted in the primary tank, even though fairly long exposures are recommended. The antibiotic could have a severe impact on the bacterial community of the tank. Instead, prepare a treatment tank that can appropriately maintain the specimens you wish to treat for several days. The tolerance of different corals for this treatment varies considerably. *Acropora* spp., including the staghorn coral, seem to tolerate the treatments well, but finger corals (*Stylophora* spp.), pencil corals (*Madracis* spp.), and cluster corals (*Pocillopora* spp.) do not tolerate even brief exposures. Some authors precede the chloramphenicol bath with a fairly severe 30-min exposure to a 5–10 drop per liter strength of Lugol's iodine bath, others follow the chloramphenicol bath with a short 10 drop per liter Lugol's iodine dip, and others employ all three treatment regimens for severe cases. The recommended strength of the chloramphenicol bath also varies by author, at between 10 and 50 mg chloramphenicol per liter of seawater (Sprung and Delbeek, 1997; Borneman 2001). The bath can be conducted for several days, but a complete 100% water change with freshly made antibiotic-enriched seawater is recommended each day. Most treatments are conducted for 24 h or less. As with all baths and dips, it is important that the animal being treated is observed frequently and removed from the medicated water when signs of distress appear. At the higher dose levels, most specimens can only tolerate 2 or 3 days of treatment at best. Lowering the metabolic rate of corals by reducing light levels is thought by some to reduce the stress and

improve tolerance of long bath treatments. Upon removal from the treatment water, it is best to rinse the treated coral in seawater before returning it to its husbandry or quarantine tank. Because of the potential environmental impact of potent antibiotics, the bathwater should always be treated to destroy the drug before it is discarded. Adding ½ cup (60 mL) of full-strength chlorine bleach per 5 gallons (20 L) of treatment water and allowing it to sit for several hours before discarding it is reported to be effective in inactivating chloramphenicol (Sprung and Delbeek, 1997; Borneman 2001). This precaution has the advantage of at least partially disinfecting the bathwater before it is returned to the environment.

Levamisole Baths

Levamisole, which is an anthelmintic drug that is used to treat a wide variety of metazoan infestations in terrestrial species, has been used in a 24-h bath to treat infestations of unidentified flatworms at a dose of 8 mg/L (A. Tuttle, personal communication, 2003). This level of treatment was well tolerated by velvet finger coral (*Montipora digitata*), whorled montipora (*M. capricornis*), *Acropora* spp., bird's nest coral (*Seriatopora histrix*), and club finger coral (*Stylophora pistillata*).

Direct Topical Applications
Lugol's Iodine

Full-strength 5% Lugol's iodine solution can be swabbed directly onto the edges of lesions to cauterize and disinfect wounds. This is accomplished by removing the specimen from the tank and applying a cotton or synthetic soft swab saturated with Lugol's iodine to the exposed wound. The procedure should not extend beyond 20–30 s without replacing the specimen in seawater, even if the wounds are extensive. More prolonged treatment risks severe tissue burns in the areas treated first during the procedure. Rinsing the specimen in seawater before return to the tank is apparently not required, but recommended.

Antibiotic Pastes

Many books on coral husbandry mention the application of antibiotic pastes directly to wounds. The pastes referred to are made by taking a tablet or capsule of the drug formulated for oral administration in mammals and crushing, or mixing, the contents of the capsule with a small amount of seawater until the drug is the consistency of library paste. This is then applied directly to wounds or incisions. Drugs used in this manner include neomycin and kanamycin. This approach facilitates application, particularly to corals, but drug delivery should be enhanced by using a compounding base rather than seawater. Several compounding bases are marketed for use by dentists concerned with applying topical drugs in the mouth. One example is the product Orabase (Colgate-Palmolive). These water-resistant compounding bases adhere well to wet surfaces and would be expected to stay on the treated wound or incision longer, potentially providing a more effective treatment.

Slow-Release Compounds

In an extension to the concept of formulating drug pastes with compounding bases for more consistent and longer drug delivery at the site of injury, it is appropriate to consider the possibility of placing drugs into methacrylates, cyanoacrylates, and other compounds used for sealing wounds on corals. Most of the work on the kinetics and feasibility of this approach has been developed in the orthopedic discipline, where long-term antibiotic delivery in orthopedic implant sites offers several advantages (Bayston and Milner, 1982; Henry et al., 1991a, 1991b). The technique has also been used for single-dose long-term delivery of antibiotics and antifungal agents to birds (Stetter et al., 1996). With some fairly basic kinetic studies, this could prove a valuable approach to treating coral diseases caused by infectious agents.

Medicated Feed

Fortified Live Food

Relatively little is known about the efficacy of fortifying brine shrimp (*Artemia* spp.) or live rotifers with pharmaceuticals. The basic concept is to soak or bathe the live food in a solution of the desired drug on the assumption that the live food will ingest or otherwise absorb enough to deliver effective doses as the animal being treated consumes them. Challenges center largely on unknown quantities. Part of the concept includes the need to use as high a concentration of drug bath as possible without causing toxicity to the live food being fortified. Rarely is this known. Similarly, the rate of accumulation is unknown for any drug into most any prey item, making treatment duration a matter of convenience and speculation. The final concentration of drug in the treated prey is not known, so how much to feed to achieve an effective dose is also unknown. With that said, the technique has promise. Relatively simple kinetic studies are needed to determine exactly how it should be done. The risks of administering wrong doses varies with the drug being given, but basically consists of the potential to give toxic amounts unintentionally and the risk of giving an ineffective dose that can greatly increase the chance of developing drug-resistant strains of microorganisms.

Injected Food

Food for large polyp species, larger anemones, and many jellies is large enough to allow the injection of medications in known doses before feeding. This can be accomplished in live foods as well as dead or cut foods.

Gelatinized Food

Another approach to delivering medications to marine species is to make suitable gel or slurry foods that can accommodate the drug desired. Unfortunately, the time to start experimenting with these foods is not when specimens have broken with overt disease. The approach is practical only if the specimens are adapted to and take the artificial food.

Transport and Handling

Transport and handling are key issues for successful health management of these species. Considerable morbidity and mortality are associated with shipment and transport. Mobile forms are very susceptible to trauma. In addition, some species produce toxins that can accumulate in the shipping container and harm the specimens themselves or even people unpacking the boxes (e.g., *Palythoa* spp. produce palytoxins). In addition to toxins, massive production of mucus and metabolic by-products can foul water and suffocate or poison specimens. The lack of light in shipping containers puts extra stress on zooxanthellae-bearing species. In the containers, the symbionts go into dark mode, consuming rather than producing oxygen and increasing the potential to suffocate a specimen.

One key to successful transport is proper preparation of specimens in advance. Ideally, they should be held in high-quality water conditions for at least 4 days prior to transport. They should not be fed for as long before transport as is compatible with their metabolic rate. Those that live on particulate substrates should be rinsed to flush out all sand and debris. Attached sponges and other organisms that tend to die and foul shipping containers should be removed.

The second key to successful transport is proper handling after the shipment. On arrival, specimens should be unpacked and placed in well-aerated fresh seawater baths for 10–15 min to rinse off accumulated mucus and purge toxins prior to being placed in their quarantine tanks. Swelling and edema are signs of oxygen depletion and, if not too severe, will resolve when the specimens are placed in well-oxygenated water. The issue of postshipment acclimation remains controversial. I adhere to the school of getting the animals out of the shipping water "cesspool" and into good water conditions immediately without concern about slow acclimation. It is difficult to assess the finer points of health in a specimen swollen from oxygen depletion and covered with protective mucus. A quarantine period is an important tool both to acclimate specimens and to be able to examine them for early signs of contagious disease. The length of the quarantine period is relatively arbitrary because we do not know the prepatent periods of any infectious diseases of coelenterates. For now, the criteria should be sufficient time for the organisms to resume normal postures and behaviors and to enable their careful examination.

Many anemones, including the anemone fish hosts *Heteractis malu*, *H. crispa*, and *Macrodactyla doreensis*, ship very well dry in a bag without water. On the other hand, the closely related *Heteractis magnifica* present a very tough problem. Survival is not good whether it is shipped dry or wet (Sprung and Delbeek, 1997).

Most corallimorphs are best shipped in just enough water to cover them, though some can be successfully shipped without water (*Discosoma* spp.). Corallimorphs are very sensitive to heat but tolerate cold well. Packing in ice (without their direct contact with the ice) can greatly enhance shipping success.

Gorgonians and leather corals are often shipped in just enough water to cover the specimens. Some species are best shipped dry wrapped in paper towels moist with saltwater. In either case, it is important to limit the packing to a single species in a bag. This eliminates the potential problem of interspecies incompatibilities adding to the normal distress of shipping. If shipping specimens out of water, it is important to not use pure oxygen as the atmosphere in the shipping container. The oxidative nature of a pure oxygen atmosphere can cause expulsion of zooxanthellae (Figure 3.19). When shipping specimens in water, it is appropriate and beneficial to use a pure oxygen atmosphere. In general, smaller specimens tolerate shipping and handling better than do large specimens.

Shipping of hard and soft corals is considerably more successful for many species if the corals are kept out of water. Nitrogenous and excreted waste products (including defense molecules) accumulate rapidly in shipping water, which causes severe compromise and death of corals. The key is to avoid the pooling of water in the transport container and preventing that water from contacting the coral. Removing the coral from water and allowing it to drain prior to packing facilitates a good shipment. Coral can be drained out of the water for up to 45 min prior to packing, without deleterious impact. Packing should minimize the risk of contact between corals and reduce the potential for movement during transport. A successful method for accomplishing this has been to nestle the corals on nylon stockings filled with Perlite or Vermiculite. These porous sausages hold the coral up off of the bottom of the shipping container and away from contact with pooling water. Polystyrene boxes with an extra bottom grid to further ensure distance from pooled water are used for long transports.

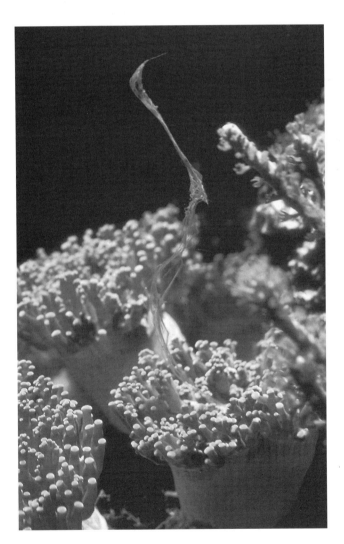

Figure 3.19. Photo of zooxanthellae release by *Euphylia* sp. Photos courtesy of www.biophoto.net.

References

Alker AP, Smith GW, Kim K. 2001. Characterization of *Aspergillus sydowii* (Thom et Church), a fungal pathogen of Caribbean sea fan corals. Hydrobiologia 460:105–111.

Alutoin S, Boberg J, Nystrom M, Tedengren M. 2001. Effects of the multiple stressors copper and reduced salinity on the metabolism of the hermatypic coral *Porites lutea*. Mar Environ Res 52:289–299.

Banin E, Israely T, Fine M, Loya Y, Rosenberg E. 2001. Role of endosymbiotic zooxanthellae and coral mucus in the adhesion of the coral-bleaching pathogen *Vibrio shiloi* to its host. FEMS Microbiol Lett 199:33–37.

Banin E, Israely T, Kushmaro A, Loya Y, Orr E, Rosenberg E. 2000. Penetration of the coral-bleaching bacterium *Vibrio shiloi* into *Oculina patagonica*. Appl Environ Microbiol 66:3031–3036.

Barnes RD. 1980. Invertebrate Zoology, 4th ed. Saunders College, Philadelphia, p. 158.

Bayston R, Milner RD. 1982. The sustained release of antimicrobial drugs from bone cement. J Bone Joint Surg [Br] 64:460–464.

Ben-Haim Y, Banim E, Kushmaro A, Loya Y, Rosenberg E. 1999. Inhibition of photosynthesis and bleaching of zooxanthellae by the coral pathogen *Vibrio shiloi*. Environ Microbiol 1:223–229.

Bentis CJ, Kaufman L, Golubic S. 2000. Endolithic fungi in reef-building corals (order: Scleractinia) are common, cosmopolitan, and potentially pathogenic. Biol Bull 198:254–260.

Blackband SJ, Stoskopf MK. 1990. In vivo nuclear magnetic resonance imaging and spectroscopy of aquatic organisms. Magn Reson Imaging 8:191–198.

Borneman EH. 2001. Aquarium Corals: Selection, Husbandry, and Natural History. TFH, Neptune City, NJ.

Bruckner A, Bruckner R. 1998. Rapid-wasting disease: Pathogen or predator? Science 279:2019–2025.

Bythell JC, Barer MR, Cooney RP, Guest JR, O'Donnell AG, Pantos O, Le Tissier MD. 2002. Histopathological methods for the investigation of microbial communities associated with disease lesions in reef corals. Lett Appl Microbiol 34:359–364.

Cooney RP, Pantos O, Le Tissier MD, Barer MR, O'Donnell AG, Bythell JC. 2002. Characterization of the bacterial consortium associated with black band disease in coral using molecular microbiological techniques. Environ Microbiol 4:401–413.

Denner EBM, Smith GW, Busse H-J, Schumann P, Narzt T, Polson SW, Lubitz W, Richardson LL. 2003. *Aurantimonas coralicida* gen. nov., sp. nov., the causative agent of white plague type II on Caribbean scleractinian corals. Int J Syst Evol Microbiol 53:1115–1122.

Downs CA, Fauth JE, Halas JC, Dustan P, Bemiss J, Woodley CM. 2002. Oxidative stress and seasonal coral bleaching. Free Radic Biol Med 33:533–543.

Ducklow HW, Mitchell R. 1979. Bacterial populations and adaptations in the mucus layers on living corals. Limnol Oceanogr 24:715–725.

Edmunds PJ, Carpenter RC. 2001. Recovery of *Diadema antillarum* reduces macroalgal cover and increases abundance of juvenile corals on a Caribbean reef. Proc Natl Acad Sci USA 98:4822–4824 and 5067–5071.

Edwards AJ, Clark S, Zahir H, Rajasuriya A, Naseer A, Rubens J. 2001. Coral bleaching and mortality on artificial and natural reefs in Maldives in 1998, sea surface temperature anomalies and initial recovery. Mar Pollut Bull 42:7–15.

Fine M, Banin E, Israely T, Rosenberg E, Loya Y. 2002. Ultraviolet (UV) radiation prevents bacterial bleaching of the Mediterranean coral *Oculina patagonica*. Mar Ecol Prog Ser 226:249–254.

Frias-Lopez J, Zerkle AL, Bonheyo GT, Fouke BW. 2002. Partitioning of bacterial communities between seawater and healthy, black band diseased, and dead coral surfaces. Appl Environ Microbiol 68:2214–2228.

Garrett P, Ducklow P. 1975. Coral disease in Bermuda. Nature 253:349–350.

Geiser D, Taylor J, Ritchie K, Smith G. 1998. Cause of sea fan death in the West Indies. Nature 394:137–138.

Gilman AG, Rall TW, Nies AS, Taylor P, eds. 1990. Goodman and Gilman's The Pharmacological Basis of Therapeutics, 8th edition. Pergamon, New York.

Goodson MS, Whitehead LF, Douglas AE. 2001. Microbial aquatic symbioses: From phylogeny to biotechnology. Hydrobiologica 461:79–82.

Harvell CD, Kim K, Burkholder JM, Colwell RR, Epstein PR, Grimes DJ, Hofmann EE, Lipp EK, Osterhaus ADME, Overstreet RM, Porter JW, Smith GW, Vasta GR. 1999. Emerging marine diseases: Climate links and anthropogenic factors. Science 285:1505–1510.

Harvell CD, Mitchell CE, Ward JR, Altizer S, Dobson AP, Ostfeld RS, Samuel MD. 2002. Climate warming and disease risks for terrestrial and marine biota. Science 296:2158–2162 [gorgonian aspergillosis image].

Henry SL, Seligson D, Mangino P, Popham JG. 1991a. Antibiotic-impregnated beads. Part I: Bead implantation versus systemic therapy. Orthop Rev 20:242–245.

Henry SL, Seligson D, Mangino P, Popham JG. 1991b. Antibiotic-impregnated beads. Part II: Factors in antibiotic selection. Orthop Rev 20:331–337.

Hodgson G. 1990. Tetracycline reduces sedimentation damage to corals. Mar Biol 104:493–496.

Kim K, Harvell CD, Kim PD, Smith GW, Merkel SM. 2000. Fungal disease resistance of Caribbean sea fan corals (*Gorgonia* spp.). Mar Biol 136:259–267.

Kopecky EJ, Ostrander GK. 1999. Isolation and primary culture of viable multicellular endothelial isolates from hard corals. In Vitro Cell Dev Biol Anim 35:616–624.

Korrubel JL, Riegl B. 1998. A new coral disease from the Southern Arabian Gulf. Coral Reefs 17:22.

Kuta KG, Richardson LL. 1997. Black band disease and the fate of the diseased coral colonies in the Florida Keys. In: Lessios HA, Macintyre IG, eds. Proceedings of the Eighth International Coral Reef Symposium, volume 1. Smithsonian Tropical Research Institute, Balboa, Panama, pp 575–578.

Littler MM, Littler DS. 1995. Impact of CLOD pathogen in Pacific coral reefs. Science 267:1356–1360.

Mills CE. 1998–present. Phylum Ctenophora: List of all valid species names. Document available at http://faculty.washington.edu/cemills/Ctenolist.html. Web page last updated November 2003.

Mills CE, Miller RL. 1984. Ingestion of a medusae (*Aegina citrea*) by the nematocyst-containing ctenophore *Haekelia rubra* (formerly *Euchlora rubra*): Phylogenetic implications. Mar Biol 78:215–221.

Mitchelmore CL, Schwarz JA, Weis VM. 2002. Development of symbiosis-specific genes as biomarkers for the early detection of cnidarian–algal symbiosis breakdown. Mar Environ Res 54:345–349.

Muller WA. 2002. Autoaggressive, multi-headed and other mutant phenotypes in *Hydractinia echinata* (Cnidaria: Hydrozoa). Int J Dev Biol 46:1023–1033.

Muller WE, Muller I, Zahn RK, Maidhof A. 1984. Intraspecific recognition system in scleractinian corals: Morphological and cytochemical description of the autolysis mechanism. J Histochem Cytochem 32:285–288.

Nagelkerken I, Buchan K, Smith GW, Bonair K, Bush P, Garzón-Ferreira J, Botero L, Gayle P, Harvell CD, Heberer C, Kim K, Petrovic C, Pors L, Yoshioka P. 1997. Widespread disease in Caribbean sea fans. II. Patterns of infection and tissue loss. Mar Ecol Prog Ser 160:255–263.

Negri AP, Smith LD, Webster NS, Heyward AJ. 2002. Understanding ship-grounding impacts on a coral reef: Potential effects of anti-foulant paint contamination on coral recruitment. Mar Pollut Bull 44:111–117.

Novak PL, Lenhoff HM. 1981. Asexual reproduction and regeneration properties of a nonbudding mutant of *Hydra viridis*. J Exp Zool 217:213–223.

Olutiola P, Cole O. 1977. Some environmental and nutritional factors affecting growth and sporulation of *Aspergillus sydowii*. Physiol Plant 39:239–242.

Ostrander GK, Armstrong KM, Knobbe ET, Gerace D, Scully EP. 2000. Rapid transition in the structure of a coral reef community: The effects of coral bleaching and physical disturbance. Proc Natl Acad Sci USA 97:5297–5302.

Paletta M. 1990. Coral aggression in reef aquaria. SeaScope 7(4):1–2.

Patterson KL, Porter JW, Ritchie KB, Polson SW, Mueller E, Peters EC, Santavy DL, Smith GW. 2002. The etiology of white pox, a lethal disease of the Caribbean elkhorn coral, *Acropora palmata*. Proc Natl Acad Sci USA 99:8725–8730.

Peters EC, Halas JC, McCarty HB. 1986. Caliocoblastic neoplasms in *Acropora palmata*, with a review of reports on anomalies of growth and form in corals. J Natl Cancer Inst 76:895–912.

Podar M, Haddock SHD, Sogin ML, Harbison GR. 2001. A molecular phylogenetic framework for the phylum Ctenophora using 18S rRNA genes. Mol Phylogenet Evol 21:218–230.

Ravindran J, Raghukumar C, Raghukumar S. 2001. Fungi in *Porites lutea*: Association with healthy and diseased corals. Dis Aquat Org 47:219–228.

Raymundo LHH, Harvell CD, Reynolds TL. 2003. Porites ulcerative white spot disease: Description, prevalence, and host range of a new coral disease affecting Indo-Pacific reefs. Dis Aquat Org 56:95–104.

Richardson LL. 1996. Horizontal and vertical migration patterns of *Phormidium corallyticum* and *Beggiatoa* spp. associated with black-band disease of corals. Microb Ecol 32:323–335.

Richardson LL, Goldberg WM, Kuta KG, Aronson RB, Smith GW, Ritchie KB, Halas JC, Feingold JS, Miller SL. 1998. Florida's mystery coral-killer identified. Nature 392:557–558.

River GF, Edmunds PJ. 2001. Mechanisms of interaction between macroalgae and scleractinians on a coral reef in Jamaica. 261:159–172.

Rodriguez-Martinez RE, Banaszak AT, Jordan-Dahlgren E. 2001. Necrotic patches affect *Acropora palmata* (Scleractinia: Acroporidae) in the Mexican Caribbean. Dis Aquat Org 47:229–234.

Rosenberg E, Ben-Haim Y. 2002. Microbial diseases of corals and global warming. Environ Microbiol 4:318–326.

Rowan R, Knowlton N, Baker A, Jara J. 1997. Landscape ecology of algal symbionts creates variation in episodes of coral bleaching. Nature 388:265–269.

Ruppert EE, Fox RS, Barnes RD. 2004. Invertebrate Zoology: A Functional Evolutionary Approach, 7th edition. Brooks/Cole—Thomson Learning, Belmont, CA, 963 pp.

Rützler K, Santavy DL. 1983. The black band disease of Atlantic reef corals. I. Description of the cyanophyte pathogen. Mar Ecol 4:301–319.

Rützler K, Santavy DL, Antonius A. 1983. The black band disease of Atlantic reef corals. III. Distribution, ecology, and development. Mar Ecol 4:329–358.

Salih A, Larkum A, Cox G, Kuhl M, Hoegh-Guldberg O. 2000. Fluorescent pigments in corals are photoprotective. Nature 408:850–853.

Shinn EA, Smith GW, Prospero JM, Betzer P, Hayes ML, Garrison V, Barber RT. 2000. African dust and the demise of Caribbean coral reefs. Geophys Res Lett 27:3029–3032.

Smith GW, Harvell CD, Kim K. 1998. Response of sea fans to infection with *Aspergillus* sp. (fungi). Rev Biol Trop 46:205–208.

Sprung J. 2002. Algae: A Problem Solver Guide. Ricordea, Miami.

Sprung J, Delbeek JC. 1994. The Reef Aquarium: A Comprehensive Guide to the Identification and Care of Tropical Marine Invertebrates, volume 1. Ricordea, Coconut Grove, FL.

Sprung J, Delbeek JC. 1997. The Reef Aquarium: A Comprehensive Guide to the Identification and Care of Tropical Marine Invertebrates, volume 2. Ricordea, Coconut Grove, FL.

Stetter MD, Sheppard C, Cook RA. 1996. Itraconazole-impregnated synthetic grit for sustained dosing in avian species. In: Proceedings American Association of Zoo Veterinarians, pp 181–185.

Sugiyama T, Fujisawa T. 1977. Genetic analysis of developmental mechanisms in hydra. I. Sexual reproduction of *Hydra magnipapillata* and isolation of mutants. Dev Growth Differ 19:187–200.

Thiel AJ. 1989. Small Reef Aquarium Basics: The Optimum Aquarium for the Reef Hobbyist. Aardvark Press, Bridgeport, CT. 175 pp.

Toller WW, Rowan R, Knowlton N. 2001. Repopulation of zooxanthellae in the Caribbean corals *Montastraea annularis* and *M. faveolata* following experimental and disease-associated bleaching. Biol Bull 201:360–373.

Upton SJ, Peters EC. 1986. A new and unusual species of coccidium (Apicomplexa: Agammococcidorida) from Caribbean scleractinian corals. J Invertebr Pathol 47:184–193.

Van Etten JL, Meints RH, Kuczmarski D, Burbank DE, Lee K. 1982. *Hydra* virus. Proc Natl Acad Sci USA 79:3867–3871.

Veron J. 2000. Corals of the World, volumes 1–3. Australian Institute of Marine Science, Townsville.

Warner ME, Fitt WK, Schmidt GW. 1999. Damage to photosystem II in symbiotic dinoflagellates: A determinant of coral bleaching. Proc Natl Acad Sci USA 96:8007–8012.

Wilsanand V, Wagh AB, Bapuji M. 1999. Antibacterial activities of anthozoan corals on some marine microfoulers. Microbios 99:137–145.

Zhang X, Huff JK, Hudson BG, Sarras MP Jr. 1990. A non-mammalian in vivo model for cellular and molecular analysis of glucose-mediated thickening of basement membranes. Diabetologia 33:704–707.

Chapter 4

TURBELLARIANS

Michael S. Bodri

Natural History and Taxonomy

The standard treatment for the Platyhelminthes divides the phylum into four classes: Turbellaria, Monogenea, Trematoda (Digenea), and Cestoda (Cestoidea). They are a much-studied, yet controversial, group, with disagreement regarding their structure, life history, method of reproduction, and zoological status. With 20,000 known species, members of the Platyhelminthes have a broad range of lifestyles. The dominant emphasis is on symbiosis, with the majority of species ectoparasitic or entoparasitic on or in other animals (Jennings, 1997). These four classes artificially correspond with the free-living flatworms, ectoparasitic single-host flukes, endoparasitic multiple host flukes, and the tapeworms. The name *Turbellaria* is based on the observation of minute vortical currents of water generated by ciliary action at the anterior end of the animal. The incorporation of molecular biological techniques and cladistic analysis into the systematics of this diverse group of organisms has resulted in a restructuring of the phylogeny. The classification that follows is based on the scheme outlined by Roberts and Janovy (2000).

The basal taxon (sister group) of the platyhelminth cladogram is the subphylum Catenulida. Rhabdocoel flatworms (e.g., the gut is a simple sac), the catenulids, are primarily a freshwater group, with some marine representatives. This is a relatively aberrant group, with a ciliated, saclike intestine, simple pharynx, and unpaired gonads. The Catenulida are distinguished from the remaining platyhelminths, the Euplatyhelminthes, by lacking a frontal organ and having monociliated epidermal cells. A frontal organ is a terminal or subterminal pit with mucoid gland cells and (sometimes) cilia.

In addition to frontal organs, the Euplatyhelminthes possess dense epidermal ciliature. Three superclasses are recognized within the Euplatyhelminthes: the Acoelomorpha, Rhabditophora, and the Neodermata. Acoelomorpha, the acoel flatworms, are typically small species with a reduced or absent permanent gut. Almost all are less than 2 mm long, free-living marine organisms. Some may act as symbionts with other invertebrates, and a few members have symbiotic algae living beneath their epidermis. The most famous example of this is found with *Convoluta roscoffensis*, on the channel coast of France. This species of acoel flatworm is colored green by the photosynthetic flagellate *Tetraselmis convolutae*. As is true of all acoels, there is no digestive cavity or gut. In *C. roscoffensis*, there are no distinct gonads, the gametes originating directly from the mesenchyme. In general, acoels feed on algae, protozoa, bacteria, and microscopic organisms. A temporary gut appears when food is ingested, and digestion occurs intracellularly and in temporary cavities, with the gut disappearing following digestion. Acoels also lack an excretory system, with a reduction and loss of protonephridia (*flame cells*).

The members of the Rhabditophora generally have numerous rodlike bodies (*rhabdites*) embedded in the tegument. Rhabdites may assist in lubrication, adhesion, and possibly predator deterrence. The flame cells of rhabditophorans, components of the excretory system, are multiflagellated. Within the rhabditophorans is the class Rhabdocoela. Worms in this class possess a bulbous pharynx and simple intestine.

The remaining superclass, the Neodermata, contains the following classes: the Trematoda, the Monogenea, and the Cestoidea. These worms have ectolecithal eggs (egg yolk is supplied by cells other than the ovum), and the ciliated epidermis of the larva is lost as an adult, with the formation of a syncytial adult tegument. Certain rhabdocoele-like rhabditophorans most likely became parasites during Cambrian time and may have given rise to parasitic flatworms: the Cestoda and the malacobothriid trematodes (Stunkard, 1975).

The former classification system that recognized the class Turbellaria now consists of the acoels and some of the rhabditophorans. The turbellarians had long been recognized as a class, but it is clear from recent research (based on ribosomal RNA sequences and reassessments of morphological features) that the class is not really monophyletic. However, the grouping persists and, until a new taxonomy has been established, it will continue to be used as a convenient way of combining a large group of mainly free-living platyhelminths and therefore here I refer to these superclasses as turbellarians. Tyler and Bush (2002) maintain a database of platyhelminth taxonomy that includes a number of important flatworm groups in addition to the Acoelomorpha. These recognized rhabditophoran groups include the Macrostomida (containing three families), the Prolecithophora (containing 11 families), the Lecithoepitheliata (containing two families), the Polycladida (containing 13 families) and, the most recognizable order, the Seriata.

Macrostomids are freshwater or marine turbellarians with a simple ciliated saclike intestine and a simple pharynx. These, rather than the more primitive Acoela, are thought to be closest to the ancestral turbellarians. Prolecithophorans are found in marine and freshwater environments. They have a bulbous pharynx. Lecithoepitheliatans are alleocoel turbellarians with a relatively simple saclike intestine. There are both marine and freshwater species. The penis is in the form of a stylet. Polycladidans are rhabdocoel turbellarians, mostly free-living marine flatworms with a few commensal and a few freshwater representatives. They have greatly flattened, oval, often brightly colored bodies, usually ranging from between 3 and 20 mm in length. They often have numerous eyes.

Two additional groups of disputed status deserve mention: the Neorhabdocoela and the Temnocephalida. Neorhabdocoelans are rhabdocoel turbellarians. A highly diverse group, there are many free-living representatives, many commensal species, and some true parasites in marine crustaceans. These have a bulbous pharynx. Temnocephalidans are also rhabdocoel turbellarians. These are commensal flatworms of marine crustaceans and vertebrates such as turtles. They cling to their hosts by using an adhesive disc on the posterior ventral surface and adhesive tentacles.

The Seriata are a diverse and important group containing the suborders Bothrioplanida, Proseriata, and Tricladida. Some taxonomists elevate each of these to the rank of order. The pharynx is folded, and the gut is alleocoel in form, with many diverticulae. The bothrioplanids contain one family. Suborder Proseriata contains marine and interstitial species. In these, the gut is not branched. The word *planaria* itself is used synonymously with Tricladida, which was at one time an order of the class Turbellaria (Brøndsted, 1969). These are mostly free-living, often actively predacious, flatworms. A few marine planarians may act as commensals, for example, *Bdelloura* sp. in the horseshoe crab. Identification of planarians to genus, particularly triclads, relies on living, mature specimens. Beyond generic identification, species identification of all nontriclads and of some triclads depends on serial sections, particularly of the reproductive system (Pennak, 1978; Gremigni, 1979). Within the Tricladida are the families best known for their free-living members: the Dendrocoelidae; the Dugessidae; the Planariidae, from which the namesake *planarian* is derived (the name planaria refers to the body form); the Bipallidae, with large introduced terrestrial species well established in the United States and other countries (Klots, 1960); the Geoplanidae; and the Rhynchodemidae.

The vast majority of the turbellarians are free-living organisms, mostly living in water, either marine or freshwater. Freshwater planarians can be found in ponds, streams, and marshy areas that have a good supply of organic matter on which they feed. There are exceptions to this general rule, however, among the terrestrial representatives, particularly the triclads. In the Turbellaria, most species are free living, with either microphagous or predatory habits. Symbiotic relationships have evolved in a significant minority, from simple facultative shelter associations to obligate entoparasitisms (Jennings, 1997).

Prey items range from bacteria and unicellular algae through protozoa and virtually all types of invertebrates, to the eggs and young stages of fishes and amphibians. Mucus laid down by free-living turbellarians can impede or trap many species of prey and lead to their capture (Calow, 1979). Several individuals of one species may, under dense populations, act together for more efficient prey capture and result in communal feeding (Pickavance, 1971; Young, 1973). Exploitation of this diverse range of prey relies on the elaboration of the embryonic stomodeal invagination into a muscular suctorial pharynx. The pharynx is capable of protrusion, extension, or eversion and can be inserted into, applied to, or extended over food items to swallow in their entirety or to withdraw body contents for subsequent extracellular and intracellular digestion in the alimentary tract (Jennings, 1997).

Symbiotic turbellarians may be ectosymbiotic or entosymbiotic. Ectosymbiotes may be considered epizoic predators that use their hosts as feeding platforms. Many entosymbiotes have a greater diversity of nutritional strategies than ectosymbiotes, with a concomitant increase in metabolic dependence on their hosts. In addition, many turbellarians have close symbiotic, commensal, or mutualistic associations with other organisms, particularly with other invertebrates, although some may act as ectocommensals to marine vertebrates such as turtles.

These commensal and parasitic forms are very similar to their free-living cousins but may have adaptations to their epidermis, such as the formation of a syncytium; loss of rhabdoids, mucous glands, and cilia; and a loss of their eyes or their reduction. Apart from these parasitic and commensal representatives, they are mostly predacious, although some may feed on algae, and many feed on diatoms as juveniles, before becoming fully carnivorous as adults.

Laboratory populations with stable temperature and feeding regimens are regulated primarily by intraspecific competition for food (Boddington and Mettrick, 1977). In the freshwater planarian *Dugesia tigrina*, individuals experience a trophic benefit from group membership, with an optimum group size that maximizes per capita ingestion rates (Cash et al., 1993). Asexual populations of *D. tigrina* increase to an equilibrium size that is maintained without loss or replacement of individuals (Armstrong, 1964).

Animals become reduced in size and their metabolic rate increases when starved. When fed again, many species are capable of renewed growth and of repeating their life cycle (physiological youth) (Stewart, 1972).

The majority of turbellarian species are hermaphroditic and reproduce sexually. Asexual reproduction occurs by budding, fission, or fragmentation. Regeneration capacity is related to asexual reproduction and decreases with sexuality (Palmberg, 1986). Perennial triclads adopt a different reproductive strategy during disturbances in food supply than do the annual species (Calow and Woollhead, 1977). The perennial *Dugesia lugubris* ceases capsule production under conditions of complete starvation, with a concomitant effect on degrowth. The annual *Dendrocoelum lacteum* continues capsule production, with a pronounced degrowth and greater tendency toward mortality because of a direct relationship between adult mortality and reproductive effort (reproductive effort increases in this species when food supply is decreased).

Asexual reproduction by fragmentation occurs in terrestrial species such as *Bipalium fuscatum* and *B. multilineatum*, with the number of regeneration fragments directly related to body length (Makino and Shirasawa, 1986). Two to four pieces of approximately equal size are produced from the body segment posterior to the mouth. Large fragments can further divide into equal-sized secondary pieces. Depending on the species, all fragmentation may occur at once or in a stepwise fashion. Starvation may initiate fragmentation in these species. Sexually reproducing and asexually reproducing turbellarian species have their lifetime defined as time from hatching until death, or fission to fission, respectively (Lange, 1968). The longest recorded turbellarian life span is 21 years (Lange, 1968). The tissue density of stem cells decreases with increase in size and age.

Turbellarians in large numbers are best reared by mechanical sectioning rather than reliance on cocoon (egg) production (Callahan and Morris, 1989). In this manner, *D. tigrina* averaging 8 mm in length can be sectioned into 600 segments, and with 94% of the segments regenerating within 8 days, if the sectioning is performed properly.

Anatomy and Physiology

The larger freshwater flatworms are rather characteristic in shape and quite familiar in appearance. They are more or less elongated, frequently flattened, and leaflike, cylindrical, or spindle shaped (Figure 4.1, Color Plate 4.1). The ventral surface is almost always flattened to some degree. In many species, the anterior end is differentiated and specialized to resemble a head. Two, or more, darkly pigmented eyespots are usually present near the anterior end and give the animal a cross-eyed appearance (Figures 4.2 and 4.3).

The free-living flatworms are conjectured to be the first group of animals to have evolved bilateral symmetry, dorsoventral asymmetry, encephalization, and a true brain. Thirteen basic cell types are described for planarians, with neoblasts,

nerve, epidermal, and fixed parenchymal cells constituting about 75% of the total cell number (Baguñá and Romero, 1981).

Most of the body of turbellarians is made up of parenchyma. Parenchyma architecture and formation was a source of conflict for years until the advent of electron microscopy and modern

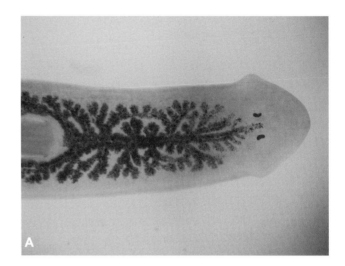

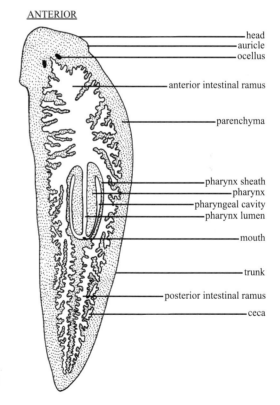

Figure 4.2. **A:** Stained whole mount of the aquatic planarian *Dugesia tigrina*, anterior end. Note the cephalization, paired eyespots, and gastrovascular system. A portion of the protrusible pharynx is visible at the left side of the photomicrograph. **B:** Drawing of *Dugesia* sp. indicating key anatomical features. Reproduced from Richard Fox, Lander University, by Alison Schroeer.

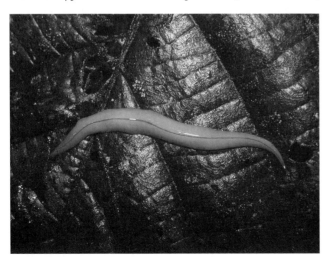

Figure 4.1. An unidentified terrestrial planarian from Ecuador, likely a *Bipalium* sp. Some tropical species approach 50–60 cm in length. This retracted specimen was approximately 10 cm.

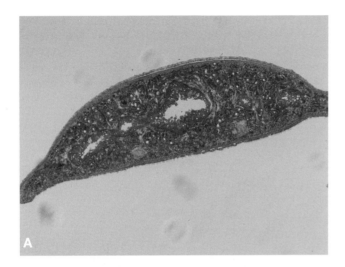

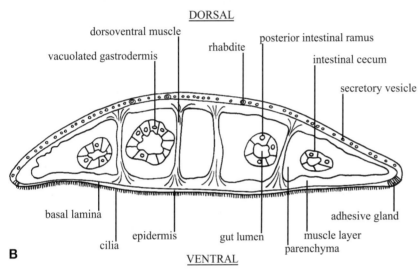

Figure 4.3. **A:** Cross section of the aquatic planarian *Dugesia tigrina*. Note the monolayered secretory epidermis. Only the ventral cells are ciliated, to assist in locomotion. The basal lamina underlies the epidermis and is visible as a *dark line*. A cluster of adhesive gland cells is just visible at the lateral edge of the ventral epidermis. Beneath the basal lamina is a layer of body wall muscle inside of which is mesenchymal tissue. The irregular cavities are intestinal rami and their ceca are lined by gastrodermis. **B:** Drawing of *Dugesia* sp. in cross section indicating key anatomical features. Reproduced from Richard Fox, Lander University, by Alison Schroeer.

histochemical techniques. Overall, the parenchyma is a loosely arranged mass of fibers and cells of several types. Previously, it was believed the parenchymal cells formed a syncytium, and this assumption was supported by the internal organs being so embedded in the parenchyma that dissecting them out is almost impossible. The parenchyma binds the epidermis with the gastrodermis and provides firm, yet pliable support for the internal organs. There are two primary cell types: the neoblast and fixed parenchymal cell (*myocyton*). Myocytons, in addition to containing a nucleus, have rough endoplasmic reticulum, free ribosomes, a vesicular Golgi apparatus, few mitochondria, and abundant glycogen. They may store lipids, as well. They are large cells with complex interdigitations and are supplied with numerous irregularly attenuated processes that are insinuated into nearly all the very narrow intercellular spaces (Brøndsted, 1969).

Neoblasts are totipotent regenerative cells, important in asexual reproduction or in the repair of damage from fragmentation or surgery. A resting neoblast, a cell not migrating to a wound or in the process of differentiation in the blastema, is roundish or spindle shaped, with an ovoid nucleus containing

1–3 nucleoli. Cytoplasm is scanty, making up only about half the cell volume. The bulk of ribosomes are free, not bound to an endoplasmic reticulum, and are associated with a large amount of RNA. The large numbers of ribosomes and proteins containing sulfhydral groups give credence to the embryonic character of these cells. Mitosis is restricted to neoblasts. Regenerative ability can be abolished by x-radiation, which selectively kills the neoblasts.

The outer surface of Platyhelminthes varies to some degree, but, by comparison between different platyhelminth groups, shows a development toward the syncytial tegument seen in the digenean and cestode parasites. In the free-living turbellarians, the epidermis consists of a monolayered ciliated cuboidal, squamous, or columnar epithelium with microvilli. Dorsal cells tend to be columnar whereas ventral cells are cuboid or somewhat flattened. Subepidermal glands, as well as the dendrites of sensory cells, may pass between or through the epithelial cells, if present (Jennings et al., 1992). The cilia are particularly abundant on the ventral surface, where they provide motility for the organism, especially in the smaller species. Muscular undulations are probably more important for the larger land planarians.

Sensory cilia may be found projecting from sensory cells within the epidermis. Most gland cells, of several types, lie just beneath the subepidermal basement membrane buried within the mesenchyme or are located within the outer epidermis, with their necks pushed through the outer layers. These gland cells secrete a number of substances that may be used in trapping prey, as an adhesive substrate, or to aid in the motility of the organism. The cells may form glandular adhesive organs ventral to the head in some species. Mucus is provided by the rhabdites deposited in epidermal gland cells.

Rhabdites, which are generally rod-shaped, strongly acidophilic bodies, are thought to be used for defense as well as secreting a slimy coat over the animal. When rhabdites are expelled, they swell enormously in water and form a heavy mucoid mass. In some turbellarians, nematocysts (stinging cells) may be found in the tegument. The nematocysts are not made by the worm but are derived from hydroids that the worm has ingested. The nematocysts are not digested but are transported from the gut to the epidermis, where they are then recycled for the organism's self-defense. Finally, in some marine species, the outer epidermis may be armed with numerous calcareous spicules, which may have a structural role.

Mesenchymal pigment, which is responsible for the color of planarians, may be contained in cells but more frequently occurs as pigment spots or vesicles. The pigment, in most species, lies just below the epidermis. Newly formed regeneration blastema is devoid of pigment, indicating that that the neoblasts have not yet developed into fixed mesenchymal cells (Brøndsted, 1969).

The muscular system is divided into a subepidermal part and a parenchymal, organ-specific part (Brøndsted, 1969). Situated beneath the basement membrane of the epidermis, the subepidermal muscular system consists of circular, longitudinal, and diagonal fibers. The parenchymal part traverses the body with longitudinal, transverse, and dorsoventral fibers. Combined, the subepidermal and parenchymal systems provide the animal with a great deal of morphological plasticity. The organ-specific muscular system is particularly well developed in the pharynx and copulatory organs. Cross-striations may be seen in the fibers attending these structures.

The majority of planarians are zoophagous, feeding on small living invertebrates. Planarians possess a muscular mouth, typically located midventrally, that leads to a pouchlike stomodeum or pharyngeal cavity. The pharyngeal cavity is plicate and capable of distension. Attached to the anterior end of the pharyngeal cavity is a muscular, protrusable pharynx, which points backward in the pharyngeal cavity. The walls of the pharynx are composed of three muscular layers, with fibers running circularly, longitudinally, and diagonally. The muscles are innervated by fine nerve plexuses. The pharynx is protruded out the mouth as a white, flexible cylinder with a trumpet-shaped lip. It may be as long as half the body length. With the ventral surface of the body and the tip of the pharynx in contact with the food source, soft or disintegrating tissues are sucked up into the gastrovascular cavity by the muscular action of the pharynx.

Extracellular digestion may take place during feeding by terrestrial planarians such as *Bipalium adventitium*, a predator of earthworms (Dindal, 1970). Food enters the intestine by first passing through the pharynx and then through a short esophagus. The gut can vary from a blind pouch to a highly branched tube that ramifies and anastomoses. The intestinal wall, called the *gastroderm*, consists of glandular cells, Minotian gland cells, and gastrodermal cells. The latter are phagocytic and are filled with food vacuoles in nonfasting animals (Brøndsted, 1969). Undigested wastes, as well as secretory products from the gastrodermis, are eliminated through the mouth.

The turbellarian brain is generally bilobed but may trend toward globular if surrounded by a capsule. Nerve strands connect dorsal trunks and, in most cases, the lateral trunks as well (Kotikova, 1986). The remainder of the animal is innervated by several plexuses, or a nerve net, that resemble those of cnidarians (Blair and Anderson, 1993). Glia have been reported that form well-developed sheaths enwrapping the neurons (Golubev, 1988). All or most of the neuronal and glial cell bodies are located in the cortex (Best and Morita, 1982). The brain exerts rostral control over reflexes organized in the segmental nervous system (Best and Morita, 1982). The brain also mediates control of asexual reproduction and sexual maturation. The medulla is formed from fibers projected from neuronal bodies in the cortex, the fibers in the cell-free neuropil forming the dorsal two-thirds and the longitudinal tracts of relatively large neurons forming the ventral third. Synaptic connections between brain neurons occur between neuropil fibers in the medulla. Turbellarians, because of the degree of development of the brain, can be classically conditioned (Kimmel and Garrigan, 1973).

The acoel turbellarians have a simple nervous system with a central component and peripheral component. The central nervous system consists of ganglia around a single sensory statocyst and the peripheral system consisting of networks of nerves supplying the parenchyma and sensory structures.

In summary, members of the Tricladida are considered the lowest species to have a mammalian-like brain and "spinal cord," with the brain consisting of centralized and clustered nerve cell bodies at the cephalic end while two ventral nerves run the length of the body and send out branches from ganglia in a ladderlike design, similar to the spinal nerves (Raffa and Valdez, 2001).

Sensory structures, including tactile cells, chemoreceptors, eyespots, and statocysts, are abundant and may be distributed in a variety of patterns. In most species, paired eyespots lie dorsally and anterior over the head ganglia. Each eyespot is bean or cup shaped, and contains translucent light-sensitive receptor cells, which are attached to nerve fibers. From the head ganglia, nerves radiate into the anterior tip of the body into the *auricles*, which are sensory pits, often ciliated, that are presumably chemoreceptors (Brøndsted, 1969; Pennak, 1978). These may be rounded, oblong, or slitlike and shallow or deep. Sensory cilia, particularly at the anterior and posterior ends, move independently of one another and the short cilia. They may be relatively stiff and resemble spines in some species. Other receptors for the detection of currents, aiding in olfaction, and for contact may be present, especially on the pharynx and anterior end of the animal.

The excretory system is of the protonephridial type. Running down both sides of the entire length of the body are a pair (usually) of tubules that branch repeatedly. Each branch, or *capillary*, terminates blindly and is enclosed by cells provided with ciliary tufts. The tubules have external outlets: the *nephridiopores*. The ciliated cells are known as flame cells or *protonephridia*. The flame cell's flagellar tuft extends into the capillary, which may interdigitate with another flame cell. At least three types of flame cells exist along with at least three types of tubule cells (Roberts and Janovy, 2000). The excretory system may be involved in osmoregulation, the excess water possibly containing nitrogenous wastes. Filtration occurs through minute slits formed by rods, or extensions of the cell, collectively called a *weir* (Roberts and Janovy, 2000). A bladder and *ampullae* may be present. Many of the excretory waste products are likely disposed of through the epidermal surface and, to a lesser degree, the gastrodermis. Some excretory granules are retained in the tissues until the animal has died.

Respiration is via the general epidermis and, to a lesser degree, the gastrodermis. Planarians all require high concentrations of oxygen and only occur in well-oxygenated habitats, although they are tolerant of anaerobic conditions for variable periods. Symbiotic algae, *zoochlorellae*, occur in the parenchyma and gastrodermis of many microturbellarians. Photosynthesis produces oxygen for use by the turbellarian, while the worm contributes carbon dioxide and nitrogenous compounds for algal metabolism. Algae may be passed to offspring via eggs (Pennak, 1978).

Reproduction in turbellarians occurs in one of three basic forms: strictly asexual reproduction via budding, fragmentation, or fission; strictly sexual; and species that can reproduce by either means, depending on genetic or physiological strain and environmental conditions.

Fragmentation is usually preceded by a degeneration of the internal organs. The entire worm fragments into pieces that secrete mucus, which then hardens to form a small cyst within the slime mass. Following an inactive period of a few weeks to the entire winter, a whole miniature individual emerges from the cyst.

Transverse fission begins with an elongation of the body, followed by pinching in of the tissue at approximately the midpoint of the body. The pinching proceeds rapidly until the animal is separated. The posterior of the anterior end develops a new tail, and the anterior of the posterior segment develops a new head. Two new but smaller animals are the result of fission. Microturbellarians may have fission occur simultaneously along several transverse planes, resulting in a series or chain of 2–8 zooids. Divisions can occur as frequently as 5–10 days.

In sexual reproduction, hermaphroditic animals differentiate both ovaries and testes from undifferentiated parenchymal cells. Development of sexual organs may depend on environmental conditions. The male sexual organs consist of numerous roundish testes connected to one of the two symmetrical and longitudinal vasa deferentia arising from near the head and extending to just behind the genital pore. The vasa deferentia widen caudally and become convoluted, forming the spermiducal vesicles, where ripe sperm are stored. A muscular penis is the termination of the spermiducal vesicles, often connected to these by a united duct. The penis consists of a bulbous base that is muscular and may contain several gland cells. These cells may secrete a granular material vital to the sperm. The bulb terminates in the penis papilla, which projects into a cavity, the *male atrium*, which unites with the female atrium. In some species, the tip of the penis is modified to form a stylet. Together these atria open externally as the common genital pore. Cement glands, copulatory glands, and accessory reproductive structures may be present.

Situated near the head is a pair of roundish or ovoid ovaries. The yolk cells are collected in follicles situated bilaterally in the body from the level of the ovaries to the genital pore. The yolk cells are deposited directly into the oviducts, or *ovovitelline ducts*, which lead to the copulatory organs. The ducts unite near the midline posterior to the mouth and enter the female atrium. Anterior to the penis bulb is a saclike bursa copulatrix that unites with the female atrium by means of a bursal canal.

Sexually mature individuals copulate with other mature individuals of the same species. Copulation occurs by elongation and protrusion of the penis out the genital pore and through the genital pore of the other animal. Sperm is discharged into the bursal canal. Copious amounts of mucus are secreted from the genital pore region during copulation. Sperm are stored in the bursa copulatrix and then migrate up the oviducts. Eggs are fertilized as they leave the ovaries. Yolk cells aggregate around the fertilized egg as it traverses the oviduct, and in the male antrium the aggregates are surrounded by a proteinaceous capsule forming a cocoon. Cocoons can contain several to twenty zygotes and thousands of yolk cells. The cocoon, when laid, may be sessile or stalked. Microturbellarians generally lay single eggs, each enclosed in a capsule or shell that may be stalked. Summer eggs (thin-shelled, rapidly developing eggs) or winter eggs (thicker-shelled eggs with delayed hatching) may be produced. Winter eggs may be retained within the body and are not liberated until the adult dies.

The cocoons will hatch into small offspring identical in appearance to the adults. Cocoons are resistant to low temperatures but not to desiccation. Hypodermic impregnation, in which the sperm are transferred through the piercing of the body, occurs in species with a penile stylet. It is unknown how the sperm find their way into the female reproductive system. Mature eggs are liberated by the rupturing of the body wall.

Environmental Disorders and Preventive Medicine

Temperature

Temperature plays a role in the distribution of freshwater triclad species (Reynoldson et al., 1965). *Dugesia polychroa* and *D. tigrina* are relatively thermophilous species that can complete their life cycle only in a temperature range of 10°–23°C (Van der Velde et al., 1986). *Planaria torva* is eurythermal, completing its life cycle over a temperature range of 3.5°–20°C (Sefton and Reynoldson, 1972). Four common British lake-dwelling species have similar life-cycle lengths at 10°C but show distinct contrasts above and below this temperature (Reynoldson et al., 1965; Sefton and Reynoldson, 1972). Temperature has also been identified as a significant factor influencing the distribution of stream-dwelling triclads (Reynoldson et al., 1965). There is a marked effect on rate of development, with a linear relationship between speed of development and temperature. Turbellarians kept at high temperatures tend to decrease in size and fecundity. Failure to breed at low temperatures is, in part, due to retardation of testes development. Similarly, at high temperatures, both testes and ovaries are adversely affected. Distribution is directly related to the prevalence of prey, with temperature effects secondary.

Survival of planaria, terrestrial or aquatic, is influenced by temperature. The longest recorded survival of *Artioposthia triangulata*, a terrestrial planarian that feeds on earthworms, was 60 weeks at 5°C. Starved planarians kept at 23°C failed to survive for 1 week, and no individual at 20°C survived beyond 3 weeks, regardless of the size of the planarian at the start of environmental manipulation (Blackshaw, 1992). Time to death depends on the rate of weight loss, which increases with temperature. Degrowth of turbellarians has three distinct phases: (a) breakdown of pigment granules, exhaustion of intracellular lipid reserves, and a reduction in glycogen; (b) dedifferentiation of gland and pigment cells, suppressed gland secretions, digestion of muscle fibers, breakdown of parts of the gut, and a general decrease in cell size; and (c) gross histolysis of portions of the gut, followed, in turn, by a breakdown of the reproductive system (Blackshaw, 1992). The pharyngeal musculature and innervation remain largely intact to ensure a functional means of predation. Degrowth reverses the process of growth but creates a reserve of stem cells that can enable growth and development to commence should food be encountered.

Salinity

Occurrence of wild populations of triclad species depends on their osmoregulatory capacity. Salinity greatly influences survivorship, and continual survival of *D. lugubris* and *D. polychroa* is possible only at a chlorinity level below 3.8 ppt, with higher chlorinities tolerated for a limited time (Van der Velde et al., 1986).

Ultraviolet Radiation

Shortwave ultraviolet light (254 nm = $7.83 \times 10 - 19$ J = 4.89 eV) either stimulates the release of some unidentified substance in a wavelength-dependent manner or disrupts dopaminergic binding or transduction processes (Raffa et al., 2000).

Chemicals

Freshwater triclads are susceptible to heavy-metal ions of lead and copper, with the toxicities varying based on the metal's association with different anions (Kapu and Schaeffer, 1991; Pyatt et al., 1991). In the study by Pyatt et al. (1991), detrimental effects caused by lead chloride and lead nitrate were limited, with decreased mucus production above 100 ppm and constant re-

coiling and uncoordinated movement. Copper chloride at 10 ppm and copper sulfate at 5 ppm induced behavioral changes and excess mucus production. Fatalities occurred in copper chloride concentrations as low as 20 ppm. Behavioral changes were observed for all cations at concentrations of 5 ppm. Mucus secretions effectively trap lead cations and may provide a degree of protection from the toxins. Lead nitrate and copper sulfate act synergistically, enhancing toxicity for lead nitrate relative to its direct cation effect and decreased toxicity for copper sulfate. Kapu and Schaeffer (1991) found that patterns of response for boron, nickel, selenium, zinc, chromium, copper, and lead (but not iron) changed over time, suggesting a concentration-response effect of individual metals. As duration of exposure increased, more animals exhibited shape changes and labored movement, with toxicity generally increasing with concentration and with exposure time. Water hardness was also found to affect the toxicity of metals, specifically copper, lead, and zinc. In the case of copper sulfate, the chemical exerts a genotoxic effect. Copper-induced strand breakage occurs, with copper (and possibly iron) playing a catalytic role in the initiation of free radicals in the presence of available cellular reductants (Guecheva et al., 2001). DNA could be attacked by these reactive oxygen species, leading to base damage and DNA-strand excision.

Zinc exposure causes metallothionein and protein concentrations to increase and hemocyanin concentrations to decrease in *D. dorotocephala* exposed to zinc-spiked natural sediments (Martinez-Tabche et al., 2002). The 96-h EC_{50} (median effective concentration) for zinc was 12.52 mg zinc/kg of sediment. Metallothionein production could be an effective defense mechanism in planaria.

Cadmium levels (cadmic ion) of 0.1 ppm or greater suppress fissioning. Higher concentrations in the range of 0.7 ppm produce varying amounts of head resorption (Best and Morita, 1982).

Mercury, as methylmercuric chloride, causes morphologically abnormal heads in decapitated planarians at various concentrations (Best and Morita, 1982). At concentrations of 0.08 ppm or less, behavioral abnormalities were induced. Neurotoxic effects, such as fissioning suppression, can be induced with concentrations as low as 0.1 ppb.

Actinomycin D inhibits mRNA transcription. It affects regenerating adult and immature turbellarians in slightly different fashion, with the animals showing critical periods of sensitivity. Regenerating adults demonstrate teratogenic affects, whereas immature worms regenerate smaller heads but are otherwise normal. These observations suggest de novo mRNA is necessary for adults, whereas mRNA for immature turbellarian regeneration is already present (Best and Morita, 1982).

Disturbances to cephalic regeneration are attributed to exposure to colchicines, colcemide, and puromycin. Puromycin, a protein-synthesis inhibitor, in conjunction with colcemide produces polarity reversals (head growing out of the caudal end of an animal), as does exposure to colchicine alone. Axial gradients of colcemide can induce differentiation of supernumerary heads at the caudal end (Best and Morita, 1982).

Exaggerated extension, uncoordinated writhing, enhanced fissioning at low concentrations, and inhibited fissioning at higher concentrations are indicative of chlordane exposure, which, in the range of 0.7 ppm, causes dissolution of the head (Best and Morita, 1982).

Concentrations of 50 or 100 ppm of caffeine act as a mild locomotor stimulant. At higher concentrations, 100–200 ppm, caffeine suppresses locomotor activity and produces a high incidence of head lesions and head resorption (Best and Morita, 1982).

Saturated aqueous solutions, approximately 60 ppm, of thalidomide produce a significant, time-dependent interference with RNA synthesis and cellular differentiation (Best and Morita, 1982).

Dimethylbenzthracene (DMBA), benzanthracene (BA), and benzpyrene (BP) were fed to intact asexual turbellarians in an egg-yolk carrier. Groups administered DMBA developed a high incidence of supernumerary eyes or heads, tumorlike growths, or supernumerary heads growing from a tumor mass, generally appearing in the second and third month after administration. BP-fed and BA-fed groups had high mortality (Foster, 1969; Best and Morita, 1982).

Methylcholanthrene induces tumors and supernumerary heads upon exposure of localized regions, with a latency order of approximately 3 months (Foster, 1969).

Infectious Diseases

J.B. Jennings stated (personal communication),

In over forty years' experience in working with these fascinating animals I have noted repeatedly their extraordinary health and vigor! This is in spite of the very wide range of habitats, diets, modes of life and geographical locations exploited by these supposedly simple animals.

Overall, turbellarians are hardy animals with few infectious diseases. No reports of infectious diseases affecting laboratory populations were found in the literature. The bulk of turbellarians with reported health problems came from wild-collected individuals or wild populations manipulated in the laboratory.

Viruses

Electron microscopy has revealed the presence of viruses in turbellarians with no report of disease. Readers are referred to Kishida and Asai (1977), Le Moigne and Sauzin-Monnot (1971), Oschman (1969), and Reuter (1975).

Bacteria

No reports of bacterial infections were found in the literature, although poor husbandry practices, such as not removing food and infrequent water changes, would promote the growth of bacteria in laboratory cultures.

Protozoans

Codreanu and Balcesco (1971), de Puytorac and Grain (1960), Fuhrmann (1916), and Holmquist (1967) all report the occurrence of gregarines from a number of planarian hosts, including terrestrial and freshwater species.

Aseptate gregarine parasites of the genus *Monocystella* (Lecudinidae), consisting of approximately 10 species, are infective to turbellarians. In *M. epibatis*, gamonts liberated from oocysts grow within the host tissue and associate in pairs when mature (syzygy). A cyst wall develops around the pair, which undergo reduction divisions to form isogametes or anisogametes. Within the gametocyst, fusion of the gametes leads to the formation of oocysts, each of which contains eight sporozoites (Cannon and Jennings, 1988). Sporozoites liberated from oocysts are ingested with food and most likely gain entry to gut cells of their marine host directly or through phagocytosis. There is no asexual reproduction known.

Tetrahymena pyriformis and *T. corlissi*, common freshwater ciliates, have been recognized as parasites of freshwater triclad turbellarians (Wright, 1981; Armitage and Young, 1990). Experimental data indicate that infection is due to ingestion of the ciliate with food rather than exposure to the ciliate in water. Subsequent development can be fast, with substantial mortality at temperatures greater than 15°C. Prevalence of this parasite in laboratory populations exceeds 50% and can attain levels of 85%, with mean intensities of 500 ciliates per infected triclad. Up to this level of parasitemia, the animals generally appear healthy. At high temperatures, ciliate numbers increase and sudden and substantial mortality occurs, with subsequent tissue breakdown. It is likely that the ciliate penetrates the mesenchyme after its entry into the gut (Wright, 1968).

The peritrich *Urceolaria mitra* is a naturally occurring ectoparasite epizoic on flatworms, particularly *Polycelis tenuis* (Reynoldson, 1951).

Euglenoidina have also been reported as parasites of turbellarians (Beauchamp, 1911; Kolasa, 1982).

Nematodes

Unidentified nematodes were found infecting the pharyngeal muscles of freshwater triclads collected throughout the year. No seasonal patterns or temperature correlations were noted (Armitage and Young, 1990). Prevalence in wild-collected triclads varied from 2% to 6%, with a maximum of two nematodes in an individual triclad. The low prevalence and healthy appearance of the triclads suggest the nematodes may not be an important mortality factor in the population dynamics of wild triclads.

Other

Orthonectids are mesozoans that have been reported as parasites of marine turbellarians (Stunkard, 1954).

Neoplasia

Whether lesions referred to as tumors are truly autonomous growths comparable to vertebrate neoplasms is open to conjecture (Tehseen et al., 1992). Neoblasts are the only cells in planaria that divide mitotically during regeneration. As such, it has been suggested (Lange, 1966) that the abnormal lethal growths that arise spontaneously (Goldsmith, 1939, 1941; Stéphan, 1962; Lange, 1966) or via exposure to carcinogens (Foster, 1963, 1969; Hall, 1986; Hall et al., 1986a), insecticides (An der Lan, 1962; Villar et al., 1993), or metabolic antagonists (Henderson and Eakin, 1961) are the result of faulty differentiation control rather than neoplasia.

Studies with carcinogens and teratogens have demonstrated that responses in planarians are similar to those in mammals (Tehseen et al., 1992). Unlike mammals, however, the growths (tumors) can appear, develop, and disappear in as little as 48 h due to death of the animals or shedding of the affected body part by fragmentation. Analysis of malformations, spontaneous and teratological, could preferably be classified as hyperplasia, dysplasia, necroses, or teratogenic remodelings rather than as true tumors associated with neoplastic transformation (Hall et al., 1986a). Benign and malignant tumorlike lesions, with growths consisting of proliferating neoblast-like cells exhibiting varying levels of differentiation and a derivative population of cells resembling amitotic reticulocytes, have been observed by Hall and colleagues (Hall, 1986; Hall et al., 1986a, 1986b) in turbellarians exposed to a phorbol ester alone and in combination with cadmium. Transformed stem cells paralleled the pathogenesis of a variety of mammalian neoplastic stem-cell diseases, with malignant reticuloma cells found to differentiate from mitotically active (presumably transformed) stem cells that proliferate within the infiltrating tissue formations. Metastasis was confirmed by transplantation into healthy animals that subsequently exhibited identical histopathology and progression to lethality. Tumors that persisted but did not spread were considered benign.

Treatment of *D. dorotocephala* with polyaromatic hydrocarbons induced progressive lethal tumors with morphologic and physiological characteristics of malignant tumors in vertebrates. The growths were composed of primarily primitive cells (Foster, 1963, 1969). In one study (Tehseen et al., 1992), exposure to cadmium and polychlorinated biphenols (PCBs) resulted in three types of tumors localized in different body regions. Highly invasive, progressive, and rapidly growing tumors were reported at post-head (located at a region just behind the head) or round tail tip (a single proliferation at the tip of the tail). Pigmented rose thorn tumors, a pigmented, thorn-shaped outgrowth near the end of the tail, grew slowly and were nonlethal.

Spontaneous and induced tumors in several fissiparous species have been recorded by Goldsmith (1939, 1941), Stéphan (1962), and Lange (1966), with the development of supernumerary eyes in the tumors observed by the former two authors. Lange (1966) considered these differentiation errors rather than neoplastic, because the cells and tissues did not appear abnormal, but rather their position in relation to the rest of the animal was abnormal. Of the tumors Lange observed, one type manifested at the posterior tip as slowly growing, darkly pigmented lumps that eventually developed clear white tubes from which mucus was occasionally expelled. A less common form

initiated in the midregion of the dorsum assumed a wide craterlike shape with a clear ring of tissue forming a rim around the apex of the mound. Histological observations demonstrated the masses consisted of papillary and cryptlike structures covered and lined, respectively, by mucus-producing epithelium and a broken or perforated basement membrane. The craterlike tumors demonstrated a high degree of differentiation of some of their tissues (nervous, parenchymal, and epithelial), and the epithelium-lined crypts were otherwise morphologically similar to advanced stages of the form found on the posterior tip.

Miscellaneous Disorders

Radiation

Turbellarians exposed to 2 roentgens of radiation from cobalt 60 exhibited changes in behavior but no observable physical changes (Corbridge, 1967). There was no response of irradiated turbellarians to electrical shock, and conditioned responses could not be elicited nor could irradiated turbellarians be trained to give a conditioned response. With exposure to 4000 or 20,000 rads of radiation, most turbellarians die, with physical damage appearing after 5 days.

Irradiated food (2 and 4.8 megarads) fed to turbellarians for 6 months inhibited growth or caused a decrease in size, eventually resulting in death (Corbridge, 1967).

Cannibalism

Cannibalistic individuals were noted to arise spontaneously in laboratory cultures of asexual *D. tigrina*, representing a genetically distinct clone or a nongenetic but persistent phenotypic phase induced by conditions favoring intraspecific predation (Armstrong, 1964).

Analgesia, Anesthesia, and Surgery

Turbellarians have been popular animals in the arena of experimental zoology because of their ability to undergo regeneration. Sectioning, the typical surgical procedure performed on these animals, is typically executed without anesthesia and can be done using a scalpel or the edge of a microscope coverslip. A slicing motion is not necessary, gentle pressure being enough to produce the desired result (Callahan and Morris, 1989).

Morphallactic and epimorphic events are involved in turbellarian regeneration (Palmberg, 1986). Turbellarians sectioned bilaterally regenerate in such a manner that the anteroposterior axis coincides with that of the sectioned worm. The regulatory process is always preceded by a temporary asymmetry of some structural characteristics (Kiang and Chow, 1945). Initially, the cut surface rapidly contracts, and a thin film of epidermal cells from the stretched old epidermis covers it (Baguñà et al., 1988). An accumulation of undifferentiated cells, the regenerative blastema, appears below the wound epithelium at day 1 of regeneration. This multilayered accumulation of cells appears by the addition of new undifferentiated cells formed by cell division in the underlying parenchyma. Blastema cells do not divide, but growth of the blastema is exponential due to increase in cell size and the continuous entrance of undifferentiated cells from the stump (postblastema) to the base of the blastema. Healing of turbellarians is complete within 30 min of cutting (Baguñà et al., 1988).

Autografts and allografts are common surgical procedures in turbellarians. Implants are made by simply creating holes in the host into which the transplanted material is placed. Sometimes the grafts may migrate or are resorbed. Graft and recipient fuse to yield a morphologically and functionally integrated individual, even when host and graft are different species.

Anesthesia is generally performed on turbellarians to relax specimens prior to killing them for taxonomic studies. Anesthetics may also be used when sectioning for regenerative studies and must be very precise or to assist in surgical transplantations. A number of protocols have been reported: Narcotizing in strychnine water for several minutes was an accepted methodology for relaxation prior to killing and fixation of planarians (Pennak, 1978). Nontriclad planarians can be anesthetized with 0.1% chloretone, 1% hydroxylamine hydrochloride, chilling in cold water, or 10% ethanol (Pennak, 1978). Lethality may be the primary response in decapitated *D. dorotocephala* at levels as low as 1.0% ethanol (Best and Morita, 1982). Intact turbellarians exposed to 0.3%–0.5% ethanol may display indications of neurotoxicity (decreased fissioning and locomotor activity) with prolonged exposure.

Specimens of the terrestrial turbellarians *B. fuscatum* and *B. multilineatum* have been successfully anesthetized with carbon dioxide (Makino and Shirasawa, 1986). Blair and Anderson (1993) anesthetized *Bdelloura candida*, an ectoparasitic marine triclad, with a 1:1 solution of isotonic $MgCl_2$ and natural seawater. Prolonged exposure for 15–20 min was not detrimental to recovery.

Turbellarians also respond with characteristic behaviors to dopaminergic agonists and antagonists (Raffa and Valdez, 2001). Dopaminergic agonists induce hyperkinesias that can be antagonized by dopaminergic blocking agents (Palladini et al., 1996). Specimens treated with low levels of cocaine become motionless.

Exposure to 6-hydroxydopamine produces hypokinesia in *Dugesia gonocephala*, due to damage to presynaptic dopamine terminals (Caronti et al., 1999).

Treatment Protocols and Formulary

Antiprotozoal Agents

Chromic acid: 0.02% for several minutes to treat *Urceolaria* (Reynoldson, 1951).

Anesthetics

Carbon dioxide: gas, blown over terrestrial species (Makino and Shirasawa, 1986).
Chloretone: 0.1% (Pennak, 1978).

Ethanol: 10% (Pennak, 1978; Best and Morita, 1982).
Hydroxylamine hydrochloride: Aqueous solution of 1.0% (Pennak, 1978).
Magnesium chloride: 1:1 isotonic salt and seawater for marine species (Blair and Anderson, 1993).
Water: cold, used to effect (Pennak, 1978).

References

An der Lan, H. 1962. Histopathologische Auswirkungen von Insektiziden (DDT und Sevin) bei Wirbellosen und ihre cancerogene Beurteilung [Histopathological effects of insecticides (DDT and Sevin) on invertebrates and their cancerogenic evaluation]. Mikroskopie 17:85–112.

Armitage, M.J., and J.O. Young. 1990. A field and laboratory study of the parasites of the triclad *Phagocata vitta* (Dugès). Freshwater Biol. 24:101–107.

Armstrong, J.T. 1964. The population dynamics of the planarian, *Dugesia tigrina*. Ecology 45:361–365.

Baguñá, J., and R. Romero. 1981. Quantitative analysis of cell types during growth, de-growth, and regeneration in the planarians *Dugesia mediterranea* and *Dugesia tigrina*. Hydrobiologia 84:181–194.

Baguñà, J., E. Saló, J. Collet, M.C. Auladell, and M. Ribas. 1988. Cellular, molecular and genetic approaches to regeneration and pattern formation in planarians. Prog. Zool. 36:65–78.

Beauchamp, P. de. 1911. *Astasia captiva* n. sp. Euglenien parasite de *Catenula lemnae* Ant. Dug. Arch. Zool. Exp. Gen. 6:52–58.

Best, J.B., and M. Morita. 1982. Planarians as a model system for in vitro teratogenesis studies. Teratogenesis Carcinog. Mutagen. 2:277–291.

Blackshaw, R.P. 1992. The effect of starvation on size and survival of the terrestrial planarian *Artioposthia triangulata* (Dendy) (Tricladida: Terricola). Ann. Appl. Biol. 120:573–578.

Blair, K.L., and P.A.V. Anderson. 1993. Properties of voltage-activated ionic currents in cells from the brains of the triclad flatworm *Bdelloura candida*. J. Exp. Biol. 185:267–286.

Boddington, M.J., and D.F. Mettrick. 1977. A laboratory study of the population dynamics and productivity of *Dugesia polychroa* (Turbellaria: Tricladida). Ecology 58:109–118.

Brøndsted, H.V. 1969. Planarian Regeneration. (International Series of Monographs in Pure and Applied Biology, volume 42.) Pergamon, London, 276 pp.

Callahan, J.L., and C.D. Morris. 1989. Production and maintenance of large numbers of *Dugesia tigrina* (Turbellaria: Tricladida) for the control of mosquitoes in the field. J. Am. Mosq. Control Assoc. 5:10–14.

Calow, P. 1979. Why some metazoan mucus secretions are more susceptible to microbial attack than others. American Naturalist 114:149–152.

Calow, P., and A.S. Woollhead. 1977. The relationship between ration, reproductive effort and age-specific mortality in the evolution of life-history strategies: Some observations on freshwater triclads. J. Anim. Ecol. 46:765–781.

Cannon, L.R.G., and J.B. Jennings. 1988. *Monocystella epibatis* n. sp., a new aseptate gregarine hyperparasite of rhabdocoel turbellarians parasitic in the crown of thorns starfish, *Acanthaster planci* Linnaeus, from the Great Barrier Reef. Arch. Protistenkd. 136:267–272.

Caronti, B., V. Margotta, A. Merante, F.E. Pontieri, and G. Palladini. 1999. Treatment with 6-hydroxydopamine in planaria (*Dugesia gonocephala* s.l.): Morphological and behavioral study. Comp. Biochem. Physiol. [C] 123:201–207.

Cash, K.J., M.H. McKee, and F.J. Wrona. 1993. Short- and long-term consequences of grouping and group foraging in the free-living flatworm *Dugesia tigrina*. J. Anim. Ecol. 62:529–535.

Codreanu, R., and D. Balcesco. 1971. Sur une nouvelle grégarine, *Monocystella spelaea* n. sp. parasite d'un dendrocoelide cavernicole de Roumanie et la systématique des acéphalines des turbellariés. Protistologica 7:145–152.

Corbridge, A. 1967. Planaria: How they are effected by direct radiation and by irradiated food. J. Colo. Dent. Assoc. 45:22–25.

Dindal, D.L. 1970. Feeding behavior of a terrestrial turbellarian *Bipalium adventitium*. Am. Midl. Nat. 83:635–637.

Foster, J. 1963. Induction of neoplasms in planarians with carcinogens. Cancer Res. 23:300–303.

Foster, J. 1969. Malformations and lethal growths in planarians treated with carcinogens. Natl. Cancer Inst. Monogr. 31:683–691.

Fuhrmann, O. 1916. Eine in *Geoplana* parasitierende Gregarine. Centralbl. Bakteriol. Parasitenkd. Infectionskr. 77:482–485.

Goldsmith, E.D. 1939. Spontaneous outgrowths in *Dugesia tigrina*. Anat. Rec. 75(Suppl.):158–159.

Goldsmith, E.D. 1941. Further observations of supernumerary structures in individuals of an artificially produced clone of *Dugesia tigrina*. Anat. Rec. 81:108–109.

Golubev, A.L. 1988. Glia and neuroglia relationships in the central nervous system of the *Turbellaria* (electron microscopic data). Prog. Zool. 36:185–190.

Gremigni, V. 1979. An ultrastructural approach to planarian taxonomy. Syst. Zool. 28:345–355.

Guecheva, T., J.A.P. Henriques, and B. Erdtmann. 2001. Genotoxic effects of copper sulphate in freshwater planarian in vivo, studied with the single-cell gel test (comet assay). Mutat. Res. 497:19–27.

Hall, F.L. 1986. Cadmium in the planarian: Neurotoxicity, carcinogenesis, mitochondriogenesis, and enzyme activity. Diss. Abstr. Int. [B] 47:1884.

Hall, F., M. Morita, and J.B. Best. 1986a. Neoplastic transformation in the planarian. I. Cocarcinogenesis and histopathology. J. Exp. Zool. 240:211–228.

Hall, F., M. Morita, and J.B. Best. 1986b. Neoplastic transformation in the planarian. II. Ultrastructure of malignant reticuloma. J. Exp. Zool. 240:229–244.

Henderson, T.R., and R.E. Eakin. 1961. Irreversible alterations of differentiated tissues in planaria by purine analogues. J. Exp. Zool. 164:253–264.

Holmquist, C. 1967. *Dendrocoelopsis pyriformis* (Turbellaria Tricladida) and its parasites from Northern Alaska. Arch. Hydrobiol. 62:453–466.

Jennings, J.B. 1997. Nutritional and respiratory pathways to parasitism exemplified in the Turbellaria. Int. J. Parasitol. 27:679–691.

Jennings, J.B., L.R.G. Cannon, and A.J. Hick. 1992. The nature and origin of the epidermal scales of *Notodactylus handschini*: An unusual temnocephalid turbellarian ectosymbiotic on crayfish from Northern Queensland. Biol. Bull. 182:117–128.

Kapu, M.M., and D.J. Schaeffer. 1991. Planarians in toxicology: Responses of asexual *Dugesia dorotocephala* to selected metals. Bull. Environ. Contam. Toxicol. 47:302–307.

Kiang, H.M., and P.S. Chow. 1945. A note on lateral piece regeneration in *Planaria gonocephala*. Am. Nat. 79:474–478.

Kimmel, H.D., and H.A. Garrigan. 1973. Resistance to extinction in planaria. J. Exp. Psychol. 101:343–347.

Kishida, Y., and E. Asai. 1977. Les cristeaux intranucleaires des cellules pharyngiennes chez la Planaire, *Dugesia japonica* Ichikawa et Kawakatsu. J. Electron Microsc. 26:145–147.

Klots, A.B. 1960. A terrestrial flatworm well established outdoors in the Northeastern United States. Syst. Zool. 9:33–34.

Kolasa, J. 1982. Records of parasitic Euglenoidina in lower invertebrates. Przegl. Zool. 26:111–114.

Kotikova, E.A. 1986. Comparative characterization of the nervous system of the Turbellaria. Hydrobiologia 132:89–92.

Lange, C.S. 1966. Observations on some tumours found in two species of planaria: *Dugesia etrusca* and *D. ilvana*. J. Embryol. Exp. Morphol. 15:125–130.

Lange, C.S. 1968. A possible explanation in cellular terms of the physiological ageing of the planaria. Exp. Gerontol. 3:219–230.

Le Moigne, A., and M.J. Sauzin-Monnot. 1971. Etude au microscope electronique d'inclusions nucleaires chez des Planaires (Turbellaries, Triclades). J. Microsc. (Paris) 10:107–112.

Makino, N., and Y. Shirasawa. 1986. Biology of long slender land planarians (Turbellaria) in Tokyo and environs. Hydrobiologia 132:229–232.

Martinez-Tabche, L., C.M. Acosta, M.G. Martinez, E.L. Lopez, and J.B.P. Najera. 2002. Toxicity and uptake of zinc in the planarian *Dugesia dorotocephala* in natural sediments. J. Freshwater Ecol. 17:415–421.

Oschman, J.L. 1969. Endonuclear viruslike bodies in *Convoluta roscoffensis* (Turbellaria, Acoela). J. Invertebr. Pathol. 13:147–148.

Palladini, G., S. Ruggeri, F. Stocchi, M.F. DePandis, G. Venturini, and V. Margotta. 1996. A pharmacological study of cocaine activity in planaria. Comp. Biochem. Physiol. [C] 115:41–45.

Palmberg, I. 1986. Cell migration and differentiation during wound healing and regeneration in *Microstomum lineare* (Turbellaria). Hydrobiologia 132:181–188.

Pennak, R.W. 1978. Turbellaria (Flatworms). In: Freshwater Invertebrates of the United States, 2nd edition. John Wiley and Sons, New York, pp. 114–141.

Pickavance, J.R. 1971. The diet of the immigrant planarian *Dugesia tigrina* (Girard). I. Feeding in the laboratory. J. Anim. Ecol. 40:623–635.

Puytorac, P. de, and J. Grain. 1960. Sur deux gregarines du genre *Monocystella* endoparasites des planaires ochridiennes *Fonticola ochridana* Stankovi_ et *Neodendrocoelum sanctinaumi* Stankovi_. Ann. Parasitol. Hum. Comp. 35:197–208.

Pyatt, F.B., C. Gadd, J.B. Sykes, and D.M. Storey. 1991. An introductory appraisal of some effects of copper and lead salts on *Polycelis* spp. Environ. Educ. Information 10:25–36.

Raffa, R.B., and J.M. Valdez. 2001. Cocaine withdrawal in Planaria. Eur. J. Pharmacol. 430:143–145.

Raffa, R.B., J.M. Valdez, L.J. Holland, and R.J. Schulingkamp. 2000. Energy-dependent UV light-induced disruption of (−)sulpiride antagonism of dopamine. Eur. J. Pharmacol. 406:R11–R12.

Reuter, M. 1975. Viruslike particles in *Gyratrix hermaphroditus* (Turbellaria: Rhabdocoela). J. Invertebr. Pathol. 25:79–95.

Reynoldson, T.B. 1951. The dispersal of *Urceolaria mitra* (Peritricha) epizoic on flatworms. J. Anim. Ecol. 20:123–131.

Reynoldson, T.B., J.O. Young, and M.C. Taylor. 1965. The effect of temperature on the life-cycle of four species of lake-dwelling triclads. J. Anim. Ecol. 34:23–43.

Roberts, L.S., and J. Janovy Jr. 2000. Introduction to the phylum Platyhelminthes. In: Gerald D. Schmidt and Larry S. Roberts' Foundations of Parasitology, 6th edition. McGraw Hill, New York, pp. 189–197.

Sefton, A.D., and T.B. Reynoldson. 1972. The effect of temperature and water chemistry on the life-cycle of *Planaria torva* (Müller) (Turbellaria: Tricladida). J. Anim. Ecol. 41:487–494.

Stéphan, F. 1962. Tumeurs spontenees chez la planaire *Dugesia tigrina*. C.R. Seanc. Soc. Biol. Fil. 156:920–922.

Stewart, A.M. 1972. Life cycle and phenotypic variation in the eyes of *Procotyla fluviatilis* (Leidy) (Tricladida, Dendrocoelidae). Am. Midl. Nat. 87:538–543.

Stunkard, H.W. 1954. The life-history and systematic relations of the Mesozoa. Q. Rev. Biol. 29:230–244.

Stunkard, H.W. 1975. Life-histories and systematics of parasitic flatworms. Syst. Zool. 24:378–385.

Tehseen, W.M, L.G. Hansen, D.J. Schaeffer, and H.A. Reynolds. 1992. A scientific basis for proposed quality assurance of a new screening method for tumor-like growths in the planarian, *Dugesia dorotocephala*. Quality Assurance Good Pract. Regul. Law 1:217–229.

Tyler, S., and L.F. Bush, comp. (2002). Turbellarian taxonomic database. Version 1.0. http://devbio.umesci.maine.edu/styler/turbellaria.

Van der Velde, G., F. Hüsken, and L. Van Welie. 1986. Salinity-temperature tolerance of two closely related triclad species, *Dugesia lugubris* and *D. polychroa* (Turbellaria), in relation to their distribution in the Netherlands. Hydrobiologia 132:279–286.

Villar, D., M.-H. Li, and D.J. Schaeffer. 1993. Toxicity of organophosphorus pesticides to *Dugesia dorotocephala*. Bull. Environ. Contam. Toxicol. 51:80–87.

Wright, J.F. 1968. The ecology of stream-dwelling triclads. Unpublished Ph.D. thesis, University of Wales.

Wright, J.F. 1981. *Tetrahymena pyriformis* (Ehrenberg) and *T. corlissi* Thompson parasitic in stream-dwelling triclads (Platyhelminthes: Turbellaria). J. Parasitol. 67:131–133.

Young, J.O. 1973. The prey and predators of *Phaenocora typhlops* (Vejdovsky) (Turbellaria: Neorhabdocoela) living in a small pond. J. Anim. Ecol. 42:637–643.

Chapter 5

GASTROPODS

Roxanna Smolowitz

Natural History and Taxonomy

The gastropods (class Gastropoda, phylum Mollusca) are made up of over 80,000 species in marine, freshwater, and terrestrial environments. All gastropods have a ventrally flattened foot that provides locomotion along the various surfaces of their habitats. They are divided into three subclasses: Prosobranchia, Opistobranchia, and Pulmonata (Table 5.1) and are differentiated from other molluskan classes by the evolution of a torsed body. In the subclass Prosobranchia, the single valve (or shell) has taken on a diverse number of spiraled forms (Figure 5.1, Color Plate 5.1). Over time, members of two subclasses have detorted to varying degrees (subclasses Opistobranchia and Pulmonata). Many of the members of these two subclasses have evolutionarily discarded the shell or have retained only a remnant within their soft tissues.

The use of gastropods as laboratory animals, and in aquaculture, is limited. One genus of the Prosobranchia, the abalone (*Haliotis* sp.), is cultured extensively for food on the West Coast of the United States (Figure 5.2). Members of the Prosobranchia and Pulmonata are often found in home aquaria. *Buccinum* sp. (Dakin, 1912), *Littorina littorea* (Fretter and Graham, 1962, 1976), as well as other members of the Prosobranchia (Hyman, 1967; Hughes, 1986), are the examples used when describing the characteristics most commonly identified with the subclass. Members of both the Prosobranchia and Pulmonata serve as intermediate hosts for important animal and human parasites and for this reason are used in research.

Two opistobranch mollusks have played a major role in neurobiological research for many decades. *Aplysia californica* (a sea hare) (Figure 5.4, Color Plate 5.4) and *Hermissenda crassicornis* (a sea slug) (Figure 5.3) are used to study learning and memory. The National Resource for *Aplysia* (National Institutes of Health/University of Miami, Division of Marine Biology and Fisheries, Rosenstiel School of Marine and Atmospheric Science, 4600 Rickenbacker Causeway, Miami, FL 33149) provides cultured sea hares to other researchers across the United States.

Anatomy and Physiology

Shell

The typical shell of this class is an elongated cone, containing a visceral mass that spirals around a central shell axis, the *columella*. Turns of the spiraled shell are termed *whorls*. The head and foot protrude from the aperture of the final whorl (Figure 5.5). The apex and the oldest part of the shell is called the *spire*. Most gastropod shells demonstrate right-handed or dextral rotation (with apex held away from the observer).

All gastropods have a well-developed head with bilaterally symmetrical tentacles and eyes. At an early embryonic stage (*veliger*), the visceral mass, covered by the shell, is consolidated dorsally, elongated, and torsed 180°. This results in the visceral mass (covered by the spiral shell) lying directly over the head and closely adjacent foot. A palladial cavity is formed by the anatomical juxtaposition of the head and foot resulting in placement of the rectum in close proximity to the gill.

Palladial Cavity

The palladial cavity lies within the final whorl of the shell, is lined by mantle, and contains the gill, anus, head, and reproductive ostia. As part of the evolutionarily based torsion process, most gastropods have lost the auricle, gill, and kidney from the left side of the body (Fretter and Graham, 1962). Mild detorsion occurs in the maturation process of some species in later developmental stages, but all gastropods contain moderate degrees of nonsymmetry.

In pulmonates, a pulmonary sac is formed by the fusion of the mantle edges along the animal's back. Air enters the sac through a contractile opening termed a *pneumostome*. The roof of the sac contains a respiratory network of blood sinuses that are responsible for air exchange. In aquatic pulmonates, a small adaptive gill termed a *pseudobranch* (Luchtel et al., 1997) is present in this area.

Formation of the shell of gastropods by the mantle epithelium is explained in detail by several texts (Dakin, 1912; Hyman, 1967; Luchtel et al., 1997). In summary, the mantle ep-

Table 5.1. Taxonomic outline of the Gastropoda

Phylum Mollusca
Class Gastropoda
Subclasses
1. Prosobranchia: Torted gastropods with the mantle cavity containing the pallial complex anteriorly located, dioecious, marine, freshwater, or terrestrial.

    Order Archaeogastropoda: Mostly herbivorous, radula with many teeth, bipectinate gill or gills. *Megathura* sp. (keyhole limpets) and *Haliotis* sp. (abalone).

    Order Mesogastropoda: Herbivorous, carnivorous, and filter feeding, radula with fewer teeth, monopectinate gill (filaments on only one side of the gill axis). *Littorina* (periwinkle), *Crepidula* sp. and *Crepipatella* sp. (slipper snails), *Polinices* sp. (moon snail), *Lambis* sp. (spider conch), *Strombus* sp. (conch), and *Cypraea* sp. (cowrie).

    Order Neogastropoda: Mostly carnivorous, narrow radula with very few teeth, monopectinate gill. *Nucella* sp. (dog winkle), *Urosalpinx* sp. (oyster drill), *Buccinum* sp. and *Busycon* sp. (whelks), and *Illanassa* sp. (mud snail).
2. Opistobranchia: Torted or detorted gastropods with mantle cavity often lost; rotated to the right side; facing anteriorly; shell without ornamentation, often reduced or wanting, when present often covered with mantle or pedal folds; usually without operculum; nervous ganglia concentrated with shortening and detorsion of the visceral loop; hermaphroditic; exclusively marine. Two of the five orders have these representative genera:

    Order Anaspidea: *Aplysia* sp. and *Bursatella* sp. (sea hares).
    Order Nudibranchia (sea slugs): *Tritonia* sp., *Aeolidia* sp., and *Hermissenda* sp.
    Order Onchidiacea
    Order Cephalaspidea
    Order Pteropoda
    Order Acochlidiacea
    Order Philinoglossacea
    Order Notaspidea
    Order Sacoglossa
    Order Notaspidea
    Order Rhodopacea
    Order Pyramidellacea
    Order Parasita
3. Pulmonata: Detorted gastropods; with or without shell; mantle cavity transformed into a pulmonary sac with narrowed pore on the right side anteriorly; hermaphroditic; primarily freshwater or terrestrial; a few marine members.

    Order Basommatophora: Aquatic pulmonates—*Lymnaea* sp. and *Siphonaria* sp.
    Order Stylommatophora: Terrestrial pulmonates—*Helix* sp. (garden snail).

From Hyman (1967).

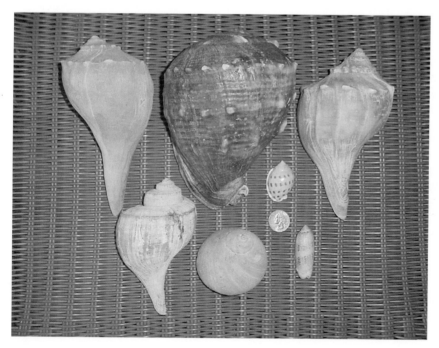

Figure 5.1. Spiral shell forms: seven species of Western Atlantic marine gastropods from North Carolina (**clockwise from bottom:** Moon snail, *Polinices duplicatus*; channeled whelk, *Busycon canaliculatum*; lightning whelk, *Busycon contrarium*; helmet, *Cassis* sp.; Scotch bonnet, *Phalium granulatum*; knobbed whelk, *Busycon carica*; and lettered olive, *Oliva sayana*. Note that all have dextral whorls (opening to the *right* when the animal's soft parts are facing the observer) except the lightning whelk, which has a sinistral opening. (Coin, U.S. quarter)

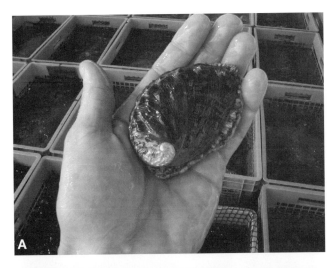

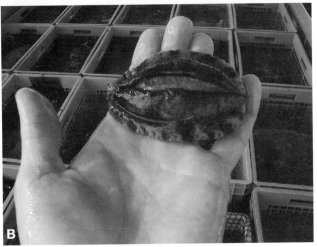

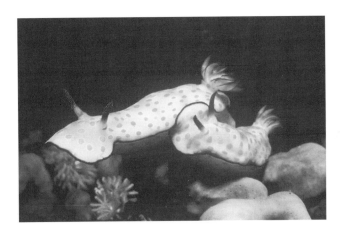

Figure 5.2. Healthy examples of cultured red abalone, *Haliotis discus hannai*. Note the full, fleshy foot of this healthy animal (**B**). Both photos courtesy of Mike Buchal, Big Island Abalone Corporation, Kailua Kona, HI.

Figure 5.3. Normal nudibranch (*Hermissenda crassicornis*).

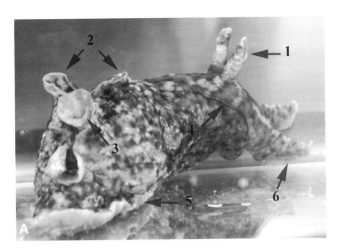

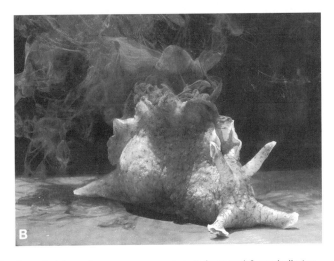

Figure 5.4. **A:** Healthy *Aplysia californica*: *1*, rhinophores; *2*, parapodia; *3*, anal siphon; *4*, open sperm groove; *5*, foot; and *6*, cephalic tentacles). **B:** Healthy animal inking. Photo B courtesy of Genevieve Anderson, Santa Barbara City College, Santa Barbara, CA.

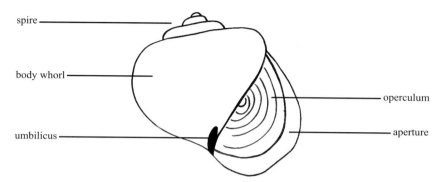

Figure 5.5. Major anatomical features of a gastropod shell. Reproduced from Richard Fox, Lander University, by Alison Schroeer.

ithelium is composed of simple columnar cells. At the mantle edge (the junction between the epithelium covering the exposed body and foot, and the epithelium that extends beneath the shell), a periostracal groove exists. At the base of this groove are periostracal cells that produce the outer layer of the shell, the *periostricum*, which is composed of fibrous, quinone-tanned proteins. As the periostricum is produced, it is pushed dorsally from the groove over the mantle epithelium underlying the shell and covering the visceral mass of the body (and away from the foot). The columnar epithelium of the mantle, over which the periostricum flows, forms a mantle-edge gland that adds a calcified, multilayered ostracum under the periostricum. The ostracum of a mature shell consists of outer prismatic and inner nacreous layers. The arrangement and number of layers of these two secretions in the mature shell vary with species. Injuries to the shell that are not adjacent to the mantle edge are repaired by deposition of inner nacreous-like shell layers by the underlying mantle epithelium (Hyman, 1967; Luchtel et al., 1997).

The operculum (trapdoor) is formed by the metapodium at the posterior portion of the foot. The metapodium is composed of a hornylike material secreted by epithelial glands in the foot. It is present only in some species of Prosobranchia (Hyman, 1967).

In many opistobranch mollusks, the shell has been greatly reduced or is no longer present. In these animals, the visceral mass also has been partially detorted. In *Aplysia californica*, a remnant shell is covered by the mantle lobes, which are only partially torsed and are oriented toward the right side of the animal. Between the lobes are the gill, anus, and gonopore. Large leaflike parapodia extend dorsally on either side of the mantle (Figure 5.4, Color Plate 5.4). Within subepidermal tissues of the inner mantle epithelium that lines the external surface of the body between the parapodia are Blochmann's glands, which are unicellular or multicellular dermal glands responsible for production of the purple, inky, thick fluid discharged when the animal is irritated (thought to be a concealment tactic). In the order Nudibranchia, of which *Hermissenda crassicornis* is a member, the mantle cavity, mantle, and gill have been lost. Instead, cerata project from the dorsal surface and are thought to function at least partially as gills (Figure 5.4).

Digestive Tract

The digestive tract of a typical gastropod consists of a muscular buccal mass found usually on a snout or proboscis that can be ei-

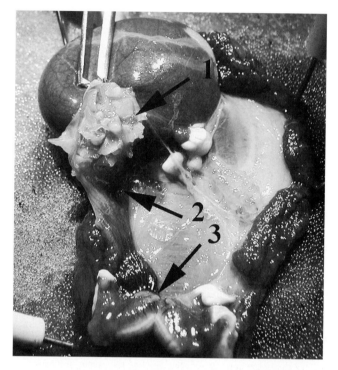

Figure 5.6. *Aplysia californica* dissection: *1*, opened gizzard showing chitinized teeth; *2*, opened crop; and *3*, opened buccal mass.

ther completely or partly retracted into the cuticular lined, buccal cavity. The lateral walls of the pharynx are lined by the *odontophore* (a hardened plate that forms the jaw) that is covered by a *radula*, which is made up of a membrane lined by chitinized teeth produced in a diverticulum off the pharynx (the radular sheath). Teeth are continuously produced in the cavity and move up the membrane to lie on the odontophore, where they are worn away with use. The odontophore can be extended into the buccal cavity by movement of the attached muscles, resulting in protrusion of the radula from the buccal cavity when eating. Specific characteristics of the teeth produced reflect the diet of each species.

Within the visceral mass are the remaining parts of the digestive system. In the prosobranch, the mouth leads to a spherical buccal cavity from the posterior end of which the esophagus begins. Long bilateral salivary glands empty into the buccal cavity in this area. The esophagus may have lateral outpouchings along

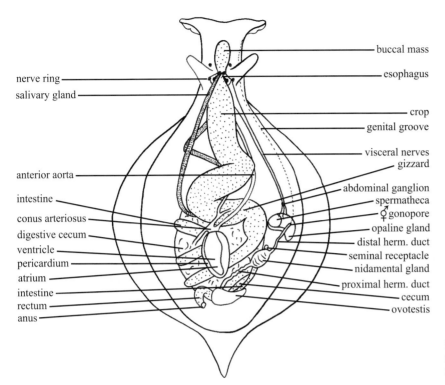

nerve ring

salivary gland

anterior aorta

intestine

conus arteriosus

digestive cecum

ventricle

pericardium

atrium

intestine

rectum

anus

buccal mass

esophagus

crop

genital groove

visceral nerves

gizzard

abdominal ganglion

spermatheca

♂ gonopore

opaline gland

distal herm. duct

seminal receptacle

nidamental gland

proximal herm. duct

cecum

ovotestis

Figure 5.7.   Detailed drawing of *Aplysia* internal anatomy. Reproduced from R. Fox, Lander University, by Alison Schroeer.

its length (*crop*) before it enters into a complicated stomach. Ducts from the digestive gland open into the stomach. The intestine leads from the stomach and loops through the body adjacent to the kidney and finally through the heart to the rectum, which empties into the palladial cavity adjacent to the gill (thus the need for good water flow through the palladial cavity). In herbivorous species, the crystalline style, a gelatinous-like rod, is produced by epithelium lining an outpouching of the stomach (termed the *style sac*). The style projects into the gastric lumen, where it abuts a heavily cuticularized area of the stomach termed the *gastric shield*. The style mechanically mixes contents of the stomach and provides digestive enzymes to break down food.

In opistobranch and pulmonate gastropods, the gastrointestinal tract is composed of an esophagus, a crop, a scleritized gizzard, a pyloric stomach (which receives digestive enzymes via ducts from the extensive digestive midgut glands), a cecum, and the intestine leading to the anus (Figures 5.6–5.8).

The Nudibranchia do not have a gizzard, and, in contrast to other gastropods, the digestive gland is highly branched and extends into cerata (fingerlike extensions of the dorsal surface of the animal). Nudibranchs, which feed on coelenterates, have developed the ability to store undischarged nematocysts in the tips of the cerata in a structure termed a *cnidosac*. Predators that attempt to feed on the cerata are stung by expulsion of the nematocyst through an opening in the cnidosac. Cerata can undergo autotomy and quickly regenerate.

Circulatory System

The open circulatory system in gastropods consists of a heart with one ventricle that lies in a pericardial sac (Figures 5.7 and

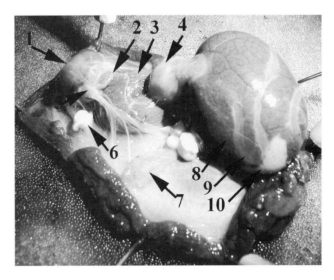

Figure 5.8.   *Aplysia californica* dissection: *1*, buccal mass; *2*, salivary gland; *3*, crop; *4*, gizzard; *5*, pleural ganglion and nerves; *6*, penial sheath; *7*, crystalline gland; *8*, digestive gland; *9*, intestine; and *10*, ovotestis.

5.9). The aorta divides into posterior and anterior branches that further divide and eventually empty into sinusoids that surround and permeate the tissues of the body. Most of the hemolymph (blood) is collected in ventral venous sinuses and directed to the gill and/or the nephridium (depending on species) and then back to the auricle of the heart. The pericardial surfaces of portions of the heart auricle contain specialized cells that project into the pericardial sac as fimbriations forming a pericardial gland.

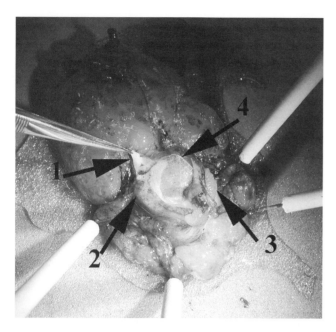

Figure 5.9.   Open mantle in *Aplysia californica*: *1*, heart pulled from pericardial sac; *2*, kidney in renal sac; *3*, gill; and *4*, shell edge.

Oxygen is carried by hemocyanin globulins that circulate free in the hemolymph. The hemolymph (blood) cells are divided into amebocytes and hyalinocytes. Phagocytosis and walling-off reactions have been attributed to amoebocytes only. No function is suggested for hyalinocytes, but they may be immature amoebocytes (Fretter and Graham, 1976; Luchtel et al., 1997).

Excretory System

Gastropods contain metanephridia composed of numerous trabeculae lined by cuboidal to columnar cells. The folds project into the nephridial lumen and are supported by sparse connective tissue in which are the hemolymph sinuses. The origin of the nephridial lumen is the renopericardial pore in the pericardial sac. The excretory lumen of the kidney leads to a nephridiopore that exits into the palladial cavity adjacent to the anus. Depending on the species, the left kidney may be absent or greatly reduced in size, and the right kidney may be divided into two anatomically distinct lobes (Hyman, 1967). In opistobranchs, the metanephridial folds that project into the lumen are often anastomosed.

Nervous and Sensory Systems

In prosobranchs, the nervous system is composed of aggregates of paired ganglia consisting of cerebral, pleural, pedal, and buccal ganglia. The first three pairs are part of a circumenteric ring that circles the pharynx/radular mass. A long visceral loop nerve that connects bilaterally to the pleural ganglia innervates the visceral mass and torses with it.

Statocysts (partially responsible for maintaining balance) are present bilaterally and are neurologically supplied by branches of the cerebral ganglia (Fretter and Graham, 1962, 1976; Hyman, 1967).

The *osphradium*, which resembles a gill, is usually identified only in aquatic prosobranchs and is present in the palladial space at the base of the siphon, adjacent to the gills. Its proposed function is chemoreception (Dakin, 1912; Hyman, 1967).

In opistobranchs, the nervous system is similar to, but more advanced than, that in prosobranchs. It is not usually torsed, and additional minor ganglia participate in and form a pronounced circumenteric ring around the buccal mass. In many opistobranchs, including *Aplysia* and *Hermissenda*, giant nerve cell bodies (up to 800 µm in diameter), so important in neural research, are in the pleural ganglion (Hyman, 1967; Thompson, 1976; Dagan and Levitan, 1981).

The rhinophores (sometimes resembling rabbit ears in opistobranchs) are lined by epithelium similar to that of the rest of the dermis and are innervated by paired ganglia that in turn connect to the cerebral ganglia. The exact function of the rhinophores, while thought to be sensory, is not known. The eyes are found on the head, but in some species are present on the tips of tentacles. When in this location, their structure is more rudimentary (Hyman, 1967).

Reproductive System

Haliotis spp., a less evolved prosobranch that lacks copulatory organs or accessory glandular structures, releases eggs and sperm by way of the right nephridiopore into the sea, where external fertilization occurs (Hyman, 1967). However, most prosobranchs are dioecious, with females usually being larger. Fertilization is usually internal, and eggs are laid in long gelatinous strands or capsules produced by a special gland, of varying complexities, depending on the species.

Most opistobranchs are hermaphroditic. In *Aplysia* sp., the large ovotestis is in the visceral mass (Figure 5.10). A thin proximal hermaphroditic duct leads from the ovotestis to an ampulla where fertilization can occur by allosperm stored in the adjacent seminal receptacle. Fertilized eggs are coated by albumen secreted from the albumen gland as they transverse the winding gland (part of the nidamental gland complex). From there, they enter the mucous gland and transverse a pathway through the nidamental gland. Along the way, a multilayered thick mucous coat is applied to the eggs to form gelatinous chains. The resulting egg chains enter the oviductal portion of the distal hermaphroditic duct and are extruded into the water column from the gonadal pore. During copulation, autosperms leave the ovotestis and travel the thin (proximal) hermaphroditic duct to the ampulla. From there, they enter the autosperm canal in the distal hermaphroditic duct and are conducted to the gonadopore. From the gonadopore, the autosperm are directed into the autosperm groove found externally on the right dorsal lateral surface of the body. Sperm travel in this groove to the tip of the penis. During copulation, the penis deposits the autosperm (which now become allosperm) into the vaginal channel of the distal hermaphroditic duct of another animal.

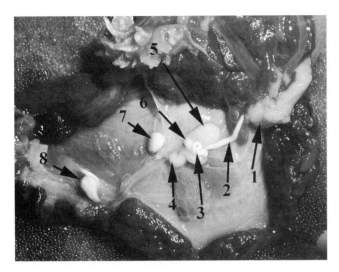

Figure 5.10. Reproduction system of *Aplysia californica*: *1*, ovotestis; *2*, proximal hermaphroditic duct; *3*, ampulla; *4*, distal hermaphroditic duct; *5*, nidamental gland (mucous and albumin glands); *6*, seminal receptacle; *7*, gametolytic gland; and *8*, penile sac.

The allosperm then travel to the spermatotheca. Some allosperm travel from the spermatotheca to the seminal receptacle, where the allosperm mature (Thompson, 1976).

Environmental Disorders and Preventive Medicine

As with all aquatic animals, the quality of the water and the food provided is of primary importance in the health of freshwater and marine gastropods. Aeration must also be provided. In general, gastropods do not appear to protect territories (are not aggressive) but do have a need for flat surfaces on which to cling (these can be vertical as well as horizontal). Space provided per animal depends on the animal's size and the mechanical ability of the system to maintain appropriate water quality. Since many gastropods are in constant contact with a substrate, the bottom and sides of the tank must be kept clean.

With such a diverse class as the gastropods, sweeping recommendations on nutrition, water temperature, and aquarium/terrarium design are not appropriate. Investigators and clinicians are encouraged to become familiar with the particular species or taxa being considered.

Infectious Diseases

Few diseases have been described in gastropods. This is probably not a reflection of the lack of disease but rather the lack of observations. An account of some known diseases follows. Although many of these diseases have not been identified in gastropods presently used as laboratory animals, it is worthwhile understanding the diseases common to this group of animals for future comparative purposes.

Bacteria Diseases

Candidatus Xenohaliotis californiensis, a Rickettsiales-like prokaryote, is responsible for a condition termed withering syndrome in abalone (Figure 5.11). The organisms invade the digestive gland epithelium, causing epithelial hypertrophy, necrosis, and low cuboidal to squamous metaplasia. Grossly, the animals exhibit decreased condition indices and foot-muscle atrophy. Laboratory-based studies showed that time from infection to overt signs of disease was 245 days. Mortality also differed between the two strains of black abalone used in the experiment (85% or 100% mortality). *Haliotis cracherodii* (black abalone) is more severely affected than is *H. rufescens* (red abalone). The disease has been described in abalone collected off the coasts of Central and Southern California (Moore et al., 2000; Finley et al., 2001; Friedman et al., 2002, 2003). Oxytetracycline injections have been shown to effectively halt progression of the disease in treated animals (Friedman et al., 2003).

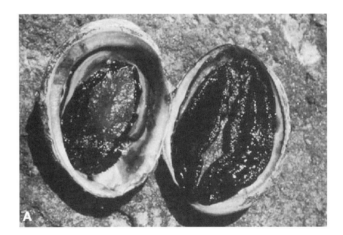

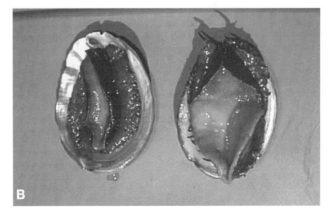

Figure 5.11. Withering syndrome in **(A)** the black abalone, *Haliotis cracherodii*, and **(B)** the red abalone, *Haliotis rufescens*. In both A and B, the diseased animal is on the *left* and a normal specimen is at *right*. Affected animals lose the ability to grasp the substratum when the foot literally withers away due to infection with *Candidatus Xenohaliotis californiensis*. Photo A courtesy of Melissa Miner and the Partnership for Interdisciplinary Studies of Coastal Oceans (PISCO) project at University of California–Santa Cruz. Photo B courtesy of Jim Moore, University of California–Davis.

Vibrio carchariae has caused severe mortality in abalone (*Haliotis tuberculata* L.) on the coast of France since 1977 and has also been identified as the cause of mortality in a Japanese abalone (*Sulculus diversicolor supratexta*). Mortality of up to 80% was noted in the 1997 event on the coast of France. The bacteria were isolated from dead abalone, and the disease was successfully reproduced both by inoculation and by exposure in the water column (Nicolas et al., 2002).

Parasitic Diseases

Labyrinthula

Mortality was noted in post set juvenile abalone (less than 190 days old) (*H. kamtschatkana* and *H. rufescens*) cultured in a facility in British Columbia. The parasite invaded the muscle and nerve tissues, causing mortality in 5 days at 12°C. Although older animals could become infected, they did not die (Bower, 1987)

Sporozoa

Coccidia (*Merocystis kathae*) have been observed in the kidney epithelium of dog whelks (*Buccinum undatum*; Prosobranchia). Epithelial cells hypertrophy when infected, but no associated necrosis or degeneration of the epithelium has been reported. Coccidia (*Pseudoklossia patellae*) have also been identified in the epithelial cells of the kidney, intestine, and digestive gland of limpets (*Patella vulgata*) that also are prosobranchs (Lauckner, 1980).

No treatment has been reported, and the intermediate hosts are not known (Lauckner, 1980).

Ciliata

While various ciliates have been identified on the gills of gastropods, their potential to cause disease is generally unknown. However, *Licnophora*, a ciliate with a tubalike outline (Figures 5.12 and 5.13), has been identified as one of the causes of *parapodial mantle–gill complex* and has been associated with branchitis and dermal ulcers in *Aplysia* and *Hermissenda* (Leibovitz and Capo, 1988).

Turbellaria

Turbellaria infections of gastropods have been reported in *Hermissenda crassicornis* held in aquaria (Leibovitz et al., 1983). Sausage-shaped, motile, white to yellow rhabdocoeles (from 1 mm to over 1 cm long) (family Fecampidae, order Neorhabdocoela) were identified in the *hemocoel* (body cavity) of this sea slug. Multiple flatworms were commonly found in the slugs and could occupy up to one-third of the body cavity. The infected slugs exhibited inanition, degeneration of the internal organs, and thinning of the body wall. The slugs died when the body wall was ruptured, releasing the flatworm. Once free from the hemocoel, the flatworm undergoes reproductive metamorphosis and forms a cocoon that attaches to a surface of the

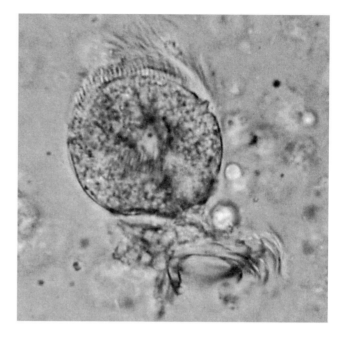

Figure 5.12. *Licnophora* ciliate from a gill clip. ×650.

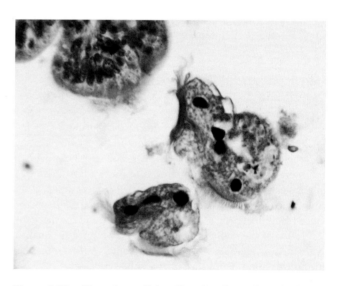

Figure 5.13. *Licnophora* ciliates. Hematoxylin–eosin-stained paraffin slide of gill. ×650.

aquarium. Larvae hatch from the cocoon and directly infect the host through the digestive system (Figure 5.14).

Turbellaria infections have also been reported in the dog whelk in the North Sea. Flatworms are found in the dilated renal lumen and in the mantle cavity in these instances (Lauckner, 1980).

Trematoda

Gastropods, especially the marine snails, are the most common first intermediate host for the digenetic trematodes (Figure

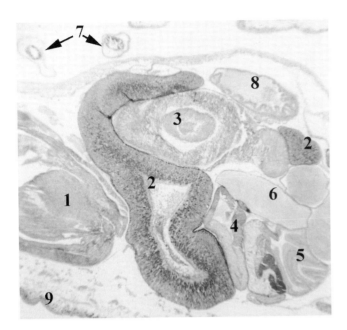

Figure 5.14. Turbellariad worm infection of *Hermissenda crassicornis*: *1*, buccal mass; *2*, turbellariad worm; *3*, penis; *4*, mucus gland; *5*, albumen gland; *6*, ampulla; *7*, cerata; and *8*, renal lumen; and 9.

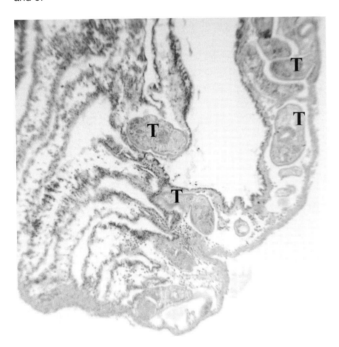

Figure 5.15. Trematodal infestation of the gill's vascular sinus. *T*, cercariae.

5.15). While many different trematodes (and their various forms consisting of sporocysts, cercariae, redia, and germinal balls) have been found and named in the tissues of gastropods, the second and final hosts are not known for most of these trematodes. Various conditions have been observed in infected gastropods (Fretter and Graham, 1962; Lauckner, 1980), including (a) giganticism, thought to result from increased food intake caused

by the infection; (b) orange/brown discoloration of the foot, due to liberation of carotenoid pigments dispersed throughout the hemolymph upon degeneration of the infected digestive gland; (c) parasitic castration; (d) behavioral changes (for example, crawling into the open where the host snail can be predated); (e) extensive areas of necrosis and discoloration of the tissues, causing an infestation boils in the body; and (f) variation in the shell shape due to asymmetrical formation of the shell's spire.

Although infected gastropods often do not exhibit obvious mortality as a result of infection, they do exhibit decreased tolerance to high temperatures and an inability to move long distances or to thermally appropriate waters. There is often great variation in the severity of infection, the number of animals infected, the sex infected, and the season of highest infection rate.

Rarely, gastropods can serve as the final host for digenetic trematodes. If present, the trematodes may be found in the lumens of the digestive gland or in the kidney. *Proctoeces buccini* infections are found in the nephridial lumen of the dog whelk (Loos-Frank, 1969; Lauckner, 1980).

Annelida

Polydora sp, a (spionid) polychaete, commonly infests the shells of prosobranchs. Larvae of these worms burrow into the shells, destroy the mineralized matrix, and can substantially weaken the shells. In such infections, the most severely affected areas of the shell are the oldest (the uppermost shell whorls), and shell loss in these areas may expose the underlying inner shell surface to the environment (Lauckner, 1980).

Haliotis rufescens is infested by a sabellid polychaete that inserts itself between the mantle edge and the shell edge and covers itself with a thin membrane. In response, the abalone mantle draws away slightly and begins to secrete a ventrally directed new shell edge instead of a laterally directed new shell. The larvae of this parasite exit the adult's tunnel in the shell and then infest the newly formed edge, causing continued downturning of the shell. This hermaphroditic, self-fertilizing, but nonplanktonic, polychaete can quickly infect a population of abalone, causing malformed shells. The abalone themselves do not appear to be significantly (clinically) affected (Oakes and Fields, 1996).

Copepoda

Numerous species of copepoda infect gastropods (Monod and Dollfus, 1932). Only a few species infect the shelled gastropods. *Panaietis haliotis* infects the mouth cavity of the abalone *Haliotis gigantean* and causes lesions (Lauckner, 1980). Similarly, *Nucellicola holmanae*, another highly modified copepod, infects the soft tissues of the dog whelk (*Nucella lapillus*). Although the infecting copepod is often well described, the lesions produced in the infected gastropod are not (Lamb et al., 1998).

Many species of copepods infect the opistobranchs. Externally attached copepods are not highly modified. However, the numerous members of the copepod genus *Splanchnotrophus*, which live within the body cavity of nudibranchs, are greatly modified. These endoparasitic copepods produce egg sacs that

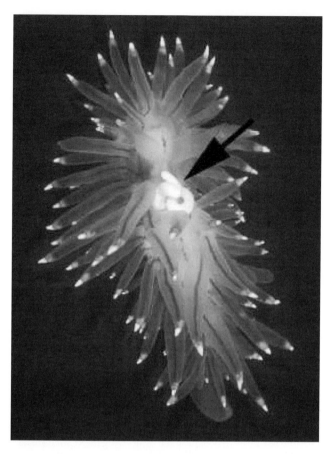

Figure 5.16. Paired egg masses (*arrow*) of the endoparasitic splanchnotrophid copepod, *Ismaila belciki*, in the nudibranch, *Janolus fuscus*.

form protruberances visible under the external body wall (Figure 5.16), or egg sacs that project through the body wall, and thus are easily identified in many cases. Apposition of the egg sacs in this position is thought to allow for easy access to the seawater upon hatching by rupture through the nudibranch's external surface or by directly hatching into the surrounding waters (www.seaslugforum.net/ismaila.htm [Lauckner, 1980]). Unfortunately, detailed descriptions of lesions and resulting mortality caused by these parasites, as well as the life cycle of most of these parasitic copepods, are lacking. As an example, the peocilostomatoid copepod *Ismaila occulata* is endoparasitic in the giant red nudibranch (*Dendronoius iris*). The male copepod floats free in the digestive gland, and the posterior extremity of the female attaches to the walls of the diverticular branches in the cerata, penetrating the body wall and projecting to the surrounding seawater. Egg sacs laid by the female protrude through the hole and appear to be attached to the surface of the cerata (Ho, 1981).

Miscellaneous Disorders

To metamorphose successfully into their adult form, *Aplysia* must be fed one of six species of algae (although other untested types

may also be effective). As with many invertebrates, nutrition of gastropods is poorly understood, but research with *Aplysia* points to the great differences in health and growth that result when appropriate food is provided (Capo and Stommes, 1998).

Gas-bubble disease of opistobranchs was described by Leibovitz and Capo (1988) in *Aplysia* and has been reported in *Hermissenda* by others. Affected *Aplysia* floated and contained observable gas bubbles in the tissues and gills. In the case of air-bubble accumulation in *Aplysia*, the internal gas was caused by exposure to seawater supersaturated with air. Once the water supply loop was repaired, the problem disappeared. Air bubbles have also been identified in the body and cerata of captive *Hermissenda*. The cause is not known but appears to be associated with movement of animals from one body of water to another. Death (probably caused by pressure necrosis of vital organs by the air bubbles) often results (www.seaslugforum.net/ hermcras.htm#m10465).

Shell lesions of unknown etiology have been reported in the New Zealand blackfoot abalone, *Haliotis iris* (Nollens et al., 2003). These lesions contribute to decreased growth rate in affected animals (Figure 5.17, Color Plate 5.17). Nollens et al. (2002) found that radiography, ultrasonography, and endoscopy (the most accurate of the three) could all be used to diagnose the internal shell lesion disease. Endoscopy required anesthesia with sodium pentobarbitone (60 mg/L at 23°C [Aquilina and Roberts, 2000]). A subsequent study evaluated heart rate (which decreased with increased exposure time to the anesthetic) and recovery times of the same species when using sodium pentobarbitone at the same concentration as previously mentioned (Sharma et al., 2003). The investigators found that larger animals took longer to relax and recover. The shell lesion disease problem in *Haliotis iris* has resulted in hematological research on this species (Nollens et al., 2004). Table 5.2 contains reference range values for a number of clinical pathology parameters in this species. Figure 5.18 illustrates bleeding an abalone from the branchial vein.

Anesthesia, Analgesia, and Surgery

Little work has been done to identify appropriate anesthetic agents. Analgesia has not been addressed in the literature, and gastropods are euthanized by long-term immersion in an anesthetic agent, followed by fixation or exsanguination. See Table 5.3 for a list of anesthetic agents used in gastropods.

Fractured gastropod shells can be repaired by external fixation (Figure 5.19). The use of surgical epoxy and an adhesive transparent bandage was used to repair an apple snail (Lewbart and Christian, 2003).

Treatment Protocols and Formulary

Bath treatments of antibiotics (at the same level as for fish) can be used because the exposed epithelium and gills are very porous (White et al., 1996). Injection into the hemocoel may be used in treatment of opistobranchs, and injections into the foot muscle have been shown to be effective for many of the gas-

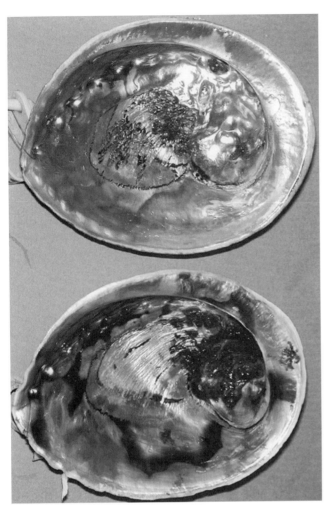

Table 5.2. *Haliotis iris* clinical pathology reference ranges: sample size, total number of circulating hemocytes (total HC), differential hemocyte count,[a] and levels of hemolymph analytes (± standard error) of clinically healthy blackfoot abalone (*Haliotis iris*)

Analyte[b]	Mean	Reference Ranges
N	**70**	
Total HC ($\times 10^6$/mL)	10.2 ± 0.8	8.8–11.6
Type 1 (%)	22 ± 1	19–25
Type 2 (%)	46 ± 2	42–51
Type 3 (%)	31 ± 3	26–36
Glucose	18 ± 1	16–20
Total protein	19.9 ± 0.7	18.6–21.2
LDH	8.51 ± 0.60	6.93–10.44
ALT	2.78 ± 0.43	1.95–3.96
AST	5.47 ± 0.55	4.38–6.56
Amylase	0.247 ± 0.042	0.158–0.389
Ca++	11.89 ± 0.13	11.64–12.15
Fe++	6.13 ± 0.28	5.58–6.69
N	**34**	
Muscle glycogen	0.98 ± 0.18	(0.84–1.15)
Urea	0.37 ± 0.04	(0.29–0.45)
N	**19**	
Na+	461 ± 6	(450–474)
K+	10.9 ± 0.2	(10.6–11.3)

[a]Criteria based on description of hemocyte morphology in Shields et al. (1996) and Sminia et al. (1983).
[b]Units of measurement are g/L (protein), U/L (LDH, ALT, AST, and amylase), μmol/L (Fe++), mmol/L (Ca++, Na+, K+, and urea), μg/L (glucose), and mg/g (glycogen).
Adapted from Nollens, et al., 2004.

Figure 5.17. Shells from the New Zealand black abalone showing grossly visible shell disease. The shell at the **top** displays the mineralized form of the disease, whereas the shell at the **bottom** contains the gelatinous form. Photos courtesy of Hendrick Nollens, University of Florida, Gainesville, FL, and Inter-Research.

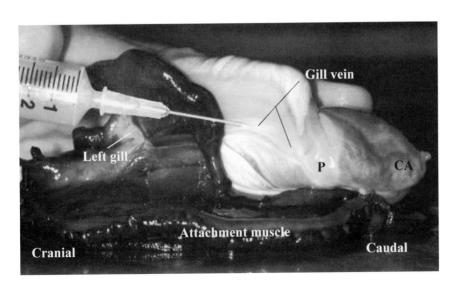

Figure 5.18. Collecting blood from a New Zealand black abalone (*Haliotis iris*) by using the branchial vein. *CA*, conical appendage; and *P*, pericardium. From Nollens et al., 2004.

Table 5.3. Anesthetic agents for gastropods

Agent	Common Name	Procedure	References
1. Magnesium sulfate	Abalone	4%–22% (wt/vol), 5–8 min	White et al., 1996
2. 2-Phenoxyethanol	Abalone	0.05%–0.3% (vol/vol) 1–2 min	White et al., 1996
3. Chloral hydrate	Limpet	Dilute solution for swimming larvae	Costello and Henley, 1971
4. Ethanol (95%)	Mollusks	5%–15% solution 2–8 min	Ross and Ross, 1999
5. Clove Oil (eugenol)	Pulmonates	0.6% in water	Araujo et al., 1995.
6. Magnesium chloride	Sea hare	0.4 M $MgCl_2$ in seawater with 2 mM Hepes (ph 7.7) injected into hemocoel through the foot	F. Strumwasser (personal communication)
7. Sodium pentobarbitone	Abalone	60 mg/L of seawater at 23°C	Aquilina and Roberts, 2000; Sharma et al., 2003

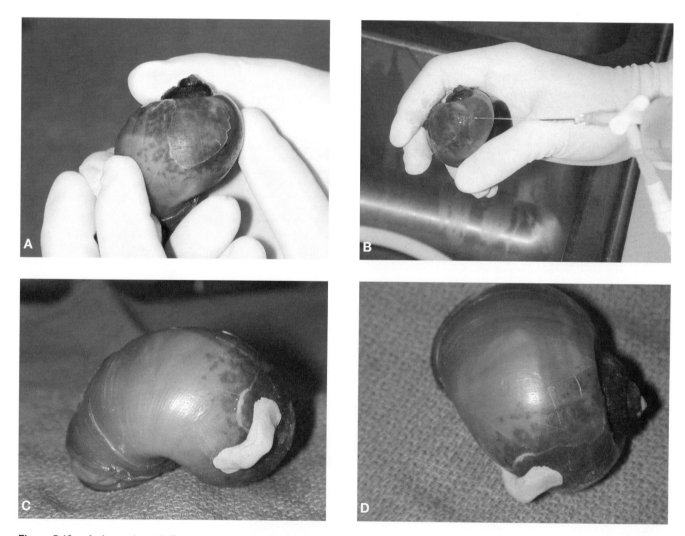

Figure 5.19. **A:** An apple snail (*Pomacea* sp.) sustained a shell fracture after crawling out of its aquarium. **B:** Sterile saline was used to cleanse the wound. **C:** Surgical epoxy was used to stabilize the fracture site, and the periostricum was roughened with a Dremel sanding bit. **D:** Povidone iodine-impregnated Tegaderm (3M, St. Paul, MN) (ventral to the apex and spirals) was used to cover the depression defect.

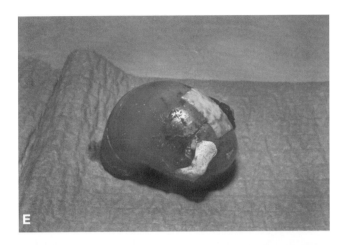

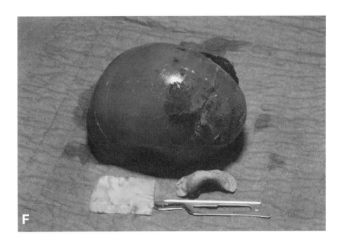

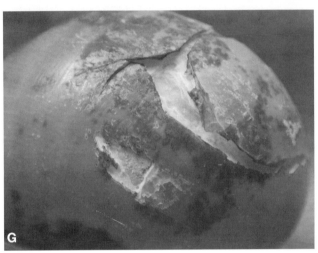

Figure 5.19. **E:** The appearance of the snail several months after shell repair. **F:** The external fixators have been removed. **G:** The shell is stable after new mineralized tissue was produced by the mantle. From Lewbart and Christian, 2003.

tropods (Lellis et al., 2000; Friedman et al., 2003; F. Strumwasser [Marine Biological Laboratory], personnel communication). Feed additives have also been used successfully (Friedman et al., 2003; Smolowitz, personal communication).

Bath treatments with formalin or copper-based products are toxic to most invertebrates and should not be attempted.

References

Aquilina B, Roberts R (2000). A method for inducing muscle relaxation in the abalone, *Haliotis iris*. Aquaculture 190:403–408.

Araujo R, Remon JM, Moreno D, Ramos MA (1995). Relaxing techniques of freshwater molluscs: Trials for evaluation of different methods. Malacologia 36:29–41.

Bower SM (1987). The life cycle and ultrastructure of a new species of thraustochytrid (Protozoa: Labyrinthomorpha) pathogenic to small abalone. Aquaculture 67:269–270.

Capo T, Stommes D. (1998). Feeding the laboratory model: Dietary induced variability in *Aplysia* growth. In: Slime Lines, volume 4. University of Miami–NIH National Resource for *Aplysia*, Miami, Florida. www.rsmas.miami.edu/groups/sea-hares/slimelines4/ Access date, 24 June 2005.

Costello DP, Henley C (1971). Methods for Obtaining and Handling Marine Eggs and Embryos, 2nd edition. Marine Biological Laboratory, Woods Hole, MA, 247 pp.

Dagan D, Levitan IB (1981). Isolated identified *Aplysia* neurons in cell culture. J Neurosci 1:736–740.

Dakin WJ (1912). Buccinum (the whelk). In: Herdman WA, ed. LMBC Memoirs on Typical British Marine Plants and Animals, volume 20. Williams and Norgate, London, 115 pp.

Finley CA, Wendell F, Friedman CS (2001). Geographic distribution of *Candidatus* Xenohaliotis californiensis in northern California abalone. In: Aquaculture 2001: Book of Abstracts. World Aquaculture Society, Louisiana State University, Baton Rouge, LA, 225 pp.

Friedman CS, Biggs W, Shield JD, Hedrick RP (2002). Transmission of withering syndrome in black abalone, *Haliotis cracherodii* Leach. J. Shellfish Res 21:817–824.

Friedman CS, Trevelyan G, Robbins TT, Mulder EP, Fields R (2003). Development of an oral administration of oxytetracycline to control losses due to withering syndrome in cultured red abalone *Haliotis rufescens*. Aquaculture 224:1–23.

Fretter V, Graham A (1962). British Prosobranch Molluscs. Adlard and Son, Dorking, London, 755 pp.

Fretter V, Graham A (1976). A functional anatomy of invertebrates. Academic, London, 589 pp.

Ho J (1981). *Ismaila occulta*, a new species of poecilostomatoid copepod parasitic in a dendronotid nudibranch from California. J Crustacean Biol 1:130–136.

Hughes RN (1986). A functional biology of marine gastropods. John Hopkins University Press, Baltimore, 245 pp.

Hyman LB (1967). The Invertebrates, volume 6: Mollusca I. McGraw-Hill, New York, 792 pp.

Lamb EJ, Boxshall GA, Mill PJ, Grahame J (1998). Postembryonic stages of *Nucellicola holmanae* Lamb et al., 1996 (Copepoda: Poecilostomatoida), and endoparasite of the dog whelk *Nucella lapillus* (Gastropoda). J Mar Syst 15:261–267.

Lauckner G (1980). Diseases of mollusca: Gastropoda. In: Kinne O, ed. Diseases of Marine Animals. John Wiley and Sons, New York, pp 311–424.

Leibovitz L, Capo TR (1988). Diseases of a mass cultured marine laboratory animal, the sea hare, *Aplysia californica*. In: Perkins FO and Cheng TC, eds. Third International Colloquium on Pathology of Marine Aquaculture. Virginia Institute of Marine Science, Gloucester Point.

Leibovitz L, Lederhendler I, Harris L (1983). Endoparasitic turbellarid infestations of captive laboratory-maintained *Hermissenda crassicornis*, and eolid nudibranch. Presented at the Annual Meeting of the Society for Invertebrate Pathology at Cornell University, Ithaca, New York, 7–11 August 1983.

Lellis WA, Plerhoples TA, Lellis KA (2000). Evaluation of potential anesthetics for freshwater mussel *Elliptio complanta*. J Shellfish Res 19:983–990.

Lewbart GA, Christian L (2003). Repair of a fractured shell in an apple snail. Exotic DVM Vet Mag 5(2):8–9.

Loos-Frank FB (1969). Zwei adulte trematoden aus Nordseemollusken: *Proctoeces buccini* n. sp. und *P. scrobiculariae* n. sp. Z Parasitkde 32:324–340.

Luchtel DL, Martin AW, Deyrup-Olsen I, Boer HH (1997). Gastropoda: Pulmonata. In: Harrison FW, Kohn AJ, eds. Microscopic Anatomy of Invertebrates, volume 6B: Mollusca II. Wiley-Liss, New York, pp 459–718.

Moore JD, Robbins TT, Friedman CS (2000). The role of a Rickettsia-like prokaryote in withering syndrome in California red alabone, *Haliotis refescens*. J Shellfish Res 19:525–526.

Nicolas JL, Basuyaux O, Mazurie J, Thebault A (2002). *Vibrio carchariae*, a pathogen of the abalone *Haliotis tuberculata*. Dis Aquat Org 50:35–43.

Nollens HH, Keogh JA, Probert PK (2003). Effects of shell lesions on survival, growth, condition and reproduction in the New Zealand blackfoot abalone *Haliotis iris*. Dis Aquat Org 57:127–133.

Nollens HH, Keogh JA, Probert PK (2004). Haematological pathology of shell lesions in the New Zealand abalone, *Haliotis iris* (Mollusca: Gastropoda). Comp Clin Pathol 12:211–216.

Nollens HH, Schofield JC, Keogh JA, Probert PK (2002). Evaluation of radiography, ultrasonography and endoscopy for the detection of shell lesions in live abalone *Haliotis iris* (Mollusca: Gastropoda). Dis Aquat Org 50:145–152.

Oakes FR, Fields RC (1996). Infestation of *Haliotis rufescens* shells by a sabellid polychaete. Aquaculture 140:139–143.

Ross LG, Ross B (1999). Anaesthetic and Sedative Techniques for Aquatic Animals. Blackwell Science, Oxford, pp 48–49.

Sharma P, Nollens HH, Keogh JA, Probert PK (2003). Sodium pentobarbitone-induced relaxation in the abalone *Haliotis iris* (Gastropoda): Effects of animal size and exposure time. Aquaculture 218:589–599.

Shields JD, Perkins FO, Friedman CS (1996) Hematological pathology of wasting syndrome in black abalone. J Shellfish Res 15:498.

Sminia T, Van Der Knaap WPW, Van Asselt LA (1983) Blood cell types and blood cell formation in gastropod mollusks. Dev Comp Immunol 7:665–668.

Thompson TE (1976). Biology of Opisthobranch Molluscs, volume 1. John Wright and Sons, Bristol, UK, 207 pp.

White HI, Hecht T, Potgieter B (1996). The effect of four anaesthetics on *Haliotis midae* and their suitability for application in commercial abalone culture. Aquaculture 140:145–151.

Chapter 6

CEPHALOPODS

Joseph M. Scimeca

Introduction

Cephalopods are among the most fascinating animals in the oceans. They make up approximately 4% of the world's food (FAO, 2003) for human consumption and are essential to the world's finfish food chain. With increasing frequency, many cephalopods are displayed in large institutional and public aquarium exhibits, and some are used for the home aquarium. These animals are important to many laboratories worldwide, with the biomedical community using them for research (Lee, 1994). Cephalopods, specifically octopus, squid, and cuttlefish, have commercial value for their use in restaurants, cuttlebones for the pet bird industry, and unfortunately the *Nautilus* for the collectable value of its chambered shell. With the exception of the *Nautilus*, cephalopods are generally top-line ocean predators. They hunt their prey and are very active feeders (Boyle, 1991).

Natural History and Taxonomy

Cephalopods are members of the phylum Mollusca and share basic body organizational features with the gastropods, bivalves, and other mollusks. Cephalopods vary considerably in size; most are large, but some, such as the pygmy octopus (*Octopus joubini*), weigh in at 30 g, compared with the giant Pacific octopus (*Octopus dofleini*), whose weight is often over 50 kg. Recently, a colossal squid was reported in New Zealand. This 150-kg, 5-m, immature female *Mesonychoteuthis hamilotoni* was caught on the surface of the Ross Sea (Sackton, 2003).

Cephalopods are well represented in the fossil record and, as a class, arose with a heavy external shell early in the Silurian period. Modern cephalopods have only a shell remnant that is greatly modified or completely absent. Over 780 species of living cephalopods are known (Wood and Day, 2005), a relatively small number compared with the over 10,000 fossil groups described (Voss, 1977). Much of the higher classification of recent cephalopods is unstable. CephBase (Wood and Day, 2005) is the suggested source of information on cephalopod classification, species images, and worldwide distribution (Wood et al., 2000).

The subclass Nautiloidea are cephalopods with a heavy external chambered shell that may be straight or coiled; these ani-

mals have two pairs of gills and nephridia with numerous unsuckered appendages. The *Nautilus* is a representative of this subclass. In the subclass Coleoidea, the shell is internal and reduced, and in the order Sepioidea, the calcareous chambered shell is present internally, functioning as a buoyancy organ. Representatives of this subclass include the genera *Sepia* and *Euprymna*. *Sepia officinalis*, the common cuttlefish, is pictured in Figure 6.1. *Euprymna scolopes* can become an easily reared cephalopod for laboratory research projects. Numerous laboratory studies have investigated its symbiotic bacterium, *Vibrio fischeri*, which lives in the sepiolid's light organ to produce a weak light under the body of the animal. This gives it countershading and camouflage from predators (Figure 6.2) (Anderson and Mather, 1996).

In the order Teuthoidea, the shell is reduced to a chitinous pen lying dorsally. The body is elongated and usually finned, with eight suckered arms and two long tentacles. The squids, including *Lolliguncula brevis*, belong to this group (Figure 6.3). The order Octopoda (the octopuses) has a shell that is markedly reduced and split into two lateral rods. The globular body is with or without fins. *Octopus bimaculoides* is a representative example of the octopuses. Note the false eyes or ocelli on either side of the head (Figure 6.4).

The few species of *Nautilus* occur in the Indo-Pacific region, are relatively sluggish, and rely on their shell for protection against predators. It is believed they spend most of their life near the bottom. Saunders and Landman (1987) give a detailed account of their biology.

The cuttlefish are characteristic of coastal waters and distributed mainly in the Eastern Hemisphere and in temperate and tropical zones, but are absent from waters of North, South, and Central America (Wood and Day, 2005). They are bottom-dwelling predators that often bury themselves in sand or sediment by using their lateral fins to dig and place the sediment on their bodies. Cuttlefish, with the aid of their cuttlebone, can achieve neutral buoyancy and hover and blend in with their environment.

The octopuses are represented by a number of families and have a worldwide distribution. They are *epibenthic*, which means they live near or on the bottom. They are associated with stony or rocky habitats where they can find good shelter and food but have been found in muddy or sandy bottoms.

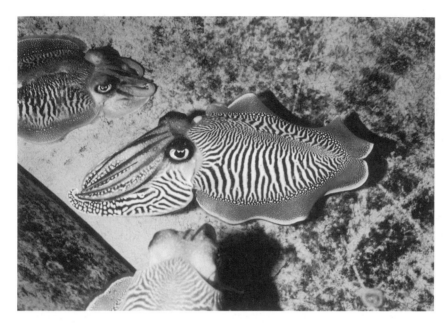

Figure 6.1. *Sepia officinalis*, the common cuttlefish. Note the prominent zebra pattern of the male (*center*) surrounded by two females. Photo courtesy of the NIH National Resource Center for Cephalopods, UTMB, Galveston, TX.

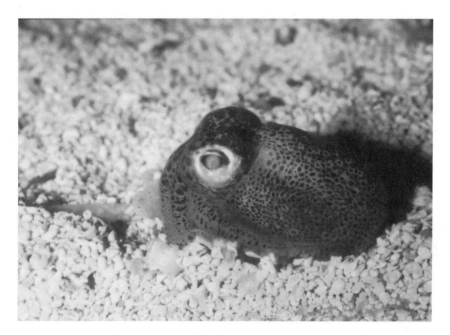

Figure 6.2. *Euprymna scolopes* (the Hawaiian bobtail squid) has a symbiotic bacterium, *Vibrio fischeri*, that lives in the light organ to produce a weak light under the body of the animal. The chromatophores in the skin are prominent. Photo courtesy of the NIH National Resource Center for Cephalopods, UTMB, Galveston, TX.

The squids (order Teuthoidea) are a large and diverse group of families differing widely in habitat and distribution. Two suborders important in commercial enterprises are the Myopsida (squids of the genus *Loligo*, which are shoaling animals and complete their life cycle in coastal waters) and the Oegopsida (families of deep-water genera including *Todaredes* and *Illex*, which dwell at the edges of the continental shelf).

Class: Cephalopoda
  Subclass: Nautiloidea
    Order: Nautilida
      Family: Nautilidae

Subclass: Coleoidea
  Division: Neocoleoidea
    Superorder: Octopodiformes
      Order: Octopoda
        Suborder: Cirrina
          Family: Cirroteuthidae
          Family: Opisthoteuthidae
          Family: Grimpoteuthidae
          Family: Luteuthidae
          Family: Stauroteuthidae
        Suborder: Incirrina
          Family: Alloposidae

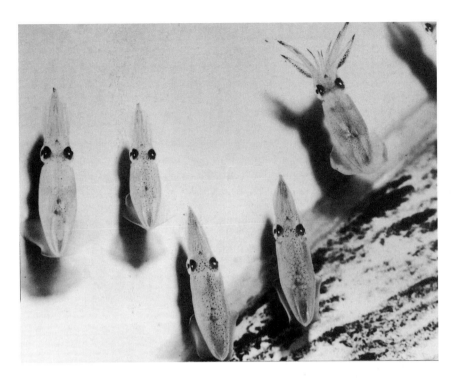

Figure 6.3. *Lolliguncula brevis* is a representative example of squids. Note that these are young or recently hatched. Photo courtesy of the NIH National Resource Center for Cephalopods, UTMB, Gavelston, TX.

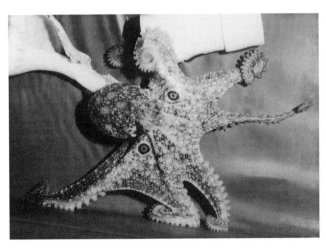

Figure 6.4. *Octopus bimaculoides* (common two-spotted octopus) with the two prominent false eyes or ocelli. Photo courtesy of the NIH National Resource Center for Cephalopods, UTMB, Gavelston, TX.

        Family: Amphitretidae
        Family: Argonautidae
        Family: Bolitaenidae
        Family: Idioctopodidae
        Family: Octopodidae
        Family: Ocythoidae
        Family: Tremoctopodidae
        Family: Vitreledonellidae
     Order: Vampyromorphida
        Family: Vampyroteuthidae
  Superorder: Decapodiformes
    Order: Tuethida
      Suborder: Oegopsina

        27 Families
      Suborder: Myopsina
        Family: Loliginidae
    Order: Sepiidea
        Family: Sepiadariidae
        Family: Sepiidae
    Order: Sepioloda
        Family: Idiosepiidae
        Family: Sepiolidae
           Subfamily: Sepiolinae
           Subfamily: Rossiinae
          Subfamily: Heteroteuthinae
    Order: Spirulida
        Family Spirilidae

Like other mollusks, cephalopods are bilaterally symmetrical and have a well-developed coelomic cavity.

Cephalopods have a semelparous life history, which means they grow rapidly to sexual maturity, spawn once, and die (Hanlon, 1987). Life span and growth rate in laboratories are temperature dependent and usually last 1 year for most, with the exception of the *Nautilus*, which is long lived. The giant Pacific octopus has been documented to live 3–5 years. Hatchlings display true exponential growth for the first third of the life cycle, growing at rates of 6%–12% of wet body weight per day. To support such growth, squids and cuttlefishes consume an almost pure protein diet from their prey of fishes, shrimps, and crabs, converting 30%–50% of the diet into growth (DeRusha et al., 1989; Hanlon et al., 1991; Lee, 1994). This high-protein diet results in the production of large quantities of nitrogenous waste in the form of ammonia. Cephalopods excrete 2–3 times the amount of ammonia per kilogram of body weight compared with fishes (Lee, 1994).

Anatomy and Physiology

The general anatomy of the cephalopods has been graphically portrayed (Boyle, 1991; Boyle, 1999). Figures 6.5–6.8 outline the anatomy of the *Nautilus*, octopus, cuttlefish, and squid. The *Nautilus* has a chambered shell divided into partitions to help with protection and assist in buoyancy. The squids do not have gas-filled spaces, and the shell is reduced to a chitinous rod, or pen, which is also called the gladius. This structure lies dorsally in the mantle, giving the animal rigidity. Sepioids, particularly the cuttlefish, have a cuttlebone that serves for support and buoyancy. Octopuses do not have a shell remnant although there is a stylet along either side of the mantle.

Since all cephalopods actively catch and eat live prey, a wide range of food items have been documented (Boletzky and Hanlon, 1983; Nixon, 1987; Castro and Lee, 1994; Lee, 1994). Squids and cuttlefish maneuver so they can strike their prey with extension of their tentacles and rapid body propulsion. Once trapped within the tentacles, the prey is drawn toward the mouth and bitten by the chitinous beak. Smaller pieces of flesh are swallowed. After the pieces of flesh are ingested, the food passes through the digestive tract consisting of a crop, stomach, cecum, and intestine. Some of the digestion takes place in the lumen of the intestine, but most takes place in the large digestive gland. Two short ducts connect the digestive gland to the junction of the stomach and cecum. The feces (pigmented depending on the diet) are bound with mucus and expelled through the anus into the water.

The respiratory system consists of well-vascularized gills suspended in the mantle cavity. The water flows over the gill lamellae in the opposite direction of blood flow, a countercurrent system maximizing the exchange of gases (Wells and Wells, 1982). The *Nautilus* has two pair of gills, whereas all other cephalopods possess just a single pair. The oxygen-carrying pigment in cephalopods is hemocyanin. This blue blood traverses a complex arrangement of vessels, and the cardiovascular tissues, including the branchial hearts, vena cavae, and auricles, have a contractile component.

The cephalopod cellular immune system consists of one type of blood cell, or hemocyte, which functions in basic cellular immunity but is not phagocytic (Ratcliffe and Rowley, 1981). Humoral immunity involves lectinlike proteins that bind or

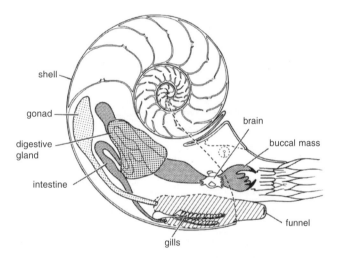

Figure 6.5.   Generalized anatomy of a *Nautilus*.

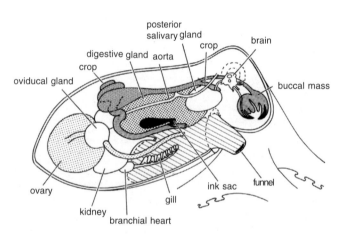

Figure 6.6.   Generalized anatomy of a female octopus.

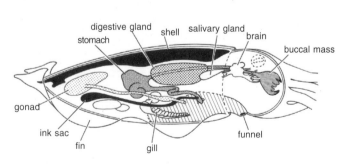

Figure 6.7.   Generalized anatomy of a cuttlefish.
Figures 6.5–6.8 from Boyle 1999.

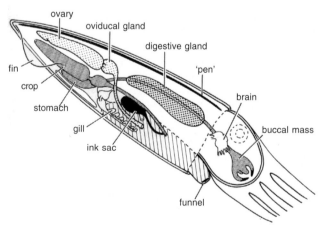

Figure 6.8.   Generalized anatomy of a squid.

clump foreign antigens. Clumping of cephalopod hemocytes has been associated with septicemia (Russo and Tringali, 1983; Olafson, 1988).

Cephalopods have a well-developed nervous system that is organized around a central core of nerve cells. In the octopus, the brain is centered between the eyes in a tough cartilaginous cranium. Numerous divisions of the brain have been well described (Wells, 1978). In general, subesophageal regions of the brain control the muscle groups. The octopus has well-developed optic and ocular nerves, and, interestingly, some autonomy of the movements in its arms, mantle, and buccal cavity isolated from the central nervous system (Boyle et al., 1979). Of particular interest to neurophysiologists is the giant axon of the squid. These axons may be more than 1 mm in diameter and up to 18 cm long. These characteristics have enabled much basic research and many advances in our understanding of neural transmission (Martin, 1977).

The integumentary system is comprised of a delicate one-cell layer of epidermis consisting of columnar epithelial cells with a microvillous border and a deeper dermis containing chromatophores, iridophores, and leucophores (Hanlon and Messenger, 1996). The chromatophores have black, yellow, red, and orange pigments. Much research has been done on the neural control of chromatophores (Dubas and Boyle, 1985; Hanlon and Messenger, 1988). The chromatophore organ consists of an elastic pigmented structure with a series of muscle fibers radially arranged (Cloney and Florey, 1968). When the muscles contract, the pigmented sac is expanded and imparts color to the surface of the skin. When the muscles relax, the color is sequestered and the animal appears white to grayish white.

Luminescent organs, which are known for many species of cephalopods, have been used to study symbiosis. These organs use a symbiotic relationship of bacteria and the animal to produce light. The luminescence is thought to have a role in camouflage and signaling. Recently, a protein called reflectin was discovered in the squid *Euprymna scolopes*. Reflectin is a family of unusual proteins that are deposited in flat, structural platelets in reflective tissues of the squid. These proteins are encoded by at least six genes in three subfamilies and have no reported homologs outside of squids (Crookes et al., 2004).

The coleoids have an ink sac composed of a muscular bladder with an opening into the exhalent water flow at the base of the funnel. When a cephalopod is startled or chased by a predator, the ink is discharged into the water as a cloudlike mass. The purpose of the diversion is not to set up a screen but to appear as an object (pseudomorph) to hold the attention of the pursuer while the cephalopod rapidly changes direction, giving it a few extra seconds to escape (Boyle, 1991). In captivity, if enough cephalopods secrete ink, the tank will become black until the filtration system removes the pigment. This must be removed by using protein skimmers or activated carbon (Lee et al., 1994b; Oestmann et al., 1997; Walsh et al., 2002).

Males and females may be discerned externally by the modifications of the arm used for sperm transfer by the mature male. In octopods, it is the third right arm or *hectocotylus*. In the myopsid squid, it is the fourth left. In mature cuttlefish, the male guard arm has striking zebra stripes.

Many cephalopod species will lay eggs in captivity. The cuttlefishes will lay small numbers of eggs deposited together in clumps—fewer than 1000 over a few weeks. They are individually deposited, fixed firmly to a hard substrate, and range in size from 1 to 10 mm in diameter. Each egg is enclosed in a tough sheath. Squids have several different types of eggs, depending on the species. Large embryo species lay groups of egg strands having 3–10 large embryos per strand. Small embryo species lay either groups of egg strands having hundreds of small embryos per strand or large egg masses containing thousands of small embryos. Captive octopuses may lay eggs, ranging from 12 to 15 mm in length. The eggs are organized into strings attached to the roof of their den or overhangs in the wild or to objects within the tank. Females brood the egg mass, ventilating eggs with seawater and protecting them from predators.

Environmental Disorders and Preventive Medicine

Cephalopods have been cultured in the laboratory at the National Resource Center for Cephalopods (NRCC) in the United States for close to 30 years (Forsythe, 2005). This resource is supported by the National Institutes of Health's National Center for Research Resources (NCRR) (www.ncrr.nih.gov). The squid, *Sepioteuthis lessoniana*, has been cultured through seven successive generations in the NRCC laboratory (Walsh et al., 2002). The pharaoh cuttlefish, *Sepia pharaonis*, was cultured through five consecutive generations in the laboratory (Minton et al., 2001) by using closed, recirculating water filtration systems. The cuttlefish, *Sepia officinalis*, has been cultured through seven generations in a recirculating marine system (Forsythe et al., 1994).

The cephalopod immune system can be compromised easily with poor water quality, overcrowding, and/or increased bacterial load on the aquatic system. Environmental disturbances can lead animals to aggressive behavior or cause trauma via bumping into the tank sides when reacting to stress or abrupt disturbances.

Tanks and filtration design are variable, and the layouts of the filtration apparatus are adaptable to space availability and the type of cephalopod maintained (Yang et al., 1989; Forsythe et al., 1994; Walsh et al., 2002). Excellent water quality and monitoring of animals are essential for a good health care program (Oestmann et al., 1997).

A typical cephalopod system filtration process begins when the water leaves the tank or holding area and then passes through a foam fractionator (protein skimmer), which removes organic and large molecular proteins from the water, including ink. The water passes on through a mechanical filter, removing particles 100 μm or larger, then through a high-grade activated carbon, and finally through a biological filter that uses nitrifying bacteria to break down ammonia to less toxic forms.

Temperature range for temperate species is 15°–22°C and 25°–32°C for tropical species. In general, the salinity is 27–36 parts per thousand, pH 7.7–8.2, ammonia and nitrites <0.1 mg/L, and nitrates <20.0 mg/L (Hanlon, 1987; Lee et al., 1994b; Sherrill et al., 2000).

Disease management of captive cephalopods depends on careful and attentive husbandry with high-quality nutrition, frequent clinical assessment and observation of animals, and appropriate use of antibiotics. Prevention of traumatic lesions by proper tank design, excellent water quality, creating hiding places, and reducing stress factors like overcrowding and increased human activity will enhance the overall health program. Cephalopod caregivers should keep excellent records of water quality, examinations, growth, nutrition, and evaluations of unexpected deaths. Freshly dead animals should receive thorough necropsies, including microbial culture and sensitivity tests. An aggressive preventive medicine program can help prevent large losses (Oestmann et al., 1997).

Octopuses, and in some cases squid and cuttlefish, can pose a health hazard to human handlers. Many species of octopod are known to bite with their beaks and can inflict a large wound. The anterior salivary gland contains poison and pharmacologically active compounds having toxic effects (Halstead, 1965). The results of a bite are painful and often described as being like bee stings. In some cases, partial paralysis extending beyond the site of the bite has been reported. Maculotoxin, the salivary compound from the Australian blue-ringed octopus *Hapalochlaeona maculosa*, has indistinguishable effects from the puffer-fish venom tetrodrotoxin. The blue-ringed octopus has caused human fatalities (Flecker and Cotton, 1955). In humans, maculotoxin action blocks sodium channels and causes motor paralysis and occasionally respiratory failure.

When undisturbed, the blue-ringed octopus has dark brown ochre bands over its arms and body, with blue circles superimposed on these bands. When the animal is disturbed in any way, or removed from the water, the colors darken and the rings turn a brilliant electric blue. This dramatic and beautiful color change and the animal's small size help to identify it. The blue-ringed octopus should not be picked up or touched in any way except by those properly trained. Symptoms of the bite include numbness of the mouth and tongue, blurring of vision, loss of tactile sensation, difficulty with speech and swallowing, paralysis of the legs, and nausea. If the patient is not treated, paralysis may occur within minutes, followed by unconsciousness. Death can follow from heart failure due to lack of oxygen. Even with fixed, dilated pupils, the senses of the patient are often intact. The victims are aware but unable to respond. There is no known antidote for the toxin.

Infectious Diseases

In the wild, cephalopods can often survive major trauma. Healthy individuals that have been captured had several regenerating arms (Boyle, 1991). In the literature, numerous disease states have been reported in which cephalopods carry a wide variety of parasites and symbions (Hanlon et al., 1988; Hanlon and Forsythe, 1990), including viruses, bacteria, fungi, protozoans, nematodes, monogeans, digeneans, cestodes, acanthocephalans, polychaetes, hirudineans, branchiuran crustaceans, copepods, and isopods (Hochberg, 1983). The common diseases of each group will be discussed relating to laboratory culture and captive care of cephalopods. Table 6.1 lists some common pathogenic agents encountered in the laboratory.

Viruses may be common, but identification and reporting of them is uncommon. When evaluating a disease process, one should consider that the squid, octopus, and cuttlefish are short-lived animals in culture. One has to take into account the age of the animal and its history in the overall clinical picture before developing extensive diagnostic regimens. Its immune function, as in many animals, can diminish with the aging process.

Wild-caught animals are prone to mechanical damage. One has to keep in mind the semelparous life-cycle challenges in the management of cephalopods with life spans of 12–14 months (Sherrill et al., 2000). Cuts and abrasions of the animal's skin

Table 6.1. Some common pathogens encountered in cephalopods

Category	Species	References
Bacteria		
Vibrio sp.	Multiple cephalopods	Reimschuessel et al., 1990; Sherrill et al., 2000
Aeromonas hydrophila	Multiple cephalopods	Sherrill et al., 2000
Citrobacter freundi	Multiple cephalopods	Sherrill et al., 2000
Pseudomonas sp.	Multiple cephalopods	Stoskopf et al., 1987
Acinebacter anitratus	Multiple cephalopods	Stoskopf et al., 1987
Viruses		
Virus particles: arm musculature	Octopus	Farley, 1978
Virus particles: stomach epithelium	Cuttlefish	Devauchelle and Vago, 1971
Fungi		
Fusarium sp.	*Nautilus*	Scimeca, 1994
Cladosporium sp.	Octopus	Scimeca and Oestmann, 1995
Protozoans		
Icthyobodo sp.	Octopus	Forsythe et al., 1988
Aggregata sp.	Multiple cephalopods	Scimeca and Oestmann, 1995
Microspora sp.	Cuttlefish	Hochberg, 1983
Chromidina sp.	Multiple cephalopods	Hochberg, 1983

from nets and handling are a frequent cause of morbidity and eventual mortality. The epidermal microvillous skin layer is one cell thick and contains many delicate mucous and columnar epithelial cells. The skin is easily damaged and, in captivity, cuttlefish can jet across the tank and damage the skin, eventually leading to septicemia and death (Scimeca and Oestmann, 1995). Mantle lesions are typically preceded by abnormal swimming behavior and commonly lead to secondary bacterial infections affecting multiple organ systems and leading to rapid death (Sherrill et al., 2000) (Figure 6.9). If the force of the animals' propulsion against the side of the tank is great, as in the case of cuttlefish, the result may be cuttlebone fracture, as represented in Figure 6.10. Occasionally, if an air stone is in the tank, they can hover in the stream of bubbles and eventually an air/gas pocket will form beneath the skin in the head region. This air pocket will break, causing an ulcer that will become septic and their death shortly afterward.

Cuttlefish can sustain skin abrasions and cuts if there is crowding and competition between growing males that are displaying territorial rights. In a retrospective study of 186 common cuttlefish, the top-ranked clinical disease syndromes were anorexia, mantle lesions, ocular lesions, and lethargy (Sherrill et al., 2000). Septic conditions can lead to ocular opacities, but not all ocular opacities are related to infectious processes. The early treatment of lesions is useful, but not all lesions heal in a display or production tank. Cuttlefish with a fractured cuttlebone usually do not grow well and are best removed from the colony.

Bacterial infections are a predominant clinical problem in captive and laboratory-reared cuttlefish (Sherrill et al., 2000). *Vibrio* sp. was isolated on postmortem from hemolymph, abdominal fluid, and eyes of four captive cuttlefish with myocarditis (Reimschuessel et al., 1990). Of the 36 bacteria species found associated with diseased cephalopods, over half have belonged to the genus *Vibrio*. The bacteria were cultured from the skin, muscle, hemolymph, eye, and ovary (Hanlon et al., 1983).

In the *Nautilus*, skin abrasions and septic conditions have been noted. One case involving the dorsal mantle with pigment loss was due to a deep infection by the fungal organism *Fusarium* sp.

An indirect fluorescent antibody test was positive for hyphal elements in the *Fusarium* group. The elements extended from the deep ulcer into the musculature of the mantle (Scimeca, 1994). The octopus is prone to skin penetrations and abrasions with deep ulcers leading to septicemia and eventual death (Hanlon et al., 1983) (Figure 6.11). With good water quality, some of the ulcerative dermatitis may heal with antibiotic therapy whereas others will proceed to septicemia and death. Ocular lesions and lens opacities can be observed both from wild and in cultured ani-

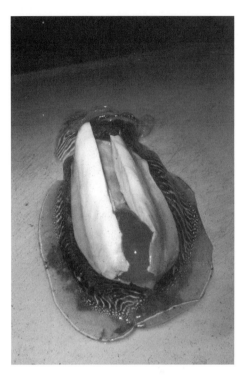

Figure 6.10. Close-up of a severe cuttlebone fracture in *Sepia officinalis*. Trauma can cause these lesions. Photo courtesy of the NIH National Resource Center for Cephalopods, UTMB, Galveston, TX.

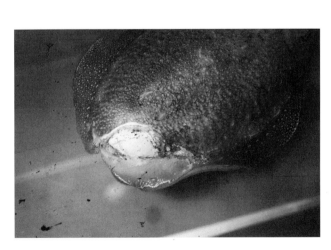

Figure 6.9. Close-up of the distal mantle tip demonstrating an early ulcer and underlying cuttlebone in the common cuttlefish *Sepia officinalis*. Photo courtesy of the NIH National Resource Center for Cephalopods, UTMB, Galveston, TX.

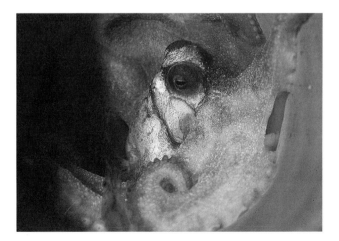

Figure 6.11. Close-up of *Octopus briareus* with an ulcer in front of the left eye. Photo courtesy of the NIH National Resource Center for Cephalopods, UTMB, Galveston, TX.

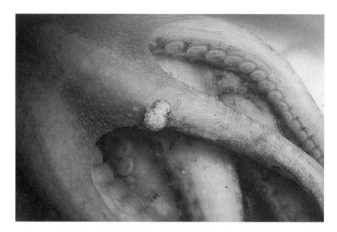

Figure 6.12. The lesions on the arm of this *Octopus bimaculoides* were caused by a coccidian (*Aggregata* sp.) within the dermis and epidermis. Photo courtesy of the NIH National Resource Center for Cephalopods, UTMB, Galveston, TX.

mals. Wild-caught octopods can have coccidian parasites within the intestinal tract. These coccidians are often in the genus *Aggregata* (Staruch et al., 1993). One of the three reported *Aggregata* species is pathogenic. Multiple white, raised hyperplastic vesicles caused by this parasite have been observed on an arm of *Octopus bimaculoides* (Figure 6.12). Several octopuses have been diagnosed with inanition and upon necropsy have had gastric ulcers, an uncommon condition (Scimeca and Oestmann, 1995). *Octopus rubescens* has been observed to have ulcerative lesions on the distal mantle. The exact etiology is not known but is thought to be in part due to trauma from bumping into the tank wall or from infection of the small papilla in this region (J.W. Forsythe, personal communication, 2004).

Captive squid have had minimal disease problems, although skin ulcerations and traumatic lesions can occur in overcrowded conditions. Squids have been observed with tears in their cornea and conjunctiva on occasion, but these have healed.

Neoplasia

The incidence of neoplasia is extremely low. A few reports have been noted, but this author has not observed any neoplastic lesions, and those case reports may have been describing hyperplastic lesions. Jullien and Jullien (1951) reported several tumors on the ventral mandible in cuttlefish. An iridophoroma has been reported by the National Zoo and is on file at the Registry of Tumors in Lower Animals (Drs. Esther Peters and Marilyn Wolfe, personal communication, 2004). The National Resource Center for Cephalopods has not verified any tumors, including the iridophoroma (Lee et al., 1994a). In summary, neoplasia in cephalopods appears to be extremely rare.

Miscellaneous Disorders

An entity sometimes encountered in octopuses is *autophagy* ("self-eating") of the arms and is a well-known form of self-mutilation or self-destruction. Stress and hunger are assumed to cause autophagy but may not be the primary cause of the condition. There is no conclusive evidence that the primary cause is an infectious agent, but autophagy can cause an entire population of animals in a closed water system to die. The agent can be transmitted through a closed system of recirculating seawater with biological and sand filters. The agent seems to affect the nervous system, and animals die within 1–2 days (Budelmann, 1998).

Analgesia, Anesthesia, and Surgery

Magnesium chloride ($MgCl_2$) is a suitable anesthetic agent because it is easy to obtain, inexpensive, stable, nontoxic, and

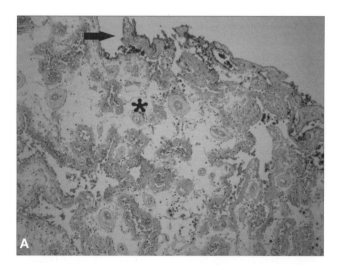

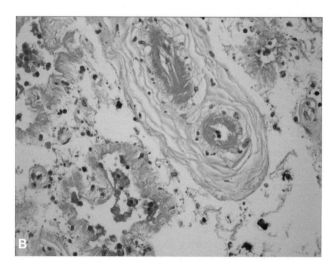

Figure 6.13. Ink sacculitis, hemocytic, diffuse, mild, with marked edema in an octopus. **A:** The ink-sac mucosa (*arrow*) is covered by black pigment, and there is edema of the submucosa (*star*). Hemocytes are scattered throughout. **B:** Perivascular edema and sloughing of ink-sac mucosal cells. Photos courtesy of David Rotstein.

the solution is easy to prepare (Messenger et al., 1985). A standard solution of 75 g of MgCl^2 dissolved into 1 L of distilled water and then mixed with an equal volume of seawater is the most effective means of anesthesia (Scimeca and Forsythe, 1999). A 1:1 mixture is used for surgical anesthesia and some invasive clinical procedures; a 1:3 or 1:4 dilution has been adequate for handling and examinations, and a 1:9 dilution is used for sedation and shipping. A surgical plane of anesthesia can be obtained in octopuses by using this preparation with the addition of an ethanol push consisting of a 1% solution (by volume) of ethanol added to the MgCl^2 mixture (about 10 mL of ethanol is added to each liter of the seawater–magnesium chloride mixture). Ethanol alone (3% for induction and 1.5% for recirculating maintenance) has been used for a cuttlefish (*S. officinalis*) surgical procedure with good success (C. Harms, personal communication, 2005). Magnesium chloride has been preliminarily evaluated in cephalopods across five different genera, and all were effectively anaesthetized. The site of action for MgCl^2 is thought to be the central nervous system, because stimulation of the fin nerve in anesthetized cuttlefish elicits a motor response; it is believed that MgCl^2 works at the postsynaptic membrane of the nerve–muscle junction in crustaceans and vertebrates. Extracellular recording from the fin nerve reveals no efferent activity. The age, gender, size, and species have to be considered before cephalopods are anesthetized.

The gill and major blood vessels of octopods can be accessed in anesthetized animals by cutting the median pallial adductor muscles and inverting the mantle musculature. The animals recover with no side affects from this procedure (J.W. Forsythe, personal communication, 2004).

Recovery rates and performance with the placement of arterial and venous catheters have been good. These catheterizations did not last long—only a matter of hours. Sutures are frequently not required but, when used, should be placed in the underlying connective tissue and opposed lightly (Boyle, 1991).

Euthanasia is via terminal anesthesia, and death is assured with separation of the brain in the case of the octopus (by using a blade or sharp scissors to bisect the brain between the eyes). In squids, anesthesia followed by decapitation assures a humane death.

Treatment Protocols and Formulary

The best approach in the treatment of cephalopods is the careful monitoring and control of water quality. Since the high surface area skin has a microvillous border, drugs may be absorbed at toxic levels. The formulary is empirical but has been helpful with a wide variety of cephalopods. Close monitoring is essential in the clinical treatment of these animals. While most treatment protocols involve the immersion route (the animal is immersed in water containing the chemotherapeutant), intramuscular (IM), and even intravenous (IV) routes are possible (Figure 6.14).

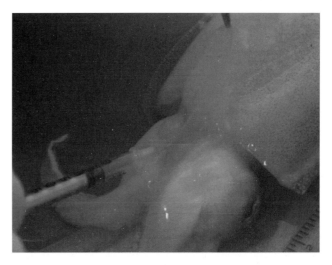

Figure 6.14. Removing hemolymph with needle and syringe from the cephalic vein of the European cuttlefish (*Sepia officinalis*). Photo courtesy of Stacey Gore.

Antibiotics	Dose		
Chloramphenicol	75 mg/kg PO or IM	q 12 h	6 days
Enrofloxacin*	10 mg/kg PO	q 8–12 h	
	5 mg/kg IV	q 8–12 h	
	2.5 mg/L bath for 5 h	q 4–6 h	
Gentamicin	20 mg/kg IM	q 24 h	
Tetracycline	10 mg/kg IM	q 24 h	
Nitrofuran	(Tank treatment)		
Furazolidone (Furoxone)	50 mg/L for 10 min	q 12 h	
Nitrofurazone (Furacin)	25 mg/L for 1 h	q 12 hr	
	1.5 mg/L for 72 h		
Metronidazole	100 mg/L for 16 h		

Euthanasia		
Ethanol	10% in seawater	
Magnesium chloride	10% in seawater	

*Based on a study by Gore et al. (2004). IM, intramuscular; IV, intravenous; and PO, per os (orally).

References

Anderson RC and Mather JA (1996). Escape responses of *Euprymna scolopes* Berry, 1911 (Cephalopoda: Sepiolidae). J Molluscan Stud 62:543–545.

Boletzky SV and Hanlon R (1983). A review of the laboratory maintenance, rearing, and culture of cephalopod mollusks. Mem Mus Vic 44:147–187.

Boyle PR. 1999. Cephalopods. In UFAW Handbook on the Care and Management of Laboratory Animals, 7th ed. (Poole T., ed.). Blackwell Science Ltd. pp. 119–120.

Boyle PR (1991). The Care and Management of Cephalopods in the Laboratory. UFAW Handbook. Longman, Harlow, UK, 63 pp.

Boyle PR, Mangold K, and Froesch D (1979). The mandibular movements of *Octopus vulgaris*. J Zool (Lond) 188:53–67.

Budelmann BU (1998). Autophagy in octopus. S Afr J Mar Sci 20:101–108.

Castro BG and Lee PG (1994). The effects of semi-purified diets on growth and condition of *Sepia officinalis* L. (Mollusca: Cephalopoda). Comp Biochem Physiol [A] 109:1007–1016.

Cloney RA and Florey E (1968). Ultrastructure of cephalopod chromatophore organs. Z Zellforsh Mikrosk Anat 89:250–280.

Crookes WJ, Ding L, Huang QL, Kimbell JR, Horwitz J, and McFall-Ngai MJ (2004). Reflectins: The unusual proteins of squid reflective tissues. Science 303:235–238.

DeRusha RH, Forsythe JW, DiMarco FP, and Hanlon RT (1989). Alternative diets for maintaining and rearing cephalopods in captivity. Lab Anim Sci 39:306–312.

Devauchelle G and Vago C (1971). Particules d'allure virale dans les cellules de l'estomac de la seiche, *Sepia officialis* L. (Mollusques, Cephalopods). C R Hebd Seances Acad Sci Paris 272:894–896.

Dubas F and Boyle PR (1985). Chromatophore units in *Eledone cirrhosa* (Cephalopoda). J Exp Biol 117:415–431.

FAO (Food and Agricultural Organization of the United Nations) (2003). FAO Yearbook of Fishery Statistics, volume 92/1. FAO, Rome (www.fao.org).

Farley CA (1978). Viruses and viruslike lesions in marine mollusks. Mar Fish Rev 40:18–20.

Flecker H and Cotton BC (1955). Fatal bite from octopus. Med J Aust 2:329–331.

Forsythe JW (2005). National Resource Center for Cephalopods, University of Texas Marine Branch: www.nrcc.utmb.edu; access date, 19 June.

Forsythe JW, Hanlon R, and DeRusha R (1988). First observation of an ectoparasitic bodonid flagellate on a marine invertebrate host [Abstract]. In: Perkins FO and Cheng TC, eds. Third International Colloquium on Pathology in Marine Aquaculture. Virginia Institute of Marine Science, Gloucester Point, 2 pp.

Forsythe JW, DeRusha RH, and Hanlon RT (1994). Growth, reproduction and life span of *Sepia officinaalis* (Cephalopoda: Mollusca) cultured through seven consecutive generations. J Zool (Lond) 233:175–192.

Gore SR, Harms CA, Papich MG, Lewbart GA, Kukanich B, and Forsythe J. (2004). A pharmocokinetic study of enrofloxacin in the European cuttlefish (*Sepia officinalis*) after single intravenous injections and bath administration. Proc Int Assoc Aquat Anim Med 35:122–123.

Halstead BW (1965). Poisonous and Venomous Marine Animals of the World, volume 1. US Government Document Printing Office, Washington, DC, pp 663–770.

Hanlon RT (1987). Mariculture. In: Boyle PR, ed. Cephalopod Life Cycles, volume 2: Comparative reviews. Academic, London, pp. 291–305.

Hanlon RT and Forsythe JW (1990). 1. Diseases of Mollusca: Cephalopoda. 1.1. Diseases caused by microorganisms. In: Kinne O, ed. Diseases of Marine Animals, volume 3. Biologische Anstalt Helgoland, Hamburg, pp 23–46.

Hanlon RT and Messenger JB (1988). Adaptive coloration in young cuttlefish (*Sepia officinalis* L.): The morphology and development of body patterns and their relation to behaviour. Philos Trans R Soc Lond [B] 320:437–487.

Hanlon RT and Messenger JB (1996). Cephalopod Behavior. Cambridge University Press, Cambridge, 232 pp.

Hanlon RT, Forsythe FW, Cooper KM, DiNuzzo AR, Folse DS, and Kelly MT (1983). Fatal penetrating skin ulcers in laboratory reared octopuses. Am Malacol Bull 2:93–94.

Hanlon RT, Forsythe JW, and Lee PG (1988). External pathologies of cephalopods in captivity. Proc Int Colloq Pathol Mar Aquacult 3:17–18.

Hanlon RT, Turk PE, and Lee PG (1991). Squid and cuttlefish mariculture: An updated perspective. J Ceph Biol 2:31–40.

Hochberg FG (1983). The parasites of cephalopods: A review. Mem Natl Mus Vic 44:109–145.

Jullien A and Jullien A-P (1951). Sur un type de tumeur non provoquee experimentalement et observee chez la Seiche. C R Hebd Seances Acad Sci Paris 233:1322–1334.

Lee PG (1994). Nutrition of cephalopods: Fueling the system. Mar. Freshwater Behav Physiol 25:35–51.

Lee PG, Lu L-JW, Salazar JJ, and Holoubek V (1994a). Absence of formation of benzo[a]pyrene/DNA adducts in the cuttlefish (*Sepia officinalis*, Mollusca, Cephalopoda). Environ Mol Mutagen 23:70–73.

Lee PG, Turk PE, Yang WT, and Hanlon RT (1994b). Biological characteristics and biomedical applications of the squid *Sepioteuthis lessoniana* cultured through multiple generations. Biol Bull 186:328–341.

Martin R (1977). The giant nerve fibre system of cephalopods: Recent structural findings. Symp Zool Soc Lond 38:261–275.

Messenger JB, Nixon M, and Ryan KP (1985). Magnesium chloride as an anaesthetic for cephalopods. Comp Biochem Physiol [C1] 82:203–205.

Minton JW, Walsh LS, Lee PG, and Forsythe JW (2001). First multigeneration culture of the tropical cuttlefish *Sepia pharaonis* Ehrenberg, 1831. Aquacult Int 9:379–392.

Nixon M (1987). Cephalopod diets. In: Boyle PR, ed. Cephalopod Life Cycles, volume 2: Comparative Reviews. Academic, New York, pp 201–219.

Oestmann DJ, Scimeca JM, Forsythe JW, Hanlon RT, and Lee PG (1997). Special considerations for keeping cephalopods in laboratory facilities. Contemp Top Assoc Lab Anim Sci 36:89–93.

Olafson JA (1988). Role of lectins in invertebrate humoral defense. Am Fish Soc Spec Publ 18:189–205.

Ratcliffe NA and Rowley AF (1981). Invertebrate Blood Cells. Academic, New York, pp 301–323.

Reimschuessel RM, Stoskopf MK, and Bennett RO (1990). Myocarditis in the common cuttlefish (*Sepia officinalis*). J Comp Pathol 102:291–298.

Russo G and Tringali G (1983). Hemagglutinating and antibacterial activity in hemolymph of *Octopus vulgaris*. Rev Int Oceanogr Med 70/71:49–54.

Sackton J, ed (2003). Giant squid caught on surface near New Zealand, only second specimen captured. Midland Independent Newspaper, 8 April. www.Seafood.com News.

Saunders WB and Landman NH, eds (1987). *Nautilus*: The Biology and Paleobiology of a Living Fossil. Plenum, New York, 632 pp.

Scimeca JM (1994). What's your diagnosis? Pigmentation loss in the *Nautilus, Nautilus pompilius*. Texas Branch of the American Association of Laboratory Animal Science, Dallas.

Scimeca JM and Forsythe JW (1999). The use of anesthetic agents in cephalopods. Proc Int Assoc Aquat Anim Med 30:94.

Scimeca JM and Oestmann DJ (1995). Selected diseases of captive and laboratory reared cephalopods. Proc Int Assoc Aquat Anim Med 27:88.

Sherrill J, Spelman LH, Reidel CL, and Montali RJ (2000). Common cuttlefish (*Sepia officinalis*) mortality at the National Zoological Park: Implications for clinical management. J Zoo Wildl Med 31:523–531.

Staruch MH, Gillette D, Lewbart GA, and Poynton S (1993). The occurrence of a coccidian parasite in the gastrointestinal tract of the Atlantic octopus, *Octopus vulgaris*. Proc Int Assoc Aquat Anim Med 24:75–77.

Stoskopf MK, Nevy S, and Flynn S (1987). Treatment of ulcerative mantel disease due to *Pseudomonas* spp. in *Octopus dofleini* and *Octopus bimaculoides* with oxytetracycline [Poster]. Proc Int Assoc Aquat Anim Med 1:102.

Voss GL (1977). Present status and new trends in cephalopod systematics. Symp Zool Soc Lond 38:49–60.

Walsh LS, Turk PE, Forsythe JW, and Lee PG (2002). Mariculture of the loliginid squid *Sepioteuthis lessoniana* through seven successive generations. Aquaculture 212:245–262.

Wells MJ (1978). Octopus: Physiology and Behaviour of an Advanced Invertebrate. Chapman and Hall, London, 417 pp.

Wells MJ and Wells J (1982). Ventilatory currents in the mantle of cephalopods. J Exp Biol 99:315–330.

Wood JW and Day CL (2005). CephBase. University of Texas Marine Branch: www.cephbase.utmb.edu; access date, 19 June.

Wood JW, Day CL, Lee PG, and O'Dor RK (2000). CephBase: Testing ideas for cephalopod and other species-level databases. Oceanography 13:14–20.

Yang WT, Hanlon RT, Lee PG, and Turk PE (1989). Design and function of closed seawater systems for culturing loliginid squids. Aquacult Eng 8:47–65.

Chapter 7

BIVALVES

Jay F. Levine, Mac Law, and Flavio Corsin

Introduction

Oysters, clams, mussels, and other bivalves are vertically compressed mollusks within the class Bivalvia (Lamellibranchia), which numerically is the second largest class of mollusks (Healy, 2001). There are more than 10,000 species recognized worldwide, found in freshwater, estuarine, and marine surface waters. Within aquatic ecosystems, bivalves fill a critical niche, the majority functioning as living filters that remove suspended particulates, detritus, phytoplankton, and bacteria from the water column (Kohata et al., 2003). In this manner, they are important in sustaining water quality. Other bivalve species, the protobranch bivalves, are deposit feeders living beneath the sediment, where their movement and feeding help the degradation of organic materials (Stasek, 1965; Zardus, 2002). Bivalves also serve as a source of food for a variety of other aquatic and terrestrial fauna, and as a substrate for the colonization of fauna that adhere to bivalve shells or invade the shell cavity. Although their ecological relevance is significant, they are best recognized for the roles they play as commercial seafood products. Bivalves harvested from commercial fisheries or aquaculture leases have played a profound role in the economic development of coastal communities. In addition, bivalves comprise a large portion of the shell fauna collected by amateur or professional conchologists on our beaches and freshwater stream banks, and historically have played a significant role in the apparel industry as a source of buttons, or pearls, and as a frequent item on the shelves of novelty shops.

Bivalve aquaculture is a global enterprise providing a vast array of products for human consumption and the continued perpetuation of the cultured pearl industry. Marine oysters (Ostreidae), clams (Myiidae and Veneridae), mussels (Mytilidae), scallops (Pectinidae), and cockles (Cardiidae) support the bulk of the cultured bivalve harvest for human consumption and for apparel (Pteriidae). Indeed, the annual total tonnage of cultured oysters alone routinely exceeds 3 million metric and has an economic value of more than 3 billion dollars (Wijkstrom et al., 1998).

Bivalves are increasingly being included as display animals in homes and public aquaria, and as invertebrate alternatives for biomedical research studies. This chapter is an introduction to their basic anatomy and physiology, their maintenance require-

ments, and standard aquaculture techniques. Detailed descriptions of three distinct economically relevant bivalve diseases are provided as examples of the types of problems that may affect bivalve health in both closed recirculating and open systems. Due to their commercial importance, bivalve diseases have been studied extensively for more than a century, and the bivalve disease research literature includes thousands of peer-reviewed articles and numerous texts. Consequently, this review is a brief introduction for veterinarians. Readers interested in a more comprehensive review of bivalve anatomy and physiology and bivalve diseases have a wealth of outstanding journals (e.g., *Journal of Shellfish Diseases* and *Diseases of Aquatic Organisms*), monographs (e.g., Fisher, 1988), review articles (Bower et al., 1994), and texts (e.g., Kennedy et al., 1996) from which to further their understanding of issues that impact bivalve health.

Basic Anatomy and Physiology

The Shell

Commercially important bivalves are lamellibranch (subclass Lamellibranchia) mollusks, with a calcareous shell secreted by underlying mantle tissue that is embryonically divided into right and left lobes (McMahon, 1991). Although the shell matrix is visually and functionally divided into right and left valves, the valves originate from a single external structure joined by an elastic hinged ligament that connects the valves. Shells are covered by a water-resistant organic layer of scleroprotein secreted by the edge of the mantle (Figure 7.1), which forms a thin periostracum. In many species, the periostracum is often partially eroded. The shell matrix is primarily crystalline calcium carbonate and shell protein (McMahon, 1991) secreted by the mantle and deposited in fairly uniform outer and inner layers. The physical point of origin of shell deposition is the *umbo* (beak or point of origin of growth), which generally protrudes above the hinge line (Barnes, 1968). The inner layer of the majority of bivalve species (e.g., Mytilidae, marine mussels; and Unionidae, freshwater mussels) is a visually attractive, often colorful matrix of aragonite and conchiolin called the *nacre* (Figure 7.2), which is secreted by the mantle surface (Healy, 2001). Pearls are formed when irritating granules (e.g., sand) are trapped between the outer and inner layers of shell and covered by nacre.

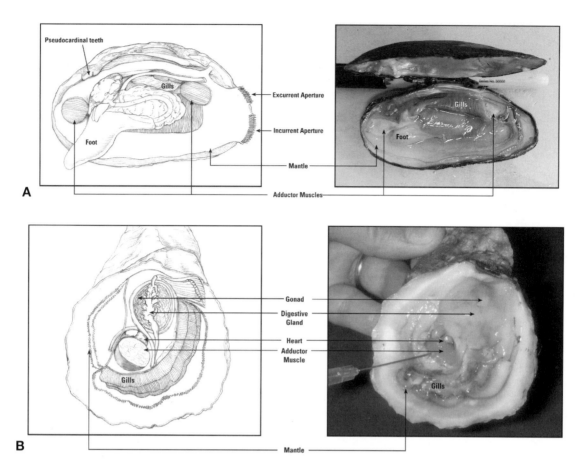

Figure 7.1. Half-shell views and diagrammatic representations of **(A)** the common elliptio (*Elliptio complanata*), a freshwater bivalve in the family Unionidae, and **(B)** the eastern oyster (*Crassostrea virginica*), a marine bivalve in the family Ostreidae. Illustrations by Brenda Bunch.

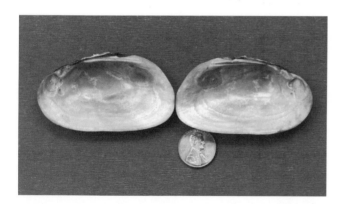

Figure 7.2. The point of attachment of the adductor muscles is readily apparent (*oval indentation* in the nacre) on the interior surface of a bivalve shell. The interior shell matrix—the nacre—is also readily apparent in this photo of the two valves of a freshwater mussel.

Interlocking toothlike protrusions on the shell edge along the hinge line are present in many bivalve families. The number, size, and orientation of these *hinge teeth* often serve as species-distinguishing characteristics (Figure 7.1). Additional projections, *lateral teeth*, pseudocardinal teeth (Unionidae), and other

variable external features, that define the visual appearance of shells, ridges, color, and pigmentation, also assist with species identification (Bogan, 1993). Shells can be relatively symmetrical and uniform (clams and scallops) or asymmetrical (oysters) and markedly variable in shape and appearance. The physical condition, shape, and contour of the valves of bivalve species often reflect the physical environmental forces that define the habitat in which they are located (Carriker, 1996). In their simplest form, these shell surface features are reflected in erosions at the umbo of freshwater mussels resulting from the erosive forces of suspended materials in flowing water. In contrast, the phenotypic plasticity of oysters is evident in the asymmetrical marked variation in the length, width, height, and physical contour of their shells, which is often determined by oyster density and the physical conditions that define the substrate to which they are attached (Kennedy et al., 1996) (Figure 7.3).

Shell movement (opening and closing) is controlled by strong adductor muscles (Figure 7.1). Embryonically, bivalves have two adducter muscles (anterior and posterior), but the anterior adductor of sessile bivalves (e.g., oysters) regresses during development and only a single adductor muscle controls shell movement (Eble and Scro, 1996). Estimates from the study of oysters indicate that the adductor muscle of some species can withstand a pulling force of 10 kg before separating from the

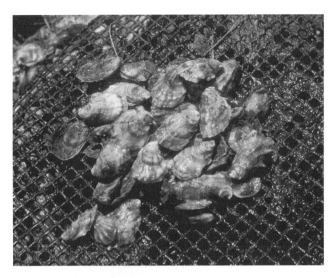

Figure 7.3.   The physical appearance of oysters in their intertidal habitat generally reflects environmental forces that affect shell growth. Variation in size and shape is readily apparent in this group of cultured oysters.

shell (Galtsoff, 1964). Adductor muscle points of attachment are readily apparent on the nacre of either valve after removal (Figure 7.2). Loss of muscle turgor is a common clinical finding in bivalves with health problems.

Internal Anatomy and Physiology

Circulatory System

The circulatory system of bivalves is open. Eble (1996) provides an outstanding review of the intricacy of hemolymph circulation in oysters. In most bivalves, hemolymph is pumped from a muscular heart through arteries to open sinuses (*hemocoels*), where it circulates through other bivalve tissues. The heart in freshwater mussels is wrapped around the rectum (McMahon, 1991) (Figure 7.1), whereas in oysters it is located between the rectum and the adjacent adductor muscle (Eble, 1996). Bivalve hearts have a single ventricle and two atria. Many species possess accessory hearts that help circulate hemolymph through the mantle and renal tissue (Eble, 1996).

Heart function, including rate and intraventricular pressure in oysters and other bivalves, has been studied extensively. Heart rate is responsive to ambient changes in temperature, salinity, the mechanical effect of shell closure, and changes in pH (Eble, 1996). Heart rates in oysters of 47 beats/min have been reported at 25°C (Federighi, 1929) and 20 beats/min at 20°C (Koehring, 1937), and at 2–6/min when the valves were closed at 17.5°C (Eble, 1996) and 14–16 beats/min with the valves open. Heart rate also seems to vary with pumping and filtration rates (Eble, 1996) and may be partially driven by oxygen tension of fluid in the mantle cavity in some species (Bayne et al., 1976; Eble, 1996). In one study of *Crassostrea gigas*, mean intraventricular systolic pressure was recorded to be 32.5 ± 7.0 mm water, and mean intraventricular diastolic was 3.0 ± 2.0 mm water (Hevert, 1984).

Hemolymph

This is the bivalve equivalent of vertebrate blood (Jones, 1983). Although the biochemical composition of bivalve hemolymph varies widely between the orders of bivalves, the basic constituents of hemolymph are fairly uniform. As already noted, in addition to its role in respiration and host defense, hemolymph plays an important role in bivalve locomotion. Bivalve hemolymph is comprised of proteins, phagocytic cells, and the biochemical products of organ function (e.g., enzymes) and respiration. Although the hemolymph of marine ark shells (*Anadara trapezia*) contains a respiratory pigment, the majority of bivalves lack an oxygen-binding protein pigment (hemoglobin) (Healy, 2001), and oxygen is dissolved directly into hemolymph (McMahon, 1991). In one study conducted with *Rangia cuneata*, Marsh (1990) documented that calcium-binding phosphoproteins are abundant in clam hemolymph and apparently produced by granular hemocytes.

Hemocytes

Bivalve hemocytes are relatively uniform, with one cell type predominating and one or more additional morphological forms potentially apparent. Hemocytes actively engage in phagocytosis as a defense against pathogens and foreign substances, as well as play a role in bivalve nutrition and waste-product excretion (Cheng, 1996). Different hemocyte cell forms display variable degrees of chemotaxic ability. Marked seasonal changes in hemocyte number and bactericidal activity have been observed in oysters (Canesi et al., 2002).

Complete blood counts and serum chemistry panels are routine components of vertebrate health examinations. Similarly, hemolymph analysis can provide a window to understanding the health status of bivalves. Hemocytes are active participants in maintaining homeostasis. Their absolute number and the proportion of morphologically distinct forms can potentially play a similar role to that of a differential cell count in the health examination of vertebrates.

Fisher and Ford (1988) proposed the use of flow cytometry to quantify different morphological subtypes of hemocytes as a tool in bivalve health assessments and research.

Gas Exchange and Respiration

The gills and mantle are the primary organs of respiration. In the majority of bivalve species, they perform multiple functions, and their actual structure and function in different families of bivalves are markedly variable. Cilia of protruding ctenidia filaments on the gills of some species maintain water flow across the gills and help disperse fouling materials (Healy, 2001). In other species (e.g., unionids), the gills are elongated and folded into demibranchs. The folding substantially increases the gill surface area. The gills along with the palps in these species play a role in particle filtration and sorting. In unionids, the gills also serve as broad chambers for larvae (*glochidia*) (Tankersley and Dimock, 1993). These multiple roles in unionids have energy costs. Although pumping rate does not appear to be affected (Tankersley,

1996), larval brooding impacts respiration and oxygen consumption in gravid female *Pyganodon cataracta* and possibly other unionid species (Tankersley and Dimock, 1993).

In addition to its role in respiration, like the gills, the mantle of many bivalves serves multiple functions. The mantle is the primary organ of shell deposition, and in some species it also plays a role in particle collection, retention, and sorting (Stasek, 1965; McMahon, 1991; Zardus, 2002).

Bivalves are benthic organisms, and life in the benthos is subject to marked oxygen changes that are daily, seasonal, and event driven (e.g., hurricanes). In systems impacted by eutrophication, water-column stratification can result in bottom oxygen demands for organic particle degradation that exceed bottom dissolved oxygen availability (Pandian, 1999). Unlike mobile aquatic vertebrates, bivalves have limited dispersal capabilities during periods of hypoxia. Extended periods of bottom hypoxia and anoxia routinely result in the transient and sometimes persistent loss of invertebrates from the benthos. Although new bivalves and other invertebrates may be recruited during the spring, anoxia often results in the complete loss of the benthic community in the summer.

In intertidal areas, some bivalves sustain daily periods of air emersion. Individual species of bivalves display varying degrees of tolerance for bottom hypoxia and air emersion (Figure 7.4). The majority of bivalves are facultative anaerobic succinate-producing species (Friedl, 1996) and alter predominant metabolic pathways in response to changes in oxygen availability. Hypoxia has been associated with lower filtration rates, lower ingestion rates, and decreased feces production in a clam (*Ruditapes decussatus*). This capacity for anaerobic respiration sustains respiratory metabolism during periods of hypoxia (Sobral and Widdows, 1997). Tolerance to hypoxic conditions appears temperature dependent (Hicks and McMahon, 2002). Sobral and Widdows (1997) suggest that these reductions in metabolic activity help prevent the depletion of energy reserves during periods of hypoxia. In one study, Simpfendoerfer and coworkers (1995) compared aerial respiration in two bivalves: *Perumytilus purpuratus*, which inhabits the intermediate tidal zone, and *Mytilus chilensis*, which predominantly inhabits the lower tidal zone. The aerial oxygen-uptake capability of *Perumytilus purpuratus* (30%–50%) was more than double that of *M. chilensis* (5%–15%).

Estuarine bivalves are also subject to routine changes in salinity and temperature. In studies conducted with sea scallops (*Placopecten magellanicus*), both salinity and temperature appeared to impact clearance rate and oxygen utilization (Frenette et al., 2002). Similar changes in oxygen consumption were apparent in three bivalves—the Baltic tellin (*Macoma balthica*), the common cockle (*C. edule*), and the thin tellin (*Tellina tenuis*)—in response to changing salinities between 1 and 33 ppt. Respiration was significantly different when the animals were held at the upper and lower extremes of salinity tolerance for each species (Wilson, 1984). Wilson and Elkaim (1991) described four factors that determine temperature tolerance of burrowing (*infaunal*) bivalve species: general location on the shore, burrowing depth (for those that burrow), geographic range, and seasonal cycles.

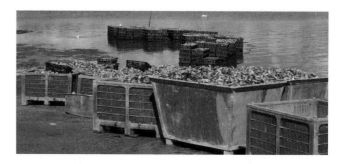

Figure 7.4. Oysters on a dock harvested from deep-water leases. Bivalves vary in their tolerance to air emersion. Some industries use periods of air emersion after harvest to harden oysters prior to market.

Fluid Balance and Excretion

Bivalves live in both estuarine and freshwater environments. Osmoregulation in bivalves mirrors that of their vertebrate counterparts. Freshwater species must contend with a constant gain in water and loss of ions, and salt-tolerant species contend with a continual loss of water and net gain of ions (McMahon, 1991). Freshwater bivalves continuously excrete the cations ammonia (NH_4) and hydrogen ion (H^+) from the hemolymph. Chloride is exchanged for bicarbonate (HCO_3-) and hydroxide ($OH-$) (McMahon, 1991), and net Ca^{2+} uptake supports shell deposition. Cellular and hemolymph osmotic concentrations of unionids are 25%–50% of other freshwater species (McMahon, 1991). Dietz (1985) documented that the gills are the main site of sodium and chloride uptake in unionids. In freshwater bivalves, the kidneys are the main route of water excretion, and there is a net loss of ions to surrounding freshwater (McMahon, 1991). Martin (1983) estimates that one species (*Anodonta cygnea*) excretes 0.03 mL/g wet tissue daily. Reduced filtration particle retention has been observed in gravid *Pyganodon cataracta* (Tankersley and Dimock, 1993; Tankersley, 1996), and this reduction may be due to changes in the functional processing of particles by demibranch cilia.

The closure of valves provides osmotic protection for freshwater mussels when water levels have diminished in transient headwater streams and for intertidal marine species when tides recede. Although water loss is curtailed when valves are closed, extended periods of closure impact respiration. Oxygen exchange is impeded and can result in extended periods of hypoxia and eventual anoxia (McMahon and Williams, 1984). *Corbicula* spp. use a mucus plug to cover their siphons to prevent desiccation (McMahon, 1991).

Feeding, Diet, and Digestion

Bivalves are predominantly filter feeders (suspension feeders) that remove bacteria, algae, and detritus from the water column (Langdon and Newell, 1990). In this manner, they are important in sustaining water quality in surface waters (Bachmann and Usseglio-Polatera, 1999) and are viable beneficial additions to aquaria. In suspension-feeding bivalves, the gills and palps (Figure 7.1) assist in removing particles from the water column and in particle sorting. In contrast, the protobranch bivalves, a subclass that includes more than 600 species, are deposit feeders (Stasek, 1965; Zardus 2002). They feed on organic sediments and help process organic materials for degradation by other benthic organisms. The gills of protobranch bivalves are comparatively smaller and used only for respiration. Particle retrieval is the job of the mantle and palpal tentacles (Stasek, 1965). The postmetamorphic juveniles of many unionids use a form of foot, or pedal, feeding to ingest particles in the sediment (Reid et al., 1992; Hakenkamp and Palmer, 1999). Tankersley and coworkers (1996) found that different feeding strategies are used during the life history of the unionid, *Utterbachia imbecilis*. Recently metamorphosed juveniles rely predominantly on pedal feeding, and adults rely more on suspension feeding. Feeding and the gastrointestinal anatomy of both freshwater and marine species have been reviewed extensively (McMahon, 1991).

In unionids, water enters through an inhalant aperture formed by mantle tissue. However, in the majority of marine bivalves, the valves open producing a narrow slit between the valves. Water flowing into the mantle cavity is filtered by cilia on the surface of the gills and often the palps. The processing of particles by the gills in some bivalves is markedly complex; particles are sorted, and those selected pass through a cilia-lined esophagus into the stomach. The interior of the bivalve stomach is lined with cilia, which continue the sorting of particles. Unionids have a style sac that contains a hardened rod of mucopolysaccharides: the *crystalline style* (McMahon, 1991). Cilia in the style sac rotate the rod against a hardened plate: the *gastric shield*, which is composed of chitin, with underlying epithelial cells that secrete enzymes aiding digestion. The style has a mixing function and drives food toward the gastric enzymes of the gastric shield. At this point, undigested particles are either passed along to the midgut, hindgut, and rectum for expulsion as pseudofeces, or are redirected back into the style sac, processed further, and moved into a digestive diverticulum, where further digestion and assimilation continues. Tankersley and Dimock (1993) conducted elegant studies employing fiberoptics to track particle movement through unionids and found marked differences in particle progression and sorting in unionids and marine bivalves.

Glucose metabolism is apparently metabolically regulated by the production of insulinlike substances by gut epithelium (Jadhav and Lomte, 1982; Joose and Geraerts, 1983). Insulinlike-substance secretion is modulated by hemolymph glucose concentrations.

The diets of filter-feeding bivalves are primarily comprised of materials suspended in the water column, such as organic detritus, bacteria, and algae. Actual diets are variable and depend on habitat characteristics, primary productivity, nutrient input, and other natural and anthropogenic factors that ultimately determine the suspended organic content of the water. The subclass Protobranchia includes species that feed beneath the sediment by using their labial palps (Zardus, 2002).

Growth and Metabolism

The evolution of each bivalve species has juggled the trade-offs between body size, shell thickness, and growth rate. Larger body size provides enhanced protection against predation for most aquatic species. The comparative rapid growth of some species enhances the likelihood of survival to reproductive age. Bivalves allocate approximately one-third of their metabolic energy to shell deposition (Wilbur and Saleuddin, 1983). Rapid-growing, thin-shelled species devote less energy to shell growth than do slow-growing, thick-shelled species. However, thin-shelled species are comparatively more susceptible to predation (McMahon, 1991).

Many species of bivalves are long-lived, and bivalve longevity ranges from relatively brief, as observed with fingernail clams (pea clams, Sphaeriidae), to decades, as seen in the Margaritiferidae (e.g., *Margaritifera margaritifera*) and Unionidae (e.g., *Anadonta anatina*) (Zotin and Vladimirova, 2001).

Bivalves display marked species, habitat, and seasonal variation in filtering, feeding, basic metabolic processes like oxygen utilization, and tissue biochemical composition (McMahon, 1991). As with the majority of other ectothermic aquatic species, metabolite activity increases during warmer periods and declines during cooler periods. In one study, the surf clam, *Paphias donacina*, displayed changes in filtration rate and oxygen uptake in response to seasonal changes in temperature (Marsden, 1999). However, even at low temperatures ($-1°C$), many bivalves continue to filter and remove particles from the water column (Loo, 1992). In studies conducted with the giant scallop, *Placopecten magellanicus*, seasonal changes in oxygen consumption were related to changes in gametogenesis (Shumway et al., 1988). Individual species like *Pisidium* spp., which are mud burrowers, have a reduced gill surface area and have lower overall metabolic requirements that provide greater tolerance to extended periods of hypoxia (Lopez and Holopainen, 1987). Factors such as pH can impact bivalve growth profoundly. In one study, Ringwood and Keppler (2002) documented a greater than 50% reduction in the growth of the hard clam, *Mercenaria mercenaria*, when minimum pH levels decreased to below 7.2 and mean pH levels to below 7.5.

Feeding and overall metabolic function can also be profoundly affected by the presence of contaminants in water. The increased release of fine-grain sediments into surface waters in association with riparian development can disrupt normal gill respiratory and filtering activity (Aldridge et al., 1987). Various pesticides alter bivalve respiration (Mane et al., 1986), and some bivalves may shift from aerobic to anaerobic processes in response to heavy-metal contamination (Brown et al., 1996). Marine biotoxins may also impact bivalve respiration and filtration (Li et al., 2002).

Nervous System

Unlike other mollusks, bivalves lack a centralized nervous system and cephalic sensory organs. The bivalve nervous system is comprised predominantly of distributed ganglia, sensory tentacles or papillae in the mantle, photoreceptors, cilia that serve as tactile sensors, chemosensors, and statocysts (Kraemer, 1978) that play a role in body orientation and positioning (Healy, 2001).

Reproduction

Bivalves are largely functionally dioecious. Sexual dimorphism is apparent in some species (e.g., *Villosa constricta*), but the sex of the majority of bivalve species cannot be readily distinguished from external morphological features. Some bivalve families possess the ability for sex reversal (are alternate hermaphrodites) (e.g., oysters), whereas others are functionally hermaphroditic (e.g., *Corbicula* spp.), sustaining both sexes simultaneously, and capable of self-fertilization (Wilbur and Gaffney, 1991). The gonads of oysters and other bivalve families that can undergo sex reversal remain undifferentiated until spawning. The reproductive organs of others are generally paired, but pairing may not be readily apparent in some species (McMahon, 1991). During spawning, the gonads are readily apparent and comprise a large proportion of the visceral mass.

Bivalve sperm are released into the surrounding water. Fertilization generally occurs within the confines of the two valves of females (e.g., in unionids) or surrounding water (e.g., in scallops and zebra mussels) (Healy, 2001). Sperm of different bivalve families vary substantially in size and functional morphology, and sperm morphology can be used to determine family and sometimes genus. Early life stages are mobile veliger larvae that either are free swimming or possess minimal locomotor capabilities and depend primarily on water currents for dispersal. Unionids (freshwater mussels) are ovoviviparous; embryos are held within marsupial sacs (brood chambers) of the gills (McMahon, 1991). These swollen marsupia are readily apparent if the valves are opened during brooding. Larval forms often have morphological features that can be differentiated for taxonomic purposes.

The free-swimming larvae of sessile bivalves (e.g., oysters) attach to a suitable substrate, undergo metamorphosis into juveniles, and remain in place for the duration of their lives (Thompson et al., 1996). Environmental factors and possible chemical composition of various substrates serve as triggers for larval adherence (*spat fall*) and attachment (*set*) (Kennedy, 1996). The larvae of other species undergo a direct metamorphosis into mobile juveniles, with active pedal locomotion that aids in their movement toward appropriate substrates and food resources. In unionids, a group that comprises nearly 300 taxa in North America, the glochidia must attach to the gills or fins of a fish to complete their metamorphosis into juveniles. This relationship is often species specific, with a particular species of fish required for attachment and successful metamorphosis (Williams et al., 1993). Many unionids have functional *lures* that are used to attract fish prior to dispersal. Some species possess morphologically distinct mantle flaps that resemble small species of fish, fish fry, insects, or other invertebrates (Kraemer, 1970). The mantle flaps are used to lure the appropriate hosts for the glochidia (Haag and Warren, 2003). When the fish strikes the mantle flap, the fish are showered with glochidia that readily attach predominantly to the gills and sometimes the fins. Other unionids release their glochidia in masses of eggs (*conglutinates*). A portion of the eggs in conglutinates are often nonviable and create color-pattern differences that give conglutinates the appearance of fish prey (e.g., oligochaetes, or fish fry). Others exude mucus threads that also serve as lures.

Various environmental cues induce spawning. Changes in temperature, food availability, salinity, and day length serve as environmental signals that spawning can begin. Consequently, the timing of spawning in individual bivalve families, genera, and species is geographically variable (Thompson et al., 1996). The spawning of *Crassostrea virginica*, the Eastern oyster, appears to be driven by temperature changes and is markedly variable within its home range (Shumway, 1996). In some species, gradual temperature increases induce gametogenesis, and major temperature changes induce spawning. Temperature is clearly an important inducement to spawning of the bay scallop (*Aequipecten irradians concentricus*) (Sastry, 1966). Reproduction appears to be induced by a combination of temperature changes and changes in the availability of phytoplankton. However, little is known about the hormonal modulation of gametogenesis and spawning in bivalves. Marked changes in body condition can be observed throughout the reproductive season, and the dynamics of protein metabolism and of glycogen storage and utilization have been studied in only a few commercially relevant species. Miac and coworkers (1997) found lipid levels of *Mya arenaria* in Puck Bay to be higher in autumn, when gonad development begins, and in early spring, just prior to spawning. Sterols and polyunsaturated fatty acids (PUFAs) play a key role in bivalve reproduction. The species and chemical composition of algal diets, and particularly their lipid content, can impact the reproductive health of cultured bivalves (Soudant et al., 2000). Microalgae sterol and PUFA levels have been equated with the sterol and lipid content of hatchery-reared larval oysters (*C. virginica* and *C. gigas*) and scallops (*P. maximus*). Dietary deficiencies of specific PUFAs have been associated with impaired gametogenesis in scallops (*Pecten maximus*) (Soudant et al., 2000).

Mechanical stimulation with flowing seawater and chemical stimulation with serotonin injections have both been used effectively to induce synchronous spawning in sea scallops (*Placopecten malellanicus*) (Desrosiers and Dube, 1993). Serotonin and other biochemicals have been extensively examined for their value in inducing spawning for hatchery production of *Mytilus edulis*, *Ruditapes philippinarum* (Liu and Xiang, 1994), *Crassostrea virginica*, and other bivalves of commercial relevance (Gibbons and Castagna, 1984; Tanaka and Murakoshi, 1985). Many species that spawn in the spring will also spawn in the fall, and spawning in some species persists throughout the spring, summer, and fall.

Behavior

Bivalve species are either sessile or mobile. Oysters and other sessile bivalves remain in place after larval forms attach to habitat substrate, unless they are physically moved by external forces (e.g., fishermen). Sessile bivalves are at the complete mercy of the surrounding environment, with no mechanism to avoid chemical and physical disturbances. When undisturbed the valves are routinely parted for feeding. The sole physical response available to sessile bivalves is shell closure and a cessation of filtering and feeding. Shell opening and closing are generally asynchronous between individuals in a population or aquarium. However, external chemical or physical stimuli may result in synchronous closure of all individuals in a population. This nonspecific response to noxious stimuli has been exploited by field biologists to monitor the presence of pollutants entering surface waters by using devices that monitor shell movement with mechanical sensors (e.g., a Mussel Monitor [Ansto, Mensai, NSW]) (Rajagopal et al. 1997). Valve closure in freshwater mussels (unionids) has been documented in response to hypoxia (Heinonen et al., 1997) and a broad array of compounds, such as aluminum (Kadar et al., 2001), chlorine (Rajagopal et al., 1997), and suspended particulates (Aldridge et al., 1987). Doherty and coworkers (1987) examined the effect of zinc and cadmium on the valve activity of the freshwater bivalve *Corbicula flumenia*. Duration of valve closure increased as heavy-metal concentrations increased. Similar responses have been observed in oysters (e.g., to associated marine biotoxins [Matsuyama et al., 1999]) and green mussels (to chlorine [Gunasingh-Masilamoni et al., 2002]), as well as other marine bivalves in response to a broad range of compounds (e.g., tributyl tin and wood preservatives).

The foot is the main means of locomotion of burrowing bivalves. It provides a means of dispersal away from noxious influences and movement for feeding or reproduction. Trueman (1983) described the series of events that support the pedal movement of freshwater mussels (unionids). The process begins with the relaxation of the adductor muscles, expansion of the hinge ligament and the opening of the valves, and the physical anchoring of the animal. The foot decreases in diameter, lengthens and moves the animal forward as musculature tightens around a large circulatory sinus that lies within the adductor muscle. Hemolymph then flows into the end of the foot and expands the foot into the substratum. The adductor muscle then contracts, closes the valves, and forces water out of the shell, loosening the surrounding substratum. Retractor muscles then pull the shell forward into the loosened sediment. Trueman and Brown (1985) documented a standing pressure of 3 kPa in the pedal sinus during burrowing by the saw donax (*Donax serra*).

Various species are capable of surface movement above sediments (Imlay, 1982) and vertically on rocks and other hard surfaces (Cleland et al., 1986). In addition to feeding, these surface movements provide some opportunity to relocate locally in response to changing water depths and food availability and for reproductive purposes. Some species (e.g., *Corbicula* spp. and *Dreissena* spp.) attach byssal threads to surrounding substrate as anchors (Rajagopal et al., 2002) to support pedal movement (McMahon, 1991).

Bivalves as Biological Filters

Bivalves have been exploited to help sustain water quality within aquaculture ponds (Zmora and Shpigel, 2001) and in ecosystem restoration. By functioning as biological filters, they can have positive environmental effects (Levine, 2003). Indeed, Soto and Mena (1999) demonstrated that the freshwater mussel, *Diplodon chilensis*, could be used to reduce total algal biomass and proposed their potential use to reduce the hypereutrophic impact of salmon aquaculture. In addition to the benefits of total particle removal by bivalves, the surface of bivalve shells serve as substrates for decomposers (e.g., nitrifying bacteria) that can help sustain water quality in natural aquatic systems, aquaculture facilities, and closed or flow-through aquaria. In one study in research ponds conducted with *Ruditapes philippinarium* and *Crassostrea gigas*, Kohata and coworkers (2003) demonstrated that bivalve presence and filtration markedly reduced total organic load.

Bivalves as Bioindicators

As suspension feeders, bivalves ingest and accumulate numerous compounds in the water column. Some compounds are metabolized by hepatopancreatic enzymes and other processes, with the metabolites being excreted. Other compounds are accumulated without processing, with some reaching steady state with the surrounding water or sediment. The propensity for bivalves to filter and concentrate chemicals and pathogens has prompted their extensive use for environmental monitoring. Bivalve harvesting and chemical assessment was the backbone of the National Mussel Watch Program in the United States (Beliaeff et al., 1997) and of similar programs in other regions (Sericano, 2000). Bivalves have been used to monitor surface waters for pesticides, metals, and enteric pathogens.

Bivalve feeding in a population is induced by the presence of suitable particles for ingestion in the water column. In the absence of food being introduced in a bolus, bivalve feeding should be relatively asynchronous. At any single time in a large group of bivalves, some will be open and others will be siphoning. However, in response to a bolus of any form of environmental irritant, bivalves will close synchronously. This behavior has facilitated the development of a number of devices that are designed to measure bivalve feeding and use synchronous shell closure as an early-warning device for detecting the introduction of noxious materials into the water column.

Culture

The culture of bivalves for human consumption is a global enterprise. *Crassostrea gigas* is the predominant species in culture; more than 2.9 million tonnes are harvested annually (Rana and Immink, 1998). The techniques used for bivalve culture are quite variable based on the species being reared, regional and local differences in product preferences, local farming habits and traditions, and environmental factors that limit the range of culture alternatives. Oyster seed for culture is either collected using juvenile oyster (*spat*) collectors (Figure 7.5) that are placed in spawning areas or purchased from hatcheries. Regardless of the source, juvenile oysters ranging from approx-

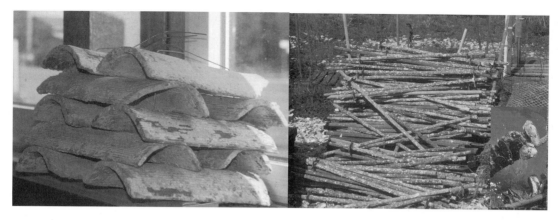

Figure 7.5. Spat collectors (tiles coated with lime, polyvinylchloride tubes, and other collectors) are used to provide substrate for juvenile oysters that are then harvested and cultured for human consumption. In the **inset**, the oysters were not removed from the spat collectors.

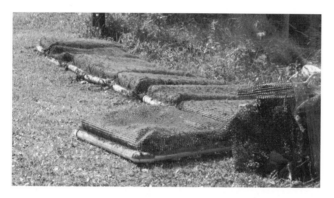

Figure 7.6. Bags used for oyster culture. Bags containing oysters can be floated in the water column by using Styrofoam floats supported on racks or suspended from ropes. Oysters are also cultured while held in tiered baskets (lanterns) or seeded directly into the benthos for bottom culture.

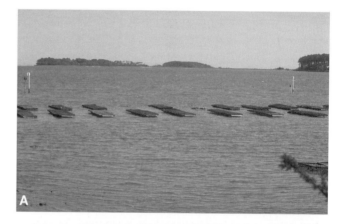

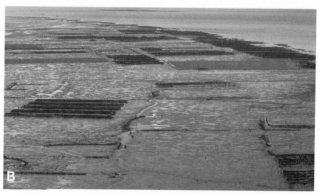

Figure 7.7. Table culture of oysters in bags. Oysters held in mesh bags are supported in the water column by rebar or polyvinylchloride racks. **A:** Eastern North Carolina. **B:** The Atlantic Coast of France. In both photos, the water has receded and the bags are readily apparent.

imately 12–25 mm are then either dispersed for bottom culture or held in the water column by using bags (Figure 7.6), lanterns, or trays (Matthiessen, 2000). Lanterns commonly used in Asia and the Pacific are strung and hung vertically in series in the water column. Bags are either wrapped around posts, suspended in the water column from a lattice of support timbers, floated on the surface, or placed on metal or plastic supports (*table culture*) (Figure 7.7). Maintenance requirements are variable and depend on the specific techniques used for grow out and environmental conditions. Local fouling with algae and other organic debris increases maintenance requirements. Oysters are harvested when they reach market size, which varies with local and regional marketing preferences. In some regions, oysters are held after harvest in either open or closed recirculating aquaria for 24 h to remove grit or debris. Oysters are also held in ponds after harvest from primary growing areas to enhance product value. In France, oysters are frequently placed in ponds prior to marketing to effect a color change induced by the presence of the diatom *Haslea ostrearia* that provides a green tint to oyster meat (Turpin et al., 2001). These animals receive a premium price in local markets. In other areas, animals

with similar green meat are discarded because there is no local market for *green oysters*. Oysters are often held in closed or open aquaria (e.g., raceways or troughs) after harvest for *depuration* (the clearing of pathogens). However, depuration is not universally successful. It may not readily remove specific pathogens such as noroviruses, the agents most frequently associated with

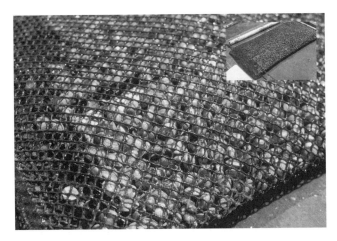

Figure 7.8. Hard clams are grown in tented bags or hard mesh bags like this one and are placed on the estuary bottom.

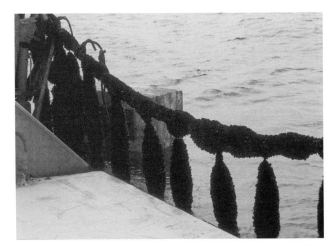

Figure 7.9. Long-line mussel culture in coastal France. Bags of juvenile mussels are suspended from long lines and harvested after the mussels mature.

human illness after oyster consumption. Alternative means of pathogen elimination, by chemical or other methods, either have not been universally effective or have not been well received by consumers.

Clams are traditionally grown using some form of bottom culture, frequently in tented bags or in mesh bags staked to the estuary bottom (Figure 7.8) (Castagna, 1985; Vaughan, 1988). Cultured clams are relatively uniform in size, and sorting is easily mechanized. In some European regions, clam culture somewhat reflects the planting of crops with tractors. Tractors are used to bury clam bags, and street-sweeper-like devices are used to harvest marketable animals. Tray culture is also used in some regions.

Blue mussels, *Mytilus* spp., are reared in bags wrapped around posts or directly on posts (*bouchot-type culture*) on the bottom of, or suspended in, the water column (Prou and Goulletquer, 2002). In some areas, newly recruited juveniles are collected on shells held in bags in intertidal areas and then transferred to deep-water locations for grow out, where they are suspended on long lines (Figure 7.9). Post culture in some areas has become highly mechanized, and amphibious vehicles have been developed that strip the bags containing market-sized mussels from posts.

Scallop culture has been locally successful in some regions. Both bay scallops and the large sea scallops have been cultured. Scallops are either reared in trays or bags or seeded on bottom leases (Rucai and Lian-chen, 1991; Grant et al., 2003). Other species of marine bivalves, such as cockles and other traditional regional species, have been cultured for human consumption. Freshwater culture historically focused on the culture of mussels for the button industry, but the advent of synthetic buttons has essentially eliminated this industry. Culture of the species previously used for button culture, however, now supports a stable market in mussel shells. The shells are sold for use in pearl culture. The nacre is used to seed pearl production in pearl oysters by placing small pieces of nacre between the inner and outer layers of shell being produced by pearl oysters.

Health Requirements

Introduction

Bivalve culture for human consumption is a global enterprise. Although the specific growth requirements of individual species vary, three universal basic requirements drive the effective selection of rearing locations: (a) water quality, (b) physical and chemical conditions that define the rearing site, and (c) adequate diet. Taken together, this makes site selection a primary factor determining the success of aquaculture leases. These requirements have been described extensively for individual species in numerous books and monographs (e.g., see Kennedy et al., 1996). We provide a few basic parameters for clinicians to consider when assessing the quality of the bivalve rearing environment.

Water Quality

Temperature, salinity, dissolved oxygen, pH, alkalinity, and hardness must reflect the specific growth requirements of the species reared. When talking with clients with problems rearing bivalves for commercial sale in aquaculture leases, ensure that they possess the needed equipment to monitor these physical parameters, or that they use a local information resource (e.g., federal or state agency, or growers' cooperative) that provides the information. Determine whether these factors were considered when the lease location was selected, and how these factors are being monitored. Has the area been evaluated for potential contaminants associated with adjacent land use? If substantial development is apparent in the area around the lease, what means are used by local agencies to monitor surface waters and potential groundwater sources? Are historical municipal, state, federal, or grower cooperative records available that provide a historical profile of the growing area? If a sudden loss of a large number of animals has occurred, could marine biotoxins be present?

In hobbyist or display closed recirculating aquaria, clinicians should determine whether the level of nitrogenous waste is routinely evaluated and how often. Are the chemicals being used to conduct these analyses up to date? Ask to see the records, if any are maintained. Does the owner understand the cycle of nitrogenous waste within closed recirculating aquaria?

Dietary Concerns

The majority of bivalve species are suspension feeders. The primary exception are the giant clams (*Tridacna* spp.). *Tridacna* can use commensal algae as a food source. The residing primary producers require well-lit aquaria, but as long as lighting is adequate, trace minerals are available, and water quality is maintained, they do reasonably well in closed recirculating aquaria. Other bivalves, however, require regular feeding with natural sources of algae, detritus, and bacteria, or whole-food supplements. Sustaining algal feeding is difficult for many hobbyists, and the failure of suspension-feeding bivalves to thrive in closed recirculating aquaria is frequently related to starvation. When talking with aquaculturists rearing commercial crops, or hobbyists, determine whether they understand the dietary requirements of the species being reared. Have phytoplankton analyses been conducted to determine the species of algae present? What is the diversity of species present? Due to the difficulty of sustaining algal cultures, display aquariums and hobbyists may be feeding a single species rather than providing a diverse diet that accommodates all of the maintenance and growth requirements of a species.

Other Considerations

Each rearing situation, whether an aquaculture lease or home aquarium, is unique due to the dynamic nature of aquatic ecosystems. Whether in live culture in an estuary or a home aquarium, additional considerations may include (a) the rearing substrate, (b) flow dynamics, and (c) site security. Some species have markedly specific substrate requirements. Grain size, organic content, chemical content, and substrate depth should be considered. The flow dynamics of a site may determine the availability of resident algae and other dietary components. Flow is a particularly important consideration for aquaculture leases and must be sufficient to ensure that delivery of algae and other dietary constituents is adequate and that waste removal is satisfactory. Large populations of bivalves held in aquaculture leases can be literally residing in their own waste if flow is not adequate for clearing the nitrogenous and solid waste from the rearing environment. An additional consideration is the security of the lease. Has any dumping been conducted at or near the site of the aquaculture lease? Has anyone placed something in the aquarium (e.g., a piece of scrap metal) that could pose a hazard to resident species?

Diagnosing Health Problems

The basic steps for clinical problem solving with bivalves are no different than the steps used by veterinarians to approach clinical problems in vertebrates. Whether the clinician is working with a single display specimen or a large captive population, a thorough history serves as the foundation, followed by visual and physical examination, tissue sampling, laboratory assessment of sampled tissues, and a review of all clinical findings. Although opportunities for pharmacological intervention are minimal, a thorough history and clinical examination can provide clues to correctable husbandry-related factors. Euthanasia and a thorough gross and histopathological examination can provide a definitive diagnosis, but the initial intent should be to provide recommendations to correct a problem without sacrificing an individual in the bivalve population being evaluated. Many bivalves, particularly freshwater bivalves, are endangered or are threatened and protected by the Endangered Species Act (see Chapter 20). When state or federally listed species are involved, euthanasia may not be an option. Consequently, the clinician will have to rely solely on clinical history, physical examination, and a review of water quality and other environmental factors to make recommendations for resolving a problem. A recently deceased specimen may be available for histopathological evaluation, but decomposition is rapid and there may be little viable tissue for preservation, processing, and examination.

History: Origin, Holding Environment, and Transport

The oral clinical history that can be provided by aquaculturists responsible for the care of bivalves is generally limited. A thorough history about the origin of the animals should be obtained (Table 7.1). This is particularly important when a private aquaculturist is involved and the animals being evaluated are freshwater bivalves. At least 70 of the estimated 300 species in the family Unionidae in North America are listed as federally endangered and are protected by the Endangered Species Act. As already noted, these animals cannot be sacrificed for necropsy and histopathological evaluation without a special permit.

Clinical History

History taking for bivalve populations must be tailored to address the particular habitat: surface waters, aquaculture lease, closed or open recirculating holding facility for harvested crops, or individual or large display aquaria. The basic elements, however, are similar, focused on a description of the population or individual, its basic location and habitat, and the temporal course of the health problem being evaluated. Is the animal a freshwater, estuarine, or marine species? What is the holding or rearing environment? Is the animal a representative of a larger cohort (aquaculture crop or natural bed) or a single display specimen? Are other species or potential predators present? Were multiple animals collected for examination? Are animals being held at other locations experiencing similar problems (e.g., different aquaculture leases)? Were the animals collected in the same location? For animals harvested from natural systems, or aquaculture leases, what is the character of adjacent land use (e.g. agricultural, industrial, or residential)? Are there

Table 7.1.   Basic questions about a bivalve's origin, original holding, and transport

Question	Utility
Was the animal captive reared in a hatchery or wild caught?	Captive-reared animals may be less likely to be experiencing pathogen-associated illnesses but may lack innate resistance to local pathogens.
	Captive-reared animals held in closed recirculating systems may have experienced extended periods of poor water quality.
How long has the animal been in captivity?	If the animal was recently collected, an infectious agent of wild origin may be more likely.
	The animal may not be accustomed to the captive-rearing environment.
How long has the animal been in the current aquarium?	The animal may not have been appropriately acclimated to the rearing environment when transferred from the wild or prior rearing environment.
	If transport was recent, transport conditions may have been less than optimum.
Has the animal been transported recently?	New environmental conditions may be markedly different: salinity, temperature, pH, hardness, and dissolved oxygen saturation.
If the animal was previously held in captivity, was it a flow-through or closed recirculating system?	Flow-through systems may subject captive animals to pathogens and contaminants.
If the animal was wild caught, how was it collected?	Injury or damage may have occurred during collection and transport.
Was the bivalve out of water for an extended period?	There are marked species differences in the tolerance to periods of air emersion.
For hatchery-reared animals, were there prior health problems?	It could be the perpetuation of a prior health problem.
If wild caught, what is the animal's geographic origin?	There can be marked geographic and regional differences in pathogen distribution, based on the environmental conditions needed for their growth.
	The problem could be due to transboundary pathogens (foreign-animal pathogens)

potential point sources of anthropogenic contamination? How were the animals collected (e.g., type of gear)? How were the animals transported? Thoroughness is often the key to diagnostic success. For oysters harvested and sold in the United States for human consumption, there should be chain of custody information documenting the point of collection, date of collection, and the individual that harvested the animals.

A few basic questions focused on the visual description of the animal's behavior can provide an impression of the severity of the health problem. These initial queries should focus on an individual animal's feeding behavior, valve activity, and physical appearance. When a larger group of animals is involved, an assessment of the synchrony of valve activity can provide some helpful clues. For clams and other bivalves with a foot and some degree of mobility, movement patterns may also be helpful. After a review of the primary problem identified by the owner (Table 7.2), researcher, or keeper in a display aquarium, a complete review of the aquaria is essential.

The primary presenting complaint when no deaths have occurred will generally be a delayed response to feeding, or delayed closure after the animal is disturbed. Bivalves should begin siphoning shortly after food is introduced unless there is some other chemical or physical disruption to its habitat. Valve closure is generally rapid in response to any physical disturbance or the introduction of a noxious chemical. If more than one animal is present, even if it is a different species, the majority of individuals should respond by siphoning if appropriate food is introduced.

Unfortunately, the first recognition of a clinical problem is often an empty shell resulting from the death and decomposition of an animal. Your physical examination should begin with the shells of any animals that have died and a visual examination of the external surface. The shell exterior should be examined for erosions, holes, and organisms. The interior of the shell should be examined for discoloration, erosion, and tracts and tunnels through the nacre. If the animal is a freshwater mussel, and the aquarist does not have a strong background in freshwater mollusk taxonomy, the shell should be retained for taxonomic evaluation by a malacologist to ensure it is not a state or federally listed species.

Aquatic systems are dynamic and complex, reflecting the interactions of all biotic and abiotic components. Water quality that meets the basic life-sustaining requirements of a particular species is the primary ingredient for success when rearing aquatic species in closed aquaria. It is also the primary target of a veterinary assessment of the bivalve-rearing environment.

Using Hemolymph to Assess Health

Hemolymph collection and analysis for pathogen detection has been a routine component of the health assessment of oysters for decades (Ford, 1986; Yanick and Heath, 2000) (Figure 7.10). Procedures for hemolymph collection have also been adapted for freshwater mussels, and routine hemolymph evaluation may play a role in assessing the health, conservation, and use of mussels as environmental sentinels. Sample collection technique

Table 7.2. Primary clinical history and physical examination of bivalve health

Siphoning/feeding	Does the animal begin to siphon within 1 min of feed being placed in the water?
	Has the duration of siphoning changed?
	How often does the animal siphon?
	Are the valves continually closed?
Response to tactile contact	Does the shell close when the animal is touched or disturbed?
	How quickly does it respond: immediately, delayed, not at all?
Valve resilience (turgor)	Do the valves gape and remain open?
	Can the valves be easily parted?
Mobility (for bivalves with a foot)	Has the animal's movement within the aquaria increased or decreased?
	Has another species moved the bivalve (in aquaria with multiple species)?
Growth at leading edge of valves	Is new valve growth evident?
Examination of shell surface	
External surface	Are there erosions, holes, discolorations, or epiphytic organisms (e.g., oyster drills or boring sponges)?
Internal surface (nacre)	Are there discolorations, holes erosions, tunnels, or tracts?
	If tracts through the nacre are apparent, does a hole extend to the exterior surface?

Table 7.3. Reference range hemolymph values for the freshwater mussel, *Elliptio complanata*

Parameter	Number	Range
Weight (g)	n = 380	18.8–104.6
Cell count (cells/µL)	n = 377	250–2300
Ammonia (µmol/L)	n = 380	<10–138
AST (U/L)	n = 374	<4–38
Bicarbonate (mmol/L)	n = 375	<5–12
Calcium (mg/dL)	n = 375	13.1–23.7
Glucose (mg/dL)	n = 372	<2–0.77
Magnesium (mg/dL)	n = 374	1.6–3.8
Phosphorus (mg/dL)	n = 374	<0.3–0.9
Protein (mg/dL)	n = 378	19.5–142.8

Adapted from Gustafson et al. (2005b).

and reference ranges for hemolymph of *Elliptio complanata*, a widely distributed freshwater mussel species east of the Mississippi, have been developed (Gustafson et al., 2005a and 2005b) (Table 7.3). Corporeau and Auffret (2003) developed markers in oyster hemolymph for quantifying stress-protein activity. Hemolymph has also been used for quantifying cholinesterase activity in scallops (Owen et al., 2002), vitellins in freshwater mussels (Gagne et al., 2001), immune function in mussels (Luengen et al., 2004), phenoloxidase activity in several species of marine bivalves (Deaton et al., 1999), and to detect and quantify numerous other compounds in a variety of bivalve species. Additional work is needed to make hemolymph evaluation a routine tool for veterinarians. Species-specific reference ranges are needed for hemolymph compounds. Hemolymph could also serve as a nonlethal means of obtaining cells as a source of DNA for genetic analysis.

Diagnostic Pathology

Disease surveillance as well as diagnostics for specific disease problems are usually performed by histopathology or a combination of histopathology and assays for specific pathogens.

Although this chapter is not intended to provide an exhaustive treatment of bivalve histopathology, we discuss recommended techniques for routine sampling, preservation, and submission of tissues, using examples of several major bivalve diseases.

Gross Examination of Specimens

Prior to opening a bivalve, examine the valves for external damage or for evidence of predation. Standard meristics taken at the time of examination include length, width, and height (depth) measurements. Check the outermost edges of the valves for evidence of new shell growth. Prior to opening, bivalves can be relaxed and euthanized by submersion in water containing tricaine methanesulfonate (MS-222) (300 mg/L). Bivalves need to be opened very carefully to prevent personal injury and damage to the specimen. A pair of Kevlar, heavy canvas or leather gloves should be worn to prevent injury when opening bivalves. Shucking knives can be purchased commercially. With the bivalve held pressed down on a hard surface, the shucking knife should be inserted into the space between the valves to sever the hinged ligament (Figure 7.11). As the valves are separating, the instrument can be carefully used to pry them apart and then to cut the adductor muscles, holding the valves closed. A scalpel, if used carefully, can also be used to sever the adductor muscle and is generally less disruptive to internal tissues.

After opening a bivalve, the initial impression should be that the visceral mass fills the mantle cavity. In healthy animals, the gills should glisten and have a uniform structure. Serous atrophy is associated with inadequate and/or poor nutrition, or with wasting caused by chronic disease conditions, and is readily apparent when contrasting a healthy animal with a sick one. After careful gross examination of the specimen, the remaining adductor muscle, if still intact (second adductor, if present), should be severed as close to its attachment on the shell as possible with a sharp blade, taking care not to damage the internal tissue. The rectum may then be excised with scissors and placed into an appropriate culture tube containing transport media for microbiology, if needed. The soft tissues should then be placed on a clean cutting board for dissection using a sharp razor blade or scalpel. The first transverse cut is made at the junction of the

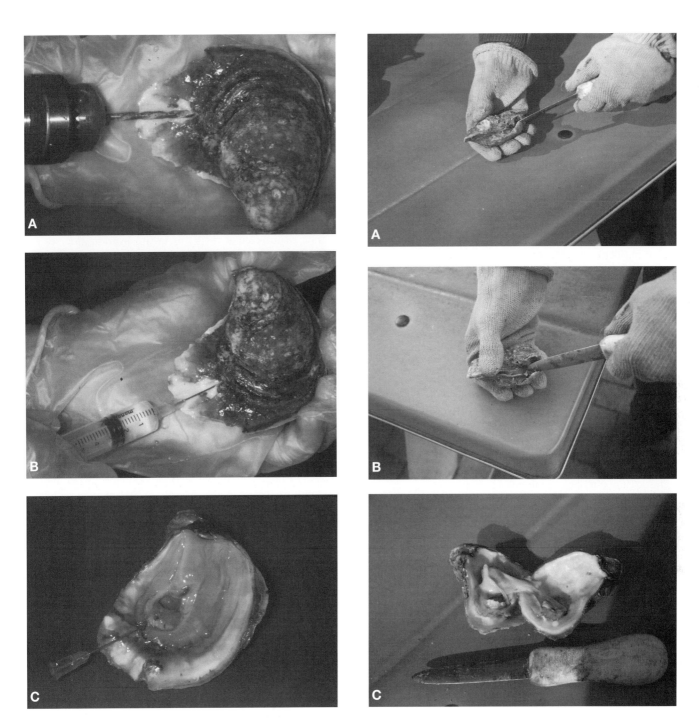

Figure 7.10A–C.   Procedure for harvesting hemolymph from oysters: Kevlar, leather, or thick canvas gloves are recommended. A small hole is drilled through the shell, and a small-gauge needle is passed through the adductor muscle into the pericardial sinus.

Figure 7.11A–C.   Procedure for opening an oyster for gross necropsy and sampling tissues for histopathology. Kevlar, leather, or thick canvas gloves are recommended. A shucking knife, or another steel utensil (e.g., a screwdriver), is placed at the beak between the two valves, turned to separate the valves, and slid forward to cut the adductor muscle. In species with two adductor muscles, the second adductor muscle is then cut with the knife or a scalpel blade. The valves are then separated, and the viscera examined in situ.

labial palps and the gills, across the body through the digestive diverticula. The second cut is made 4 to 5 mm from and approximately parallel to the first. Third and fourth cuts or more, as needed, create additional approximately 5-mm-thick tissue segments and enable microscopic examination of all tissues (National Marine Fisheries Service, 1983; Howard, et al., 2004). It is important not to make the samples too thick, because fixatives such as formalin may not penetrate to the inside of the tissue in time to prevent significant postmortem autolysis. Conversely, care must be taken not to create tissue artifacts by attempting to cut unfixed specimens too small. Use of a new, very sharp blade will help. Handle specimens with fine, toothed forceps to avoid crushed artifacts.

The irregular, anterior portion containing the labial palps is placed in filtered seawater or other appropriate isotonic solution and used to make fresh squash preparations for parasite examination. As with gill or fin clips from fish, examination of fresh squash preparations is an important part of the diagnostic regimen, because many parasites can become detached and washed away during fixation and histological processing.

The 5-mm-thick samples are placed in appropriate fixative, such as Helly's, and the remaining portion below the last cut is saved frozen for future diagnostics. Small glass or plastic screw-cap vials are useful for transport and/or mailing of diagnostic specimens. An adequate amount of fixative should always be used. A good rule of thumb is to use about 10 parts fixative to 1 part tissue. Some diagnosticians may prefer that bivalves be submitted whole, i.e., without transection, so that gross examination may be done prior to sectioning. Always contact your diagnostic laboratory before submitting specimens.

If bacterial cultures are not required, an alternative method for fixation is to open the shell slightly and inject the specimen with fixative before transport. The diagnostician may then fully open the shell for examination and sectioning for histopathology (National Marine Fisheries Service, 1983; Howard et al., 2004).

Tissue Imprints

Tissue imprints of mantle, gill, or digestive gland can sometimes provide a simple, rapid, and inexpensive means of identification of several protozoan parasites (e.g., the genera *Marteilia*, *Haplosporidium*, *Bonamia*, and *Mikrocytos*). A section of the target organ is taken, and excess water is removed using blotting paper. The section is then put on a slide, fixed with 70% methanol for about 2–3 min, and stained with any commercially available cytological blood-staining kit. Sections are then gently rinsed with tap water and dried completely, and a coverslip is applied using a synthetic resin medium. At this point, slides can be microscopically examined for the presence of the target parasite.

Fixation

Proper fixation is critical to obtain the most benefit from histopathological examination of bivalve specimens. Helly's fluid with zinc chloride in place of mercuric chloride has been the fixative of choice because it gives good cellular detail and preserves the nucleoplasm of the nuclei of ova and granules of secretory cells and amebocytes (see Chapter 19).

Davidson's fixative, which is also used, can be prepared with filtered seawater for marine bivalves such as oysters. Dietrich's fixative provides good cellular detail and little shrinkage or cell distortion. However, like any acetic acid-containing fixative, these two cause loss of the nucleoplasm from ova, as well as loss of secretions and granules. Ten percent neutral buffered formalin or buffered zinc formalin can be used and are readily available, but they do not produce as high a quality section as the other fixatives described. Carson's solution has been used by some workers when later examination by transmission electron microscopy is a consideration (National Marine Fisheries Service, 1983).

Other, more RNA-friendly fixatives are being developed as more advanced molecular diagnostic techniques such as polymerase chain reaction (PCR) or in situ hybridization see increased use in the diagnosis of marine animal diseases. The recommendations by RNAlater (Ambion, Austin, TX) for properly preserving RNA for genomic probe analysis in histological sections are described on their Web site and noted in Table 7.4.

Additional Diagnostic Assays

A variety of new diagnostic assays have been developed that increase the speed and accuracy of pathogen detection and serve as valuable tools in the diagnosis of bivalve diseases. PCR-based assays are now available for the detection of *Marteilia refringens* (Pernas et al., 2001), *Haplosporidium nelsoni*, and other bivalve diseases, but these assays are not readily available to veterinarians unless they are working in a region with strong bivalve-industry laboratory support services. Consequently, to make a presumptive diagnosis, the majority of veterinarians will have to rely on their clinical problem-solving skills, procedures like wet mounts (as already noted), and histopathological review of harvested tissues.

Control and Treatment of Diseases

The therapeutic armamentarium of veterinarians for treating bivalve diseases is rather limited. Since many bivalves are reared in open-water leases, bivalve crops are continuously at risk of exposure to pathogens introduced by native fauna. In addition, bivalve farmers have little control of environmental factors that could potentially predispose bivalves to disease. Aquaculturists rearing bivalve stock for human consumption or pearl production raise animals in high density. High-density monoculture produces conditions that accelerate the transmission of introduced pathogens. Efforts to mitigate these problems begin prior to the introduction of any bivalve seed for culture. Careful site selection is essential and should involve consideration of

1. Flow dynamics and nutrient availability
2. Presence or absence of predators (e.g., oyster drill)
3. Physical environmental factors that facilitate or retard growth (e.g., salinity)
4. Presence of native fauna and potential pathogens
5. Water quality
6. Adjacent land use

Table 7.4.   Fixatives

RNA-friendly
349 mL 37% Formaldehyde
407 mL 95% Ethanol
222 mL Distilled water (it will take ca. 22 mL of ammonium
    hydroxide to bring the pH to 6–7)
*pH to ca. 6.5 with concentrated (29%) ammonium hydroxide

Final volume = 1 L

Helly's Solution
Zinc chloride	1000 g
Potassium dichromate	500 g
Distilled water	20 L

Add 5 mL of 37%–40% formaldehyde per 100 mL of fixative, just prior to use.

Dietrich's fixative
Distilled water	9000 mL
95% Ethyl alcohol	4500 mL
Glacial acetic acid	300 mL

Davidson's fixative
95% Ethyl alcohol	330 mL
37% Formaldehyde	1500 mL
Glacial acetic acid	115 mL
Distilled (or tap) water**	335 mL

*pH should be determined by using pH paper and not an electronic meter because the alcohol content of the fixative inhibits an accurate pH reading from being obtained with the latter device. From Hasson et al. (1997).
**Filtered seawater may be substituted for use with marine species.

Hatchery operators producing bivalve stock for grow out have substantial control of the hatchery environment. The use of sound biosecurity measures in the hatchery can reduce the likelihood that a hatchery operator will experience problems such as larval vibriosis, a disease affecting oyster larvae (Elston, 1984; Ford and Tripp, 1996). However, bivalve farmers rarely practice simple biosecurity practices used by other agricultural industries. Prudent measures such as the quarantining of new stock offer a degree of protection from the introduction of pathogens. At times, entire industries have been placed at risk by pathogens introduced with nonnative species or by the introduction of cohorts from other rearing areas.

Veterinary intervention begins with the accurate diagnosis of bivalve diseases and a clear understanding of the dynamics of disease transmission. At times, depopulation and restocking after a washout period is the sole control option. However, a variety of therapeutic measures have been attempted. Efforts to reduce the risk of disease focus on alternative rearing practices such as altering planting schedules (e.g., in juvenile oyster disease) and harvesting schedules (e.g., in disease caused by *Haplosporidium nelsoni*). Efforts to control infections with *Perkinsus marinus*, a protozoan that has devastated oyster production of *Crassostrea virginica* along the U.S. Atlantic Coast, have focused on depopulation, avoiding the introduction of

stock from infected areas, and abandoning leases for 1–2 years after depopulation (Andrews and Ray, 1988). Chemical treatments have proved ineffective (Ford and Tripp, 1996), and emersion of the animals in low-salinity water has resulted in transient benefits.

In closed aquaria, the likelihood of infection with infectious agents is minimal unless infected individuals are introduced. The principal factors contributing to the loss of bivalves in captivity are poor diet and starvation.

Diets should be carefully selected to meet the particle-utilization capabilities and nutritional needs of individual species. Efforts should be encouraged for aquarists to select a diverse diet for the species and avoid feeding a monoculture of algae (Beck and Neves, 2003). Dietary failures have been most apparent in efforts to rear juvenile freshwater mussels and sustain adult freshwater mussels in captivity.

Selected Diseases

The list of pathogens affecting bivalves is extensive, and a comprehensive review of bivalve pathogens is beyond the scope of this chapter. Clinicians, however, can benefit from a wealth of online Internet resources (Office International des Epizooties [OIE], 2002), digitized libraries, monographs, and book chapters (e.g., Bower et al., 1994; Ford and Tripp, 1996) focused on bivalve diseases. We present examples of three diseases of international relevance to commercial bivalve culture—marteiliosis and bonamiosis—that have had global importance to the oyster industry, and a disease of clams—brown ring disease.

Marteiliosis

Marteiliosis (aka Aber disease, digestive gland disease, or QX disease) is a disease of bivalves that is associated with infection with organisms of the genus *Marteilia* (phylum Paramyxea). Two species—*M. refringens* and *M. sydney*—have contributed to substantial economic losses within the global oyster industry. Another member of the genus—*M. maurini*—has been reported to affect *Mytilus galloprovincialis* and *Mytilus edulis*. Studies by Le Roux and coworkers (2001) suggest it is phylogenetically distinct from *M. refringens*. Other *Marteilia* spp. (*M. lengehi* and *M. christenseni*) have been detected (OIE, 2002). Both *M. refringens* and *M. sydney* are considered reportable diseases by the OIE.

Marteilia refringens has a broad host range and has been observed in European oysters (*Ostrea edulis*), Foveaux Strait oysters (*Ostrea chilensis*), American or Eastern oysters (*Crassostrea virginica*) when reared in France, common blue mussels (*Mytilus edulis*), and common cockles (*Cardium edule*), as well as other bivalves (OIE, 2002). *Marteilia refringens* devastated *O. edulis* production in France (Heral, 1989; Legraien and Crosaz, 1999), has been detected throughout Europe in the southern United Kingdom, France, Spain, Portugal, Italy, Croatia, and Greece, and has been reported in Morocco (Zrncic et al., 2001; OIE, 2002). The host range of *M. sydney* is comparatively narrow, and the pathogen has been detected in Sydney rock oysters

(*Saccostrea glomerata* [= *commercialis*]), as well as black-lip oysters (*Saccostrea echinata*) and Thailand rock oysters (*Saccostrea forskali*) (Hine and Thorne, 2000). *Marteilia sydney* has affected oyster production predominantly in Queensland, New South Wales, and Western Australia.

Marteilia enters the host through the epithelia of the palps and gills. The protozoan initially develops and proliferates in the stomach, intestine, and digestive-tract epithelia (Grizel, 1974). Clinical signs are not readily apparent until late stages of infection and are characterized by poor growth, poor body-condition indices, gaping, and eventual death (Figueras and Montes, 1988). Gross pathology includes apparent resorption of the gonads and pale yellow-brown discoloration of the digestive glands that is associated with infiltration and sporulation of the parasite. Refractile bodies with sporonts can be readily detected in wet smears and tissue imprints (Figure 7.12, Color Plate 7.12) of the digestive gland. Sporonts progressively increase in size from 5 to 8 to 40 μm. *Marteilia* spp. are readily detected during histopathology examination of hematoxylin–eosin (H&E)-stained sections of the digestive glands (Bower and McGladdery, 2003) (Figure 7.13, Color Plate 7.13). A variety of molecular techniques such as in situ hybridization and PCR–restriction fragment length polymorphism have been developed to detect *Marteilia* spp. infections (Le Roux et al., 1999; Kleeman and Adlard, 2000; Kleeman et al., 2002).

Although the life cycle of *Marteilia* spp. within oysters has been well characterized and documented ultrastructurally by transmission electron microscopy, aspects of the *Marteilia* life cycle remain unclear. Direct transmission from infected to noninfected oysters has proven unsuccessful. Studies by Berthe and coworkers (1998) suggest that an intermediate host may be required for transmission. *Marteilia refringens* has been detected in the copepod *Paracartia grani*, and the copepod could play a role in sustaining transmission of the pathogen (Audemard et al., 2002).

In Bretagne, France, initial infections with *M. refringens* apparently occur between May and August during the first year of planting and over winter (Figueras and Montes, 1988). Deaths are generally first observed during the spring of the second year of growth in May and continue through August.

No specific control measures for *Marteilia* spp. infection have been developed, but efforts to develop *S. glomerata* populations resistant to the parasite look promising (Nell and Hand, 2003).

Bonamiosis

Bonamiosis (microcell disease, hemocyte disease, and winter mortality) is a disease of oysters that is associated with the haplosporidians *Bonamia ostreae*, *B. exitiosus*, and *Mikrocytos roughleyi* (Bower and McGladdery, 2003). Marked variability in bivalve genus and species susceptibility is apparent (Grizel et al., 1988; Culloty et al., 1999). *Bonamia ostreae* has been observed predominantly in oysters in the genus *Ostrea* (*O. edulis*, *O. conchaphila*, *O. puelchan*, *O. angasi*, and *O. chilensis*). Infections with *Bonamia* have also been observed in New Zealand flat oysters (*Tiostrea chilensis*) (Hine et al., 2002), and a *Bonamia*-like parasite has been detected in Suminoe oysters (*Crassostrea rivularis*) in France (Cochennec-Laureau et al., 2003). The disease

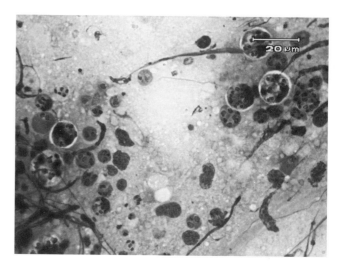

Figure 7.12.   Tissue imprint from *Ostrea edulis* infected with the protozoan, *Marteilia refringens*, the agent of Aber disease. An identifying characteristic of *Marteilia refringens* is the brightly eosinophilic inclusions or refringent bodies within the sporangia.

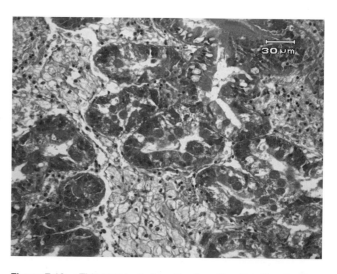

Figure 7.13.   This histological section from the digestive gland of the oyster *Ostrea edulis* illustrates the severe damage that *Marteilia refringens* can inflict on the host, particularly when large numbers of spores are released simultaneously from the digestive-gland epithelium. Multifocally, there is extensive necrosis and loss of digestive epithelial cells; the remaining cells are often swollen and have microvilli loss at the lumenal surface. Tubule lumens contain necrotic debris and scattered sloughed, swollen cells, many of which are infected with *M. refringens*. Hematoxylin–eosin stain.

has a very wide geographic range, affecting oysters in North America, Europe and Australia. *Bonamia exitiosus* and *Mikrocytos roughleyi*, are only prevalent in coastal waters of Australia and New Zealand; infections with *B. exitiosus* have been observed in the flat oyster, the Foveaux Strait oyster and *O. denselammellosa*. *Mikrocytos roughleyi* has been observed in the Sydney rock oyster (*Saccostrea glomerata*) in New South Wales (Australia) (Cochennec-Laureau et al., 2003).

Economic losses associated with bonamiosis can be profound, with mortalities reaching 80% among oysters infected with *M. roughleyi* (Smith et al., 2000) and over 90% in oysters infected with *B. exitiosus* (Bower and McGladdery, 2003). In France, production of European flat oysters was decimated by infections first with *Marteilia refringens* and then with *B. ostreae* (Boudry et al., 1996). A vibrant coastal economy driven by the oyster industry rapidly collapsed, resulting in the loss of thousands of jobs. *Bonamia* spp. infections are considered reportable by the OIE (2002).

In the Northern Hemisphere, *B. ostreae* reaches peak prevalence in the fall. Although infections can be detected in the first year of growth in areas with endemic *B. ostreae*, the prevalence of infection and mortality is markedly higher during the second year of growth (Robert et al., 1991; Culloty and Mulcahy, 1996). Hine and coworkers (2002) have suggested that coinfection with other protozoa may increase the likelihood of infection with *B. exitiosus* and observed pathology in *O. chilensis*. Both *M. refringens* and *B. ostreae* are endemic throughout portions of the Western European North Atlantic Coast, and duel infection may enhance the likelihood of *O. edulis* mortality. In studies conducted with *O. chilensis* infected with *B. exitiosus*, mortality was highest in infected oysters kept in close confinement in troughs, after transient exposure to extreme hot or cold temperatures, and when held at high salinities. Infection intensity was greater among females and after spawning (Hine et al., 2002).

Infection with *B. ostreae* and other *Bonamia* spp. is characterized by an initial decline in body condition. Gross pathology may not be readily apparent in all infected animals, but discoloration of the digestive glands, mantle, and gills may be evident in heavily infected individuals.

Bonamia spp. are distinguishable in stained hemolymph smears, tissue imprints (Figure 7.14, Color Plate 7.14), and H&E tissue sections (Figure 7.15, Color Plate 7.15) (OIE, 2002). Massive tissue hemocyte infiltration provides a point of reference and focal point for observation of the parasite in the digestive gland and other organs (Cochennec-Laureau et al., 2003). *Bonamia* spp. are 2–5 μm in size, whereas *M. roughleyi* parasites are smaller (1–2 μm) with a large nucleus (1 μm) (Diggles et al., 2003). Histologically, *M. roughleyi* parasites are characterized by bipolar or eccentric nucleolar structures and a cytoplasmatic vacuole (OIE, 2002; Bower and McGladdery, 2003). Comparisons of light-microscopic techniques for detecting *Bonamia* spp. have indicated that the organism is more readily observed in heart-tissue imprints than in standard H&E preparations and imprints of other organisms (Diggles et al., 2003). Monolayers prepared from oyster hemolymph have proven to be the most sensitive means of detecting the protozoan through light-microscopic methods that would be readily available to practicing veterinarians. In situ hybridization (Carnegie et al., 2003; Diggles et al., 2003), monoclonal antibodies for pathogen detection (Hine, 1996), and PCR-based assays have been developed that provide an effective means of specific diagnosis (Adlard and Lester, 1995; Carnegie et al., 2000; Bower and McGladdery, 2003).

Bonamia-free oysters placed in close proximity to infected oysters develop patent infections with *B. ostreae*. Consequently, depopulation and later restocking have been consistently at-

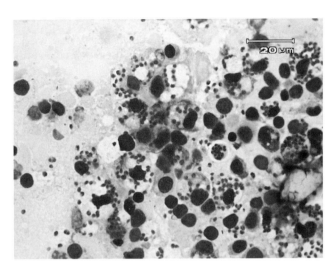

Figure 7.14. Tissue imprint from the oyster *Ostrea edulis* shows hemocytes infected with multiple cells of *Bonamia ostreae*. This parasite is round, deeply basophilic, and measures 2–3 μm in diameter. A stained direct smear (cytological preparation) is often the best way to identify specific parasite morphology, since there are minimal processing artifacts when compared with histological preparations.

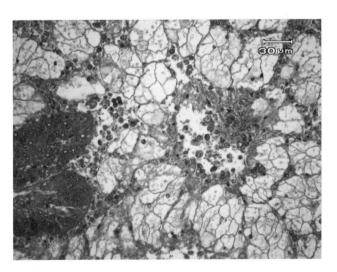

Figure 7.15. Histological section of the digestive gland of the oyster *Ostrea edulis*. The vesicular connective tissue surrounding the two digestive-gland tubules at the *left* is infiltrated with granular hemocytes, many of which are infected with multiple cells of *Bonamia ostreae*. Bonamiosis is characterized by heavy hemocytic infiltration especially around the stomach and digestive gland, but also may involve the gonad and gills. Hematoxylin–eosin stain.

tempted to limit the spread of *B. ostreae* and other *Bonamia* species. Early harvesting at 15–18 months of production (Montes et al., 2003) and subtidal culture (Bower and McGladdery, 2003) have been suggested to minimize the impact of *Bonamia* spp. infection on oyster lease productivity and profitability. Hervio and coworkers (1995) observed that the progeny of oysters that survived laboratory challenge with *B. ostreae* were more likely to survive infection. Breeding programs focused on the development of *B. ostrea*-resistant *O. edulis* stocks have been implemented to enhance the likelihood of successfully bringing cultured *O. edulis* to market in endemic areas (Baud et al., 1997). Hand and coworkers (1998) observed enhanced survival of triploid Sydney rock oysters (*Saccostrea commercialis*) grown in areas with endemic *Mikrocytos roughleyi*. Mortality among triploids was nearly two-thirds less than that observed among intact *S. commercialis*.

Brown Ring Disease

This is a disease of clams and has been observed in *Ruditapes philippinarum* and *R. decussatus* and associated with the presence of *Vibrio tapetis* (*Vibrio* P1) (Paillard and Maes, 1994). Brown ring disease was initially recognized in France in 1987 in *R. philippinarum* imported from the United States (Paillard and Maes, 1994) but has not been reported in the United States. Since its initial detection, the disease has been reported in Spain, Portugal, and England (Castro et al., 1997; Allam et al., 2000a).

Vibrio tapetis is transmitted from clam to clam (Martinez-Manzanares et al., 1998). Infected animals generally develop distinctive brown (conchiolin) deposits between the shell edge and the pallial line (Paillard and Maes, 1994). The *Vibrio* adheres to the periostracal lamina, disrupting periostracum production, and penetrates into the clam's extrapallial space, from where it invades the soft tissues (Allam et al., 2002). Proliferation of the *Vibrio* disrupts homeostasis, growth, body condition, and organ function (Paillard and Maes, 1994). Infected individuals develop a hemocytosis and increased lysozyme activity as hemocyte abundance apparently increases in both hemolymph and extrapallial fluid in response to infection (Allam et al., 2000a, 2000b). Infected clams may be more susceptible to other pathogens and less resilient to environmental extremes. Not all affected clams die of *V. tapetis* infection (Castro et al., 1997), and there are apparently species-specific differences in clam susceptibility (Allam et al., 2001), as well as differences in *V. tapetis*-strain infectivity (Novoa et al., 1998). Differences in resistance between host species and between different groups of *R. philippinarum* seem to be associated with differences in the phagocytic response of granular hemocytes to infection (Allam et al., 2001).

Brown ring disease can be diagnosed by examining the inner shell for the characteristic brown ring around the mantle edge that is associated with a disruption of periostracum production (Paillard and Maes, 1994). *Vibrio* presence can be detected by using routine bacteriologic methods. A variety of molecular tools have been developed for detecting *V. tapetis* and differentiating *V. tapetis* strains (Romalde et al., 2002).

Environmental factors may play a role in the response of clams to the pathogen. In one study, Reid and coworkers (2003) found that hemocyte count and mortality were significantly greater in experimentally infected *R. philippinarum* held at 40 ppt salinity than in *R. philippinarum* held at 20 ppt. Recovery of clams from infection with the *Vibrio* may also be supported by

higher ambient temperatures (Bower and McGladdery, 2003). Few effective specific control measures have been documented to minimize the economic effect of brown ring disease. Selection of culture sites in areas without disease may reduce the likelihood of infection, but *Vibrio* species are fairly ubiquitous in estuarine and marine environments.

Other Health Problems

Bivalves are plagued by a variety of pathogens, so the list of bivalve diseases is lengthy. The selected diseases already noted are of economic relevance, and the general bias has been to explore the diseases of commercially important bivalves. Bivalves are also challenged by the presence of predators and species like oyster drills (*Urosalpinx cinere*) and *Polydora* that damage bivalve shells (Avault, 1998; Mortensen et al., 2000) and potentially enhance their susceptibility to infection and disease. Our knowledge of health problems affecting other bivalves (e.g., freshwater mussels), however, is in its infancy because of the absence of much commercial incentive for initiating the research.

Neoplasia

A variety of neoplasias have been observed in a number of bivalve species (Mix et al., 1977; Yevich and Barszcz, 1977; Housem et al., 1998). The majority of these are hemolymph in origin. A recent article (Barber, 2004) describes two important forms of neoplasia (disseminated neoplasia and gonadal neoplasia) in a number of commercially important bivalves of the U.S. East and West Coasts. In disseminated neoplasia, circulating hemocytes can be several times larger than normal cells and are anaplastic (Barber, 2004). The small basophilic cells characteristic of gonadal neoplasia in soft-shell clams (*Mya arenaria*) and hard-shell clams (*Mercenaria* spp.) can be aggressive, invading adjacent organs and structures (Barber, 2004). Most individuals exhibiting gonadal neoplasia (also known as *germinomas*) are female (Barber, 2004). The table in Appendix 1 contains a list of bivalve neoplasms documented by the Registry of Tumors in Lower Animals (RTLA).

Additional Health Resources

A variety of Internet resources (e.g., OIE, 2002) make information about the species distribution, geographic distribution, and health effects of specific bivalve pathogens readily available to veterinary practitioners and bivalve biologists. A simple search for key terms (bivalve, diseases, and specific bivalve species) yields a wealth of information that is routinely updated. However, because Web-site addresses change frequently, their inclusion in this chapter has been generally avoided. In addition, we suggest that practitioners relying on the Internet as a source of bivalve health information seek their information from university and agency Web sites that reflect the recent overview of peer-reviewed biomedical literature.

References

Adlard, R.D., and R.J.G. Lester. 1995. Development of a diagnostic test for *Mikrocytos roughleyi*, the aetiological agent of Australian winter mortality of the commercial rock oyster, *Saccostrea commercialis* (Iredale & Roughley). Journal of Fish Diseases 18:609–614.

Aldridge, D.W., B.S. Payne, and A.C. Miller. 1987. The effects of intermittent exposure to suspended solids and turbulence on three species of freshwater mussels. Environmental Pollution 45:17–28.

Allam, B., C. Paillard, A. Howard, and M. Le Pennec. 2000a. Isolation of the pathogen *Vibrio tapetis* and defense parameters in brown ring diseased Manila clams *Ruditapes philippinarum* cultivated in England. Diseases of Aquatic Organisms 41:105–113.

Allam, B., C. Paillard, and M. Auffret. 2000b. Alternations in hemolymph and extrapallial fluid parameters in the Manila clam, *Ruditapes philippinarum*, challenged with the pathogen *Vibrio tapetis*. Journal of Invertebrate Pathology 76:63–69.

Allam, B., A. Ashton-Alcox, and S.E. Ford. 2001. Haemocyte parameters associated with resistance to brown ring disease in *Ruditapes* spp. clams. Developmental and Comparative Immunology 25:365–375.

Allam, B., C. Paillard, and S.E. Ford. 2002. Pathogenicity of *Vibrio tapetis*, the etiological agent of brown ring disease in clams. Diseases of Aquatic Organisms 48:221–231.

Andrews, J.D., and S.M. Ray. 1988. Management strategies to control the disease caused by *Perkinsus marinus*. In: W.S. Fisher, ed. Disease Processes in Marine Bivalve Molluscs. (American Fisheries Society Special Publication 18.) American Fisheries Society, Bethesda, MD, pp. 169–177.

Audemard, C., F. Le Roux, A. Barnaud, C. Collins, B. Sautour, P.-G. Sauriau, X. De Montaudouin, C. Coustau, C. Combe, and F. Berthe. 2002. Needle in a haystack: Involvement of the copepod *Paracartia grani* in the life-cycle of the oyster pathogen *Marteilia refringens*. Parasitology 124:315–323.

Avault, J.W., Jr. 1998. Predators and pests of mollusks: Oysters, clams and mussels. Aquaculture Magazine 24:56–61.

Bachmann, V., and P. Usseglio-Polatera. 1999. Contribution of the macrobenthic compartment to the oxygen budget of a large regulated river: The Mosel. Hydrobiologia 410:29–46.

Barber, B.J. 2004. Neoplastic diseases of commercially important marine bivalves. Aquatic Living Resources 17:449–466.

Barnes, R.D. 1968. The Mollusks. In: Invertebrate Zoology. W.B. Saunders, Philadelphia, pp. 321–346.

Baud, J.-P., A. Gerard, and Y. Naciri-Graven. 1997. Comparative growth and mortality of *Bonamia ostreae*-resistant and wild flat oysters, *Ostrea edulis*, in an intensive system. 1. First year of experiment. Marine Biology 130:71–79.

Bayne, B.L., J. Widdows, and R.J. Thompson. 1976. Physiology II. In: B.L. Bayne, ed. Marine Mussels: Their Ecology and Physiology. Cambridge University Press, Cambridge, pp. 207–260.

Beck, K., and R.J. Neves. 2003. An evaluation of selective feeding by three age-groups of the rainbow mussel *Villosa iris*. North American Journal of Aquaculture 65:203–209.

Beliaeff, B., T.P. O'Conner, D.K. Daskalakis, and P.J. Smith. 1997. U.S. Mussel Watch data from 1986–1994: Temporal trend detection at large spatial scales. Environmental Science and Technology 31:1411–1415.

Berthe, F.C.J., M. Pernas, M. Zerabib, P. Haffner, A. Thebault, and A.J. Figueras. 1998. Experimental transmission of *Marteilia refringens* with special consideration of its life cycle. Diseases of Aquatic Organisms 34:135–144.

Bogan, A.E. 1993. Freshwater bivalve extinctions (Mollusca: Unionoida): A search for causes. American Zoologist 33:599–609.

Bower, S.M., and S.E. McGladdery. 2003. Synopsis of infectious diseases and parasites of commercially exploited shellfish. http://www-sci.pac.dfo-mpo.gc.ca/shelldis/title_e.htm.

Bower, S.M., S.E. McGladdery, and I.M. Price. 1994. Synopsis of infectious diseases and parasites of commercially exploited shellfish. Annual Review of Fish Diseases 4:1–200.

Brown, H.J., H.W. Stokes, and R.M. Hall. 1996. Changes in oxygen consumption and biochemical composition of the marine fouling dreissinid bivalve *Mytilopsis sallei* (Recluz) exposed to mercury. Ecotoxicology and Environmental Safety 33:168–174.

Canesi, L., G. Gallo, M. Gavioli, and C. Pruzzo. 2002. Bacteria–hemocyte interactions and phagocytosis in marine bivalves. Microscopy Research and Technique 57:469–476.

Carnegie, R.B., B.J. Barber, S.C. Culloty, A.J. Figueras, and D.L. Distel. 2000. Development of a PCR assay for detection of the oyster pathogen *Bonamia ostreae* and support for its inclusion in the *Haplosporidia*. Diseases of Aquatic Organisms 42:199–206.

Carnegie, R.B., B.J. Barber, and D.L. Distel. 2003. Detection of the oyster parasite *Bonamia ostreae* by fluorescent in situ hybridization. Diseases of Aquatic Organisms 55:247–252.

Carriker, M.R. 1996. The shell and ligament. In: V.S. Kennedy, R.I.E. Newell, and A.F. Eble, eds. The Eastern Oyster *Crassostrea virginica*. Maryland Sea Grant College, College Park, MD, pp. 75–168.

Castagna, M. 1985. Farming of the northern hard clam, *Mercenaria mercenaria* (Linne) in Virginia [abstr.]. Journal of Shellfish Research 5:33.

Castro, D, J.A. Santamaria, A. Luque, E. Martinez-Manzanares, and J.J. Borrego. 1997. Determination of the etiological agent of brown ring disease in southwestern Spain. Diseases of Aquatic Organisms 29:181–188.

Cheng, T.C. 1996. Hemocytes: Forms and Functions. In: V.S. Kennedy, R.I.E. Newell, and A.F. Eble, eds. The Eastern Oyster *Crassostrea virginica*. Maryland Sea Grant College, College Park, MD, pp. 299–333.

Cleland, J.D., R.F. McMahon, and G. Elick. 1986. Physiological differences between two morphotypes of the Asian clam, *Corbicula* [abstr.]. American Zoologist 26:103A.

Cochennec-Laureau, N., K.S. Reece, F.C.J. Berthe, and P.M. Hine. 2003. *Mikrocytos roughleyi* taxonomic affiliation leads to the genus *Bonamia* (*Haplosporidia*). Diseases of Aquatic Organisms 54:209–214.

Corporeau, C. 2003. In situ hybridization for flow cytometry: A molecular method for monitoring stress-gene expression in hemolymph cells of oysters. Aquatic Toxicology 64:427–435.

Culloty, S.C., and M.F. Mulcahy. 1996. Season-, age-, and sex-related variation in the prevalence of bonamiasis in flat oysters (*Ostrea edulis* L.) on the south coast of Ireland. Aquaculture 144:53–63.

Culloty, S.C., B. Novoa, M. Pernas, M. Longshaw, M.F. Mulcahy, S.W. Feist, and A. Figueras. 1999. Susceptibility of a number of bivalve species to the protozoan parasite *Bonamia ostreae* and their ability to act as vectors for this parasite. Diseases of Aquatic Organisms 37:73–80.

Desrosiers, R.R., and F. Dube. 1993. Flowing seawater as an inducer of spawning in the sea scallop, *Placopecten magellanicus* (Gmelin, 1791). Journal of Shellfish Research 12:263–265.

Deaton, L.E., P.J. Jordan, and J.R. Dankert. 1999. Phenoloxidase activity in the hemolymph of bivalve mollusks. Journal of Shellfish Research 18:223–226.

Dietz, T.H. 1985. Ionic regulation in freshwater mussels: A brief review. American Malacological Bulletin 3:233–242.

Diggles, B.K., N. Cochennec-Laureau, and P.M. Hine. 2003. Comparison of diagnostic techniques for *Bonamia exitiosus* from flat oysters *Ostrea chilensis* in New Zealand. Aquaculture 220:145–156.

Doherty, F.D., D.S. Cherry, and J. Cairns Jr. 1987. Valve closure responses of the Asiatic clam (*Corbicula fluminea*) exposed to cadmium and zinc. Hydrobiologia 153:159–167.

Eble, A.F. 1996. The Circulatory System. In: V.S. Kennedy, R.I.E. Newell, and A.F. Eble, eds. The Eastern Oyster *Crassostrea virginica*. Maryland Sea Grant College, College Park, MD, pp. 271–298.

Eble, A.F., and R. Scro. 1996. General Anatomy. In: V.S. Kennedy, R.I.E. Newell, and A.F. Eble, eds. The Eastern Oyster *Crassostrea virginica*. Maryland Sea Grant College, College Park, MD, pp. 19–74.

Elston, R.A. 1984. Prevention and management of infectious diseases in intensive mollusc husbandry. Journal of the World Mariculture Society 14:284–300.

Federighi, H. 1929. Temperature characteristics for the frequency of heart beat in *Ostrea virginica* Gmelin. Journal of Experimental Zoology 54:89–194.

Figueras, A.J., and J. Montes. 1988. Aber disease of edible oysters caused by *Marteilia refringens*. In: W.S. Fisher, ed. Disease Processes in Marine Bivalve Molluscs. American Fisheries Society Special Publication 18:38–46.

Fisher, W.S., ed. 1988. Disease Processes in Marine Bivalve Molluscs. (American Fisheries Society Special Publication 18.) American Fisheries Society, Bethesda, MD, 315 pp.

Fisher, W.S., and S.E. Ford. 1988. Flow cytometry: A tool for cell research in bivalve pathology. In: W.S. Fisher, ed. Disease Processes in Marine Bivalve Molluscs. American Fisheries Society Special Publication 18:286–291.

Ford, S.E. 1986. Effect of repeated hemolymph sampling on growth, mortality, hemolymph protein and parasitism of oysters, *Crassostrea virginica* [abstr.]. Comparative Biochemistry and Physiology 85A:465–470.

Ford S.E., and M.R. Tripp. 1996. Diseases and defense mechanisms. In: V.S. Kennedy, R.I.E. Newell, and A.F. Eble, eds. The Eastern Oyster *Crassostrea virginica*. Maryland Sea Grant College, College Park, MD, pp. 581–660.

Frenette, B., G.J. Parsons, and L.A. Davidson. 2002. Influence of salinity and temperature on clearance rate and oxygen consumption of juvenile sea scallops *Placopecten magellanicus* (Gmelin). In: Aquaculture Canada 2001. Proceedings of the contributed papers of the 18th Annual meeting of the Aquaculture Association of Canada, no. 5, pp. 17–19.

Friedl, F.E. 1996. Oysters, oxygen metabolism, and hemocytes. Journal of Shellfish Research 15:501.

Gagne, F., D.J. Marcogliese, C. Blaise, and A.D. Gendron. 2001. Occurrence of compounds estrogenic to freshwater mussels in surface waters in an urban area. Environmental Toxicology 16:260–268.

Galtsoff, P.S. 1964. The American Oyster *Crassostrea virginica* (Gmelin). Fisheries Bulletin 64:1–480.

Gibbons, M.C., and M. Castagna. 1984. Serotonin as an inducer of spawning in six bivalve species. Aquaculture 40:189–191.

Grant, J., C.W. Emerson, A. Mallet, and C. Carver. 2003. Growth advantages of ear hanging compared to cage culture for sea scallops, *Placopecten magellanicus*. Aquaculture 217:301–323.

Grizel, H. 1974. Mollusc parasitology. Oceanis 3:190–207.

Gustafson, L.L., M.K. Stoskopf, A.E. Bogan, W. Showers, T.J. Kwak, S. Hanlon, and J.F. Levine. 2005a. Evaluation of a nonlethal technique for hemolymph collection in *Elliptio complanata*, a freshwater bivalve (Mollusca: Unionidae). Diseases of Aquatic Organisms 65:159–165.

Gustafson, L.L., M.K. Stoskopf, W. Showers, G. Cope, C. Eads, R. Linnehan, T.J. Kwak, B. Andersen, and J.F. Levine. 2005b. Reference ranges for hemolymph chemistries from *Elliptio complanata* of North Carolina. Diseases Aquatic Organisms 65:167–176.

Gunasingh-Masilamoni, J., K.S. Jesudoss, K. Nandakumar, K.K. Satapathy, J. Azariah, and K.V.K. Nair. 2002. Lethal and sub-lethal effects of chlorination on green mussel, *Perna viridis*, in the context of biofouling control in a power plant cooling water system. Marine Environmental Research 53:65–76.

Haag, W.R., and M.L. Warren Jr. 2003. Host fishes and reproductive biology of 6 freshwater mussel species from the Mobile Basin, USA. Journal of the North American Benthological Society 22:78–91.

Hakenkamp, C.C., and M.A. Palmer. 1999. Introduced bivalves in freshwater ecosystems: The impact of *Corbicula* on organic matter dynamics in a sandy stream. Oecologia (Berl.) 119:445–451.

Hand, R.E., J.A. Nell, I.R. Smith, and G.B. Maguire. 1998. Studies on triploid oysters in Australia. XI. Survival of diploid and triploid Sydney rock oysters (*Saccostrea commercialis* [Iredale and Roughley]) through outbreaks of winter mortality caused by *Mikrocytos roughley* infestation. Journal of Shellfish Research 17:1129–1135.

Hasson, K.W., J. Hasson, H. Aubert, R.M. Redman, and D.V. Lightner. 1997. A new RNA-friendly fixative for the preservation of penaeid shrimp samples for virological detection using cDNA genomic probe. Journal of Virological Methods 66:227–236.

Healy, J.M. 2001. The mollusca. In: D.T. Anderson, ed. Invertebrate Zoology. Oxford University Press, South Melbourne, pp. 147–155.

Heinonen, J., J. Kukkonen, O.-P. Penttinen, and I.J. Holopainen. 1997. Effects of hypoxia on valve-closure time and bioaccumulation of 2,4,5-trichlorophenol by the freshwater clam *Sphaerium corneum* [L.]. Ecotoxicology and Environmental Safety 36:49–56.

Hervio, D., E. Bachere, V. Boulo, N. Cochennec, V. Vuillemin, Y. Le Coguic, G. Cailleteaux, J. Mazurie, and E. Mialhe. 1995. Establishment of an experimental infection protocol for the flat oyster, *Ostrea edulis*, with the intrahemocytic protozoan parasite *Bonamia ostreae*: Application in the selection of parasite-resistant oysters. Aquaculture 132:183–184.

Hevert, F. 1984. Urine formation in the lamellibranchs: Evidence for ultrafiltration and quantitative description. Journal of Experimental Biology 111:1–12.

Hicks, D.W., and R.F. McMahon. 2002. Respiratory responses to temperature and hypoxia in the nonindigenous brown mussel, *Perna perna* (Bivalvia: Mytilidae), from the Gulf of Mexico. Journal of Experimental Marine Biology and Ecology 277:61–78.

Hine, P.M., and T. Thorne. 2000. A survey of some parasites and diseases of several species of bivalve mollusc in northern Western Australia. Diseases of Aquatic Organisms 40:67–78.

Hine, P.M., B.K. Diggles, M.J.D. Parsons, A. Pringle, and B. Bull. 2002. The effects of stressors on the dynamics of *Bonamia exitosus* Hine, Cochennec-Laureau & Berthe, infections in flat oysters *Ostrea chilensis* (Philippi). Journal of Fish Diseases 25:545–554.

Housem, M.L., C.H. Kim, and P.W. Reno. 1998. Soft-shell *Mya arenaria* with disseminated neoplasia demonstrate reverse transcriptase activity. Diseases of Aquatic Organisms 34:187–192.

Howard D.W., E.J. Lewis, B.J. Keller, and C.S. smith. 2004. Histological Techniques for Marine Bivalve Mollusks and Crustaceans. NOAA Tech. Memo. NOS NCCOS 5, 218 pp.

Imlay, M.J. 1982. Use of shells of freshwater mussels in monitoring heavy metals and environmental stresses: A review. Malacological Review 15:1–14.

Jadhav, M.L., and V.S. Lomte. 1982. Hormonal control of carbohydrate metabolism in the freshwater bivalve, *Lamellidens corrianus*. Rivista di idrobiologia Monte del Lago sul Trasimeno 21:27–36.

Jones, H.D. 1983. The circulatory system of gastropods and bivalves. In: A. Saleuddin and K. Wilbur, eds. The Mollusca, volume 5: Physiology, Part 2. Academic, New York, pp. 189–238.

Joose, J., and W.P.M Geraerts. 1983. Endocrinology. In: A. Saleuddin and K. Wilbur, eds. The Mollusca, volume 4, Part 1. Academic, New York, pp. 318–406.

Kadar, E., J. Salanki, R. Jugdaohsingh, J.J. Powell, C.R. McCrohan, and K.N. White. 2001. Avoidance responses to aluminium in the freshwater bivalve *Anodonta cygnea*. Aquatic Toxicology 55:137–148.

Kennedy, VS. 1996. Biology of larvae and spat. In: V.S. Kennedy, R.I.E. Newell, and A.F. Eble, eds. The Eastern Oyster *Crassostrea virginica*. Maryland Sea Grant College, College Park, MD, pp. 371–422.

Kennedy, V.S., R.I.E. Newell, and A.F. Eble, eds. 1996. The Eastern Oyster *Crassostrea virginica*. Maryland Sea Grant College, College Park, MD, 734 pp.

Kleeman, S.N., and R.D. Adlard. 2000. Molecular detection of *Marteilia sydneyi*, pathogen of Sydney rock oysters. Diseases of Aquatic Organisms 40:137–146.

Kleeman, S.N., F. Le Roux, A.F. Berthe, and R.D. Adlard. 2002. Specificity of PCR and in situ hybridization assays designed for detection of *Marteilia sydneyi* and *M. refringens*. Parasitology 125:131–141.

Koehring, V. 1937. The rate of heart beat in clams. Bulletin of the Mountain Desert Island Biological Laboratory 39:25–26.

Kohata, K., T. Hiwatari, and T. Hagiwara. 2003. Natural water-purification system observed in a shallow coastal lagoon: Matsukawa-ura, Japan. Marine Pollution Bulletin 47:148–154.

Kraemer, L.R. 1970. The mantle flap in three species of *Lampsilis* (Pelecypoda: Unionidae). Malacologia 10:225–282.

Kraemer, L.R. 1978. Discovery of two distinct kinds of statocysts in freshwater bivalved mollusks: Some behavioral implications. Bulletin of the American Malacological Union, pp. 24–28.

Langdon, C.J., and R.I.E. Newell. 1990. Utilization of detritus and bacteria as food sources by two bivalve suspension-feeders, the oyster *Crassostrea virginica* and the mussel *Geukensia demissa*. Marine Ecology Progress Series 58:299–310.

Legraien, E.Y.G., and O. Crosaz. 1999. Oyster Culture in Brittany: Farming Techniques and Problems. Ecole nationale veterinaire d'Alfort, Maisons Alfort, 179 pp.

Le Roux, F.C., A. Audemard, A. Barnaud, and F. Berthe. 1999. DNA probes as potential tools for the detection of *Marteilia refringens*. Marine Biotechnology 1:588–597.

Le Roux, F., G. Lorenzo, P. Peyret, C. Audemard, A. Figueras, C. Vivares, M. Gouy, and F. Berthe. 2001. Molecular evidence for the existence of two species of *Marteilia* in Europe. Journal of Eukaryotic Microbiology 48:449–454.

Levine, J.F. 2003. Aquaculture: Pre-harvest food safety. In: M. Torrence and R. Issaccson, eds. Microbial Food Safety in Animal Agriculture. Iowa State Press, Ames, pp. 369–395.

Li, S., W. Wang, and D.P.H. Hsieh. 2002. Effects of toxic dinoflagellate *Alexandrium tamarense* on the energy budgets and growth of two marine bivalves. Marine Environmental Research 53:145–160.

Liu, H., and J. Xiang. 1994. Studies on Induction of Spawning by Biochemical Signal Molecules in Several Bivalves. Marine Sciences/Haiyang Kexue, Qingdao, China, pp. 35–38.

Loo, L.O. 1992. Filtration, assimilation, respiration and growth of *Mytilus edulis* L. at low temperatures. Ophelia 35:123–131.

Lopez, G.R., and I.J. Holopainen. 1987. Interstitial suspension-feeding by *Pisidium* spp. (Pisididae: Bivalvia): A new guild in the lentic benthos? American Malacological Bulletin 5:21–30.

Luengen, A.C., C.S. Friedman, P.T. Raimondi, and A.R. Flegal. 2004. Evaluation of mussel immune responses as indicators of contamination in San Francisco Bay. Marine Environmental Research 57:197–212.

Matsuyama, Y., T. Uchida, and T. Honjo. 1999. Effects of harmful dinoflagellates, *Gymnodinium mikimotoi* and *Heterocapsa circulariasquama*, red-tide on filtering rate of bivalve molluscs. Fisheries Science 65:248–253.

Mane, U.H., S.R. Akarte, and D.A. Kulkarni. 1986. Acute toxicity of fenthion to freshwater lamellibranch mollusk, *Indonaia caeruleus* (Prashad 1918), from Godavari River at Paithan-a biochemical approach. Bulletin of Environmental Contamination and Toxicology 37:622–628.

Marsden, I.D. 1999. Respiration and feeding of the surf clam *Paphies donacina* from New Zealand. Hydrobiologia 405:179–188.

Marsh, M.E. 1990. Immunocytochemical localization of a calcium-binding phosphoprotein in hemocytes of heterodont bivalves. Journal of Experimental Zoology 253:280–286.

Martin, W.A. 1983. Excretion. In: A.S.M. Saleuddin and K.M. Wilbur, eds. The Mollusca, volume 5: Physiology, Part 2. Academic, New York, pp. 353–405.

Martinez-Manzanares, E., D. Castro, J.I. Navas, M.L. Lopez-Cortes, and J.J. Borrego. 1998. Transmission routes and treatment of brown ring disease affecting Manila clams (*Tapes philippinarum*). Journal of Shellfish Research 17:1051–1056.

Matthiessen, G. 2000. Oyster Culture. Blackwell Science, Oxford, 176 pp.

McMahon, R.F. 1991. Mollusca: Bivalvia. In: J.H. Thorp and A.P. Covich, eds. Ecology and Classification of North American Freshwater Invertebrates. Academic, San Diego, pp. 315–399.

McMahon, R.F., and C.J. Williams. 1984. A unique respiratory adaptation to emersion in the introduced Asian freshwater clam (*Corbicula fluminea* (Muller) (Lamellibranchia: Corbiculacea). Physiological Zoology 57:274–279.

Miac, J., M. Groth, and M. Wolowicz. 1997. Seasonal changes in the *Mya arenaria* (L.) population from inner Puck Bay. Oceanologia 39:177–195.

Mix, M.C., H.J. Pribble, R.T. Riley, and S.P. Tomasovic. 1977. Neoplastic disease in bivalve mollusks from Oregon estuaries with emphasis on research on proliferative disorders in Yaquina Bay oysters. Annals of the New York Academy of Sciences 298:356–373.

Montes, J., B. Ferro-Soto, R.F. Conchas, and A. Guerra. 2003. Determining culture strategies in populations of the European flat oyster, *Ostrea edulis*, affected by bonamiosis. Aquaculture 220:175–182.

National Marine Fisheries Service. 1983. Histological Techniques for Marine Bivalve Mollusks. U.S. Department of Commerce, NOAA, NMFS, Northeast Fisheries Center, Woods Hole, MA.

Nell, J.A., and R.E. Hand. 2003. Evaluation of the progeny of second-generation Sydney rock oyster *Saccostrea glomerata* (Gould, 1850) breeding lines for resistance to QX disease *Marteilia sydneyi*. Aquaculture 228:27–35.

Novoa, B., A. Luque, D. Castro, J.J. Borrego, and A. Figueras. 1998. Characterization and infectivity of four bacterial strains isolated from brown ring disease–affected clams. Journal of Invertebrate Pathology 71:34–41.

Office of International Epizootics (OIE). 2002. International Aquatic Animal Health Code and Diagnostic Manual for Aquatic Animal Diseases. OIE, Paris. http://www.oie.int/eng/normes/fmanual/A_summry.htm, Paris.

Owen, R., L. Buxton, S. Sarkis, M. Toaspern, A. Knap, and M. Depledge. 2002. An evaluation of hemolymph cholinesterase activities in the tropical scallop, *Euvola* (Pecten) *ziczac*, for the rapid assessment of pesticide exposure. Marine Pollution Bulletin 4:1010–1017.

Paillard, C., and P. Maes. 1994. Brown ring disease in the Manila clam *Ruditapes philippinarum*: Establishment of a classification system. Diseases of Aquatic Organisms 19:137–146.

Pandian, T.J. 1999. Marine organisms in hypoxia and anoxic environments. In: B.L.K. Somayajulu, ed. Ocean Science: Trends and Future Directions. Indian National Science Academy, New Delhi, pp. 177–195.

Pernas, M., B. Novoa, F. Berthe, C. Tafalla, and A. Figueras. 2001. Molecular methods for the diagnosis of *Marteilia refringens*. Bulletin of the European Association of Fish Pathologists 21:200–208.

Prou, J., and P. Goulletquer. 2002. The French mussel industry: Present status and perspectives. Bulletin of the Aquaculture Association of Canada 102:17–23.

Rajagopal, S., G. Van der Velde, and H.A. Jenner. 1997. Shell valve movement response of dark false mussel, *Mytilopsis leucophaeta*, to chlorination. Water Research 31:3187–3190.

Rajagopal, S., G. Van der Velde, and H.A. Jenner. 2002. Does status of attachment influence survival time of zebra mussel, *Dreissena polymorpha*, exposed to chlorination? Environmental Toxicology and Chemistry 21:342–346.

Rana, K., and A. Immink. 1998. Trends in Global Aquaculture Production: 1984–1996. Fishery Information, Data and Statistics Service (FIDI), Food and Agricultural Organization of the United Nations (FAO), Rome. http://www.fao.org/WAICENT/FAOINFO/ FISHERY/trends/aqtrends/aqtrend.asp.

Rana, K., M. Perotti, S. Montanaro, and A. Immink. 1998. Aquaculture production in China. FAO Aquaculture Newsletter no. 20, pp. 9210.

Reid, H.I., P. Soudant, C. Lambert, C. Paillard, and T.H. Birkbeck. 2003. Salinity effects on immune parameters of *Ruditapes philippinarum* challenged with *Vibrio tapetis*. Diseases of Aquatic Organisms 56:249–258.

Reid, R.G.B., R.F. McMahon, D.O. Foighil, and R. Finnigan. 1992. Anterior inhalant currents and pedal feeding in bivalves. Veliger 35:93–104.

Ringwood, A.H., and C.J. Keppler. 2002. Water quality variation and clam growth: Is pH really a non-issue in estuaries? Estuaries 25:901–907.

Robert, R., M. Borel, Y. Pichot, and G. Trut. 1991. Growth and mortality of the European oyster *Ostrea edulis* in the Bay of Arachon (France). Aquatic Living Resources 4:265–274.

Romalde, J.L., D. Castro, B. Magarinos, L. Lopez-Cortes, and J.J. Borrego. 2002. Comparison of ribotyping, randomly amplified polymorphic DNA, and pulse-field gel electrophoresis for molecular typing of *Vibrio tapetis*. Systematic Applied Microbiology 25:544–550.

Rucai, W., and S. Lian-chen. 1991. Culture of Farrier's scallop, *Chlamys farreri* (Jones and Preston) in China. In: W. Menzel, ed. Estuarine and Marine Bivalve Mollusk Culture. CRC, Boca Raton, FL, pp. 278–282.

Sastry, A.N. 1966. Temperature effects in reproduction of the bay scallop, *Aequipecten irradians* Lamarck. Biological Bulletin 130:118–134.

Sericano, J.L. 2000. The Mussel Watch approach and its applicability to global chemical contamination monitoring programs. International Journal of Environment and Pollution 13:1–6,340–350.

Shumway S.E. 1996. Natural environmental factors. In: V.S. Kennedy, R.I.E. Newell, and A.F. Eble, eds. The Eastern Oyster *Crassostrea virginica*. Maryland Sea Grant College, College Park, MD, pp. 467–514.

Shumway, S.E., J. Barter, and J. Stahlneccker. 1988. Seasonal changes in oxygen consumption of the giant scallop, *Placopecten magellanicus* (Gmelin). Journal of Shellfish Research 7:77–82.

Simpfendoerfer, R.W., M.V. Vial, D.A. Lopez, M. Verdala, and M.L. Gonzalez. 1995. Relationship between the aerobic and anaerobic metabolic capacities and the vertical distribution of three intertidal sessile invertebrates: *Jehlius cirratus* (Darwin) (Cirripedia), *Perumytilus purpuratus* (Lamarck) (Bivalvia) and *Mytilus chilensis*

(Hupe) (Bivalvia). Comparative Biochemistry and Physiology [B] 111:615–623.

Smith, I.R., J.A. Nell, and R. Adlard. 2000. The effect of growing level and growing method on winter mortality, *Mikrocytos roughleyi*, in diploid and triploid Sydney rock oysters, *Saccostrea glomerata*. Aquaculture 185:197–205.

Sobral, P., and J. Widdows. 1997. Influence of hypoxia and anoxia on the physiological responses of the clam *Ruditapes decussatus* from southern Portugal. Marine Biology 127:455–461.

Soto, D., and G. Mena. 1999. Filter feeding by the freshwater mussel, *Diplodon chilensis*, as a biocontrol of salmon eutrophication. Aquaculture 171:1–2,65–81.

Soudant, P., F.L. Chu, and J.F. Samain. 2000. Lipid requirements in some economically important bivalves. Journal of Shellfish Research 19:605.

Stasek, C.R. 1965. Feeding and particle sorting in *Yoldia ensifera* (Bivalvia: Protobranchia), with notes on other nuculanids. Malacologia 2:349–366.

Tanaka, Y., and M. Murakoshi. 1985. Spawning induction of the hermaphroditic scallop, *Pecten albicans*, by injection with serotonin. Bulletin of National Research Institute of Aquaculture 7:9–12.

Tankersley, R.A. 1996. Multipurpose gills: Effect of larval brooding on the feeding physiology of freshwater unionid mussels. Invertebrate Biology 115:243–255.

Tankersley, R.A., and R.V. Dimock Jr. 1993. Endoscopic visualization of the functional morphology of the ctenida of the unionid mussel *Pyganodon cataracta*. Canadian Journal of Zoology 71: 811–819.

Tankersley, R.A., J.J. Hart, and W.G. Wieber. 1996. Developmental shifts in the feeding biodynamics of juvenile *Utterbakia imbecillus* (Mollusca: Bivalvia). Journal of Shellfish Research 15:530–531.

Thompson, R.J., R.I.E. Newell, V.S. Kennedy, and R. Mann. 1996. Reproductive processes and early development. In: V.S. Kennedy, R.I.E. Newell, and A.F. Eble, eds. The Eastern Oyster *Crassostrea virginica*. Maryland Sea Grant College, College Park, MD, pp. 335–370.

Trueman, E.R. 1983. Locomotion in molluscs. In: A.S.M. Saleuddin and K.M. Wilbur, eds. The Mollusca, volume 4: Physiology, Part 4. Academic, New York, pp. 155–198.

Trueman, E.R., and A.C. Brown. 1985. Dynamics of burrowing and pedal extension in *Donax serra* (Mollusca: Bivalvia). Journal of Zoology 207:345–355.

Turpin, V., J. Robert, P. Goulletquer, G. Masse, and P. Rosa. 2001. Oyster greening by outdoor mass culture of the diatom *Haslea ostrearia* Simonsen in enriched seawater. Aquaculture Research 32:801–809.

Wilbur, A.E., and P.M. Gaffney. 1991. Self-fertilization in the bay scallop, *Argopecten irradians*. Journal of Shellfish Research 10:274.

Wijkstrom, U., A. Gumy, and R. Grainger. 1998. The State of World Fisheries and Aquaculture 1998. Food and Agricultural Organization (FAO), Rome.

Williams, J.D., M.L. Warren, K.S. Cummings, J.L. Harris, and R.J. Neves. 1993. Conservation status of freshwater mussels of the United States and Canada. Fisheries 18:6–22.

Wilson, J.G. 1984. Assessment of the effect of short-term salinity changes on the acute oxygen consumption of *Cerastoderma balthica*, and *Tellina tenuis* from Dublin Bay. Journal of Life Science Royal Dublin Society 5:57–63.

Wilson, J.G., and B. Elkaim. 1991. Tolerances to high temperature of infaunal bivalves and the effect of geographical distribution, position on the shore and season. Journal of the Marine Biological Association of the United Kingdom 71:169–177.

Yanick, J.F., and D.D. Heath. 2000. Survival and growth of mussels subsequent to haemolymph sampling for DNA. Journal of Shellfish Research 19:991–993.

Yevich, P.P., and C.A. Barszcz. 1977. Neoplasia in soft-shell clams *Mya arenaria* collected from oil-impacted sites. Annals of the New York Academy of Sciences 298:409–426.

Zardus, J.D. 2002. Protobranch bivalves. Advances in Marine Biology 42:1–65.

Zmora, O., and M. Shpigel. 2001. Filter feeders as biofilter in marine land based systems. In: Aquaculture 2001. World Aquaculture Society, Baton Rouge, LA, pp. 21–25.

Zotin, A.A., and I.G. Vladimirova. 2001. Respiration rate and species-specific lifespan in freshwater bivalves of Margaritiferidae and Unionidae families. Seriya biologicheskaya [Proceedings of the Russian Academy of Sciences] 3:331–338.

Zrncic, S., F. Le Roux, D. Oraic, B. Sostaric, and F.C.J. Berthe. 2001. First record of *Marteilia* sp. in mussels *Mytilus galloprovincialis* in Croatia. Diseases of Aquatic Organisms 44:143–148.

Chapter 8

ANNELIDS

Gregory A. Lewbart

Introduction

The annelids are a large, diverse group of segmented wormlike animals that are divided into three main classes: Polychaeta, Oligochaeta, and Hirudinea. All are characterized by regular segmentation of the trunk. It is believed this segmentation evolved as a means of burrowing via peristaltic contractions (Ruppert and Barnes, 1994). Annelids possess a coelomic cavity that is divided into segments by regular septa. The circulatory, excretory, and nervous systems are also segmented. A cuticle covers the animal, and segmented setae occur in nearly all members of the phylum. The mouth is located anteriorly and the anus posteriorly with a straight gut between the two openings (Ruppert and Barnes, 1994).

In this chapter, each of the major classes are addressed separately. The Branchiobdellida, a small class of annelids that are parasitic or commensal on crayfish crustaceans, are discussed in Chapter 12. Raftos and Cooper (1990) provide a comprehensive review of annelid diseases.

Polychaetes

Natural History and Taxonomy

The polychaetes are a diverse group of over 8000 species that belong to 86 families (Ruppert and Barnes, 1994). Nearly all are marine, and sizes vary from less than a millimeter to a meter in length. They occupy a variety of aquatic habitats, and many burrow or build tubes in or upon marine sediments and substrates. There are several excellent references on polychaete taxonomy, morphology, and natural history (Hartman, 1959, 1965; Fauchald, 1977; Ruppert et al., 2004).

Anatomy and Physiology

With the tremendous diversity of form, it is impossible to represent the entire class with a single anatomical drawing. *Nereis* sp., a common errant marine genus, is commonly used in classrooms and laboratories for polychaete-anatomy studies. These worms are widely available and frequently used as bait for coastal fishing endeavors in the United States. Figure 8.1 illustrates the basic anatomical features of *Nereis* sp. Figure 8.2 is a micrograph of an interstitial member of the family Syllidae (*Parapionosyllis manca*) that illustrates the key anatomical features of the polychaete head and anterior gut. The basic external morphological features are indicated in this micrograph.

The sensory prostomium, which typically contains eyes, antennae, and tentacles, is located anterior and above the oral opening. Just caudal to the prostomium is the peristomium, which also possesses sensory structures (cirri and palps) and forms the boundaries of the mouth (Figure 8.3). The segment following the peristomium begins a series of anatomically similar segments that usually have paired parapodia. Parapodia are unique to polychaetes and distinguish them from the oligochaetes and leeches.

The parapodia, which typically have gills and setae, are used in locomotion, respiration, and defense.

The epidermis is comprised of a thin collagenous cuticle overlying a columnar or cuboidal epithelium. Glandular mucus-secreting cells are frequently associated with this epithelium (Ruppert and Barnes, 1994). Generally, two muscle layers (circular and longitudinal, respectively) lie beneath the epidermis and above the peritoneum.

The gastrointestinal (GI) tract is typically straight and somewhat differentiated. Many polychaetes have a well-defined muscular pharynx, followed by an esophagus, stomach, intestine, rectum, and anus associated with the terminal segment, the pygidium (Ruppert and Barnes, 1994). These different sections of the GI tract can be difficult to distinguish grossly.

Polychaetes employ a wide variety of feeding strategies based on their environment, lifestyle, and morphology. Some polychaetes are predatory and feed on other invertebrates. Prey are typically captured and dispatched with an eversible proboscis and sharp jaws (Ruppert and Barnes, 1994). Other polychaetes are omnivores and are opportunistic feeders. *Nereis brandti*, a very large benthic polychaete of the Pacific Northwest (up to 1.8 m long), consumes mainly green algae (Ruppert and Barnes, 1994). Still others, like the well-studied lugworm (*Arenicola* sp.), are deposit feeders and strain nutrients from ingested and excreted substrates like sand and mud. Many burrowing polychaetes use this feeding strategy. Many species have symbiotic relationships with other marine invertebrates. Martin and

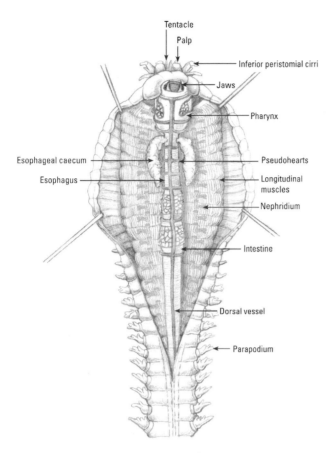

Tentacle
Palp
Inferior peristomial cirri
Jaws
Pharynx
Esophageal caecum
Pseudohearts
Esophagus
Longitudinal muscles
Nephridium
Intestine
Dorsal vessel
Parapodium

Figure 8.1.   An errant polychaete, *Nereis* sp. Drawing by Brenda Bunch.

Britayev (1998) provide a comprehensive review of the nearly 300 species of symbiotic polychaetes belonging to 28 families.

Many, but not all, polychaetes have gills for respiration. The diversity of location and structure indicates that gills may have developed independently several times within the polychaete group (Ruppert and Barnes, 1994). Whereas some polychaetes have paired branchial tissue associated with parapodia, others have the gill tissue localized at the anterior end.

Most polychaetes possess a closed circulatory system with blood flowing anteriorly in a large dorsal vessel and posteriorly in the ventral vessel. Polychaetes lack a true heart and rely on coelomic pressure and muscular contractions to push blood through the circulatory system. In some cases, heartlike pumps are present as part of the circulatory system (Ruppert and Barnes, 1994). Some smaller species lack a defined circulatory system, and the tissues are simply bathed with coelomic fluid.

Whereas the coelomic fluid contains a significant number of cells, the blood, or hemolymph, does not. Although the hemolymph of many polychaetes, especially the smaller ones, is colorless, the class does possess three of the four recognized respiratory blood pigments (Ruppert and Barnes, 1994). The majority of polychaetes with a respiratory pigment have *hemoglobin*. *Hemerythrin*, a nonheme, iron-based pigment, is found in the genus *Magelona*. This unusual blood pigment is also found in the unrelated phyla Priapulida and Sipuncula and in some

brachiopods (Ruppert and Barnes, 1994). The third polychaete circulatory pigment is called *chlorocruorin*. This pigment, unique to polychaetes, is similar to hemoglobin, but its molecular structure gives the hemolymph a green hue. Depending on species, the respiratory pigments may be used in oxygen transport, oxygen storage, or both (Ruppert and Barnes, 1994).

The excretory organs of polychaetes are paired nephridia that are generally associated with each segment (exceptions do occur). Normally, the anterior portion of the nephridial tubule is located in the segment anterior to the nephridiopore (Ruppert and Barnes, 1994). Most polychaete species have metanephridial systems, whereas those that lack a circulatory system possess protonephridial systems. Specialized tissue associated with the external lining of the intestine may contribute to excretion in polychaetes. This tissue is termed *chlorogogen tissue* and is also found in earthworms (Ruppert and Barnes, 1994).

Most polychaetes have a brain located in the prostomium. The brain innervates the sensory structures of the head, as well as the circumesophageal connective that links the ventral nerve cord with the brain. In most cases, there is a single ganglion per segment that sends nerves to the body wall (Ruppert and Barnes, 1994). Many polychaetes, especially tube dwellers, can contract rapidly and efficiently. Giant axons in the ventral nerve cord facilitate these rapid contractions, since nerve conduction is a product of axon diameter. In fact, the largest nerve axon diameter known to science is 1.7 mm and belongs to the fanworm, *Myxicola* sp. (Ruppert and Barnes, 1994).

Many polychaetes have well-developed sense organs. The eyes of polychaetes, which may number from two to four pairs, are primarily light detectors with a retinal cup (Ruppert and Barnes, 1994). Many polychaetes possess structures called *nuchal organs* located in the peristomial region of the head. These ciliated cavities are chemosensory and are believed to aid the animal in locating food.

Many polychaete species have an amazing ability to regenerate lost body parts. Some species can even regenerate their entire head. The tube dwellers and burrowing species are most adept at regeneration. In fact, *Chaetopterus*, a tube-dwelling genus, can regenerate a complete body from a single intact segment (Ruppert and Barnes, 1994).

Although there are some exceptions, most polychaetes display sexual reproduction. The sexes are usually separate and, in most cases, gametes are produced by segmented gonadal tissue. A variety of methods are employed for gamete release to the environment where fertilization occurs. In some species, the gametes exit via the nephridiopore, and others have specialized coelomoducts. One terminal strategy for the adults of some species involves rupture of the body and subsequent escape of the gametes (Ruppert and Barnes, 1994). One of the most interesting reproductive strategies, and one unique to polychaetes, is termed *epitoky*. *Epitokes* are swimming reproductive individuals that emerge from marine benthic substrates. Epitoky is found in members of the families Eunicidae, Nereidae, and Syllidae. Epitokes are either transformed adults or arise from modified segments that begin as segmental buds and separate from a benthic individual. Either way, the epitokes are modified for reproduction, and a significant portion of their body contains ga-

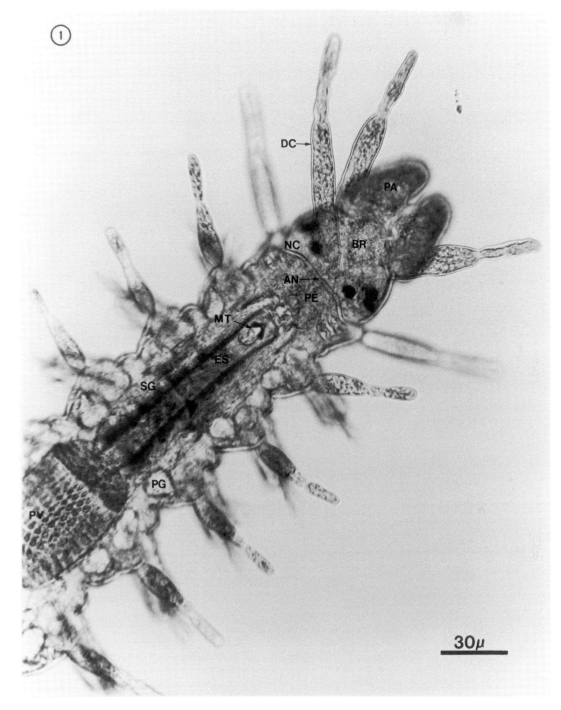

Figure 8.2. Photomicrograph of *Parapionosyllis manca*, an interstitial syllid polychaete, showing key anatomical features. *DC*, dorsal cirrus; *PA*, palps; *BR*, brain; *NC*, nuchal organ cleft; *AN*, annulus; *PE*, peristomium; *MT*, medial tooth; *ES*, esophagus; *SG*, salivary gland; *PG*, parapodial gland; and *PV*, proventriculus.

metes. Epitokes frequently swarm together during finite breeding periods and synchronously release gametes to the surrounding sea. There is strong evidence that female pheromones attract males and that the presence of sperm stimulates egg release (Ruppert and Barnes, 1994). In most cases, polychaete eggs develop into a swimming trochophore larva that metamorphoses into a juvenile resembling the adult form. Metamorphosis likely occurs due to a number of internal and external cues. Ilan et al. (1993) found that calcium concentrations in the environment induced metamorphosis in *Phragmatopoma californica* (higher concentrations led to an increased rate of metamorphosis). A puzzling, but interesting, finding of this study was that certain

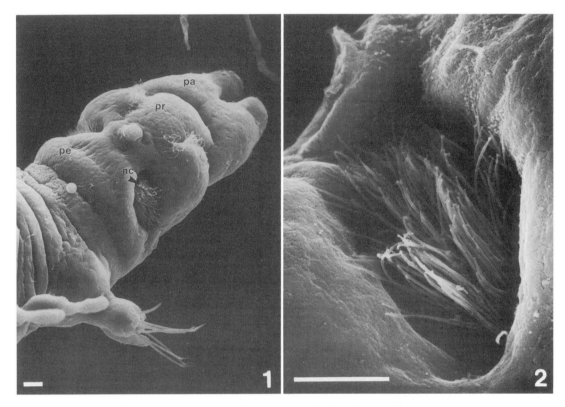

Figure 8.3. Scanning electron micrograph of *Parapionosyllis manca*. *nc*, nuchal cleft; *pe*, peristomium; *pr*, prostomium; and *pa*, palps. From Lewbart and Riser (1996), Figure 1 (p. 287).

calcium-channel blockers also induced metamorphosis in *P. californica*. Bacterial biofilms and bacterial metabolites appear to be important for inducing larval settlement in *Hydroides elegans* (Harder et al., 2002). There is good evidence that polychaete egg masses have innate antibacterial activity. Benkendorff et al. (2001) found that polychaete egg masses belonging to two species (*Eupolymnia* sp. and one unidentified species) had antibacterial activity for three human pathogens (*Escherichia coli*, *Pseudomonas aeruginosa*, and *Staphylococcus aureus*).

The annelid immune system, especially with regard to graft acceptance and rejection, has been studied in some detail. Vetvicka et al. (1994) provide a thorough review of annelid immunology. Like most invertebrates, the primary mode of defense in polychaetes is cellular via phagocytosis (Vetvicka et al., 1994) (Table 8.1). The classic early description of comparative invertebrate inflammation and phagocytosis was presented during the latter part of the 19th century (Metchnikoff, 1884).

Table 8.1. Immune reactions among major phyla*

Phyla	Phagocytosis	Graft Rejection	Complement	Natural Killer Cells	T Cells	B Cells	Antibodies
Porifera	+	+	−	+	−	−	−
Platyhelminths	+	+	−	−	−	−	−
Mollusks	+	+	−	+	−	−	−
Echinoderms	+	+	?	−	−	−	−
Annelids	+	+	?	+	−	−	−
Arthropods	+	+	?	−	−	−	−
Urochordates	+	+	−	+	−	−	−
Agnathans	+	+	+	−	?	+	+
Elasmobranchs	+	+	+	−	+	+	+
Osteichthys	+	+	+	+	+	+	+
Amphibians	+	+	+	+	+	+	+
Reptiles	+	+	+	+	+	+	+
Aves	+	+	+	+	+	+	+
Mammals	+	+	+	+	+	+	+

*From Vetvicka (1994), p. 268.

Environmental Disorders and Preventive Medicine

Being primarily aquatic, polychaetes are subject to environmental stressors and toxins. Work performed 3 years after the 1978 *Amoco Cadiz* supertanker wreck and subsequent oil spill showed that some polychaetes (cirratulids and capitellids) not only survived but became the dominant mudflat fauna (Conan, 1982).

Nereis diversicolor, a common western and eastern Atlantic polychaete, has been investigated as an invertebrate model and bioindicator species for environmental pesticide toxicity (Scaps et al., 1997; Scaps and Borot, 2000). Both carbamate and organophosphate pesticides inhibit acetylcholinesterase (AChE) activity in *N. diversicolor* (Scaps et al., 1997).

Eurythoe complanata individuals exposed to sublethal copper concentrations exhibited a decrease in immune function based on coelomocyte viability and differential counts (Nusetti et al., 1998). Normal immune function resumed following depuration of tissue copper levels. It appears that at least some polychaetes, like other marine invertebrates, are sensitive to copper. There is also strong evidence that *E. complanata* accumulates zinc in its tissues after laboratory exposure (Marcano et al., 1996). *Eudistylia vancouveri* that were exposed to 20 µg/L copper exhibited branchial (radiole) degeneration (Young and Roesijadi, 1983). These worms could regenerate damaged gill tissue by producing a copper-binding low molecular weight protein approximately 1 week after exposure to the copper. The authors believe this protein can detoxify intracellular copper.

While polychaetes are sensitive to ivermectin, one study demonstrated that those living beneath salmon net pens were not affected by salmon receiving 0.05 mg/kg ivermectin per os twice weekly for 3 months (Costelloe et al., 1998).

Endocrine disruptors can negatively impact marine invertebrates (Depledge and Billinghurst, 1999). Although most research in this area has focused on vertebrates, marine invertebrates are vulnerable to a variety of these compounds (Table 8.2). It has been shown that 4-*n*-nonylphenol increased production but decreased viability on eggs from the polychaete *Dinophilus gyrociliatus* (Price and Depledge, 1998).

Chromosomal aberrations resulted when *Neanthes arenaceodentata* larvae were exposed to ionizing radiation (Harrison et al., 1986; Anderson et al., 1990). Brood size was negatively affected in this species, even when larvae were irradiated (4.0 Gy for adults and 8.4 Gy for larvae) (Anderson et al., 1990). The effects of radiation on *N. arenaceodentata* are reviewed by Anderson and Wild (1994).

Infectious Diseases

Very little has been published about infectious diseases of polychaetes. Some information is in the literature and is included in the following paragraphs.

An iridovirus was identified in *N. diversicolor* that appeared to infect the spermocytic cells (Devauchelle and Durchon, 1973). It does appear that polychaetes can be reservoir hosts for viruses. This was supported by the detection of systemic ecto-

Table 8.2.   Endocrine disruptors of invertebrates*

Alkylphenols
  Nonylphenol
  Pentylphenol
Herbicides
  Atrazine
  Diquat dibromide
  Diuron
  Simazine
Insecticides
  DDT
  Diflubenzuron
  Endosulfan
  Endrin
  Kelthane
  MCPA
  Methoprene
  Pentachlorophenol
  Piperonyl butoxide
Metals
  Cadmium
  Lead
  Mercury
  Selenium
  Tributyltin (TBT)
  Zinc
Mixtures
  Crude oil derivatives
  Paper and pulp mill effluents
  Tannery effluent
  Sewage effluent
PCBs
  Aroclor 1242
  Clophen A50
Vertebrate Steroids
  Diethylstilbestrol
  Testosterone

*Modified from Depledge and Billinghurst (1999), p. 33.

dermal and mesodermal baculovirus (SEMBV) DNA particles in a benthic polychaete (Ruangsri and Supamattaya, 1999).

A study that surveyed seven species of marine invertebrates from the depths of the Gulf of Mexico (300–400 m) for bacterial isolates included a nereid polychaete (*Nereis* sp.). *Vibrio vulnificus* was cultured from the gut of this species, but no pathology was indicated. The authors of this study rated the counts (4.1×10^2) as "relatively low" compared with the crustaceans and echinoderms (Dilmore and Hood, 1986). Only *V. alginolyticus* was isolated from water and sediments.

The freshwater polychaete, *Manayunkia speciosa*, is known to be an alternate host for *Ceratomyxa shasta*, a myxozoan parasite of salmonid fishes (Bartholomew et al., 1997). Electron microscopy confirmed that the actinosporean life stage is found in the epidermis of the polychaete (Figure 8.4).

Species of the genus *Haplozoon*, an aberrant dinoflagellate, are known to parasitize marine polychaetes (Siebert, 1973; Leander et al., 2002). These intestinal parasites confused early researchers who incorrectly classified them as mesozoans or apicomplexans (Dogiel, 1906; Neresheimer, 1908; Poche, 1913; Calkins, 1915). It wasn't until nearly a decade later (Chatton,

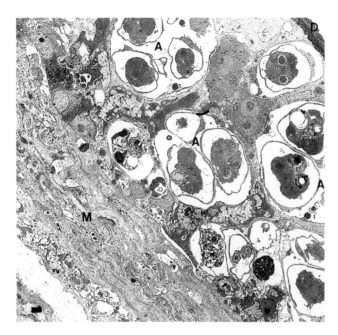

Figure 8.4. In this transmission electron micrograph, developing *Ceratomyxa shasta* actinosporean pansporoblasts (*A*) are evident between the dermis (*D*) and striated muscle (*M*) of a freshwater polychaete. Scale bar = 1.0 µm. From Bartholomew et al. (1997), Figure 6 (pp. 866–867).

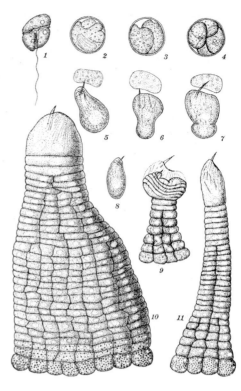

Figure 8.5. These 11 camera-lucida drawings illustrate the anatomical stages of *Haplozoon* spp. **1:** Free-swimming dinospore of *H. clymenellae*. ×2000. **2:** Encysted *H. clymenellae* dinospore prior to division. ×2000. **3:** Encysted *H. clymenellae* dinospore first division. ×2000. **4:** Encysted *H. clymenellae* dinospore second division.×2000. **5:** *Haplozoon dogieli* trophocyte attached to intestinal epithelial cell. ×450. **6:** Same as drawing 5, but 5 min later. **7:** Same as drawing 6, but 5 min later. **8:** *Haplozoon clymenellae* trophocyte. ×450. **9:** *Haplozoon dogieli* colony with trophocyte (contracted, *stippled*; and expanded, *dotted*), gonocytes, and terminal sporocytes. ×450. **10:** Pectinate colony of *H. clymenellae*. ×450. **11:** Pyramidal colony (first row of cells) of *H. clymenellae*. ×450. From Shumway (1924), Figures 1–11 (p. 74).

1920; Shumway, 1924) that *Haplozoon* was correctly placed with the dinoflagellates. *Haplozoon axiothellae*, one of the most thoroughly studied species, parasitizes *Axiothella rubrocincta*, a Pacific maldanid polychaete. These parasites are unusual in that they have a multicellular trophont life stage (Leander et al., 2002) (Figures 8.5 and 8.6). There is no evidence that these parasites cause significant clinical disease.

Gregarine parasites have been described from many polychaete species (Lankester, 1863, 1866; Ganapati, 1946; Schrével, 1969; Desportes and Théodoridès, 1986). These organisms usually parasitize the gut, but it is unclear what clinical effect they have.

Reports of ciliated protozoal parasites of polychaetes are rare. Kozloff (1961) reported and described a new genus and species (*Ignotocoma sabellarum*) of ciliate belonging to the family Ancistrocomidae. Members of this group are normally found to parasitize gastropod and pelecypod mollusks (Kozloff, 1961). *Ignotocoma sabellarum* was found on the peristomial cirri of *Schizobranchia insignis* and *Eudistylia vancouveri*, both members of the Sabellidae. Virtually all of the polychaetes examined were parasitized by these ciliates (Figure 8.7). No mention was made regarding the clinical significance of these parasites.

Orthonectids are an odd group of small, multicellular animals that appear to be strictly parasitic upon marine invertebrates. Most reported cases are from the Mediterranean Sea or the European Atlantic (Kozloff, 1965). There are only about 20 described species in this group that is sometimes given the rank of class and sometimes declared a separate phylum. Kozloff (1965) described a new genus and species (*Ciliocinta sabellar-*

iae) from the sabellid polychaete *Sabellaria cementarium* (Figure 8.8). He examined 88 polychaetes and found two infected animals, both mature males showing no clinical signs. The orthonectids were found associated with the body wall of the polychaetes.

Although polychaetes do not appear to bear significant helminth or crustacean parasitic burdens, they can serve as intermediate or primary hosts for some digenean parasites (Reimer, 1973; Zander and Reimer, 2002). In one laboratory study (McCurdy, 2001), *Pygospio elegans* individuals exposed to cercaria of the digenean *Lepocreadium setiferoides* fragmented more readily than unexposed controls. Exposure to cercaria also resulted in reduced size and survival among the experimental *P. elegans* and overall poor reproductive success.

Polychaetes (at least 28 species) can be symbiotic with or perhaps parasitic on other polychaetes (Martin and Britayev, 1998). Micaletto et al. (2002) reported a case where the dorvelleid polychaete *Veneriserva pygoclava* was found in the coelomic cavity of

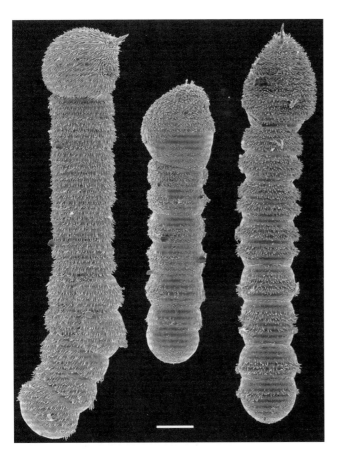

Figure 8.6. Scanning electron micrograph showing three organisms of *Haplozoon axiothellae* from the same polychaete host. Note the diversity of morphology (scale bar = 10 μm). From Leander et al. (2002), Figure 2 (pp. 290–291).

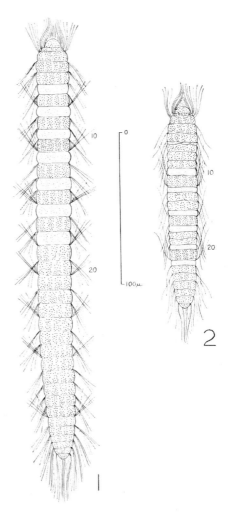

Figure 8.8. Drawings of the orthonectid mesozoan *Ciliocinta sabellariae* (**1**, female; and **2**, male) from the sabellid polychaete *Sabellaria cementarium*. Scale bar = 100 μm. From Kozloff (1965), Figures 1 and 2 (p. 39).

Laetmonice producta, a member of the family Aphroditidae. The authors examined 842 specimens of *L. producta* and found 209 symbionts/parasites in 163 host polychaetes. Despite the high prevalence, the authors did not observe any host tissue damage or deleterious effects.

Anesthesia and Analgesia

Like many marine invertebrates, polychaetes respond well to magnesium chloride in the water. Although some species might be more sensitive than others, a concentration of between 7.5% and 8.0% seems to work well for relaxation (Lewbart and Riser, 1996; Müller et al., 2003).

Surgery

Although there are no reports of veterinary surgery for polychaetes in the literature, a number of studies have looked at the

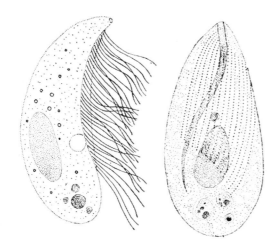

Figure 8.7. Drawings of *Ignotocoma sabellarum*, a ciliate found to parasitize the peristomial cirri of two species of sabellid polychaetes: *Schizobranchia insignis* and *Eudistylia vancouveri*. The figure on the **left** is from a living specimen, and on the **right** is a camera-lucida drawing from Hollande's fixed specimens. Living specimens ranged in size from 23 × 12 × 8.5 μm to 33 × 16 × 10 μm. From Kozloff (1961), (p. 62).

processes of autotomy and regeneration in different polychaete species (Hyman, 1940; Clark, 1968; Clavier, 1984; Eckberg and Hill, 1996; McCurdy, 2001; Müller et al., 2003). Unlike most polychaetes capable of regeneration, members of the genus *Chaetopterus* can regenerate both anterior and posterior segments (Eckberg and Hill, 1996).

Formulary

There is a paucity of published information on chemotherapeutic treatment of polychaetes. Robbins et al. (1987) used streptomycin (0.2 mg/mL) and penicillin G (0.5 mg/mL) in seawater as part of an experiment examining anaerobiosis in *Terebella lapidaria*.

Oligochaetes

Natural History and Taxonomy

There are over 3000 species of oligochaetes, with most being terrestrial or freshwater. This group includes the widely recognized and successful earthworms and night crawlers. Their size range parallels that of the polychaetes except their largest member, the giant Australian earthworm, can reach 3 m in length (Ruppert and Barnes, 1994).

Although they are related to the polychaetes, researchers believe that oligochaetes evolved independently from a common marine annelid ancestor (Ruppert and Barnes, 1994).

Anatomy and Physiology

Oligochaetes differ from polychaetes in that they lack a well-developed head and parapodia. All possess setae that are usually small in terrestrial species and well developed in aquatic forms. One of the most distinguishing features of oligochaetes is the glandular clitellum that secretes a cocoon for eggs and mucus to aid in copulation.

The general body structure of oligochaetes is similar to that of the polychaetes. They move primarily by muscular peristaltic contractions, like the burrowing polychaetes (Ruppert and Barnes, 1994).

Whereas a large number of polychaetes manufacture tubes, very few oligochaetes do. The majority move freely through a variety of substrates, including dirt, mud, sand, peat, and decaying leaves. Others can be found beneath rocks and other stationary objects. They can occur in impressively high numbers, with 8700 oligochaetes documented from a single square meter of soil (Ruppert and Barnes, 1994). It is well known that earth-dwelling oligochaetes aerate and mix the soils in which they live. Charles Darwin first described this important fact (Ruppert and Barnes, 1994).

Nearly all oligochaetes are opportunistic scavengers that feed on detritus, debris, and decomposing organic materials. Some are deposit feeders, like some polychaetes, and can sift and assimilate nutrients from ingested soil and other substrates. The GI tract is generally straight and, in the case of earthworms,

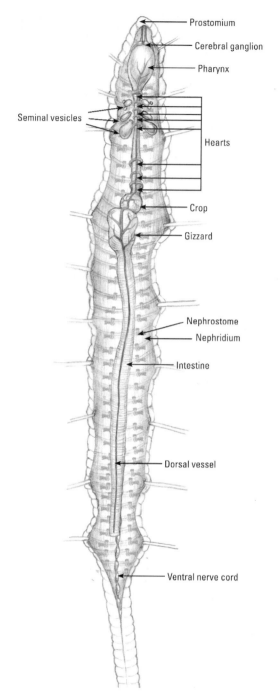

Figure 8.9. A large earthworm (*Lumbricus* sp.) with appropriate labels. Drawing by Brenda Bunch.

contains a pharynx, esophagus, gizzard and/or crop, and intestine (Figure 8.9). When present, the cuticle-lined gizzard is used for grinding ingesta and the crop for storage. A number of gutless interstitial marine oligochaetes belong to the family Tubificidae. In at least several species of the genus *Phallodrilus*, numerous intracellular bacteria are associated with the subcuticular tissues (Richards et al., 1982; Felbeck et al., 1983). It is hypothesized that these nonpathogenic, chemo-organotrophic bacteria are either mutualistic or commensal symbionts. These symbiotic bacteria are commonly found associated with the Pogonophora (which lack a gastrointestinal tract) and fix CO_2 by oxidizing sulfide (Felbeck and Somero, 1982).

Unlike the polychaetes, very few oligochaetes have gills. In this group, gas is exchanged almost exclusively by diffusion. Although there are exceptions, the oligochaete and polychaete circulatory systems are similar. Most oligochaetes use plasma hemoglobin as their oxygen-carrying pigment. Oligochaetes generally require very little oxygen and, in some cases, can survive for periods with no oxygen at all. *Tubifex tubifex*, a popular food source in the aquarium fish pet trade, is an example of an oligochaete that actually thrives in poor water conditions with little oxygen. When exposed to water with normal oxygen levels, these tubificid worms may die (Ruppert and Barnes, 1994).

Most oligochaetes excrete nitrogenous waste and maintain salt and fluid balance with a segmented metanephridial system. Earth-dwelling oligochaetes frequently secrete both ammonia and urea. Some oligochaetes modify their behavior, especially during climatic changes, to maintain fluid balance.

The oligochaete nervous system resembles that of the basic polychaete plan except the cerebral ganglion is usually more posterior in oligochaetes. Oligochaetes also have giant neurons that enable rapid muscular contractions. Well-developed sense organs are absent in oligochaetes, so they rely on dispersed photoreceptors in the integument for light detection.

Reproductive strategies are more numerous in oligochaetes compared with polychaetes. Some species reproduce asexually, some sexually, and others use both strategies. Unlike polychaetes, the majority of oligochaetes are hermaphroditic and display reciprocal sperm transfer (Ruppert and Barnes, 1994). Unfertilized eggs exit via gonopores and are deposited in the clitellum-manufactured cocoon several days after copulation. As the worm contracts, the cocoon passes cranially, and sperm are deposited into the cocoon after the eggs. Fertilization occurs in the cocoon, where direct development (no larval forms) takes place. The developmental interval is quite varied (about a week to several months) depending on species. The single common earthworm (*Lumbricus terrestris*) egg hatches in about 3 months (Ruppert and Barnes, 1994). The cocoons of many species contain more than one egg but rarely more than 20. Time to sexual maturity varies but can be close to a year. Some oligochaetes live for several years and 6-year-old captives have been documented (Ruppert and Barnes, 1994).

Infectious Diseases

As with polychaetes, the literature is not rich with infectious disease descriptions from oligochaetes. Fischer et al. (2003) proved that earthworms belonging to the family Lumbricidae can harbor and perhaps serve as a vector for several mycobacterial species. Although the infection rates by all species of mycobacteria were low among several species of earthworms (8.2% of 109 samples from 433 worms), the authors felt that the earthworms could serve as vectors for these bacteria, but that the risk was minimal, especially since mycobacteria were hard to isolate shortly after the worms ingested contaminated feces. The following organisms were isolated from earthworms sampled in close proximity to vertebrates: *Mycobacterium avium* subsp. *paratuberculosis*, *M. avium*, and *M. scrofulaceum*. There was no evidence of illness in any of the earthworms, and it has been established that earthworms protect themselves from pathogenic bacteria via phagocytosis and with coelomic fluid lytic enzymes (Stein and Cooper, 1978; Marks et al., 1981; Tuckova et al., 1986; Bilej et al., 2000).

It was reported that *L. terrestris* has at least five different coelomocyte types (acidophils, basophils, chlorogogen cells, granulocytes, and neutrophils) plus two subtypes (Stein et al., 1977; Stein and Cooper, 1978) (Table 8.3). These cells were distinguished primarily by cytochemical techniques. All of these cells have pseudopodia and are phagocytic except the chlorogogen cells (Stein et al., 1977). For detailed reviews of earthworm antimicrobial defense, immunity, and the inflammatory response, see Stein and Cooper (1983) and Bilej et al. (2000).

The crystalliferous spore-forming bacterium *Bacillus thuringiensis* has been used as an insecticide against certain lepidopteran larvae (Heimpel, 1955; Heimpel and Angus, 1960). It was discovered that, when the bacteria were applied to soil at high concentrations (30–50 × 10⁹ spores per gram), the ingested bacteria killed 100% of *Lumbricus terrestris* (Smirnoff and Heimpel, 1961). On histopathological examination bacteria were found throughout the body of the worm. The authors pro-

Table 8.3. The major coelomocyte types (Wright's stain) of *Lumbricus terrestris**

Cell type	Frequency (%)	Size (μm)	Cytoplasm	Nucleus	Granule characteristics
Acidophil I	6.2 ± 3.4	10–30	Blue	Dark red–violet; eccentric	Many; pink to red
Acidophil II	0.7 ± 0.5	10–15	Blue	Dark red–violet; eccentric or central	Moderate to many; pink to red
Basophil	63.5 ± 6.1	5–30	Blue	Dark blue–violet; eccentric or central	Few; dark blue
Chlorogogen I		10–25 × 30–60	Pale blue	Rose; eccentric	Many; medium blue
Chlorogogen II	1.4 ± 0.9	12–20	Blue	Rose; eccentric	Many; dark blue–violet
Granulocyte	8.1 ± 6.6	8–40	Blue	Dark violet; eccentric	Variable in color and number
Neutrophil	18.0 ± 5.9	12–50	Pale blue, pink or lavender	Rose; eccentric or central	Few to moderate; color variable

*Modified from Stein et al. (1977).

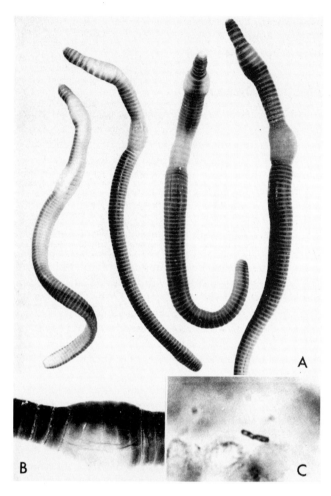

Figure 8.10. **A:** Four *Eisenia foetida* earthworms with blister disease. **B:** Magnified blister (third worm from the left). **C:** Spore former with crystal-shaped body. From Heimpel (1966), Figure 1 (p. 297).

posed that the bacteria penetrated the gut, likely anterior to the gizzard, and then became systemic. A subsequent experiment with much lower (and more applicable) concentrations of the bacteria showed *B. thuringiensis* to be safe for earthworms (Benz and Altwegg, 1975). A condition termed *blister disease* has been described in the earthworm *Eisenia foetida* (Heimpel, 1966). Although Koch's postulates were not fulfilled, *B. thuringiensis* was found to be closely associated with the lesions (Figure 8.10).

Aeromonas hydrophila was consistently isolated from the coelomic cavities of *L. terrestris* and *E. foetida*, but there is no mention of any disease or pathology associated with these cases (Marks and Cooper, 1977).

There is a brief report of a microsporidian infection in four aquatic oligochaetes (Naidu, 1959). In this report, the author identified *Mrazekia caudata* as causing mortality among the worms *Pristina longiseta longiseta* and *Nais communis* (family Naididae). Apparently, the coelomic sporocysts rupture, releasing spores, causing morbidity and mortality in the worm.

Aquatic oligochaetes are well known to be carriers of interme-

diate myxozoan parasite life stages. Intensive research has shown that the myxozoans are not protozoans at all and should be grouped with the Metazoa (Kent et al., 1994; Gilbert and Granath, 2003). In nearly all cases, the primary host for these parasites (over 1300 species) is a teleost fish (Lom and Dykova, 1992). The myxozoan stage that affects the oligochaete host is termed the *triactinomyxon* (TAM). The TAMs occur in the oligochaete gut and develop from ingested myxospores. There is no evidence that these organisms cause significant pathology to the worm (Gilbert and Granath, 2003). The TAMs are excreted in the oligochaete's feces and then attach to a fish by using polar filaments (Gilbert and Granath, 2001) (Figure 8.11). The TAMs migrate to the cartilage of the fish via the central nervous system. The parasite matures, differentiates, and feeds on the cartilage until sporogenesis. Production of myxospores completes the life cycle (Figure 8.12, Color Plate 8.12). Perhaps the most well-studied case is that of *Tubifex tubifex* as the intermediate host for salmonid whirling disease caused by *Myxobolus cerebralis* (Wolf and Markiw, 1984; Gilbert and Granath, 2003). Whirling disease

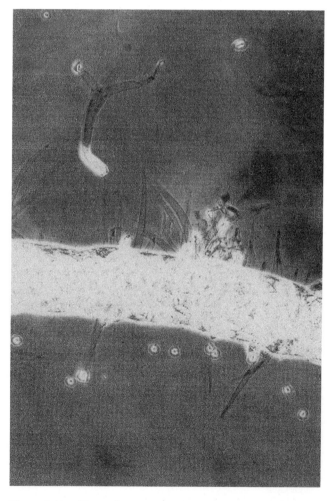

Figure 8.11. Photomicrograph of a fecal packet from *Tubifex tubifex* infected with *Myxobolus cerebralis*. A number of triactinomyxons can be seen breaking free of the packet. From Gilbert and Granath (2001), Figure 1A (p. 103).

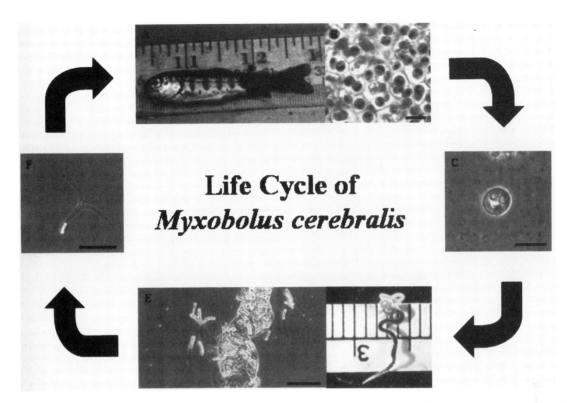

Figure 8.12.   The life cycle of *Myxobolus cerebralis*. **A:** Infected juvenile trout (millimeter scale). **B:** Photomicrograph of heavily infected (numerous myxospores) trout cartilage (scale bar = 20 μm). **C:** A single myxospore that must be ingested by an oligochaetes (scale bar = 10 μm). **D:** A single *Tubifex tubifex* (millimeter scale). **E:** *Tubifex* fecal packet containing triactinomyxons (*TAMs*). **F:** *Myxobolus cerebralis* TAM (scale bar = 150 μm). Fish become infected when a TAM attaches via its polar filaments. From Gilbert and Granath (2003), Figure 1 (p. 659).

has had a huge economic impact in that it has negatively affected both cultured and wild salmonid populations in the United States.

Another important disease of cultured fish in the United States is proliferative gill disease (PGD) of channel catfish (*Ictalurus punctatus*). The causative agent of PGD is the myxosporidian *Aurantiactinomyxon* sp. *Dero digitata*, an aquatic oligochaete, which is known to be an intermediate host for PGD (Bellerud, 1995). *Kidney enlargement disease*, also known as *polycystic kidney disease*, is a serious problem in goldfish (*Carassius auratus*) that is caused by the myxozoan *Hoferellus carassii*. The intermediate host for this parasite is a member of the family Naididae (Trouillier et al., 1996). The authors of this study described the life cycle of *H. carassii* and believe the oligochaete host to be *Nais elinguis* (Figure 8.13).

An interesting study that surveyed live European tubificid oligochaetes destined for the U.S. ornamental fish trade found seven different triactinomyxons (Lowers and Bartholomew, 2003) (Figure 8.14). This study illustrates the risk of importing and feeding live aquatic oligochaetes to fish.

Aside from the myxozoans, there are few reports of parasitic diseases of oligochaetes. Ciliated protozoans parasitize oligo-

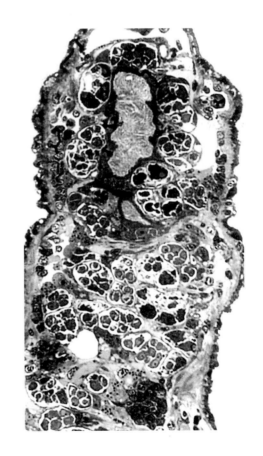

Figure 8.13.   Photomicrograph of the oligochaete *Nais* sp. infected with *Hoferellus carassii*. Multiple developing stage masses of the aurantiactinomyxon spore can be seen between intestinal epithelial cells. ×600. From Trouillier et al. (1996), Figure 24 (pp. 180–181).

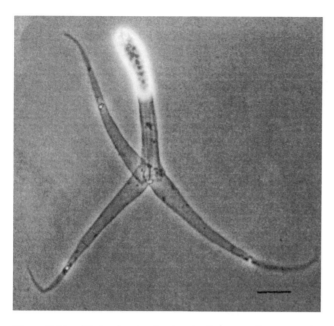

Figure 8.14. Photomicrograph of a triactinomyxon from a tubificid oligochaete destined as food for the ornamental fish hobby. Scale bar = 10 μm. From Lowers and Bartholomew (2003), Figure 8, p. 90.

chaetes. One study (Naidu, 1961) described a new species of ciliate (*Radiophyroides puytoraci*) from the freshwater oligochaete *Aeolosoma travancorense*. The author reported finding four or five ciliates in every worm examined, but did not mention pathology or morbidity.

Anesthesia and Analgesia

Cooper and Roch (1986) describe anesthetizing *Lumbricus terrestris* with a 5% alcohol (presumably ethanol) solution for 1 h prior to tissue-grafting experiments. In a set of earlier experiments, Cooper (1968) describes using 5% ethanol in Rushton's Ringer's solution until the worms (*L. terrestris* and *E. foetida*) were immobilized. Marks and Cooper (1977) employed 5% ethanol at 23°C to immobilize *L. terrestris* and *E. foetida*.

Surgery

There is abundant literature about regeneration and tissue transplantation research on oligochaetes (Cooper, 1968, 1969; Cooper and Roch, 1986). It appears that earthworms readily accept integument autografts but always reject xenografts (Cooper, 1968).

Hirudineans

Natural History and Taxonomy

There are about 500 species of leeches, and they can be found on land, in the marine environment, and in freshwater. They are

more similar to oligochaetes than polychaetes in that they lack a well-defined head and parapodia. Other characteristics they share with oligochaetes include hermaphroditism, gonads and gonadal ducts restricted to a small number of segments, and a cocoon-producing clitellum (Ruppert and Barnes, 1994).

There are no interstitial leeches, and the smallest leech measures about 1 cm in length. The largest member of the group is *Haementeria ghiliani*, an Amazonian leech that attains a length of 30 cm. Unlike polychaetes and oligochaetes, there is not much interspecies morphological variety among the leeches. The anterior and posterior segments have been modified as suckers, and the anterior end is typically more tapered. Leeches are dorsoventrally flattened and have a fixed number of segments (Figure 8.15). All species lack setae. Segmentation is not obvious, and the annular rings do not correspond with the internal segments. (The best way to observe the segmentation is to count the internal ganglia.) Hirudineans lack or have reduced internal septa and coelomic spaces. It is believed this reduction in segmentation and septation contributes to the leech's ability to swim and crawl as opposed to tunnel and burrow. The body wall is similar to that of the other annelids except for a thick layer of subepidermal connective tissue that fills much of the body cavity.

Most leeches occur in freshwater, and their numbers can be

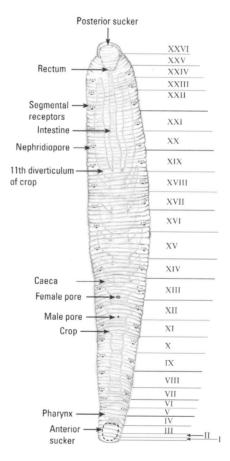

Figure 8.15. A leech with the general anatomy and segmentation illustrated. Drawing by Brenda Bunch.

quite remarkable. They prefer quiet or slow-moving water with high organic loads. One square meter of Illinois water contained over 10,000 leeches (Ruppert and Barnes, 1994).

The majority of leeches lack gills and respire through the epidermis. Some have a typical annelid circulatory system, whereas others rely on coelomic sinuses for fluid transport. Some leeches possess hemoglobin, but many species do not have an oxygen-carrying pigment.

Most leeches feed with the aid of a proboscis that can be everted from the mouth. Whether the leech has a proboscis or not, there are three bladelike teeth in the mouth that work via muscular contractions to compromise the integument of the host. Specialized salivary glands secrete an anticoagulant that helps maintain steady blood flow. A muscular pharynx lies behind the mouth and leads to the esophagus. Next come the stomach, intestine, rectum, and anus. Approximately 75% of leeches suck blood from a host, and the remainder are predaceous on other invertebrates (Ruppert and Barnes, 1994). Although leeches are not host specific, they usually attack one taxon (e.g., fishes, reptiles, or mammals). Some leeches consume the blood of mollusks, crustaceans, insects, and other invertebrates. *Hirudo medicinalis*, the well-known medicinal leech, belongs to the family Hirudinidae that parasitizes mammals. The medicinal leech is capable of making 24 cuts per second with its sharp jaws (Ruppert and Barnes, 1994). Leeches can consume blood volumes in excess of their body weight. *Hirudo* sp. can ingest three or more times its weight in blood, a meal that may take 6 months or more to digest. Leeches use very few digestive enzymes and appear to rely heavily on gut bacterial flora for digestion and assimilation of nutrients.

The leeches' ability to consume relatively large quantities of blood has made them valuable to humans for centuries. Adams (1988) provides an interesting history of the medicinal leech and its application to human medicine. The medicinal leech yields excellent clinical results when placed upon inflamed, congested, and infected human tissues (Karlovitz, 1998; Pardaev et al., 1999; Deuse et al., 2001) and can consume nearly nine times its body weight in blood (Dickinson and Lent, 1984).

Leeches are also valuable to the biomedical community for their natural anticoagulants. Hirudin, produced by the medicinal leech, is a potent thrombin inhibitor (Markwardt, 2002). In fact, research has shown that hirudin is more effective than low molecular weight heparin at preventing deep-vein thrombosis following hip replacement (Breddin, 2003). Gene technology has been used to produce recombinant forms of hirudin for clinical use (Markwardt, 2002; Schoofs et al., 2002; Breddin, 2003).

Leeches have metanephridia that secrete a hypo-osmotic urine and help maintain salt and fluid balance.

The leech nervous system resembles that of polychaetes and oligochaetes. Since there is fusion of some anterior and posterior segments (to form suckers), some of the segmental ganglia occur in close proximity to one another (Ruppert and Barnes, 1994). Leeches do not have well-developed sense organs (merely small simple eyes and sensory papillae), but they are good at detecting light, vibrations, and apparently heat.

Leeches reproduce sexually and, like oligochaetes, are generally hermaphroditic. Whereas oligochaetes are simultaneous hermaphrodites, leeches are protandric hermaphrodites. Fertilization is internal, and the penis deposits sperm into the mate's vagina. Some leeches use *hypodermic impregnation*, where a spermatophore is injected into the mate. In either case, fertilized eggs are deposited into a cocoon secreted by the clitellum. Some leeches (arhynchobdellids) have a larval stage in the cocoon (Ruppert and Barnes, 1994). Others (glossiphoniids) are known to brood their eggs and young.

Unlike some polychaetes and oligochaetes, leeches cannot regenerate (Hyman, 1940).

Infectious Diseases

There is a fair amount of interest in the gut pathogens of leeches because these annelids can serve as vectors for human infectious diseases. Leeches also transmit or have the potential to transmit a wide variety of diseases to nonhuman animals (Dickinson and Lent, 1984; Adams, 1988; Snower et al., 1989; Nehili et al., 1994). These pathogens include viruses, bacteria, and protozoal parasites. Table 8.4 includes a list of leeches and their pathogens, whether in vivo or experimental. There are most certainly many undescribed cases of leeches transmitting pathogens to their hosts. A thorough study examining a number of pathogens surviving in the leech gut found no evidence of them in the leech salivary glands (Nehili et al., 1994). The authors cautioned that leeches are still potential vectors of many pathogens, and manipulating (e.g., squeezing or salting) an attached leech could cause them to regurgitate previously ingested pathogens into the new host. Single use of farmed medicinal leeches will also reduce the risk of disease transmission to humans (Nehili et al., 1994). A technique where a small amount of salt is applied to an engorged medicinal leech (to facilitate regurgitation of a blood meal) has been described in the plastic surgery literature (Aslan et al., 2003). Once regurgitation occurs, the leech should be placed into clean water for salt removal. This technique, although ultimately fatal to the leech, seems to allow for two or three uses for a human patient.

In one study (Mo et al., 2003), *Escherichia coli*, *Proteus* sp., and *Salmonella* sp. were isolated from diseased *Witmania pigra* leeches. The clinical signs included hemorrhage, edema, and soft bodies. An in vitro pathogenicity test involving inoculation of healthy leeches found that 100% of them inoculated with *E. coli* and *Proteus* sp. died, whereas 25% of leeches challenged with *Salmonella* sp. succumbed. The authors determined that all three bacterial organisms were sensitive to a number of antimicrobials, including amikacin, chloramphenicol, and ciprofloxacin. Another study recommended prophylactic antibiotics for human patients being treated with medicinal leeches (Nonomura et al., 1996). The authors isolated *Aeromonas* spp. from the surface and homogenates of all leeches tested (*H. manillensis* and *H. medicinalis*), and *Pseudomonas fluorescens* was frequently found. Based on a sensitivity study involving 15 antimicrobial agents, it was recommended that aminoglycosides, carbapenems, or ofloxacin be used on the human patients.

Kikuchi et al. (2002) examined nine species of glossiphoniid leeches for rickettsial organisms and found them in a large per-

Table 8.4. Some gastrointestinal pathogens of leeches

Leech	Pathogen	References
	Viruses	
Hirudo nipponica	Hepatitis B (experimental)	Zhu, 1986
Piscicola salmositica	Infectious hematopoietic necrosis virus	Mulcahy et al., 1990
Cameroon toothless leech	Hepatitis B	Nehili et al., 1994
	HIV I	Nehili et al., 1994
	HIV II	Nehili et al., 1994
	Bacteria	
Batracobdelloides tricarinata	*Streptococcus* sp.	Bragg et al., 1989
Hirudo medicinalis	*Acinetobacter* sp.	Nehili et al., 1994
	Aeromonas hydrophila	Snower et al, 1989; Nehili et al., 1994
	Aeromonas spp.	Nonomura et al., 1996
	Citrobacter freundii	Nehili et al., 1994
	Escherichia coli	Nehili et al., 1994
	Flavobacterium indologenes	Nehili et al., 1994
	Klebsiella pneumoniae	Nehili et al., 1994
	Morganella morganii	Nehili et al., 1994
	Providencia sp.	Nehili et al., 1994
	Providencia alcalifaciens	Nehili et al., 1994
	Pseudomonas sp.	Nehili et al., 1994
	Pseudomonas alcaligenes	Nehili et al., 1994
	Pseudomonas fluorescens	Nonomura et al., 1996
	Escherichia coli	Mo et al., 2003
	Salmonella sp.	Mo et al., 2003
	Serratia sp.	Nehili et al., 1994
	Proteus sp.	Mo et al., 2003
Torix tagoi	*Rickettsia* sp.	Kikuchi et al., 2002
Hemicrepsis marginata	*Rickettsia* sp.	Kikuchi et al., 2002
	Protozoans	
Glossiphonia complanata	*Nosema glossiphoniae*	Spelling and Young, 1986a
Hirudo medicinalis	*Plasmodium berghei*	Nehili et al., 1994
	Toxoplasma gondii	Nehili et al., 1994
	Trypanosoma brucei	Nehili et al., 1994
Johanssonia arctica	*Trypanosoma murmanensis*	Khan et al., 1980
Malmiana scorpii	*Haemogregarina myoxocephali*	Khan et al., 1980
Oxytonostoma typica	*Haemogregarina delagei*	Siddall and Desser, 2001a
Placobdella ornata	*Haemogregarina balli*	Siddall and Desser, 2001b
	Trematoda	
Erpobdella octoculata	*Cyathocotyle opaca*	Spelling and Young, 1986b
	Apatemon gracilis	Vojtek et al., 1967
	Cotylurus sp.	Votjek et al., 1967
	Prohemistomulum opacum	Votjek et al., 1967
Erpobdella testacea	*Apatemon gracilis*	Vojtek et al., 1967
Glossiphonia complanata	*Cyathocotyle opaca*	Spelling and Young, 1986b
	Cotylurus sp.	Votjek et al., 1967
Haemopis sanguisuga	*Cyathocotyle opaca*	Vojtek et al., 1967
	Apatemon gracilis	Vojtek et al., 1967
	Cotylurus sp.	Votjek et al., 1967
	Prohemistomulum opacum	Votjek et al., 1967
	Prohemistomulum sp.	Votjek et al., 1967
Helobdella stagnalis	*Cyathocotyle opaca*	Spelling and Young, 1986b
Hemiclepsis marginata	*Cotylurus* sp.	Votjek et al., 1967
Hirudo medicinalis	*Apatemon gracilis*	Vojtek et al., 1967
	Prohemistomulum opacum	Votjek et al., 1967
	Prohemistomulum sp.	Votjek et al., 1967

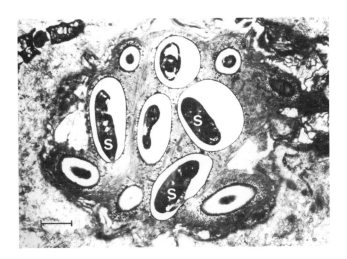

Figure 8.16. *Nosema glossiphoniae* spores infecting muscle tissue of the leech *Glossiphonia complanata*. Scale bar = 2 μm. From Spelling and Young (1986a), Figure 1 (p. 183).

centage of wild leeches from two species (Table 8.4). The authors state that the leech *Rickettsia* sp. is distinct from arthropod-associated *Rickettsia* species. This is the first published report of *Rickettsia* from an annelid.

One study (Czeczuga et al., 2003) described a variety of zoosporic fungal organisms from 17 species of leeches in Polish waters. The most common organism isolated from the leeches was *Saprolegnia* spp., followed by *Peronosporales* spp. All of the leeches tested harbored at least one species of *Saprolegnia*, and *Dictyuchus sterile* was cultured from 13 leech species.

The microsporidian *Nosema glossiphoniae* infects the muscle tissues of the leech *Glossiphonia complanata* (Spelling and Young, 1986a). Meronts and mature spores were found in the pale white lesions located ventrally on the leech (Figure 8.16).

Trematode metacercaria have been described from a number of leech species but do not seem to harm the annelids (Vojtek et al., 1967; Spelling and Young, 1986b).

Anesthesia

There is little in the literature on anesthesia of leeches. One article describes the use of saturated mephenesin (3-*o*-toloxy-1,2-propanediol) to anesthetize leeches for grafting research (Tettamanti et al., 2003).

Surgery

Little work has been performed with regard to surgery in leeches. A recent study (Tettamanti et al., 2003) examined allograft and xenograft rejection in the medicinal leech, *Hirudo medicinalis* (xenografts originated from *Glossiphonia complanata*). The authors used surgical cat gut (Johnson and Johnson, New Brunswick, NJ) to suture grafts onto the recipient leech. Postsurgically, leeches were kept in moist chambers for 24 h before their return to an aquatic system. All of the

leeches survived the anesthetic and surgical protocol. In this study, autografts resulted only in local inflammation. *Hirudo medicinalis* rejected both allografts and xenografts.

References

Adams SL. 1988. The medicinal leech: A page from the annelids of internal medicine. Ann Intern Med 109:399–405.

Anderson SL and Wild GC. 1994. Linking genotoxic responses and reproductive success in ecotoxicology. Environ Health Perspect 102(Suppl 12):9–12.

Anderson SL, Harrison FL, Chan G, and Moore DH. 1990. Comparison of whole animal and cellular bioassays in the prediction of radiation effects on marine organisms. Arch Environ Contam Toxicol 19:164–174.

Aslan G, Terzioglu A, and D Tuncali. 2003. The re-usable medicinal leech. Plast Reconstr Surg 111:1358–1359.

Bartholomew JL, Whipple MJ, Stevens DG, and Fryer JL. 1997. The life cycle of *Ceratomyxa shasta*, a myxosporean parasite of salmonids, requires a freshwater polychaete as an alternate host. J Parasitol 83:859–868.

Bellerud BL. 1995. Etiological and epizootiological factors associated with outbreaks of proliferative gill disease in channel catfish. J Aquat Anim Health 7:124–131.

Benkendorff K, Davis AR, and Bremner JB. 2001. Chemical defense in egg masses of benthic invertebrates: An assessment of antibacterial activity in 39 mollusks and 4 polychaetes. J Invertebr Pathol 78:109–118.

Benz G and Altwegg A. 1975. Safety of *Bacillus thuringiensis* for earthworms. J Invertebr Pathol 26:125–126.

Bilej M, de Baetselier P, and Beschin A. 2000. Antimicrobial defense of the earthworm. Folia Microbiol 45:283–300.

Bragg RR, Oosthuizen JH, and Lordan SM. 1989. The leech *Batracobdelloides tricarinata* Blanchard 1897, Hirudinea: Glossiphoniidae as a possible reservoir of the rainbow trout pathogenic *Streptococcus* spp. Onderstepoort J Vet Res 56:203–204.

Breddin HK. 2003. Current developments in antithrombotic therapy: The role of antithrombin agents. Pathophysiol Haemost Thromb 32(Suppl 3):1–8.

Calkins G. 1915. *Microtaeniella clymenellae*, a new genus and a new species of colonial gregarines. Biol Bull 29:46–49.

Chatton E. 1920. Les Peridiniens parasites: Morphologie, reproduction, ethologie. Arch Zool Exp Gen 59:1–475.

Clark ME. 1968. Later stages of regeneration in the polychaete, *Nephtys*. J Morphol 124:483–510.

Clavier J. 1984. Production due to regeneration by *Euclymene oerstedi* (Claparede) (Polychaeta: Maldanidae) in the maritime basin of the Rance (northern Brittany). J Exp Mar Biol Ecol 75:97–106.

Conan G. 1982. The long-term effects of the Amoco Cadiz oil spill. Philos Trans R Soc Lond [B] 297:323–333.

Cooper EL. 1968. Transplantation immunity in annelids. Transplantation 6:322–337.

Cooper EL. 1969. Specific tissue graft rejection in earthworms. Science 166:1414–1415.

Cooper EL and Roch P. 1986. Second-set allograft responses in the earthworm *Lumbricus terrestris*. Transplantation 41:514–520.

Costelloe M, Costelloe J, O'Connor B, and Smith P. 1998. Bull Eur Assoc Fish Pathol 18:22–25.

Czeczuga B, Kiziewicz B, and Godlewska A. 2003. Zoosporic fungi growing on leeches (Hirudinea). Pol J Environ Stud 12:361–369.

Depledge MH and Billinghurst Z. 1999. Ecological significance of endocrine disruption in marine invertebrates. Mar Pollut Bull 39:32–38.

Desportes I and Théodoridès J. 1986. *Cygnicollum lankesteri* n. sp., grégarine (Apicomplexa, Lecudinidae) parasite des annélides polychètes *Laetmonice hystrix* et *L. producta*: Particularités de l'appareil de fixation et implications taxonomiques. Protistologica 22:47–60.

Deuse U, Esch T, Dobos G, and Moebus S. 2001. Effects of leech therapy (*Hirudo medicinalis*) in painful osteoarthritis of the knee: A pilot study. Ann Rheum Dis 60:986.

Devauchelle G and Durchon M. 1973. Sur la presence d'un virus du type *Iridovirus* dans les cellules males de *Nereis diversicolor*. C R Acad Sci (Paris) [D] 277:463–466.

Dickinson MH and Lent CM. 1984. Feeding behavior of the medicinal leech, *Hirudo medicinalis* L. J Comp Physiol [A] 154:449–455.

Dilmore LA and Hood MA. 1986. Vibrios of some deep-water invertebrates. FEMS Microbiol Lett 35:221–224.

Dogiel V. 1906. *Haplozoon armatum*, n. gen., n. sp., der Vertreter einer neuen Mesozoa-Gruppe. Zool Anz 30:895–899.

Eckberg WR and Hill SD. 1996. *Chaetopterus*: Oocyte maturation, early development, and regeneration. Mar Mod Elect Rec, 6 Aug. Available from www.mbl.edu/Biological.Bulletin/mmer.html.

Fauchald K. 1977. The polychaete worms: Definitions and keys to the orders, families, and genera. Nat Hist Mus Los Angel Cty Sci Ser 28:1–190.

Felbeck H and Somero GN. 1982. Primary production in deep-sea hydrothermal vent organisms: Roles of sulfide-oxidizing bacteria. Trends Biochem Sci 7:201–204.

Felbeck H, Liebezeit G, Dawson R, and Giere O. 1983. CO2 fixation in tissues of marine oligochaetes (*Phallodrilus leukodermatus* and *P. planus*) containing symbiotic, chemoautotrophic bacteria. Mar Biol 75:187–191.

Fischer OA, Matlova L, Bartl J, Dvorska L, Svastova P, du Maine R, Melicharek I, Bartos M, and Pavlik I. 2003. Earthworms (Oligochaeta, Lumbricidae) and mycobacteria. Vet Microbiol 91:325–338.

Ganapati PN. 1946. Notes on some gregarines from polychaetes of the Madras coast. Proc Indian Acad Sci [B] 23:228–238.

Gilbert MA and Granath WO. 2001. Persistent infection of *Myxobolus cerebralis*, the causative agent of salmonid whirling disease, in *Tubifex tubifex*. J Parasitol 87:101–107.

Gilbert MA and Granath WO. 2003. Whirling disease of salmonid fish: Life cycle, biology, and disease. J Parasitol 89:658–667.

Harder T, Lau SC, Dahms HU, and Qian PY. 2002. Isolation of bacterial isolates as natural inducers for larval settlement in the marine polychaete *Hydroides elegans* (Haswell). J Chem Ecol 28:2029–2043.

Hartman O. 1959. Catalogue of the polychaetous annelids of the world. Occasional Papers of the Allan Hancock Foundation 23, 628 pp.

Hartman O. 1965. Supplement and index to the catalogue of the polychaetous annelids of the world, including additions and emendations since 1959. Occasional Papers of the Allan Hancock Foundation 28:1-197.

Harrison FL, Rice DW Jr, Moore DH, and Varela M. 1986. Effects of radiation on frequency of chromosomal aberrations and sister chromatid exchange in the benthic worm *Neanthes arenaceodentata*. In: Capuzzo JM and Kester DR, eds. Oceanic Processes in Marine Pollution, volume 1. Krieger, Malabar, FL, pp 145–156.

Heimpel AM. 1955. Investigations of the mode of action of strains of *Bacillus cereus* Fr. and Fr. pathogenic for the larch sawfly, *Pristiphora erichsonii* (Htg.). Can J Zool 33:311–326.

Heimpel AM. 1966. A crystalliferous bacterium associated with a "blister disease" in the earthworm, *Eisenia foetida* (Savigny). J Invertebr Pathol 8:295–298.

Heimpel AM and Angus TA. 1960. Bacterial insecticides. Bacteriol Rev 24:266–288.

Hyman LH. 1940. Aspects of regeneration in annelids. Am Nat 74:513–527.

Ilan M, Jensen RA, and Morse DE. 1993. Calcium control of metamorphosis in polychaete larvae. J Exp Zool 267:423–430.

Karlovitz A. 1998. Lingual trauma: The use of medicinal leeches in the treatment of massive lingual hematoma. J Trauma Injury Infect Crit Care 44:1083–1085.

Kent ML, Margolis L, and Corliss JO. 1994. The demise of a class of protists: Taxonomic and nomenclatural revisions proposed for the protist phylum Myxozoa Grasse, 1970. Can J Zool 72:932–937.

Khan RA, Barrett M, and Murphy J. 1980. Blood parasites of fish from the northwestern Atlantic Ocean. Can J Zool 58:770–781.

Kikuchi Y, Sameshima S, Kitade O, Kojima J, and Fukatsu T. 2002. Novel clade of *Rickettsia* spp. from leeches. Appl Environ Microbiol 68:999–1004.

Kozloff EN. 1961. A new genus and two new species of Ancistrocomid ciliates (Holotricha: Thigmotricha) from sabellid polychaetes and from a chiton. J Protozool 8:60–63.

Kozloff EN. 1965. *Ciliocincta sabellariae* gen. and sp. n., an orthonectid mesozoan from the polychaete *Sabellaria cementarium* Moore. J Parasitol 51:37–44.

Lankester RE. 1863. On our present knowledge of the Gregarinidae with description of three new species belonging to that class. Q J Microbiol Sci 3:83–96.

Lankester RE. 1866. Notes on the Gregarinida. Q J Microbiol Sci 6:23–28.

Leander BS, Saldarriaga JF, and Keeling PJ. 2002. Surface morphology of the marine parasite *Haplozoon axiothellae* Siebert (Dinoflagellata). Eur J Protistol 38:287–297.

Lewbart G and Riser N. 1996. Nuchal organs of the polychaete *Parapionosyllis manca* (Syllidae). Invertebr Biol 115:286–298.

Lom J and Dykova I. 1992. Protozoan parasites of fishes. Elsevier, Amsterdam, 314 pp.

Lowers JM and Bartholomew JL. 2003. Detection of myxozoan parasites in oligochaetes imported as food for ornamental fish. J Parasitol 89:84–91.

Marcano L, Nusetti J, Rodriguez GJ, and Vilas J. 1996. Uptake and depuration of copper and zinc in relation to metal-binding protein in the polychaete *Eurythoe complanta*. Comp Biochem Physiol [c] 114:179–184.

Marks DH and Cooper EL. 1977. *Aeromonas hydrophila* in the coelomic cavity of the earthworms *Lumbricus terrestris* and *Eisenia foetida*. J Invertebr Pathol 29:382–383.

Marks DH, Stein EA, and Cooper EL. 1981. Acid phosphatase changes associated with response to foreign tissue in the earthworm *Lumbricus terrestris*. Comp Biochem Physiol 68:681–683.

Markwardt F. 2002. Hirudin as alternative anticoagulant: A historical review. Semin Thromb Hemostasis 28:405–414.

Martin D and Britayev TA. 1998. Symbiotic polychaetes: Review of known species. Oceanogr Mar Biol Annu Rev 36:217–340.

McCurdy DG. 2001. Asexual reproduction in *Pygospio elegans claparede* (Annelida, Polychaeta) in relation to parasitism by *Lepocreadium setiferoides* (Miller and Northrup) (Platyhelminthes, Trematoda). Biol Bull 201:45–51.

Metchnikoff E. 1884. Researches on the intracellular digestion of invertebrates. Q J Microbiol Sci 24:89–111.

Micaletto G, Gambi MC, and Cantone G. 2002. A new record of the endosymbiont polychaete *Veneriserva* (Dorvilleidae), with description of a new sub-species, and relationships with its host *Laetmonice producta* (Polychaeta: Aphroditidae) in Southern Ocean waters (Antarctica). Mar Biol (Berl) 141:691–698.

Mo ML, Wei P, Zhou WG, Liao PJ, and Hua QH. 2003. Isolation and characterization of common pathogens from diseased leeches. Chin J Zool 38:2–7.

Mulcahy D, Klaybor D, and Batts WN. 1990. Isolation of infectious hematopoietic virus from a leech (*Piscicola salmositica*) and a copepod (*Salmincola* sp.), ectoparasites of sockeye salmon *Oncorhynchus nerka*. Dis Aquat Org 8:29–34.

Müller MCM, Berenzen A, and Westheide W. 2003. Experiments on anterior regeneration in *Eurythoe complanata* ("Polychaeta," Amphinomidae): Reconfiguration of the nervous system and its function for regeneration. Zoomorphology 122:95–103.

Naidu KV. 1959. Occurrence of a microsporidian (Protozoa) parasite in freshwater oligochaetes. Curr Sci 28:212.

Naidu KV. 1961. *Radiophryoides puytoraci* sp. nov.: Astomatous ciliate parasite from a fresh-water oligochaete. J Protozool 8:248–249.

Nehili M, Ilk C, Mehlhorn H, Ruhnau K, Dick W, and Njayou M. 1994. Experiments on the possible role of leeches as vectors of animal and human pathogens: A light and electron microscopy study. Parasitol Res 80:277–290.

Neresheimer E. 1908. Die Mesozoen. Zool Zentralbl 15:257–312.

Nonomura H, Kato N, Ohno Y, Itokazu M, Matsunaga T, and Watanabe K. 1996. Indigenous bacterial flora of medicinal leeches and their susceptibilities to 15 antimicrobial agents. J Med Microbiol 45:490–493.

Nusetti O, Rodriguez GJ, and Vilas J. 1998. Immune and biochemical responses of the polychaete *Eurythoe complanata* exposed to sublethal concentration of copper. Comp Biochem Physiol [C] 119:177–183.

Pardaev DE, Bakhramov SM, and Umarov KhM. 1999. Use of medicinal leeches in the treatment of nose furuncle and carbuncle. Uzbekiston Tibbiet Zhurnali 0(2):24–26.

Poche F. 1913. Das System der Protozoa. Arch Protistenkd 30:125–321.

Price LJ and Depledge MH. 1998. Effects of the xenooestrogen nonylphenol on the polychaete *Dinophilus gyrociliatus* [abstr]. In: Abstracts of the eighth annual meeting of the SETAC Europe, 3h/P008.

Raftos DA and Cooper EL. 1990. Diseases of Annelida. In: Kinne O, ed. Diseases of Marine Animals. Biologische Anstalt Helgoland, Hamburg, pp 229–243.

Reimer LW. 1973. Das Auftreten eines Fischtrematoden der Gattung *Asymphylodora* Loos, 1899, bei *Nereis diversicolor* O.F. Müller als Beispiel für einen Alternativzyklus. Zool Anz 191:187–196.

Richards KS, Fleming TP, and Jamieson BGM. 1982. An ultrastructural study of the distal epidermis and the occurrence of subcuticular bacteria in the gutless tubificid *Phallodrilus albidus* (Oligochaeta: Annelida). Aust J Zool 30:327–336.

Robbins IJ, Warren LM, Bestwick BW, and Rusin J. 1987. Functional anaerobiosis in the polychaete *Terebella lapidaria* L. Comp Biochem Physiol [A] 87:171–174.

Ruangsri J and Supamattaya K. 1999. DNA detection of suspected virus (SEMBV) carriers by PCR (polymerase chain reaction). Proceedings of the 37th Kasetsart University Annual Conference, pp 82–94.

Ruppert EE and Barnes RD. 1994. Invertebrate Zoology, 6th edition. Saunders College, Philadelphia, pp 499–595.

Ruppert EE, Fox RS, and Barnes RD. 2004. Invertebrate Zoology: A Functional Evolutionary Approach, 7th edition. Thompson-Brooks/Cole, Belmont, CA, 963 pp.

Scaps P and Borot O. 2000. Acetylcholinesterase activity of the polychaete *Nereis diversicolor*: Effects of temperature and salinity. Comp Biochem Physiol [C] 125:377–383.

Scaps P, Demuynck S, Descamps M, and Dhainaut A. 1997. Effects of organophosphate and carbamate pesticides on acetylcholinesterase and choline acetyltransferase of the polychaete *Nereis diversicolor*. Arch Environ Contam Toxicol 33:203–208.

Schoofs L, Clynen E, and Salzet M. 2002. Trypsin and chymotrypsin inhibitors in insects and gut leeches. Curr Pharm Des 8:483–491.

Schrével J. 1969. Recherches sur le cycle des Lecudinidae, Grégarines parasites d'Annélides polychètes. Protistologica 5:561–587.

Shumway W. 1924. The genus *Haplozoon*, Dogiel: Observations on the life history and systematic position. J Parasitol 11:59–74.

Siddall ME and Desser S. 2001a. Developmental stages of *Haemogregarina delagei* in the leech *Oxytonostoma typica*. Can J Zool 79:1897–1900.

Siddall ME and Desser S. 2001b. Transmission of *Haemogregarina balli* from painted turtles to snapping turtles through the leech *Placobdella ornata*. J Parasitol 87:1217–1218.

Siebert AE. 1973. A description of *Haplozoon axiothellae* n. sp., an endosymbiont of the polychaete *Axiothella rubrocincta*. J Phycol 9:185–190.

Smirnoff WA and Heimpel AM. 1961. Notes on the pathogenicity of *Bacillus thuringiensis* var. *thuringiensis* Berliner for the earthworm, *Lumbricus terrestris* Linneaus. J Insect Pathol 3:403–408.

Snower DP, Ruef C, Kuritza AP, and Edberg SC. 1989. *Aeromonas hydrophila* infection associated with the use of medicinal leeches. J Clin Microbiol 27:1421–1422.

Spelling SM and Young JO. 1986a. *Nosema glossiphoniae* Schroder rediscovered. J Parasitol 72:182–183.

Spelling SM and Young JO. 1986b. The occurrence of metacercariae of the trematode, *Cyanthocotyle opaca* (Wisniewski), in three species of lake-dwelling leeches. Freshwater Biol 16:609–613.

Stein EA and Cooper EL. 1978. Cytochemical observations of coelomocytes from the earthworm, *Lumbricus terrestris*. Histochem J 10:657–678.

Stein EA and Cooper EL. 1983. Inflammatory responses in annelids. Am Zool 23:145–156.

Stein EA, Avtalion R, and Cooper EL. 1977. The coelomocytes of the earthworm, *Lumbricus terrestris*: Morphology and phagocytic properties. J Morphol 153:467–477.

Tettamanti G, Grimaldi A, Ferrarese R, Palazzi M, Perletti G, Valvassori R, Cooper EL, Lanzavecchia G, and de Eguileor M. 2003. Leech responses to tissue transplantation. Tissue Cell 35:199–212.

Trouillier A, El-Matbouli M, and Hoffmann RW. 1996. A new look at the life-cycle of *Hoferellus carassii* in the goldfish (*Carassius auratus auratus*) and its relation to "kidney enlargement disease" (KED). Folia Parasitol (Prague) 43:173–187.

Tuckova L, Rejnek J, Sima P, and Ondrejova R. 1986. Lytic activities in coelomic fluid of *Eisenia foetida* and *Lumbricus terrestris*. Dev Comp Immunol 10:181–189.

Vetvicka V. 1994. Brief comparison of vertebrate and invertebrate defense reactions. In: Vetvicka V, Sima P, Cooper EL, Bilej M, and Roch P ed.. Immunology of Annelids. CRC Press, Boca Raton, FL, pp 263–279.

Vetvicka V, Sima P, Cooper EL, Bilej M, and Roch P, ed. 1994. Immunology of Annelids. CRC Press, Boca Raton, FL, 299 pp.

Vojtek J, Oprviolva V, and Votjtkova L. 1967. The importance of leeches in the life-cycle of the order Strigeidida (Trematoda). Folia Parasitol (Prague) 14:107–119.

Young JS and Roesijadi G. 1983. Reparatory adaptation to copper-induced injury and occurrence of a copper-binding protein in the polychaete, *Eudistylia vancouveri*. Mar Pollut Bull 14:30–32.

Zander CD and Reimer LW. 2002. Parasitism at the ecosystem level in the Baltic Sea. Parasitology 124(Suppl):S119–S135.

Zhu Z. 1986. An experimental study of carrier of hepatitis B virus in leeches. Chin J Epidemiol 7:4–5.

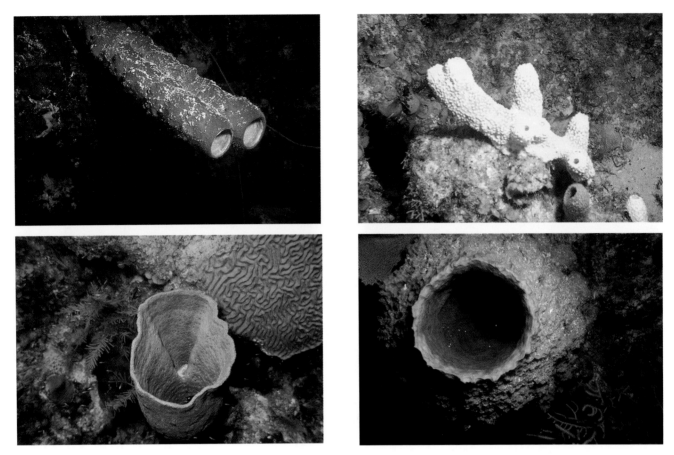

Color Plate 2.4. Four different sponges from the Turks and Caicos Islands. Symbiotic zooxanthellae can impart striking colors upon the sponge.

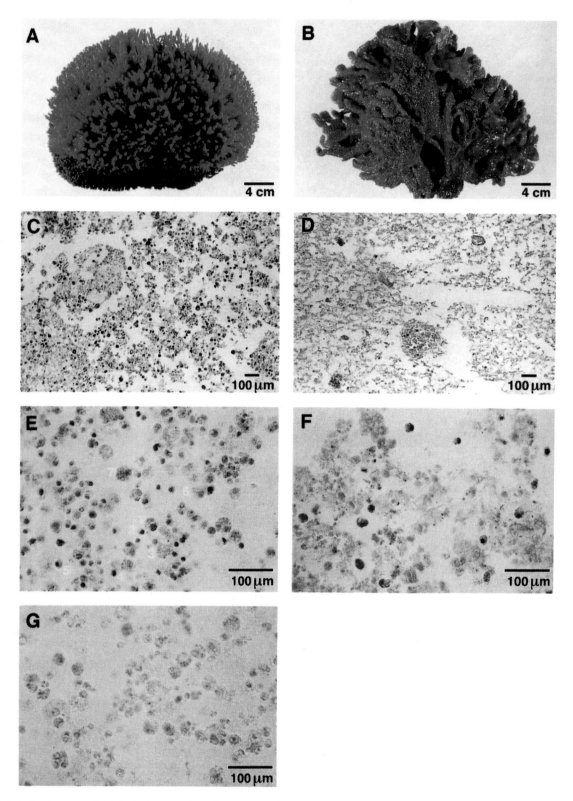

Color Plate 2.5. Gross and histological comparison of summer and winter *Microciona prolifera*: summer sponge **(A)** and winter sponge **(B)**. The winter sponge displays less color and integrity. Microscopic view of summer sponge **(C)** shows more cellularity than that of the winter sponge **(D)**. A TUNEL (terminal deoxyribonucleotidyl transferase-mediated dUTP nick end label) assay shows fragmenting nuclear DNA as brownish red **(E)**, whereas **G** is the counterstained control (no TUNEL). *Yellow numbers* are as follows: *1* and *7*, phagocytosed apoptotic cells; *2* and *5*, small apoptotic cells; and *3*, *4*, and *6*, macrophage-type (apparently healthy) and small apoptotic cells. In the winter sponge TUNEL assay **(F)**, a small number of healthy stem cells (blue nuclei) are mixed with clumps of apoptotic debris. From Kuhns et al. (1997), Figure 1 (pp. 239–240). Reprinted by permission of the Marine Biological Laboratory, Woods Hole, MA.

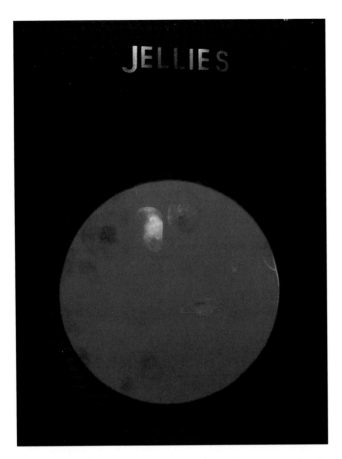

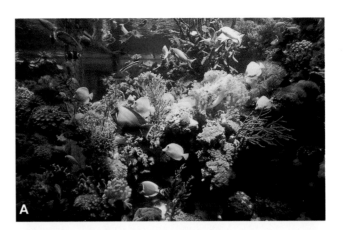

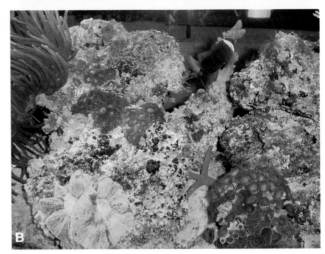

Color Plate 3.6. Jellyfish displays are becoming very popular at public aquariums and zoological parks, as well as some restaurants. Jellies are typically displayed in cylindrical tanks with carefully controlled water flow and attractive lighting. This public display contains Western Atlantic moon jellyfish (*Aurelia aurita*).

Color Plate 3.7. Private coral reef aquariums are becoming very popular throughout the world. **A:** An 11,000-L system owned by David Saxby in London. **B:** Many hobbyists are enjoying much smaller systems like the animals in this 600-L aquarium. Photo A courtesy of www.biophoto.net.

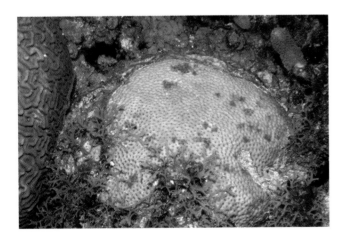

Color Plate 3.10. Dark spots disease affecting *Siderastrea sideria*. Photo courtesy of E.H. Borneman.

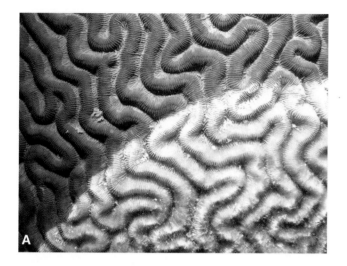

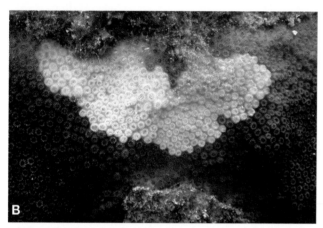

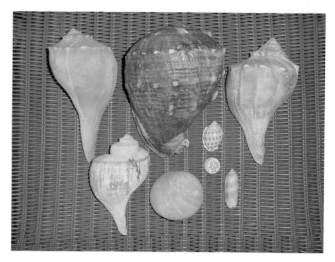

Color Plate 5.1. Spiral shell forms: seven species of Western Atlantic marine gastropods from North Carolina (**clockwise from bottom:** Moon snail, *Polinices duplicatus*; channeled whelk, *Busycon canaliculatum*; lightning whelk, *Busycon contrarium*; helmet, *Cassis* sp.; Scotch bonnet, *Phalium granulatum*; knobbed whelk, *Busycon carica*; and lettered olive, *Oliva sayana*. Note that all have dextral whorls (opening to the *right* when the animal's soft parts are facing the observer) except the lightning whelk, which has a sinistral opening. (Coin, U.S. quarter)

Color Plate 3.14. White plague disease afflicting **(A)** *Colpophyllia natans* and **(B)** *Montastrea Faveolata*. Photo courtesy of E.H. Borneman.

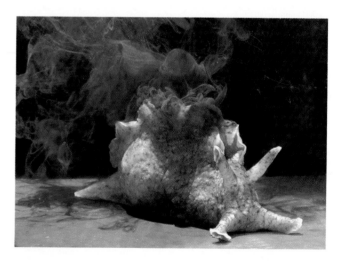

Color Plate 5.4. Healthy animal inking. Photo courtesy of Genevieve Anderson, Santa Barbara City College, Santa Barbara, CA.

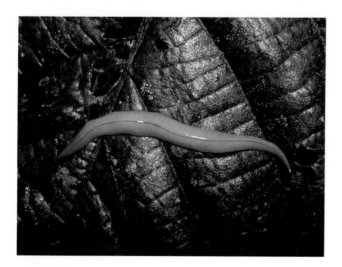

Color Plate 4.1. An unidentified terrestrial planarian from Ecuador, likely a *Bipalium* sp. Some tropical species approach 50–60 cm in length. This retracted specimen was approximately 10 cm.

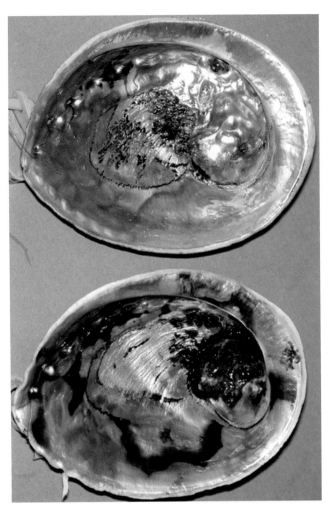

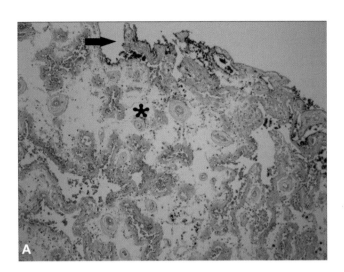

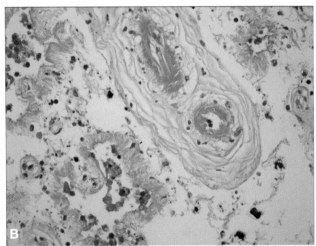

Color Plate 5.17. Shells from the New Zealand black abalone showing grossly visible shell disease. The shell at the **top** displays the mineralized form of the disease, whereas the shell at the **bottom** contains the gelatinous form. Photos courtesy of Hendrick Nollens, University of Florida, Gainesville, FL, and Inter-Research.

Color Plate 6.13. Ink sacculitis, hemocytic, diffuse, mild, with marked edema in an octopus. **A:** The ink-sac mucosa (*arrow*) is covered by black pigment, and there is edema of the submucosa (*star*). Hemocytes are scattered throughout. **B:** Perivascular edema and sloughing of ink-sac mucosal cells. Photos courtesy of David Rotstein.

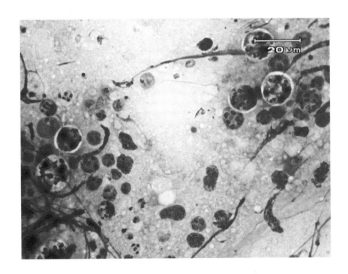

Color Plate 7.12. Tissue imprint from *Ostrea edulis* infected with the protozoan, *Marteilia refringens*, the agent of Aber disease. An identifying characteristic of *Marteilia refringens* is the brightly eosinophilic inclusions or refringent bodies within the sporangia.

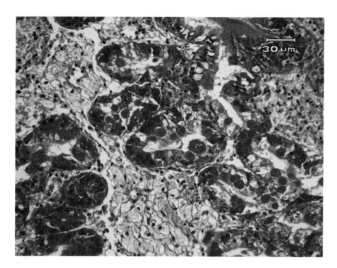

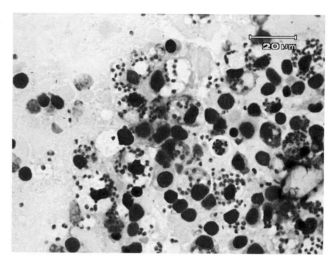

Color Plate 7.13. This histological section from the digestive gland of the oyster *Ostrea edulis* illustrates the severe damage that *Marteilia refringens* can inflict on the host, particularly when large numbers of spores are released simultaneously from the digestive-gland epithelium. Multifocally, there is extensive necrosis and loss of digestive epithelial cells; the remaining cells are often swollen and have microvilli loss at the lumenal surface. Tubule lumens contain necrotic debris and scattered sloughed, swollen cells, many of which are infected with *M. refringens*. Hematoxylin–eosin stain.

Color Plate 7.14. Tissue imprint from the oyster *Ostrea edulis* shows hemocytes infected with multiple cells of *Bonamia ostreae*. This parasite is round, deeply basophilic, and measures 2–3 μm in diameter. A stained direct smear (cytological preparation) is often the best way to identify specific parasite morphology, since there are minimal processing artifacts when compared with histological preparations

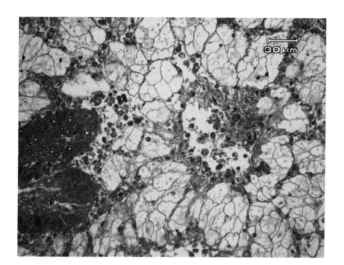

Color Plate 7.15. Histological section of the digestive gland of the oyster *Ostrea edulis*. The vesicular connective tissue surrounding the two digestive-gland tubules at the *left* is infiltrated with granular hemocytes, many of which are infected with multiple cells of *Bonamia ostreae*. Bonamiasis is characterized by heavy hemocytic infiltration especially around the stomach and digestive gland, but also may involve the gonad and gills. Hematoxylin–eosin stain.

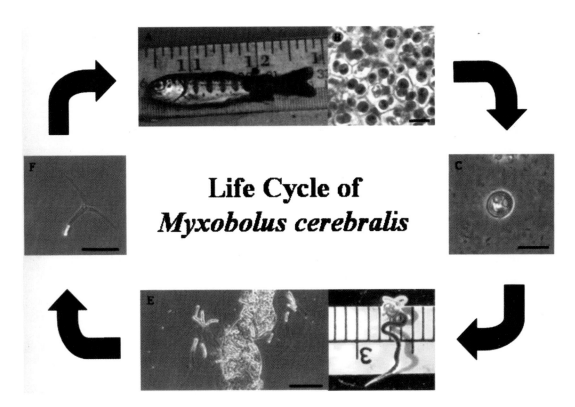

Life Cycle of
Myxobolus cerebralis

Color Plate 8.12. The life cycle of *Myxobolus cerebralis*. **A:** Infected juvenile trout (millimeter scale). **B:** Photomicrograph of heavily infected (numerous myxospores) trout cartilage (scale bar = 20 μm). **C:** A single myxospore that must be ingested by an oligochaetes (scale bar = 10 μm). **D:** A single *Tubifex tubifex* (millimeter scale). **E:** *Tubifex* fecal packet containing triactinomyxons (*TAMs*). **F:** *Myxobolus cerebralis* TAM (scale bar = 150 μm). Fish become infected when a TAM attaches via its polar filaments. From Gilbert and Granath (2003), Figure 1 (p. 659).

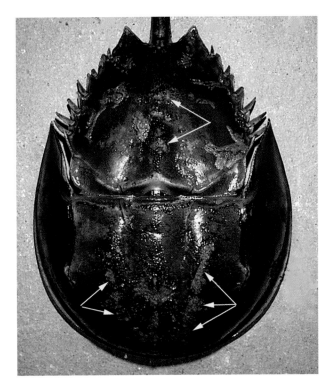

Color Plate 9.7. Typical lesion produced by green-algal infection of the carapace.

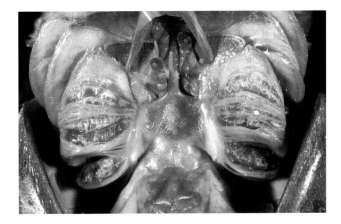

Color Plate 9.13. Hemorrhage and clotting of blue hemolymph in multiple gill leaflets.

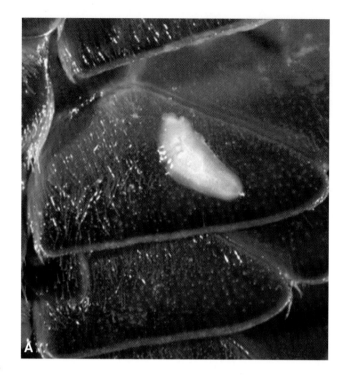

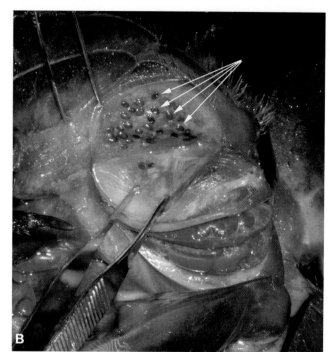

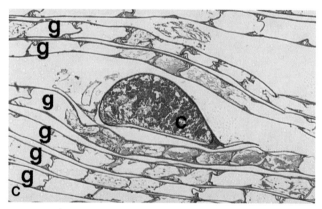

Color Plate 9.11. **A:** *Bdelloura* sp., a common external parasite, on the ventral structures of the horseshoe crab. **B:** Stalked cocoons of *Bdelloura* sp. (indicated by *arrows*) attached to the gill leaflets of a horseshoe crab. **C:** Histological preparation of the gill leaflets (g) of a horseshoe crab demonstrating the cocoon (c) and stalked attachment of *Bdelloura* sp. to the chitinous leaflets.

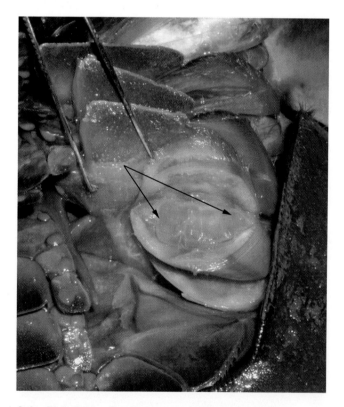

Color Plate 9.14. Emphysema of a gill leaflet (*arrows*) of a horseshoe crab as a result of supersaturation of atmospheric gases in the culture water.

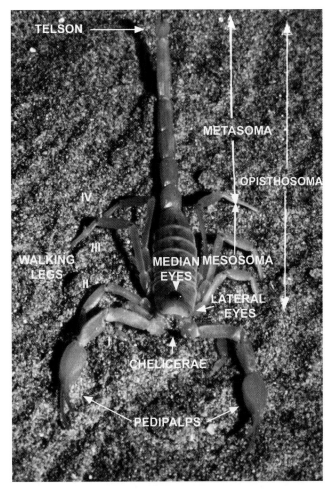

Color Plate 11.1. An adult male desert hairy scorpion, *Hadrurus hirsutus*, from the southern California desert. Note the eight walking legs; large pincerlike pedipalps; and narrow, cylindrical metasoma (tail) comprised of six segments and bearing the bulbous telson which contains paired venom glands and a hollow fanglike sting.

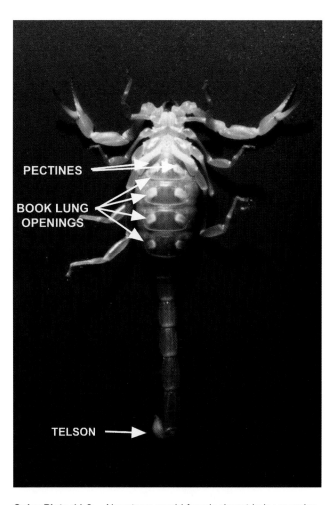

Color Plate 11.2. Near-term gravid female desert hairy scorpion, *Hadrurus hirsutus*, anesthetized to permit restraint and positioning for photography. The four pair of spiracles (book lung openings) can be seen on tergites 10–13. The paired comblike pectines are located immediately caudal to the last pair of walking legs.

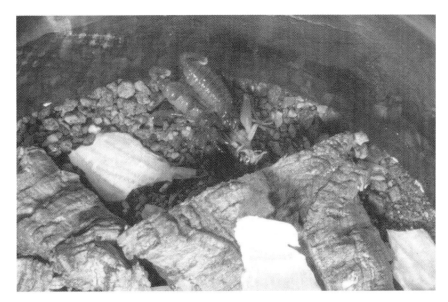

Color Plate 11.6. Two juvenile emperor scorpions, *Pandinus imperator*, sharing a single prey cricket. Note the lettuce leaves that were provided as food for any surplus crickets. It is necessary to provide food for the crickets so that they will not attack the scorpions. Young scorpions are more likely to accept the presence of their peers than are adults that are raised in isolation.

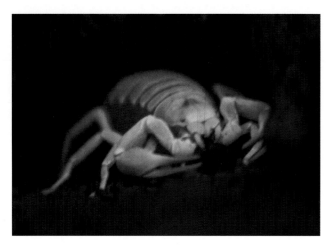

Color Plate 11.9. Adult female desert hairy scorpion, *Hadrurus hirsutus*, in her lair that is illuminated with ultraviolet light. This fluorescent reflection of the chitinous exoskeleton is characteristic of scorpions and it provides a means for locating them in the field or in a building at night.

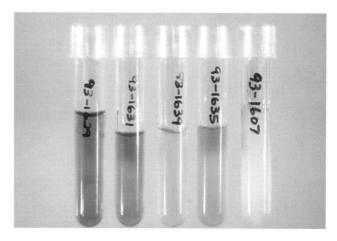

Color Plate 12.11. Appearance of various hemolymph samples from individual blue crabs (from Noga, 2000c). (Note that variations in color may be interpreted differently in various crustacean species.) (**From left to right**) *First tube:* Normal, intense blue indicating a high concentration of hemocyanin. *Second tube:* Freshly collected sample with normal, intense blue developing at the top of the tube due to the diffusion of atmospheric oxygen. *Third tube:* Pale color due to abnormally low concentration of hemocyanin. *Fourth tube:* Yellow to blue-green that is indicative of the variation in hemolymph color that can occur even among normal individuals. *Fifth tube:* Cloudy appearance, which may be associated with certain infections.

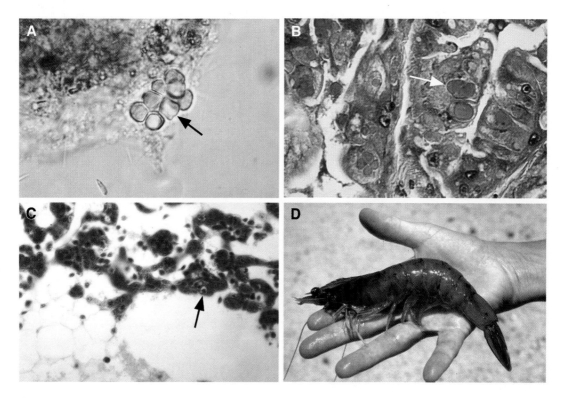

Color Plate 12.4. Diagnostic features of selected viral diseases of penaeid shrimp. **A:** Wet mount of gut squash showing monodon baculovirus occlusion bodies (*arrow*). Photo courtesy of Angelo Colorni. **B:** Histological section of gut showing monodon baculovirus occlusion bodies (*arrow*). Photo courtesy of Angelo Colorni. **C:** Histological section of hematopoietic tissue showing eosinophilic intranuclear inclusions (*arrow*) caused by infectious hypodermal and hematopoietic necrosis virus. Photo courtesy of James Brock. **D:** Melanized (black) lesions on the carapace from necrosis of the cuticular epithelium caused by Taura syndrome virus. This is characteristic of the chronic/recovery phase. Photo courtesy of James Brock.

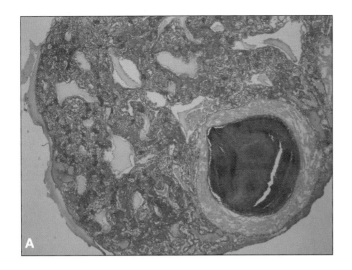

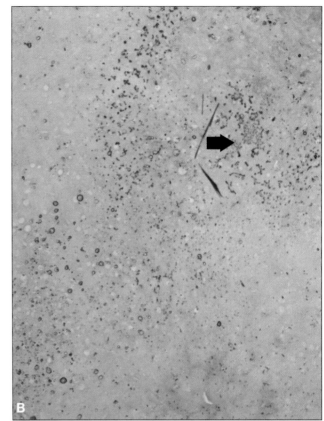

Color Plate 12.6. Gram-positive granulomatous disease in a spiny lobster (*Panulirus* sp.). **A:** Digestive gland with granulomas. H&E stain, × 40. **B:** Digestive gland. Gram-positive bacterial cocci (arrow). Gram stain, × 400. Photos courtesy of David Rotstein.

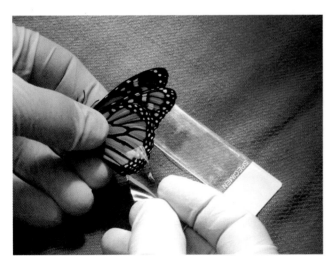

Color Plate 14.10. A small piece of clean, clear transparent tape is being used on a monarch butterfly (*Danaus plexippus*) to capture the spores of the protozoal parasite *Ophryocystis elektroscirrha*. The ventral abdomen is the ideal place to obtain a sample. The tape is then placed on a clean glass slide and examined under the microscope for the presence of small, brown or gold, football-shaped spores. This parasite is becoming common with the rapid development of butterfly houses (Figures 14.11 and 14.12) and expanding market for butterfly pupae (Dan Dombrowski, personal communication). Photo courtesy of Shane Boylan.

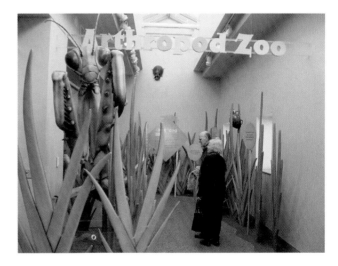

Color Plate 14.11. Butterfly houses are becoming very popular in a number of countries.

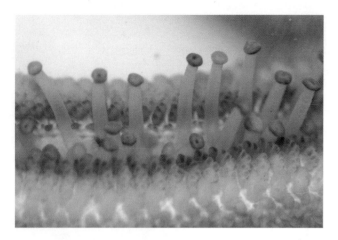

Color Plate 17.5. Magnified tube feet or podia from an asteroid. Courtesy of Kelly Krell.

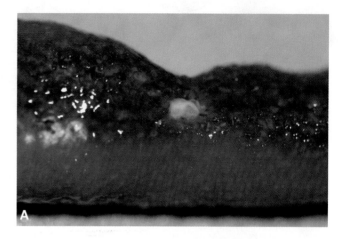

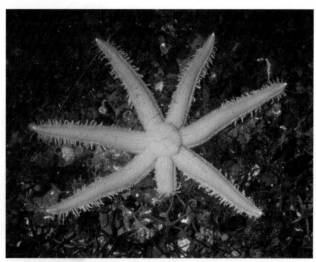

Color Plate 17.8. Limb breakage with initial regeneration in the sea star *Luidia ciliaris*, surrounded by brittle stars, Clyde Sea, Scotland. Courtesy of Richard Aronson.

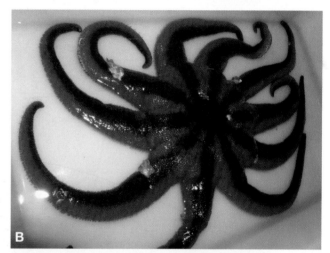

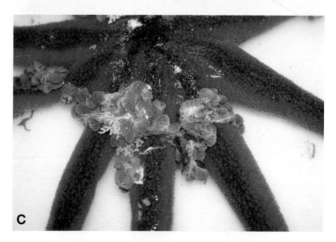

Color Plate 17.9. **A:** Mild ulcer of a sun star. **B:** Moderate ulcers. **C:** Severe ulcers resulting in multifocal evisceration in a sun star. Both the pyloric cecae (ruffled tissue) and gonad (finer, branching tissue) are clearly evident. Courtesy of Kelly Krell.

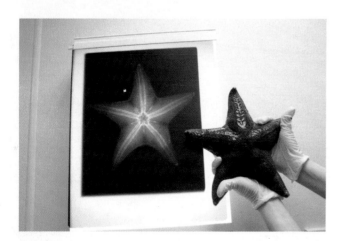

Color Plate 17.12. A helpful orientation technique used by the Shedd Aquarium is to position the animal so the madreporite is in the *top left* corner (note location of the M marker). Courtesy of Kelly Krell.

Chapter 9

HORSESHOE CRABS

Stephen A. Smith

Natural History and Taxonomy

Horseshoe crabs have persevered essentially unchanged for more than 200 million years and are the closest living relatives of the trilobites (Shuster, 1982). Fossil records of members of the family Limulidae date back as far as 500 million years. They are more closely related to the ancient sea scorpions and modern scorpions and spiders than to modern true crabs (Smith et al., 2002; Walls et al., 2002). Today, only four species of horseshoe crabs are found in two distinctly separate regions of the world. Three species—*Tachypleus tridentatus, T. gigas,* and *Carcinoscorpius rotundicauda*—are found in the coastal waters of Asia from India to Japan to the Philippine Islands. The fourth species, the so-called American horseshoe crab, *Limulus polyphemus,* occupies the western Atlantic Coast of North America from Maine south to the Yucatán Peninsula (Shuster, 1982). This chapter is concerned with the latter species.

Limulus polyphemus is a unique marine invertebrate that has and continues to serve as a multiple–use animal resource (Botton and Ropes, 1987; Berkson and Shuster, 1999; Walls et al., 2002). A recently published book thoroughly describes the biology, natural history, and biomedical value of the American horseshoe crab (Shuster et al., 2004). Culture and maintenance techniques have been reviewed and described (Smith and Berkson, 2005). Historically, the horseshoe crab was considered a bycatch nuisance item of commercial finfish fisheries that was returned to shore, pulverized, and used for fertilizer or livestock feed. Even today, the horseshoe crab's natural populations continue to be decimated by their use as bait in a commercial whelk (conch) and eel fishery (Berkson and Shuster, 1999). During the late 1990s, it is estimated that over 2.5 million horseshoe crabs were commercially harvested annually (Horseshoe Crab Technical Committee, 1998). In addition, since the early 1980s the unique relationship between spawning horseshoe crabs and migrating shorebirds has been noticed. Over a dozen species of shorebirds use horseshoe crab eggs and the carcasses of spent horseshoe crabs as a food source as the birds migrate from their South American wintering grounds to their Arctic breeding grounds (Myers, 1986). The horseshoe crab has also been used as a laboratory animal model to study the structure, physiology, and function of its large eye and simple nervous system, to study embryology of marine invertebrates, and as an inhabitant in public aquaria and coastal educational centers, and in elementary school educational programs (Cohen et al., 1979; Bonaventura et al., 1982; Walls et al., 2002). However, the horseshoe crab is probably best known for its unique *blue blood,* which contains a compound important to the human pharmaceutical industry (Norvitsky, 1984). This compound, extracted from the amebocytes of the horseshoe crab's hemolymph, is limulus amebocyte lysate (LAL) and can detect extremely minute quantities of pyrogenic endotoxin produced by Gram-negative bacteria. Purified LAL can detect one millionth of a billionth of a gram of endotoxin (Mikkelsen, 1988). Research on LAL started when it was discovered that, in the presence of certain bacteria, *Limulus* blood would quickly clot (Bang, 1953, 1956). Further studies revealed that this clotting was caused by circulating attack cells called *amebocytes* (Levin and Bang, 1964a, 1964b, 1968).

Extraction and purification of LAL is a Food and Drug Administration-regulated process that has historically required the return of the estimated 250,000 bled horseshoe crabs back to the area of harvest. Though the collection, bleeding, and transportation can be stressful on the horseshoe crabs, several studies have shown that the majority of released horseshoe crabs used in this industry survive the blood-extraction process (Rudloe, 1983; Walls and Berkson, 2000).

Taxonomic Classification

Phylum: Arthropoda
   Class: Meristomata, Subclass: Xiphosura
      Order: Xiphosurida, Suborder: Limulina
         Superfamily: Limulacea
           Family: Limulidae
              Genus: *Limulus*
                Species: *polyphemus*

Anatomy and Physiology

The external and internal anatomy of the horseshoe crab has been described by numerous authors, and readers are encouraged to examine these accounts for a more detailed narrative (Owen, 1873; Shuster, 1982, 1990; Chamberlain and Wyse,

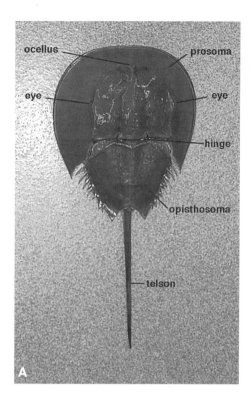

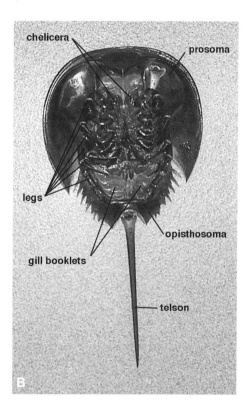

Figure 9.1. External features of the American horseshoe crab, *Limulus polyphemus*. **A:** Dorsal view showing three distinct body sections (prosoma, opisthosoma, and telson). **B:** Ventral view showing the appendages and gill booklets.

1986). Briefly, the body of this dorsoventrally flattened invertebrate is divided into three separate sections: a frontal prosoma (cephalothorax); a posterior opisthosoma (abdomen), and a telson (tail) (Figure 9.1A). The rounded prosoma has a pair of laterally located compound eyes and a centrally located ocellus, a raised midline keel, and a connecting hinge between the prosoma and opisthosoma containing a central arthrodial membrane. Ventrally, the horseshoe crab has a single pair of modified chelicera, six pairs of segmented legs, and five pairs of brachial appendages attached to the opisthosoma that bear the book gills containing the thin gill leaflets (Figure 9.1B). Not only are the book gills used for respiration and osmoregulation, they are also used for propulsion during swimming activity. Internally, the short, straight gastrointestinal tract has an anterior esophagus followed by a gizzard-like crop for macerating food items with hard shells or exoskeletons. The horseshoe crab has a large, dorsally located tubular cardiac sinus connecting to an open vascular system. Surrounding the main digestive and cardiac structures and filling the remaining cavity of the prosoma are the hepatopancreas, renal and gonadal material into which multibranched digestive diverticulae interdigitate.

There are approximately 16–17 molts over a 7- to 10-year period as the horseshoe crab reaches sexual maturity. Adult, terminal molt males, which are generally smaller than adult females, are readily identified by the first pair of chelicera that are modified into large bulbous claspers for grasping the female's opisthosoma (Figure 9.2).

Horseshoe crabs are extremely tolerant of a wide range of both wild and captive environmental conditions. They readily spawn in captivity and produce numerous viable eggs (French, 1979; Brown and Clapper, 1981). They have been reported to survive in natural waters ranging in temperatures from −5°C to 35°C, with an optimum laboratory temperature between 15°C and 21C°. Adult horseshoe crabs can endure varying salinity ranging from 5 to 35 ppt, though juvenile horseshoe crabs do not survive well at the lower ranges (Laughlin, 1982; Gonzalez-Uribe et al., 1991). All stages of the horseshoe crab are tolerant of temporary hypoxic conditions, though the short-term and long-term effects of this condition on individuals is not well studied.

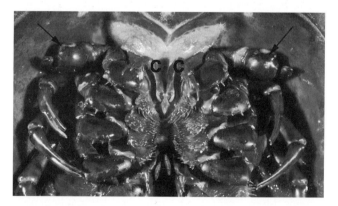

Figure 9.2. Close-up of the terminal molt male claspers (*arrows*) and chelicera (*c*).

Feeding of captive horseshoe crabs has generally not been a problem. In the wild, the adult horseshoe crab diet has been reported to include bivalve mollusks (*Mya* spp.) and marine worms such as *Nereis* spp., *Cerabratulus* spp. and *Pectinaria* spp. (Botton, 1984; Bullis, 1994). In captivity, larval stages readily feed on newly hatched brine shrimp, while juveniles and adults are commonly fed dead fish, squid, small crabs, and clams. They readily consume artificial diets, but the nutritional value of these synthetic formulations is unknown.

Environmental Diseases

Though the horseshoe crab has been used as a laboratory animal for many years, there are only scattered reports in the scientific literature of the diseases or syndromes affecting them. Noninfectious etiologies of problems of captive horseshoe crabs range from water-quality problems of ammonia toxicity, gas supersaturation, and high turbidity, to hypoproteinemic nutritional deficiencies, to molting problems of the shell, legs, or telson. In addition, traumatic injuries caused during collection (*dredging*), transport, or overcrowding during captivity can result in puncture wounds, fractures, and crushing of the exoskeleton (Figures 9.3 and 9.4). External hemorrhage from these lesions can appear significant but is rarely fatal. In some cases, surgical epoxy can be used to stabilize exoskeletal fractures (Figures 9.5 and 9.6). Wound repair in the horseshoe crab, initiated by the migration of amebocytes from the hemolymph, occurs as described by Bursey (1977) and Clare et al. (1990). A similar process was found to occur in trilobites millions of years ago (Isberg, 1917; Ludvigsen, 1977).

Lastly, only a single description of neoplasia in horseshoe crabs is reported, this being a dermoid–like tumor (Hanstrom, 1926).

Infectious Diseases

Infectious agents reported as causing health problems in horseshoe crabs include algae, fungi, colonial and filamentous cyanobacteria, Gram-negative bacteria, and a variety of parasites (Bang, 1956; Leibovitz and Lewbart, 2004). Shell disease is probably the most commonly encountered problem in wild and captive horseshoe crabs. This type of problem is usually manifested by discoloration, flaking, or more serious erosion of the exoskeleton (Bullis, 1994). A green algal (*chlorophycophytal*) in-

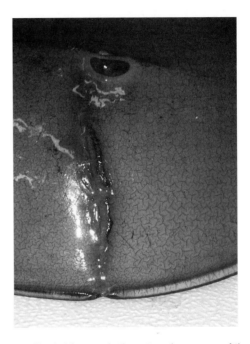
Figure 9.4. Healed fracture in the external carapace of the horseshoe crab.

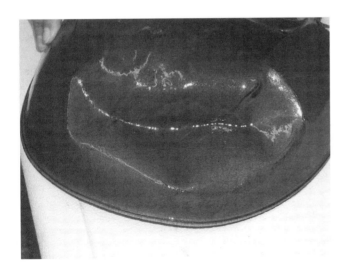
Figure 9.3. Crushed carapace from improper packing during transportation.

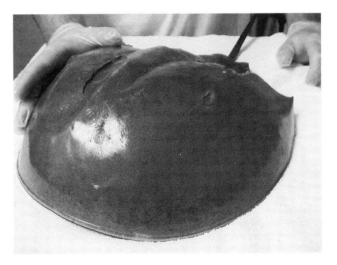
Figure 9.5. Fractured prosoma in a female horseshoe crab.

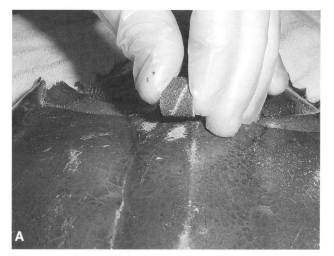

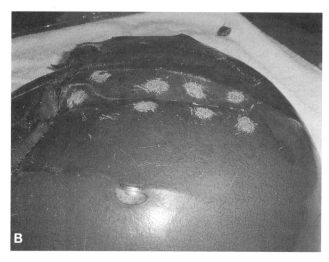

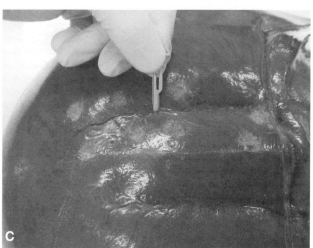

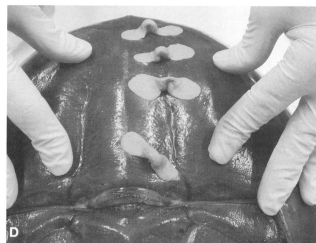

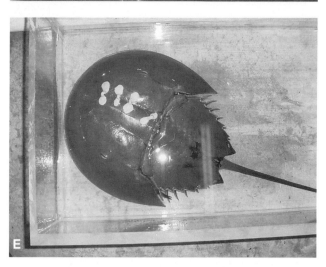

Figure 9.6. Repair of fracture in Figure 9.5 with surgical epoxy.
A and B: The exoskeleton is prepared with sandpaper or a similar
abrasive substance. **C:** The fracture is manually reduced and
stabilized. **D:** Epoxy "noodles" are rolled and then attached to the
exoskeleton. **E:** This animal was placed in shallow water for 24 h
before placement in an aquarium. The epoxy braces remained in
place for over 4 months. Unfortunately, this animal died following
transport to a new aquarium and a necropsy was not performed.
(Gregory A. Lewbart, personal communication)

fection of the dorsal surface of the prosomal exoskeleton is probably the most common infection seen in wild and captive horseshoe crabs (Leibovitz and Lewbart, 1987, 2004). Infections may manifest as a mild greenish discoloration of the superficial surfaces to a dark green-gray of the deeper prosomal tissues of the exoskeleton (Figures 9.7–9.9, Color Plate 9.7). The accessory structures of the exoskeleton, including the paired lateral eyes, the centrally located ocelli, and the medial dorsal arthrodial membrane, can also become involved.

Fungal infections of the horseshoe crab appear to be limited to captive individuals. Branchial mycosis in adult horseshoe crabs was reported by Leibovitz and Lewbart (2004), and mycotic infection of larval and juvenile horseshoe crabs appears to occur commonly, especially in those individuals housed without a sand substrate.

Another group of pathogens that commonly infect horseshoe crabs are the blue-green cyanobacteria (Leibovitz, 1986). These filamentous organisms (*Oscillatoria* spp.) colonize and penetrate the thin chitinous surfaces of the gill tissue. The disease progresses to involve the deeper tissues of the gill and vasculature sinuses, resulting in swollen and ruptured gills leaflets, tissue necrosis, and death. A similar bacteria (*Beggiatoa* spp.) also colonizes the surface of the gill leaflets, but does not appear to be as invasive as *Oscillatoria* spp. and generally results in less extensive pathology (Leibovitz and Lewbart, 2004). Young horseshoe crabs appear to be less affected by gill disease than adult, terminal molt horseshoe crabs presumably due to their periodic molting and renewal of susceptible gill tissue. Other bacteria identified from shell and gill lesions included *Leucothrix*, sp., *Vibrio* sp., *Flavobacterium* sp., *Pseudomonas* sp. and *Pasturella* sp. (Figure 9.10).

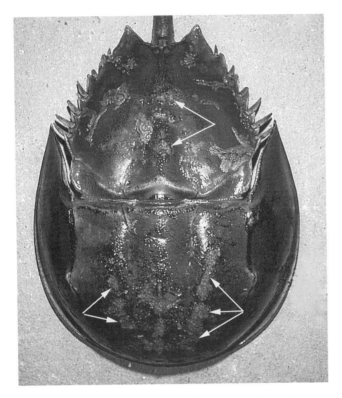

Figure 9.7. Typical lesion produced by green-algal infection of the carapace.

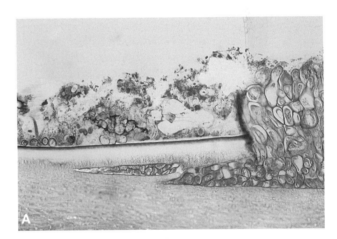

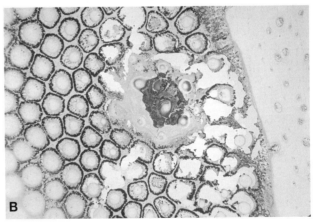

Figure 9.9. **A:** Microscopic view of green-algal filaments invading and displacing the chitinous exoskeleton. **B:** Algal filaments displacing normal lateral eye architecture (*center*). Photos by Gregory A. Lewbart and Louis Leibovitz.

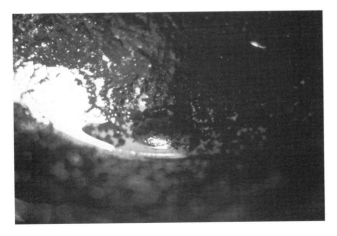

Figure 9.8. Severe green-algal infection involving the carapace and lateral eye. Photo by Louis Leibovitz.

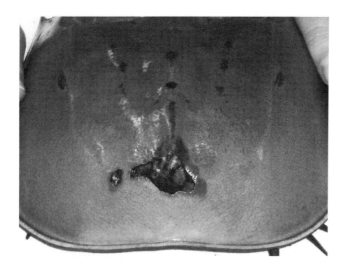

Figure 9.10. Typical lesion produced by a bacterial infection of the carapace.

A few parasites have been reported from the horseshoe crab and include a variety of protozoans, a larval digenetic trematode, a couple of nematodes, and several turbellarid worms. Juvenile and debilitated horseshoe crabs are commonly affected with protozoan species belonging to the ciliate genus *Pananophrys* spp., the flagellate genus *Hexamita* spp., or amoeba of the family Paramoebidae (Leibovitz and Lewbart, 2004). Unidentified protozoans have been reported from the hemolymph of the horseshoe crab (Chen et al., 1989). A digenetic trematode of the herring gull (*Larus argentatus*) uses the horseshoe crab as a second intermediate host for its life cycle (Stunkard, 1950, 1951, 1953, 1968). The encysted metacercarial stages can be found in large numbers in the connective tissue, muscle, brain, and eye of juvenile and subadult horseshoe crabs. No clinical significance has been reported with these parasites, though it has been postulated that they may interfere with normal body functions. There are also some species of normally free-living nematodes (*Monhysteria* spp. and *Grathponema* spp.) that have been reported to invade the carapace of the horseshoe crab (Leibovitz and Lewbart, 2004). And, finally, four or five species of triclad turbellarid worms have been described from the horseshoe crab (Ryder, 1882; Wheeler, 1894; Groff and Leibovitz, 1982; Kawakatsu, 1989). The most significant of these is *Bdelloura candida*, which commonly resides between the gill leaflets, on the ventral appendages, or on the external surface of the ventral carapace (Figure 9.11A, Color Plate 9.11A). The ectoparasite apparently derives much of its nutrition from hemolymph acquired from superficial lesions in the thin chitinous surface of the gill tissue. Stalked cocoons are deposited on the surface of the gill leaflets in which multiple embryos develop (Figure 9.11B and C, Color Plate 9.11B and C). Other species of turbellarids reported from the horseshoe crab include *B. parasitica*, *B. propinqua*, *B. wheeleri*, and *Syncoelidium pellucidum*).

In addition to the truly parasitic organisms that affect the horseshoe crab, numerous ectocommensals frequent the external surfaces of the exoskeleton. These include bryozoans, sponges, barnacles (Figure 9.12A), blue mussels, lady slippers (Figure 9.12B), snails, oysters, whelks, and a variety of coelenterates, annelids, and free-living nematodes (Botton, 1981; Turner et al., 1988; Deaton and Kempler, 1989; Grant, 2001). Rarely do any of these organisms harm the horseshoe crab, the exception being when they interfere with functions such as mobility or respiration.

Diagnostic Techniques

External examination of the horseshoe crab is easily accomplished by removing the individual from the water and either placing the horseshoe crab ventral side down on a solid surface or by manually holding the horseshoe crab. If using an examination table, care must be taken to prevent the crab from crawling off the edge of the table. Also, if individuals are placed dorsal side down, the animal will spend much of its time flexing its telson in an attempt to right itself, making examination difficult. While examining an individual, the holder should be careful to prevent fingers from being pinched between the lateral edge of the opisthosoma and the genal angle of the prosoma.

Evaluation of the health of a horseshoe crab can be very challenging because of the thick, nontransparent cuticle of the exoskeleton. In the same way, the nutritional and reproductive status of a horseshoe crab can be difficult to estimate, as gross observation and internal assessment of an individual can be problematic. However, external inspection should include visual observation of the dorsal and ventral surfaces for shell lesions and external parasites, observation of abnormalities/injuries to the ventral legs and feeding apparatus, and a thorough examination of the book gills and gill leaflets. The leaflets should be carefully examined for signs of hemorrhage (Figure 9.13, Color Plate 9.13), emphysema (Figure 9.14, Color Plate 9.14), edema, algae, bacterial, or fungal disease, and parasitic infestation. Microscopic examination of superficial scrapes of the carapace and gill leaflets can be very useful in identifying organisms residing on the surface of the exoskeleton.

Hemolymph samples may be obtained by placing the horseshoe crab in an abdominal flexure position (Figure 9.15) and inserting a hypodermic needle into the soft arthrodial membrane, the ligament at the joint between the prosoma and opisthosoma, of the medial dorsal surface (Figure 9.16A). For large quantities of hemolymph, a sterile 14-gauge trocar needle can be placed through the membrane and into the dorsal tubular cardiac sinus (Figure 9.16B). Depending on the size of the horseshoe crab, samples of 50–150 mL of hemolymph can be collected in this manner. For smaller samples of hemolymph, a 21-gauge needle can be placed into any of the intersegmental membraneous areas of the legs. Hemolymph can be analyzed for osmolality, total protein, glucose, creatinine, cholesterol, sodium, potassium, chloride, calcium, magnesium, and phosphorus concentrations, triglycerides, amylase, lipase, alkaline phosphatase (ALP), aspartate aminotransferase (AST), and γ-glutamyltransferase (GGT) activities (Table 9.1), while albumin, globulin, direct and indirect bilirubin, urea nitrogen, and creatine kinase are deemed not useful because of extremely low or nonexistent levels (Smith et al., 2002). Copper, a component of hemocyanin, the major

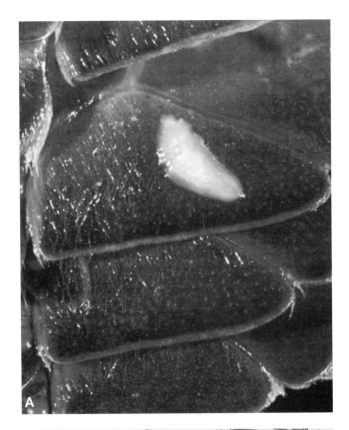

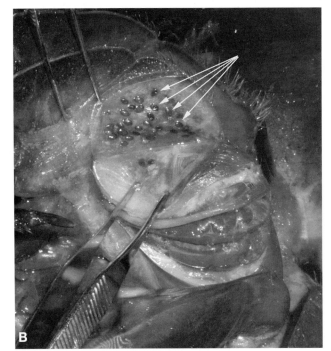

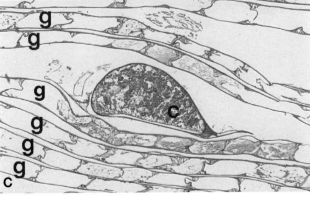

Figure 9.11. A: *Bdelloura* sp., a common external parasite, on the ventral structures of the horseshoe crab. **B:** Stalked cocoons of *Bdelloura* sp. (indicated by *arrows*) attached to the gill leaflets of a horseshoe crab. **C:** Histological preparation of the gill leaflets (g) of a horseshoe crab demonstrating the cocoon (c) and stalked attachment of *Bdelloura* sp. to the chitinous leaflets.

transport molecule for oxygen in the horseshoe crab, can also be evaluated. The intensity of the color of the hemolymph may act as an indirect indicator of oxygen saturation, with higher saturation giving a darker blue hue to the hemolymph.

Health Management

Horseshoe crabs can tolerate extremely poor water and nutritional conditions for long periods without showing obvious signs of ill-thrift. However, just because they do not show overt signs does not suggest they should be kept in anything less than optimal conditions. Again, the rigid, nontransparent exoskeleton of the horseshoe crab makes it extremely difficult to assess their health status visually. Water quality should be monitored

regularly with periodic water exchanges provided to replace minerals and ions removed by the osmoregulatory processes of the horseshoe crab from the water.

Very little has been published concerning treatment and medical management of horseshoe crabs. Acetic acid baths (3%–5% for up to 1 h of exposure) were reported by Bullis (1994) as being somewhat useful for controlling gill infections in horseshoe crabs. Freshwater baths and low-level formalin baths (1.0–1.5 ppm) have also been used to remove excessive external ectocommensal and external parasite loads (Landy and Leibovitz, 1983). This author has found antibiotic treatments for presumptive bacterial infections unrewarding. Horseshoe crabs can be humanely and quickly terminated by injecting 1–2 mL of pentobarbital or other euthanasia solution directly into the cardiac sinus.

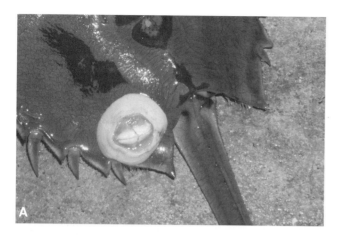

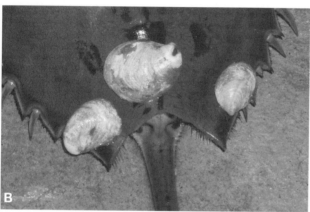

Figure 9.12. Common ectocommensals of the horseshoe crab: **(A)** barnacles and **(B)** lady slippers (*Crepidula* sp.).

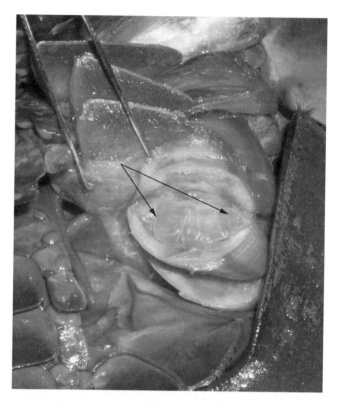

Figure 9.14. Emphysema of a gill leaflet (*arrows*) of a horseshoe crab as a result of supersaturation of atmospheric gases in the culture water.

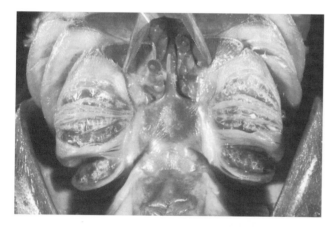

Figure 9.13. Hemorrhage and clotting of blue hemolymph in multiple gill leaflets.

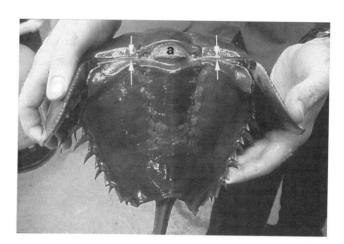

Figure 9.15. Typical abdominal flexure behavior used to examine or obtain hemolymph from the horseshoe crab.

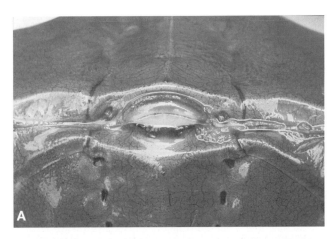

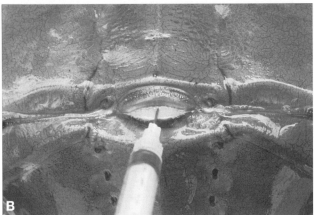

Figure 9.16. Arthrodial membrane, a median ligament at the joint between the prosoma and opisthosoma. **A:** Close-up of the arthrodial membrane used as the main site of hemolymph collection. **B:** Close-up of the arthrodial membrane with a needle inserted correctly through the ligament into the cardiac sinus.

Table 9.1. Biochemical profiles (mean) of selected hemolymph parameters of the American horseshoe crab, *Limulus polyphemus*

Osmolality	950mOsm
Total protein	8.15 g/dL
Glucose	58.5 mg/dL
Creatinine	0.7 mg/dL
Cholesterol	0.8 mg/dL
Sodium	389.5 mEq/L
Potassium	12.5 mEq/L
Chloride	445.1 mEq/L
Calcium	39.0 mg/dL
Magnesium	96.1 mg/dL
Phosphorus	3.4 mg/dL
Triglycerides	5.3 mg/dL
Amylase	9.3 U/L
Lipase	32.7 U/L
Alkaline phosphatase (ALP)	12.1 U/L
Aspartate aminotransferase (AST)	5.4 U/L
γ-Glutamyltransferase (GGT)	0.92 U/L

From Smith et al. (2002).

References

Bang, F.B. 1953. The toxic effect of a marine bacterium on *Limulus* and the formation of blood clots. Biological Bulletin (Woods Hole) 105:361–362.

Bang, F.B. 1956. A bacterial disease of *Limulus polyphemus*. Bulletin of the Johns Hopkins Hospital 98:325–351.

Berkson, J.M., and C.N. Shuster Jr. 1999. The horseshoe crab: The battle over a true multiple use resource. Fisheries 24:6–10.

Bonaventura, J., C. Bonaventura, and S. Tesh. 1982. Progress in Clinical and Biological Research, volume 18: Physiology and Biology of Horseshoe Crabs—Studies on Normal and Environmentally Stressed Animals. Alan R. Liss, New York.

Botton, M.L. 1981. The gill books of the horseshoe crab (*Limulus polyphemus*) as a substrate for the blue mussel (*Mytilus edulis*). Bulletin of the New Jersey Academy of Science 26:26–28.

Botton, M.L. 1984. Diet and food preferences of the adult horseshoe crab, *Limulus polyphemus* in Delaware Bay, New Jersey, USA. Marine Biology 81:199–207.

Botton, M.L., and J.W. Ropes. 1987. The horseshoe crab, *Limulus polyphemus*, fishery and resource in the United States. Marine Fisheries Review 49:57–60.

Brown, G.G., and D.L. Clapper. 1981. Procedures for maintaining adults, collecting gametes, and culturing embryos and juveniles of the horseshoe crab, *Limulus polyphemus* L. In: Laboratory Animal Management: Marine Invertebrates. National Academy Press, Washington, DC, pp. 268–290.

Bullis, R.A. 1994. Care and maintenance of horseshoe crabs for use in biomedical research. In: J.S. Stolen, T.C. Fletcher, A.F. Rowley, J.T. Zelikoff, S.L. Kaattari, and S.A. Smith, eds. Techniques in Fish Immunology, volume 3. SOS, Fair Haven, NJ, pp. A9–A10.

Bursey, C.R. 1977. Histological response to injury in the horseshoe crab, *Limulus polyphemus*. Canadian Journal of Zoology 55:1158–1165.

Chamberlain, S.C., and G.A. Wyse. 1986. An atlas of the brain of the horseshoe crab, *Limulus polyphemus*. Journal of Morphology 187:363–386.

Chen, S., S. Hong, Y. Chen, and Y. Yang. 1989. Cultivation of horseshoe crab amebocytes. Kaohsiung Journal of Medical Science 5:516–521.

Clare, A.S., G. Lumb, P.A. Clare, and J.D. Costlow. 1990. A morphological study of wound repair and telson regeneration in postlarval *Limulus polyphemus*. Invertebrate Reproduction and Development 17:77–87.

Cohen, E., F.B. Bang, J. Levine, J.J. Marchalonis, T.P. Pistole, R.A. Prendergast, C.N. Shuster Jr., and S.W. Watson, eds. 1979. Biomedical Applications of the Horseshoe Crab (Limulidae). Alan R. Liss, New York.

Deaton, L.E., and K.D. Kempler. 1989. Occurrence of the ribbed mussel, *Geukensia demissa*, on the book gills of the horseshoe crab, *Limulus polyphemus*. Nautilus 103(1):42.

French, K.A. 1979. Laboratory culture of embryonic and juvenile Limulus. In: E. Cohen, F.B. Bang, J. Levine, J.J. Marchalonis, T.P. Pistole, R.A. Prendergast, C.N. Shuster Jr., and S.W. Watson, eds. Biomedical Applications of the Horseshoe Crab (Limulidae). Alan R. Liss, New York, pp. 61–71.

Gonzalez-Uribe, J.F., A.A. Ortega-Salas, P. Lavens, P. Sorgeloos, E. Jaspers, and F. Ollevier. 1991. Environmental factor in rearing eggs and larva of *Limulus polyphemus* L. under laboratory conditions. Special Publication of the European Aquaculture Society 15:264–265.

Grant, D. 2001. Living on *Limulus*. In: J.T. Tanacredi, ed. *Limulus* in the Limelight: A Species 350 Million Years in the Making and in Peril? Kluwer Academic/Plenum, New York, pp. 135–145.

Groff, J.F., and L. Leibovitz. 1982. A gill disease of *Limulus polyphemus* associated with triclad turbellarid worm infections. Biological Bulletin (Woods Hole) 163:392.

Hanstrom, B. 1926. Ueber einen Fall von pathologischer Chitinbildung in Inneren des Korpers von *Limulus polyphemus*. Zoologischer Anzeiger 66:213–219.

Horseshoe Crab Technical Committee (HCTC). 1998. Status of the Horseshoe Crab (*Limulus polyphemus*) Population of the Atlantic Coast. HCTC, Atlantic State Marine Fisheries Commission, Washington, DC.

Isberg O. 1917. Ein regeneriertes Trilobitenauge. Geologiska Föreningens i Stockholm Förhandlingar 39:593–596.

Kawakatsu, M. 1989. Redescription of an ectoparasitic marine triclad, *Bdelloura candida* (Girard, 1850) (Burbellaria; Tricladida; Maricola), collected from the American horseshoe crab, *Limulus polyphemus*. Bulletin of the Biogeographic Society of Japan 44:183–198.

Landy, R.B., and L. Leibovitz. 1983. A preliminary study of the toxicity and therapeutic efficacy of formalin in the treatment of *Triclad* turbellarid worm infestations in *Limulus polyphemus*. In: Proceedings of the Annual Meeting of the Society of Invertebrate Pathology, Ithaca, New York.

Laughlin, R. 1982. The effects of temperature and salinity on larval growth of the horseshoe crab, *Limulus polyphemus*. Journal of Experimental Marine Biology and Ecology 64:93–103.

Leibovitz, L. 1986. Cyanobacterial diseases of the horseshoe crab (*Limulus polyphemus*). Biological Bulletin (Woods Hole) 171:482–483.

Leibovitz, L., and G.A. Lewbart. 1987. A green algal (chlorophycophytal) infection of the dorsal surface of the exoskeleton and associated organ structures in the horseshoe crab (*Limulus polyphemus*). Biological Bulletin (Woods Hole) 173:430.

Leibovitz, L., and G.A. Lewbart. 2004. Diseases and symbionts: Vulnerability despite tough shells. In: C.N. Shuster Jr., R.B. Barlow, and H.J. Brockmann, eds. The American Horseshoe Crab. Harvard University Press, Cambridge, pp. 245–275.

Levin, J., and F.B. Bang. 1964a. The role of endotoxin in the extracellular coagulation of *Limulus* blood. Bulletin of the Johns Hopkins Hospital 115:265–274.

Levin, J., and F.B. Bang. 1964b. A description of cellular coagulation in the *Limulus*. Bulletin of the Johns Hopkins Hospital 115:337–345.

Levin, J., and F.B. Bang. 1968. Clottable protein in *Limulus*: Its localization and kinetics of its coagulation by endotoxin. Thrombosis et Diathesis Haemorrhagica 19:186–197.

Ludvigsen R. 1977. Rapid repair of traumatic injury by an Ordovician trilobite. Lethaia 10:205–207.

Mikkelsen, T. 1988. The Secret in the Blue Blood. Science, Beijing, China, 125 pp.

Myers, J.P. 1986. Sex and gluttony on the Delaware Bay. Natural History 95:68–77.

Norvitsky, T.J. 1984. Discovery to commercialization: The blood of the horseshoe crab. Oceanus 27:13–18.

Owen, R. 1873. On the anatomy of the American king-crab (*Limulus polyphemus* Latr.). Transactions of the Linnean Society of London 28:459–506.

Rudloe, J. 1983. The effect of heavy bleeding on mortality of the horseshoe crab, *Limulus polyphemus*, in the natural environment. Journal of Invertebrate Pathology 42:167–176.

Ryder, J.A. 1882. Observations on the species of planarians on *Limulus*. American Naturalist 16:48–51.

Shuster, C.N., Jr. 1982. A pictorial review of the natural history and ecology of the horseshoe crab, *Limulus polyphemus*, with reference to other Limulidae. In: J. Bonaventura, C. Bonaventura, and S. Tesh, eds. Physiology and Biology of the Horseshoe Crabs: Studies on Normal and Environmentally Stressed Animals. Alan R. Liss, New York, pp. 1–52.

Shuster, C.N., Jr. 1990. The American horseshoe crab, *Limulus polyphemus*. In: R.B. Prior, ed. Clinical Applications of the *Limulus* Amoebocyte Lysate Test. CRC, Boca Raton, FL, pp. 15–25.

Shuster, C.N., H.J. Brockmann, R.B. Barlow. 2004. The American Horseshoe Crab. Harvard University Press, Cambridge, MA. 448 pp.

Smith, S.A., and J.M. Berkson. 2005. Laboratory culture and maintenance of the horseshoe crab (*Limulus polyphemus*). Lab Anim 34:27–34.

Smith, S.A., J.M. Berkson, and R.A. Barratt. 2002. Horseshoe crab (*Limulus polyphemus*) hemolymph, biochemical and immunological parameters. Proceedings of the International Association for Aquatic Animal Medicine 33:101–102.

Stunkard, H.W. 1950. Microphallid metacercaria encysted in *Limulus*. Biological Bulletin (Woods Hole) 99:347.

Stunkard, H.W. 1951. Observations on the morphology and life-history of *Microphallus* n. sp. (Trematoda: Microphallidae). Biological Bulletin (Woods Hole) 101:307–318.

Stunkard, H.W. 1953. Natural hosts of *Microphallus limuli*. Journal of Parasitology 39:225.

Stunkard, H.W. 1968. The asexual generation, life cycle, and systemic relations of *Microphallus limuli* (Trematoda: Digenea). Biological Bulletin (Woods Hole) 134:332–343.

Turner, L.L., C. Kammire, and M.A. Sydlik. 1988. Preliminary report: Composition of communities resident on *Limulus* carapaces. Biological Bulletin (Woods Hole) 175:312.

Walls, E.A., and J. Berkson. 2000. Effect of blood extraction on the mortality of the horseshoe crab, *Limulus polyphemus*. Virginia Journal of Science 51:195–198.

Walls, E.A., J. Berkson, and S.A. Smith. 2002. The horseshoe crab, *Limulus polyphemus*: 200 million years of existence, 100 years of study. Reviews in Fisheries Science 10:39–73.

Wheeler, W.M. 1894. *Syncoelidium pellucidum*, a new marine triclad. Journal of Morphology 9:167–194.

Chapter 10

SPIDERS

Romain Pizzi*

Introduction

Although veterinarians have generally had little to do with spiders, veterinary interest and involvement with spiders are not new (Cooper, 1987; Frye, 1992). Theraphosidae spiders in particular are increasingly popular in zoological exhibits as well as being kept as pets. Araneomorphs may also be used for research purposes. Although captive husbandry advice has been the mainstay of veterinary input, diseases are starting to become increasingly recognized and reported. There is a lack of literature dealing with arachnid diseases in standard invertebrate texts. *Brachypelma* spp., including the popular *Brachypelma smithi* (Mexican redknee tarantula), are currently in appendix II of the Convention on International Trade in Endangered Species of Wild Fauna and Flora (CITES), with *Poecilotheria* spp. likely to be added soon. Disease recognition and prevention may be important should a captive breeding and release program be needed to prevent the possible introduction of diseases into wild populations.

This chapter focuses on theraphosids, since these are the most commonly kept species, but reference is made to araneomorph species where applicable.

Taxonomy and Natural History

Taxonomy

Spiders belong to the order Araneae (phylum Arthropoda; subphylum Chelicerata; class Arachnida), which contains approximately 34,000 recognized species in about 100 families (Foelix, 1996). There are three suborders: Mesothelae, containing only one family, Liphistiidae, which are rare, primitive spiders; Araneomorphae (also called Labidognatha), containing most common spiders; and Mygalomorphae (also called Orthognatha), containing tarantulas and tarantula-like spiders.

The Mygalomorphae contains over 2200 species in 15 families. The family Theraphosidae (tarantulas) contains approximately 800 species, of which over a hundred have been kept in captivity. Other Mygalomorphae families containing species kept in captivity include Ctenizidae (trap-door spiders), Dipluridae (funnel web spiders), and Hexathelidae (Australian funnel web spiders, including the notorious Sydney funnel web spider *Atrax robustus*).

The Araneomorphae contain the bulk of spider species, but they are not as commonly kept in zoological collections or as pets. Some member families kept in captivity are Araneidae and Nephilidae (orb web spiders), Lycosidae (wolf spiders), Heteropodidae (crab spiders), and Sicariidae (sand spiders). Venomous spiders maintained in captivity include Ctenidae (which contains the extremely venomous *Phoneutria* spp.), Theriidae (*Latrodectus* sp.; widow spiders belong to this family), and Loxoscelidae (violin spiders). These venomous spiders are usually kept only by researchers and a small number of select hobbyists.

Some of the most commonly kept Theraphosidae species include the Mexican redknee tarantula (*Brachypelma smithi*); Chilean rose tarantula (*Grammostola rosea*, formerly *G. spatulata*); goliath bird eater (*Theraphosa blondi*), curlyhair tarantula (*Brachypelma albopilosum*), and pinktoe tarantula (*Avicularia avicularia*) from the Americas; as well as the Asian ornamental tarantulas (*Poecilotheria* spp.). In North America, *Aphonopelma* species such as the Texas brown tarantula (*Aphonopelma hentzi*) and desert blonde tarantula (*Aphonopelma chalcodes*) are commonly kept because of their natural occurrence in southern areas of the United States. African baboon spiders (such as *Ceratogyrus*, *Pterinochilus*, and *Hysterocrates* spp.), although less popular, are also kept, as are a large variety of other American and Asian species. Serious hobbyists may keep several thousand spiders belonging to a large number of species.

The *true tarantula*, *Lycosa tarantula*, is a European wolf spider (an Araneomorph and thus not a member of the Theraphosidae). This spider is known for the *tarantella*, the dance

*Acknowledgments. I thank Dr. R.G. Breene for kindly commenting on the script, as well as ongoing advice; Professors J.E.C. Cooper and F. Frye, who stimulated my initial interest in invertebrate medicine; Dr. John Chitty, president of the Veterinary Invertebrate Society, for advice and encouragement; Susan George of North Western Laboratories, for helping develop histological processing and staining techniques; the numerous serious keepers who kindly provided me with cases and information and, finally, my family for their endless patience and support, in spite of my strange pets.

that, during the middle ages, was believed to be the only cure for an *L. tarantula* bite. The name was later applied to the large, impressive spiders found by explorers in the New World. There are other points of confusion. Members of the genus *Tarantula* Fabricius (1793) are not even spiders. Schultz and Schultz (1998) put the *Tarantula* genus in the order Amblypygi (whip spiders), but other sources put it in the order Palpigradi (microwhip scorpions). The name *tarantula* was also applied to an arboreal lizard, perhaps belonging to the genus *Tarentola*. *Mygale* was used to refer to these spiders, but the name had already been given to a shrew species. The infraorder Mygalomorphae, of which Theraphosidae is one family, is also used in the literature. The term *bird eater* can be confusing and should be applied only to the small number of species recorded to consume birds in nature. There is an unfortunate tendency among pet shops and traders to make up imaginative names for spiders; reliance should never be placed on common names.

The American Arachnological Society's (AAS) Committee on Common Names has guidelines, but these are not universally accepted. According to AAS guidelines, the general term *tarantula* (small "t") is recognized as referring to Theraphosidae spiders, whereas *Tarantula* (large "T") is recognized as referring to the genus of tail-less whip scorpions. The AAS recognizes only the use of bird eater as applying to *Theraphosa blondi* (the goliath bird eater, the largest species of spider) (Breene, 1996). A list of the common names of theraphosids currently recognized by the AAS's Committee on Common Names is included at the end of this chapter. Latin names will be used in the text, and the terms *theraphosid* and *tarantula* are considered to be synonymous.

Many popular books on keeping tarantulas and photographic identification guides have misidentifications that this author and others have noted. Never assume a spider to be what it is named. Some species appear identical, or the same species from different localities may have markedly different coloration. The popular *Grammostola rosea* is an example of this; the brown and copper varieties have often been sold as separate species. The only truly accurate method of identification in many cases remains dissection, although examination of an excuvium may be sufficient. This can be difficult to arrange and is best undertaken through organizations such as the American Tarantula Society (ATS) and the British Tarantula Society (BTS). Contact details are listed in Resources. Accurate identification is important for captive breeding but rare with most spiders.

The large number of taxonomic revisions to species names must be considered when performing a literature search of any kind. Among the most commonly kept species, *Brachypelma* spp. were referred to as *Euthalus* spp. for a period. *Grammostola* was briefly revised to *Phrixotrichus* before being reversed. The popular Chilean rose tarantula (*Grammostola rosea*, previously *Phrixotrichus spatulata*, previously *Grammostola spatulata*) is unfortunately often still referred to by its previous Latin names, even in current literature. The genera *Rhechostica*, *Dugesiella*, *Eurypelma*, and *Aphonopelma* were regrouped in one genus, *Rhechostica*, which was later changed to *Aphonopelma*. Other generic revisions include *Haplopelma* (*Melopoeus*) and *Mygalarachne* (*Sericopelma*). Numerous articles on physiology were

published on the previous *Eurypelma* spp., and articles were published on other species that are no longer recognized, which of course is problematic.

Natural History and Captive Care

Husbandry requirements of captive animals are generally based on the current understanding of the relevant species natural history. Unfortunately, in many cases, almost nothing is known of the tarantula species in the wild. Most husbandry knowledge of tarantulas is based on accumulated experience in captivity. There are also as many sources of incorrect information on husbandry requirements as correct ones. Tarantulas are relatively photophobic and do not need ultraviolet lighting, as some sources indicate. They also do not need misting, calcium powder on their prey or, in most circumstances, external heat sources such as heating mats and bulbs.

There is also well-founded disagreement between experienced keepers over certain points. Schultz and Schultz (1998) provide an excellent synopsis of captive husbandry. Breene and O'Brien (1998) give specific requirements for over 80 Theraphosidae species. Although this author has kept a large variety of both arboreal and terrestrial theraphosids from Africa, Asia, and the New World, as well as numerous araneomorphs, there are husbandry points given here with which not all authorities may agree.

A common error committed in zoological collections is the application of herpetological husbandry directly to captive spiders. This is usually due to spiders falling under the care of the herpetological staff. Zoos with entomological staff are unfortunately the exception, so veterinarians should not assume the zookeepers to be highly knowledgeable. The vast majority of zoos buy their spiders from entomological suppliers and do not breed them, so zoos are often not a good source of information for husbandry or breeding advice.

Adult female spiders can be extraordinarily long-lived. Baerg (1958) reports a female theraphosid, collected at an estimated age of 10–12 years, living a further 16 years in captivity. Petrunkevitch (1955) mentions a female that lived in the Museum d'Histoire Naturelle, Paris, for 25 years. Very little has been published on Theraphosidae life spans. Longevity quotes vary from 6 to 12 years for some African theraphosids to over 30 years for some New World terrestrial species. Only females are long-lived; males having a terminal instar once reaching maturity. This of course makes females more desirable in the pet trade as well as for zoological display. Details of sex determination are presented later in this chapter.

Housing

The vast majority of spiders, and practically all tarantulas, must be housed individually to prevent cannibalism. Immatures from the same egg sac of *Avicularia* spp. and *Poecilotheria regalis* are sometimes kept together until adulthood. The numbers should be limited (fewer than 10 is advisable, depending on space), and cannibalism will invariably occur, even with ample provision of prey. Other *Poecilotheria* species do not appear tolerant of being housed communally.

There are some communal araneomorph species, and approximately 20 truly social spider species, cooperating in prey capture and brood care. These predominantly web spiders include the agelenids (such as *Agelena consociata*, the African funnel web spider), the eresids (*Stegodyphus* sp.), theridiids (*Anelosimus* sp. and *Achaeranea* sp.), and dictynids (*Mallos gregalis* and *Aebutina binotata*). Social, non-web-based spiders include *Diaea socialis*, a crab spider; *Delena cancerides*, a huntsman spider; and a *Tapinullus* sp. lynx spider. These spiders are not common pets.

Excessive cage height in zoos is a frequent cause of trauma and has been the most common cause of death in *Theraphosa blondi* seen by the author. With this and other large species such as *Theraphosa apophysis*, *Lasiodora parahybana*, and *Xenesthis immanis*, container height should not exceed the length of the spider's outstretched body. Providing clear plastic burrows with an exposed side allows visitors to see burrowing species and may help limit the enclosure height without creating an adverse impression. Adult (terminal instar) male tarantulas, though usually kept off display, need escape-proof containers because of their almost constant endeavors to roam in search of females. To prevent litigation, locked, escape-proof enclosures should be used for any venomous Araneomorphae species. Inclusion of cacti with spines and sharp rocks in arid-species enclosures should be avoided because such objects can cause fatal opisthosoma trauma. Aside from acting as a retreat, enclosure plants and decorations are for the viewer's and not the animal's benefit, and so should be limited. Excessive plants and rocks make cleaning difficult and tend to harbor mites.

The use of wire-mesh vivarium covers should be avoided because the claws on the end of the tarsus easily become hooked. Affected spiders may be unable to free themselves, with the result being a damaged limb or exsanguination from a ruptured joint membrane. Glass or plastic vivaria and covers are best for ease of maintenance and safety.

Substrates

Numerous substrates are recommended for captive terrestrial spiders, including vermiculite, topsoil, potting soil, and combinations of these.

Vermiculite should only be of the horticultural and not insulation type. It is inexpensive, easy to clean, and inert, and may be the best substrate for large collections because of its ease of maintenance and minimal problems. It is suitable for species needing either low or high humidity. Some spiders do not like the surface and will spend all their time attached to the enclosure walls. In such cases, the substrate should be changed. Other spiders will extensively web the surface and then appear more at ease. Vermiculite is not ideal for mating larger tarantulas because it does not provide good footing for the male to prop up the female. Spiders are usually unable to make burrows that do not collapse in vermiculite, although, in the author's experience, trap-door spiders cope well.

Potting soil should not contain fertilizers. Garden soil is not recommended because of the risk of accumulated pesticides. When using any soil or peat, water retention may be a problem, leading to fungal growth and mite problems. Breene (1998) recommends oven heating topsoil to reduce the moisture content and risk of saprophytic mites.

Sand is not recommended in recent texts (Schultz and Schultz, 1998) but is still commonly used in displays. Course particles, such as river sand, may abrade the waxy layer of the cuticle, which is important in limiting water loss. Gravel is a poor substrate because it is heavy and difficult to clean, and may be abrasive to the cuticle (Breene, 1998).

The use of carpeting should be avoided because claws may become caught and wet carpeting rots rapidly. Bark chips and wood shavings are reported to harbor mites, and aromatic woods such as cedar must be avoided, as they possess irritating volatile oils. Cat litter is not advised because it generates dust (Breene and O'Brien, 1998). Newspaper sheets or paper toweling, though not visually appealing, can be helpful as temporary substrate for some newly hatched spiderlings or ill animals. Moist paper towel is also used for packing and transporting spiders. Sphagnum moss, although prone to mites and fungal growth, is useful for rearing spiderlings of high-humidity species like *Hysterocrates gigas*.

Water and Humidity

Water should be provided in a shallow dish. Small flat jar tops are quite useful, easy to remove (with long forceps), and clean. Including a small stone or little ramp is useful for prey items such as crickets that have a tendency to drown and decompose in water dishes. Soaked balls of cotton wool should never be used, as they provide the ideal environment for microbial growth. Many terrestrial tarantulas will defecate in their water container (another reason not to use cotton wool), so containers should be cleaned and replenished at least twice weekly. Some authors recommend a raised water dish for arboreal tarantulas, but this probably is not essential. Spiders should not be misted despite numerous claims to the contrary. The majority of spiders have a strong aversion to being sprayed with water. Misting is often recommended in hobbyists' books for dysecdysis; the practice is futile since the intact cuticle is impermeable to moisture and the excuvium is separated by an endogenous subcuticular fluid layer. Newly molted spiders (even arid species) will usually have a wet appearance. Humidity in the vivarium is best altered by other means such as reducing ventilation, moistening the substrate, or providing a burrow. Genera requiring higher humidity include *Haplopelma*, *Hysterocrates*, *Lasiodora*, and *Theraphosa*.

Light

Most spiders and all tarantulas have an aversion to direct or strong lighting. Vivariums should be kept out of areas of direct sunlight and away from bright lamps. If external heating is to be supplied by lamps, these should not emit light or should be ceramic.

Temperature

Many sources recommend temperatures in the range of 74°–88°F for keeping theraphosids. For the average pet tarantula owner, no additional heating is needed despite claims to the contrary. Temperature stability appears to be more important than a precise temperature. Keeping spiders in this elevated range reportedly leads to better breeding results, but this is anecdotal. The author has observed good breeding results in collections with no external heating. In Europe, large collections are maintained with no extra heat aside from normal household winter heating. If heat is provided, thermostatic control is essential, as spiders are easily cooked. In a large collection, heating of the entire room is the best and safest option. Bottom heating via heat mats is unnatural, especially among burrowing species, and best avoided. Alternatively, heat mats may be used along the back or side of the enclosure. Employing heater bulbs dictates the use of larger and higher space-occupying enclosures so the spider does not come in contact with the heat source. Heating also leads to increased substrate desiccation. Whereas some arboreal spiders may display a sunning behavior, tarantulas do not seem to thermoselect an area in an enclosure and providing a thermal gradient is unnecessary. Some keepers maintain immatures at higher temperatures to encourage increased growth and maturation rates.

Humidity and Ventilation

Most captive tarantulas do not need much ventilation. Unlike araneomorphs, tarantulas do not have a tracheal respiratory system in addition to their book lungs. Their limited activity also means a relatively low oxygen demand. Exceptions include arboreal genera such as *Avicularia* and *Poecilotheria*, which are intolerant of overly humid conditions. Otherwise, excessive ventilation only leads to desiccation and the need to constantly top up the water dish.

Arboreals

Arboreal tarantula genera (*Avicularia*, *Poecilotheria*, *Heteroscodra*, *Iridopelma*, *Psalmopoeus*, *Stromatopelma*, and *Tapinauchenius*) do not have restrictions on cage height. The cage does not have to be very wide but should be high enough to allow climbing. Vivaria turned on one side are often suitable. The provision of climbing materials such as a wooden log, piece of cork, or bark enables spiders to build a cylindrical web retreat or nest. Substrate is not essential but may help maintain humidity, as some of these spiders need more ventilation than do terrestrial tarantulas.

Arboreal and web-spinning araneomorphs may be kept similarly, and small branches should enable web construction. Providing mesh sides may also be helpful for web construction. Orb web species can construct large and attractive webs if given the space. When keeping arboreal web-spinning araneomorphs for photographic purposes, Murphy (2000) reports building a twig frame and then covering it with clear plastic sandwich wrap. Spiders will not attach webbing to the plastic, and it can easily be removed for photography without disturbing the spiders or damaging the web.

Burrow Provision

Terrestrial species are divided into obligate and opportunistic burrowers, depending on whether they use preexisting structures (Breene and O'Brien, 1998). Many terrestrial species can be successfully kept without a burrow. Burrows can help maintain humidity and may serve as a form of environmental enrichment. Both obligate and opportunistic burrowers seem content with a retreat rather than a burrow. Retreats are strongly recommended for all terrestrial tarantulas. These are easily provided with a half-clay plant pot or similar structure (Breene, 1998). Properly placed clear plastic-tube burrows enable visitors to see burrowing species. The exposed side should be covered (most of the time) with a cardboard or wooden strip; otherwise, the spider will web over the burrow walls. If spiders are to burrow naturally, a thick layer of substrate (potting or topsoil) is needed.

Feeding

Little work has been done on spider nutritional requirements, but they are likely similar to those of predatory insects. Breene (1998) reports that *Latrodectus mactans* can be raised on a single prey species, *Drosophila*, but most captive spiders will likely benefit from some variety. Work done by Greenstone (1979) showed that several spider species took a mixture of prey to optimize the amino acid proportions in their diet. Prey species are best varied by using captive-reared invertebrates (see the section Intoxication). Some people feel that wild prey items may pose a risk to spiders. Breene (personal communication) thinks it unlikely that wild-caught invertebrates would intoxicate spiders as most modern pesticides have a rapid onset of action. To be safe, wild-caught prey may be observed for 24–48 h and/or fed a detoxifying diet as is done for edible snails (Pizzi, 2001a). Wild-caught invertebrate prey also carry a small risk of transmitting a Mermithidae nematode infection if the spider occurs naturally in the area. This has never been reported and is likely to be rare. Feeding mantids should be avoided since even small mantids may overpower and eat a captive spider.

Several North American species have been observed eating carrion in the wild. Species such as *Ceratogyrus bechuanicus* will often accept inanimate food (such as small pieces of raw chicken). So-called power feeding of ox heart and maintaining spiders under warm temperatures to encourage rapid growth are used by some *Theraphosa blondi* keepers. This type of feeding is unnatural and may predispose obese individuals to opisthosoma trauma. Although feeding of live vertebrate food such as pinkies (or even adult mice) is suggested by numerous texts, it is not recommended. Live mammalian prey items could injure the spider, and there is no evidence of nutritional benefit. There are also ethical concerns. Feeding live vertebrate prey is illegal in the United Kingdom.

A wide variety of prey invertebrates are available. *Acheta domestica* crickets make a good dietary basis for small and medium-sized spiders. *Achetta domestica* can be alternated with *Gryllus* sp. crickets for variety. Larger specimens can be fed large crickets, but *Schistocerca gregaria* and *Locusta migratoria* locusts are a better option. *Galleria mellonella* larvae (so-called *waxworms*) are a good occasional prey item and avidly consumed by most tarantulas. Waxworms are also taken by large spiderlings and even fairly small araneomorphs, posing no risk to the spiders. Even large tarantulas will usually accept them, skewering four or five on their fangs. Waxworms are useful for anorexic tarantulas, which may take them while refusing other prey. *Drosophila* sp. fruit flies are the main prey for newly hatched spiderlings. *Musca* flies, especially the curlywing flightless variety, are useful for feeding many araneomorphs and tarantula spiderlings. *Tenebrio molitor* mealworms and *Zophobas morio* super mealworms are not recommended as prey for tarantulas. Those mealworms are reportedly of low nutritional value (Bruins, 1999). More importantly, mealworms may burrow and quickly disappear into the substrate if not immediately consumed. There are anecdotal reports of these reemerging to fatally injure tarantulas undergoing ecdysis. Mealworms can be useful for web araneomorphs since there is little risk of trauma.

Handling Tarantulas

Opinions vary widely on the handling of theraphosids. Unnecessary handling of theraphosids is discouraged mainly because of the risks of injury to the spiders. Handling may be appropriate in certain circumstances, and many zoos have handling sessions for educational purposes or for treating arachnophobia. Arboreal genera such as *Avicularia*, *Poecilotheria*, *Psalmopoeus*, and *Tapinauchenius* may be nervous, fleeing before attempting to bite, and are at risk of falling even though they are arboreal. In addition to the risk to the spider, numerous New World species, such as the popular *Brachypelma smithi* and *Theraphosa blondi*, have urticating hairs that they may flicked off their dorsal opisthosoma in defense. Scanning electron micrography (Schultz and Schultz, 1998) has helped demonstrate the barbed, irritating nature of these hairs. Latex gloves are recommended for sensitive individuals, with eye protection an additional requirement in some cases. Schultz and Schultz (1998) report that surgical latex gloves are insufficient protection from the hairs of *Theraphosa blondi* and *T. apophysis*, and thicker rubber kitchen gloves may be necessary. Although many people are not sensitive to urticating hairs, some individuals have severe skin reactions, and respiratory distress has been reported in a small number of cases. Symptoms may last several days (R. Pizzi, unpublished data). The majority of African and Asian species do not have irritant hairs, which may explain why some of these species are more likely to bite in self-defense. If spiders are to be handled, this should be done over a surface such as a table to prevent falls from a height. The wearing of clothes with long sleeves (especially woolen clothes) must be avoided, as claws invariably get caught. Disposition among individual spiders within a species is variable. Spiders may often be judged by gently stroking the forelegs with a small paint-

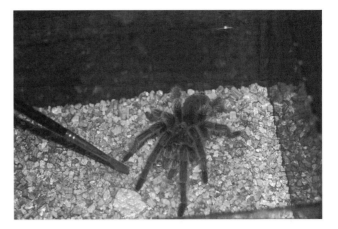

Figure 10.1. A tarantula's forelegs are gently stroked with a small brush to judge whether it is in an aggressive mood before attempted handling.

brush before handling is attempted (Figure 10.1). Spiders rearing or showing any aggressive behavior should be left alone. Spiders seem to show an increased tolerance and tameness with long-term regular handling.

Reproduction

Sexing Spiders

Gender determination of spiders at a young age is advisable in any collection where breeding is planned. In the pet trade, female spiders are more desirable and valuable because of their longer life span. The life span of an adult male may be between several weeks to over 2 years, depending on species and captive conditions (Breene, 1998). On average, most males of common theraphosid species will live 6–18 months. In contrast, adult females may live well over 20 years. Some unscrupulous dealers sell sexed females as such, but sell males as unsexed, as these may command a better price than confirmed males. Males will mature more rapidly than females when spiderlings of the same egg sac are raised to maturity. This may help prevent inbreeding in the wild.

Sex determination of adult males is fairly easy. All adult male spiders will have a thickening of the distal (tarsal) pedipalp section due to the presence of the pear-shaped palpal organ (Figure 10.2). This is occasionally described as a boxing-glove appearance. The majority of male theraphosids will also have easily visible tibial apophysis (spurs) (Figure 10.3). This hook-like appendix is visible on the ventral tibia of the first pair of legs, which are used to hold the female's fangs during mating. The most commonly encountered Theraphosidae without a tibial apophysis are *Theraphosa blondi* and the *Poecilotheria* spp. Other theraphosids without spurs are the genera *Augacephalus*, *Chilobrachys*, *Citharischius*, *Coremiocnemis*, *Heteroscodra*, *Hysterocrates*, *Metriopelma*, *Orphnaecuas*, *Phlogiellus*, *Phormigochilus*, *Phoneyusa*, *Selenocosmia*, *Sericopelma*, *Stromatopelma*, and the species *Nhandu carapoensis*.

Tarantula males will only have a palpal organ after their ter-

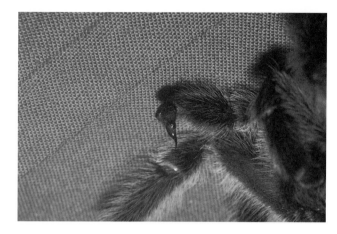

Figure 10.2. The copulatory palpal organ on the distal pedipalp of a terminal instar male Chilean rose tarantula (*Grammostola rosea*).

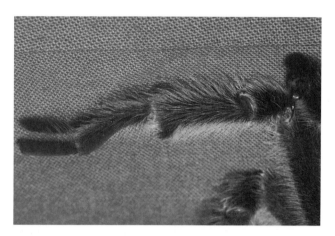

Figure 10.3. The tibial apophysis (spur) on the ventral tibia of the first pair of legs in a terminal instar male Chilean rose tarantula (*Grammostola rosea*).

minal ecdysis. In some araneomorphs, such as Lycosidae and *Polybetes* spp., palpal organs are present in juveniles and are visible as obvious swellings of the pedipalps. Male theraphosids tend to have longer legs and smaller bodies, but these features cannot be used reliably to determine sex.

Adult females often have an obviously swollen epigyne area situated between the cranial pair of book lungs on the ventral opisthosoma. This may be gently palpated as a raised area.

Theraphosids as small as the 6th instar may be sexed accurately by examination of the excuvium (shed skin) under stereomicroscopy for the presence of paired spermathecae in females (Hancock and Hancock, 1999). These spermathecae are located on the innermost surface of the excuvium along the epigastric furrow between the book lungs. Spermathecae morphology varies widely between species, but they are fairly easy to identify with practice. This is the gold standard for gender determination in spiders. Hobbyist associations often provide a postal sexing service for members (see Resources).

Other methods of gender determination include examining chelicerae shape and the presence of epiandrous glands in some males. These methods require practice and are regarded as less reliable.

Mating

Mating of spiders can be hit or miss, and, if done incorrectly, the female may not make love, but rather lunch, of the male! Even when all precautions are taken, occasionally the male may be eaten by the female. With care, an individual male may be mated with several females.

The male should always be introduced into the female's enclosure. In the wild, most adult male tarantulas search for a mate while the females remain in their burrows. The male will usually drum his palps on the substrate; this is usually clearly audible. A component of the sound is produced by stridulation of the pedipalp tibiotarsal joint. The female may respond similarly. The two spiders engage head on, and the male catches the female's fangs with his tibial apophysis and lifts her prosoma and cranial opisthosoma (Figure 10.4). He then inserts the embolus of his palpal organ into the female's spermathecae in the epigastric groove. Once the female is released, he hastily retreats. The female may occasionally chase him for a short distance. The whole process may take only a few seconds or last several minutes.

Females should be selected that have completed ecdysis in the last few months. This allows the most time for egg-sac production. The female is also less receptive when close to ecdysis. Sperm is stored in the spermathecae, so there may be a prolonged interval (months or even over a year) before an egg sac is produced. Some females may not produce egg sacs at all, even if mated several times. Wild-caught females may also produce a viable egg sac over a year after having been in captivity. Since spermathecae have a cuticular lining and are shed with the rest of the cuticle during ecdysis, females cannot produce an egg sac following ecdysis without being mated again. Bruins (1999) mentions that overly obese *Theraphosa blondi* females appear to have reduced fertility.

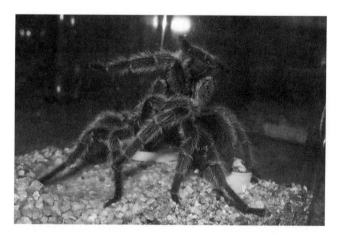

Figure 10.4. Normal mating by Chilean rose tarantulas (*Grammostola rosea*).

Although many species reproduce well in captivity, some (such as the popular *Grammostola rosea*) are difficult to breed, with most egg sacs produced by wild-caught individuals. Accurate species identification is needed since some species are quite similar. There is little funding for Theraphosidae taxonomy, with most work being undertaken by dedicated enthusiasts and part-time arachnologists.

Small enclosures may not enable the male to escape after mating or if the female is not receptive. Vermiculite as a substrate may provide inadequate footing for large species to prop up the female. It is useful to keep two thin, disposable plastic cups or plastic rulers handy to rescue a male, if necessary. In aggressive encounters the female may only remove a limb or two, with the male surviving, but bites to the prosoma are generally fatal. When males are selected for breeding, it is important to check that the most caudal pair of legs do not have the tarsus missing. These spiders cannot prop up the female adequately. Males also need their complete pedipalps and first pair of legs for copulation.

Egg Sacs

Experienced hobbyists may choose to remove the egg sac from the female and incubate it artificially, as females, if disturbed, readily cannibalize the egg sac. This yields a higher success rate compared with leaving egg sacs with the female (Schultz and Schultz, 1998). The incubator consists of a gently heated enclosure with a water container to maintain humidity and a slowly revolving chamber containing the egg sac. Readers are referred to the ATS for details on the incubator's construction. Most *Brachypelma* species egg sacs should be incubated at 25.5°–28°C (78°–82°F) with a humidity of 60%.; this is helpful in preventing fungal or parasitic infections of the egg sac. The egg sac should be opened in a large vivarium, as it may contain up to several hundred spiderlings that are otherwise easily lost.

Specific Species Requirements

Brachypelma smithi *(Mexican Redknee Tarantula)*

This is the arch-type tarantula—the species usually seen in movies because of its hardiness and attractive coloration. It is very popular and makes an excellent pet or display animal. These spiders are usually docile, and most individuals can be handled. *Brachypelma smithi* is listed in Appendix II of CITES, which contributes to the value of this spider.

The species does not have any special husbandry requirements. It is often described as an opportunistic burrower, so a retreat should be provided.

Grammostola rosea *(Chilean Rose Tarantula)*

This is one of the most common and popular species in the pet trade. Large adult specimens are more affordably priced than are *Brachypelma smithi*. There are two color morphs: a plain brown and a brighter copper (especially evident on the cara-

pace). This spider is resistant to desiccation and generally quite hardy, but is difficult to breed and occasionally becomes anorexic for several months before resuming feeding. Some authors suspect this is a wandering species, hunting at night and hiding under vegetation and rocks by day (Breene, 1998). It is generally housed in captivity as a burrowing species, and a retreat should be provided.

Theraphosa blondi *(Goliath Bird Eater Tarantula)*

This is a much sought-after and expensive species. The popularity of this spider stems from it being the largest one in the world. Size is its only redeeming characteristic, and it is not recommended for novices. It is a drab brown and can be aggressive. Goliath bird eaters also can produce airborne urticating hairs. This spider frequently assumes a moth-eaten appearance with an unattractive bald opisthosoma when on public display, because it kicks off hairs in response to visitors invariably banging on the enclosure's glass. Species such as those of *Lasiodora* and *Xenesthis* may exceed this species' average length and weight (Breene, 1998). *Lasiodora parahybana* makes an attractive large display spider, maintaining a better appearance than *T. blondi*. Goliath bird eaters are tropical and require a high level of humidity. Encouraging burrowing may assist the spider in regulating its own humidity. Otherwise, a large retreat should be provided. Spiders spending a long time over or close to the water dish need increased humidity, which may be achieved by limiting ventilation and regularly moistening the substrate. In addition to invertebrates, large *T. blondi* specimens will often accept defrosted pinkie or even adult mice, ox heart, and pieces of chicken.

Poecilotheria regalis *(Indian Ornamental Tarantula)*

This and other Asian ornamental tarantulas are popular arboreals for display and pets. They have an attractive opisthosoma pattern and striking yellow bands on the underside of the legs. This species is occasionally kept in a group display. They do not have urticating hairs. A vertical substrate, such as a piece of bark or cork sheet, is needed for the spider to build a raised-web retreat. A hole, crack, or recess is also helpful for the retreat. This is a monsoon forest species (Breene, 1998) and as such would be dry most of the year. A raised water dish is useful and will provide adequate humidity. A floor substrate is not needed although often provided for aesthetics. Other *Poecilotheria* spp. such as the equally common *P. fasciata* can be kept similarly.

Choosing Species for Pets and Display

Many species offered for sale at entomological fairs and on the Internet are not suitable for novice keepers. Some are fast or aggressive, or have particularly irritating urticating hairs. Others need specific husbandry requirements, and initial experience with easier theraphosids is advisable. Some species may be relatively easy to keep but do not make suitable display animals, as they spend most of their time hiding or in a web retreat. For the novice, *Grammostola rosea*, *Brachypelma albopilosum*, and *B. smithi* are especially good species. Other suitable spiders include *B. emilia*, *B. vagans*, and some *Aphonopelma* species, including *A. anax*, *A. hentzi*, and *A. chalcodes*. *Avicularia avicularia*, *A. versicolor*, and *Poecilotheria* species, such as *P. fasciata* and *P. regalis*, make good arboreal species once some experience with terrestrial tarantulas has been gained.

Some references list species as aggressive or not. Specimens of supposedly aggressive species may be calm and handleable, whereas an individual *Brachypelma* may bite. Aggressive species include *Ceratogyrus* spp., *Haplopelma lividum*, *H. minax*, *Harpactira* spp., *Heteroscodra* spp., *Hysterocrates* spp., *Phormictopus cancerides*, *Psalmopoeus* spp., *Pterinochilus* spp., *Stromatopelma calceata*, and *Theraphosa blondi*.

Captive Care of Other Commonly Kept Spiders

Trap-door Spiders

Several arachnid families are referred to as trap-door spiders, including Barychelidae, Ctenizidae, Nemesiidae, and Actinopodidae. *Conothele* spp. (Ctenizidae) are most commonly kept. These spiders are much smaller than tarantulas, seldom being longer than 3 cm. They are almost hairless, and many are a red or red-brown. Trap-door spiders are extremely aggressive and bite readily, so handling should not be attempted. They spin their burrow and hinged door in loose soils. A thick layer of substrate (vermiculite or potting soil) should be provided to enable construction of the burrow. These spiders are rarely seen. They catch their prey at night, and often the only signs of life are the regular disappearance of prey and the accumulation of feces in the enclosure.

Other captive Mygalomorphae include the Hexathelidae that contains the notorious *Atrax robustus* (Sydney funnel web). This species can be kept similarly to burrowing tarantulas and trap-door spiders. The Sydney funnel web spider should be kept only by experienced and cautious arachnologists.

Araneomorphs: Orb Web Spiders

Orb web spiders belonging to the families Araneidae and Nephilidae are relatively easy to care for and contribute to extremely attractive displays. Adult females are often large and brightly colored, with a body length up to 6 cm and a leg span of over 16 cm. Most species also remain in the center of their web, making them highly visible. *Argiope* species often reinforce their webs with a visible zigzag of threads. Both *Argiope* and *Nephila* spp. may be kept free in a terrarium room because they remain within their webs. Several *Nephilia* spiders may be safely kept together in a large enclosure. Provision of sidewalls of fine mesh as well as some branches will enable construction of a quality web. Water is provided via a light daily spraying of a web section. *Nephila* seems slightly more moisture dependent than *Argiope*. A small opening in the enclosure is needed for supplying food. In contrast to theraphosids, mealworms can be fed as part of the diet, as these are no threat to the spider if not eaten.

Bruins (1999) recommends a minimum enclosure size of 40 × 15 × 50 cm for *Argiope* spp. and 80 × 40 × 80 cm for adult female *Nephila* spp. Males are much smaller than females. Bruins (1999) also recommends providing a prey item before introducing a male for attempted mating. The male should be removed after a half-hour if he has not approached the female. Egg sacs may take several months to develop, and some European species may need an overwintering period.

Wolf Spiders

The best-known wolf spiders are members of the genus *Lycosa*. *Lycosa tarantula*, the true tarantulas, are the wolf spiders from Europe. These are ground-dwelling and hunting spiders. Most are shy, and many are too small for an interesting display. They carry their egg sacs with them. After hatching, the spiderlings climb onto their mother's back and travel with her before gradually dispersing.

Crab Spiders and Banana Spiders

The most commonly kept are *Heteropoda* and *Polybetes* spp., members of the Heteropodidae family. These spiders naturally occur on walls, on trees, and on banana plantations. They are flattened, with long legs, and are extremely fast, but are not aggressive and will usually try to escape. Due to their rapid movement, a small opening in the enclosure is especially helpful. This allows prey to be introduced and wastes removed (with long forceps) to prevent spiders from escaping. These spiders should be kept in enclosures with adequate wall space. Bruins (1999) recommends an enclosure five times the spider's leg span in width, height, and breadth. They also need humidity, so at least part of the substrate should be kept moist. Periodically, the enclosure walls can be gently sprayed, taking care to avoid the spiders, which may be observed to drink from the droplets formed.

The term *banana spider* is usually applied to any spider found in shipments of bananas. Although these are most often Heteropodidae, they may also be the extremely dangerous *Phoneutria* spp. For this reason, all of these spiders should be treated with caution if unidentified.

Keeping Venomous Spiders

Although all spiders, except those belonging to the Uloboridae and Holoarchaeidae families, are venomous, the World Health Organization (WHO) lists only four genera as dangerous to humans: *Atrax* (Mygalomorphae) and *Latrodectus*, *Loxosceles*, and *Phoneutria* (Araneomorphae) (Lucas and Meier, 1995). According to some authors, the WHO list is incomplete (Lucas and Meier, 1995; Breene et al., 1996). Spider venom has evolved primarily for paralysis of prey; defensive bites are secondary. Although a species may not be regarded as dangerous, nearly all spiders are venomous, and sensitive people could have a severe reaction to the venom. The majority of venoms are multicomponent in nature. Although anaphylactic reactions to a constituent of a spider's venom are rare, many severe bites have a localized and inappropriate immune response, resulting in a more clinically significant bite. An example is the development of pyoderma gangrenosum from *Loxosceles* spp. bites. Whereas most venomous spiders are not aggressive, *Atrax* and *Phoneutria* spp. are an exception.

Many precautions taken when keeping venomous species are to protect one from litigation rather than from the spiders themselves. Dangerous species should be kept in locked, escape-proof enclosures. These species should be handled as little as possible, and a second person should be present in case of an anaphylactic reaction to a bite. Zoological collections should make arrangements with a nearby hospital so the doctors are aware of the necessary treatment.

In the United Kingdom, *Latrodectus* spp. (widow spiders), *Loxosceles* spp. (violin and recluse spiders), *Atrax* spp. (including *A. robustus*, the Sydney funnel web spider), *Phoneutria* spp., and *Lycosa raptoria* are included in the Dangerous Wild Animals Act (1986). These species require a license issued by the local council, and premises are subject to inspection. A list of spider antivenoms and their suppliers are presented in Resources (Lucas and Meier, 1995). Medical opinion should be sought before considering their use.

Australian Funnel Web Spiders

The Hexathelidae family includes approximately 35 species belonging to the genera *Atrax* and *Hadronyche*. Although both sexes of *Atrax robustus* (Sydney funnel web) are venomous, the venom of male spiders is reported as 4–6 times more toxic than the female's. Fatalities have only occurred from male bites (Lucas and Meier, 1995). This may be in part due to adult males leaving their burrows in search of females. Humans and other primates seem to be especially sensitive to their venom. Unlike most venomous spiders, *Atrax* is regarded as aggressive. Most funnel web spiders are terrestrial, and housing is as for other tarantulas. These spiders, being found in temperate to subtropical areas of southeast Australia, require an increased humidity level. They do not make good display spiders, spending most of their time in a web retreat.

Widow Spiders

Latrodectus spp. widow spiders (including black widows) belonging to the Theridiidae family are well known and, while indeed venomous, are often regarded with hysteria rather than respectful caution. These species have a worldwide distribution and are often closely associated with humans. The high likelihood of contact with humans is responsible for the cases of *lactrodectism* (envenomation by widow spiders) seen. The majority of bites do not result in significant envenomation. Despite reports to the contrary, these spiders are not aggressive. All known cases of human envenomation by *Latrodectus* spp. are due to bites by females. Females rarely bite and only as a last resort when crushed, unable to escape, or defending an egg sac. *Latrodectus* spp. are regarded as the most clinically important group of spiders, and it is always best to err on the side of caution.

These spiders should not be handled directly. For litigation reasons, they should be kept in well-sealed enclosures in a locked display case. The enclosure should be cleaned by using forceps. These spiders are easy to keep, requiring only a small enclosure, a small amount of substrate, and several small branches to enable web construction. Only small invertebrates should be fed, and Breene (1998) reports *Latrodectus mactans* surviving well on a diet of *Drosophila* fruit flies. False widows (*Steatoda* spp.) are also members of the Theridiidae and should be treated and housed like widow spiders.

Violin and Recluse Spiders

The small, brown, and unimpressive *Loxosceleus* spp. spiders, like widow spiders, have an exaggerated reputation for being dangerous. They are not aggressive but often occur in close association with humans worldwide. They are easily overlooked because of their small size and reclusive nature. Cutaneous and viscerocutaneous forms of loxoscelism occur, and this spider family is regarded as the second most clinically important group. They do not make good display animals but may be kept under similar conditions as Heteropodidae crab spiders. Like other potentially dangerous species, they should not be handled and kept securely.

Phoneutria Spiders

Phoneutria is a genus whose dangerous reputation is justified. These spiders are very fast and extremely venomous. Unlike most other venomous spiders, Ctenidae family spiders such as *Phoneutria* spp. are also very aggressive. Ctenidae spiders are regarded as the most venomous spiders, and *Phoneutria* can inject large amounts of venom. They are found in South America and often occur on banana plantations. Not all banana spiders are harmless heteropodids, since any spider arriving in Europe or North America in a banana shipment is automatically called a banana spider. *Phoneutria nigriventer* has red chelicerae that can help in identification. In some areas of Brazil, *Phoneutria* bites are one of the most common causes for a trip to the hospital (White et al., 1995). Pain is reported to be the main manifestation of these bites.

Phoneutria and other Ctenidae spiders such as *Cupienius* spp. should be kept only by experienced arachnologists. To prevent delays in treatment should a bite occur, the local hospital should be advised that these spiders are being kept.

Transporting Spiders

Many countries and states have specific restrictions on live-animal transport via the mail or courier service. It is the sender's responsibility to check regulations prior to shipment. International transport will involve CITES certification if *Brachypelma* species are involved. Spiders are best mailed in strong, small plastic containers or plastic jars with moistened paper towel at each end for padding and to maintain humidity. Large containers will lead to injuries. Spiderlings are best shipped in small plastic film canisters or pill vials. Cooling the spiders for a short period in a refrigerator before packing makes handling easier. A large number of ventilation holes are not necessary because of their slow metabolic rate and diffusion method of respiration. The individual containers should be placed in a cardboard box with adequate padding such as crumpled newspaper or Styrofoam chips. This sealed box should be placed in a larger, securely closed Styrofoam-insulated box. Any necessary documentation should be duplicated and the copies enclosed in the outer box. Although labeling is necessary, the words "live tarantulas" may not be appropriate. Alternatives include "harmless live biological specimens" and "harmless live invertebrates." Shipping containers should be kept upright and protected from heat, cold, and direct sunlight. The ATS publishes a helpful booklet and Web site on shipping invertebrates (see Resources).

Anatomy and Physiology

Foelix (1996) provides a comprehensive overview of spider anatomy and physiology.

Like all arthropods, arachnids have a rigid outer protective cuticle that is secreted by the underlying epidermis. The cuticle consists of an epicuticle, an exocuticle, and an endocuticle. The epicuticle largely determines the permeability of the integument. The waxy layer of the epicuticle is important in limiting water loss. The exocuticle has a laminated composite structure consisting of polysaccharide microfibers (*chitin*) embedded in a protein matrix (*sclerotin*). This confers strength to the cuticle. The joint membranes (*pleurites*) and the opisthosoma lack an exocuticle and are predominantly endocuticle. This makes these tissues pliable but increases the risk of opisthosoma rupture if the spider is dropped. The basic arthropod segment consists of a dorsal cuticular plate or tergite, and a ventral cuticular plate or sternite, joined laterally by two flexible pleurites.

One disadvantage of having a rigid exoskeleton is limited growth. Only the opisthosoma can expand. *Ecdysis* (molting) is thus needed for growth. The body proportions change after ecdysis. Preceding ecdysis, spiders have a small prosoma, small limbs, and a large opisthosoma. After ecdysis, there is a larger prosoma and limbs, and the opisthosoma is smaller. The opisthosoma will grow larger until the next ecdysis. The new cuticle is formed in a folded state beneath the old and expands after ecdysis. Spiders will become anorexic before ecdysis and will often hide in a retreat. In tarantulas, the opisthosoma will often become darker, especially where there is alopecia. This is caused by newly formed hairs underlying the cuticle. Some araneomorphs will show darkening of the legs for the same reason. Many araneomorphs will molt in an upright position, suspended by a molting thread, whereas tarantulas will normally undergo ecdysis on their back (Figure 10.5). Molting tarantulas should not be turned upright. All spiders display three stages of ecdysis: first, the carapace lifts and detaches; second, the old opisthosoma cuticle ruptures and the opisthosoma is released; and, finally, the extremities are extracted. The process may take a few minutes for a small araneomorph to several hours for a large theraphosid. The length of the intermolt interval depends

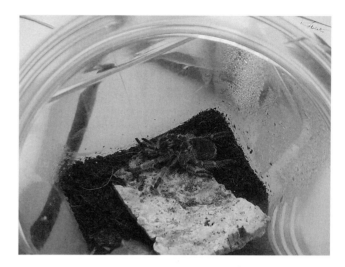

Figure 10.5.   Tarantulas on their back are usually molting and should not be disturbed. Photo by Dan Dombrowski.

on numerous variables, including the instar, nutritional status, and temperature.

Many spiders have a terminal adult instar with no further ecdysis. Whereas adult male tarantulas are a terminal instar, and do not undergo any further periods of ecdysis, adult females are not. Adult female tarantulas will continue to undergo ecdysis and can have life spans in excess of 20 years. The cuticular lining of the pharynx and sucking stomach is part of the molted excuvium, as are the spermathecae in females.

Spiders contain an endoskeleton of mesodermal origin. Most notable is the endosternite in the prosoma to which some muscles of the sucking stomach and limbs attach. Microscopically, it has a cartilage-like appearance. It differs from the cuticle in not containing chitin fibers.

The body is divided into two sections: the fused head and thorax segments, forming the prosoma (*cephalothorax*), and the caudal *opisthosoma* or abdomen. These are joined by the slender pedicel, which evolved from the first abdominal segment. Despite its small size, the pedicel contains 36 muscles (Foelix, 1996) that are important in regulating and maintaining hemolymph pressure in the prosoma. This pressure is necessary for limb extension and for expansion of the new cuticle after ecdysis.

The prosoma consists of a dorsal carapace and a ventral sternum originating from fused tergites and sternites. The carapace bears a large central depression or *carapacial apodeme*. Parts of the exoskeleton invaginating into the body are termed *apodemes*, which function as muscular and tendon insertion points. Muscles of the sucking stomach attach to the carapacial or tergal apodeme. In some African species (e.g., *Ceratogyrus* spp.), the tergal apodeme is everted to form a projection. For this reason, they are often referred to as horned baboon spiders. The coxal apodeme, situated on the ventral surface of the base of the limbs, is important in limb autotomy.

Unlike insects, spiders have simple eyes. Whereas hunting spiders such as Lycosidae, Salticidae, and Thomisidae have excellent sight, tarantulas appear to have poor vision. Some orb

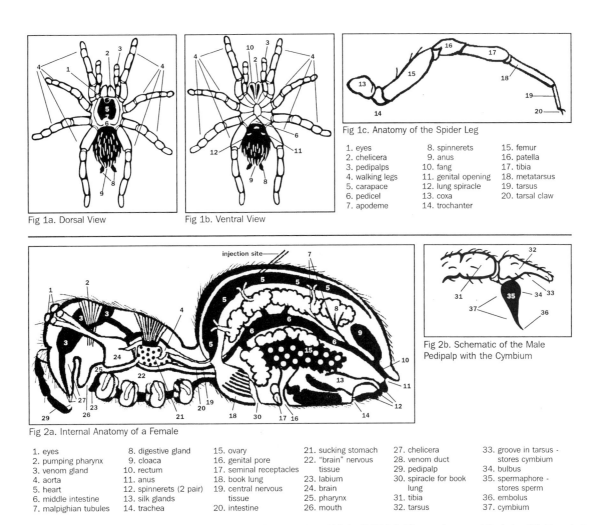

Fig 1a. Dorsal View   Fig 1b. Ventral View

Fig 1c. Anatomy of the Spider Leg

1. eyes	8. spinnerets	15. femur
2. chelicera	9. anus	16. patella
3. pedipalps	10. fang	17. tibia
4. walking legs	11. genital opening	18. metatarsus
5. carapace	12. lung spiracle	19. tarsus
6. pedicel	13. coxa	20. tarsal claw
7. apodeme	14. trochanter	

Fig 2b. Schematic of the Male Pedipalp with the Cymbium

Fig 2a. Internal Anatomy of a Female

1. eyes	8. digestive gland	15. ovary	21. sucking stomach	27. chelicera	33. groove in tarsus - stores cymbium
2. pumping pharynx	9. cloaca	16. genital pore	22. "brain" nervous tissue	28. venom duct	34. bulbus
3. venom gland	10. rectum	17. seminal receptacles	23. labium	29. pedipalp	35. spermaphore - stores sperm
4. aorta	11. anus	18. book lung	24. brain	30. spiracle for book lung	36. embolus
5. heart	12. spinnerets (2 pair)	19. central nervous tissue	25. pharynx	31. tibia	37. cymbium
6. middle intestine	13. silk glands	20. intestine	26. mouth	32. tarsus	
7. malpighian tubules	14. trachea				

Figure 10.6. External and internal tarantula anatomy. From Cappelletti and Visigalli (2004), Figures 1a–c and 2a-b (p. 41). Permission granted by the Zoological Education Network and the artist, Dr. Johnson-Delaney.

web spiders see well and will leave the center of the web when threatened. Although the majority of spiders have eight eyes, arranged in anterior and posterior rows, the number may vary from none to 12. The anterior median eyes are always the main eyes and may be much larger than the other eyes. This is especially noticeable in the Salticidae (jumping spiders).

The prosoma bears six pairs of appendages (Figure 10.6). The first are the *chelicerae*, sometimes referred to as jaws in older texts. These consist of a broad basal segment, with a distal movable fang, through which venom is injected. The chelicerae are used for grasping prey. The second pair of appendages are the *pedipalps*, which appear similar to the legs but lack the metatarsal segment. They are not used for locomotion but have a sensory role during prey capture. They are also used to manipulate prey. In adult male spiders, the copulatory organ, or *palpal organ*, is present as an obvious swelling on the distal segment. It is also present in immatures of some araneomorphs. Sperm is stored in the palpal organ and transferred to the female reproductive tract during copulation. In some species, the coxal segment of the pedipalps are modified to form chewing mouth parts. A serrated row of teeth, the *serrula*, may be present and

acts as a saw to cut into prey. Bristles on the pedipalp base act as a filter for straining ingested food.

Spiders have four pairs of legs that attach between the carapace and sternum of the prosoma. Nomenclature of the segments differs among authors. Foelix (1996) names the segments, starting proximally, as the coxa, trochanter, femur (Figure 10.6), patella, tibia, metatarsus, and tarsus, which carries 2–3 claws. Many spiders, and particularly tarantulas, have *scopulae* or dense tufts of hair on the plantar aspects of the tarsus and metatarsus that account for their ability to climb smooth vertical surfaces. The ends of each hair are split into thousands of cuticular tips. Adhesion is by a combination of numerous contact points and capillary forces from a very thin water layer on the surface of the substrate. The scopulae also play a role in holding onto captured prey.

The only appendages originating from the opisthosoma are the spinnerets (Figure 10.6). Tarantulas have two pairs, although one pair is very reduced. The various silk glands are visible in the abdomen on histology.

Spiders can autotomize and regenerate legs, spinnerets, chelicerae, and pedipalps. P. Bonnet is quoted in Foelix (1996) as autotomizing all the limbs of a spider and hand feeding it until the next ecdysis, when the limbs regenerated. Whereas the limbs contain both extensor and flexor muscles, the major joints (femur/patella and tibia/metatarsus) do not have extensor muscles and rely on hemolymph pressure for extension.

The prosoma contains the spider's central nervous system (CNS), which consists of supraesophageal and subesophageal ganglia. The prosoma also contains the paired venom glands, the sucking stomach, and extensive musculature for the limbs and sucking stomach (Figure 10.6). Diverticula of the midgut are present in the prosoma as well as the opisthosoma and may extend into the coxae of the legs.

Spiders start digestion of their food externally. After the prey has been immobilized, the spider regurgitates contents of the digestive tract onto the prey item, initiating digestion. Liquefied food is ingested through the small mouth and pharynx. Ingestion occurs through action of the sucking stomach.

The midgut enters the opisthosoma via the narrow pedicel. Large numbers of lobed diverticula originate from the midgut before the digestive tract widens and becomes the stercoral pocket. The digestive diverticula function to increase the absorptive surface area of the digestive tract and may function in food storage. A short hindgut leads to the anus. The excretory Malpighian tubules empty into the stercoral pocket, where waste is stored. The main nitrogenous waste products from spiders are guanine, uric acid, adenine, and hypoxanthine.

The heart lies in the middorsal opisthosoma (Figure 10.6) and may be visualized in large specimens with extensive opisthosoma alopecia (Figure 10.7). The book-lung folia are present in the cranio-ventral opisthosoma (Figure 10.6 and 10.8). In araneomorphs, trachea are present in the opisthosoma. The reproductive tract and various spinning glands exiting to the spinnerets are also situated in the opisthosoma. Graphic representation of a spider's organs may be misleading. Organs are by no means well demarcated, and differentiating the structures macroscopically can be difficult. Organs are usually embedded between the many midgut diverticula that occupy most of the opisthosoma.

All spider musculature is striated. Spider muscles contain fewer mitochondria (Foelix, 1996) than those of other arthropods, meaning muscles fatigue rapidly (especially in the theraphosids, which also lack tracheal respiration).

Spiders have an open venous circulatory system and a well-developed arterial system. Vessels from the heart direct hemolymph to specific organs, even reaching the tips of the tarsi. There are no capillaries. Venous return to the heart is due to a pressure gradient and follows specific pathways. The heart is surrounded by a pericardial sinus that, together with ligaments attaching to the cuticle, helps generate suction and pressure. Unlike the rest of the spider's musculature, the myocardium is relatively rich in mitochondria. The resting heart rate ranges from 30 to 40 beats/min in large theraphosids to over 100 beats/min in smaller araneomorphs. The heart rate may more than double after a small amount of activity (Foelix, 1996). A more recent study using a noninvasive technique found the resting heart rate of the tarantula *Aphonopelma hentzi* to be 5.6 ± 1.5 beats/min (Coelho and Amaya, 2000).

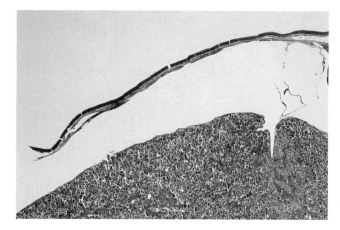

Figure 10.7. Histological section showing the heart just beneath the cuticle of the opisthosoma.

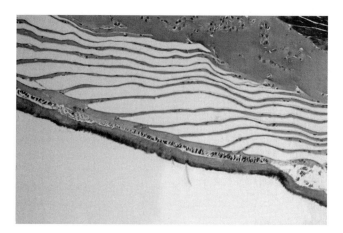

Figure 10.8. Histological section of normal tarantula book lung tissue.

Hemolymph is clear and slightly blue due to the copper in hemocyanin, the oxygen-carrying pigment. Dehydrated spiders will typically be immobile with their legs flexed beneath them. Arachnids need to maintain blood volume and pressure for leg extension.

Hemocytes appear to have analogous functions to vertebrate leukocytes, but little work has been done on their activity in spiders. Hemocytes arise directly from the myocardial cells, and, on histology, hemoblasts may occasionally be seen attached or budding from the heart lumen. This is normal and particularly evident in some spiderlings and juveniles. It has been suggested that granular hemocytes contribute to the sclerotization of the cuticle (Foelix, 1996). Accumulation of subcuticular granular hemocytes is especially evident before and after ecdysis. Other hemocytes include lebridiocytes, which contain a single large secretory vacuole, and cyanocytes, which synthesize hemocyanin. Before its release into the hemolymph, hemocyanin is found in a crystalline form in the cyanocytes. Hemocyanin has a much higher oxygen affinity than does hemoglobin and functions more as an oxygen-storage mechanism than an oxygen transporter.

The very low metabolic rate of spiders explains their ability to survive many months without food. Paul (1990) reports a tarantula's oxygen consumption being only one-hundredth that of warm-blooded vertebrates and one-fifth that of poikilothermic vertebrates. Metabolism is reduced during periods of inanition (over 80% in extreme situations), and spiders with life expectancies of 300 days have survived up to 200 days in the laboratory without food. This enables survival during naturally occurring periods of starvation (Foelix, 1996) such as overwintering.

Spider neurobiology has been better researched than many other aspects of arachnid physiology. Spiders have tactile hairs, most remarkably the trichobothrium on the legs. These are sensitive to air currents and low-frequency air vibrations, enabling the spider to detect prey. Chemosensitive hairs on distal leg segments have an open tip where numerous nerve fibers are exposed to the environment. Spiders may be seen testing, almost tasting, a substrate or prey item with the tips of their legs. Each tarsus contains a tarsal organ that acts as a humidity receptor. All large articulated hairs have a triple innervation, with only the short body hairs and scopula hairs on the tarsi lacking innervation. Remarkably, the innervation of sensory hairs is maintained during ecdysis. A dendritic connection is maintained between the base of the old hair and the tip of the newly forming hair. This connection is lost as the old cuticle is cast off.

Environmental Disorders

Trauma and Hemolymph Loss

This is one of the most common causes of captive-spider deaths. Whereas major injuries (e.g., a spider that has fallen and ruptured its opisthosoma) are obvious, small injuries (particularly of the leg joints or the bases of the legs) may not be, and exsanguination is not identified as the cause of death. The substrate usually rapidly absorbs any hemolymph, leaving little clue to the cause of death. Many so-called mysterious deaths may be from exsanguination. A 2-cm-long opisthosoma wound may lose very little hemolymph, whereas much smaller wounds can lead to rapid loss of hemolymph. Wound location is obviously important. Wounds over the dorsal opisthosoma are likely to cause rapid hemolymph loss from the heart and large vessels. Wounds at the base of appendages seem to lose hemolymph more rapidly than those more distal. A spider may take several days to gradually exsanguinate, with little more noted than a depressed attitude.

Postmating injuries occur occasionally, but these are often to the prosoma and hold a very poor prognosis. This is a normal risk of breeding. Owners interfering during ecdysis or trying to assist during a perceived dysecdysis are a common cause of trauma. This usually ends in a dismembered spider (Frye, 1992).

Treating Trauma

Although several treatment options are available, many spiders cannot be saved. The mainstay in hemostasis is cyanoacrylate adhesive. Veterinary tissue adhesives may be used, but hobbyists normally use commercial superglues. Although tissue adhesives (*n*-butyl cyanoacrylate) are reportedly less toxic, in the author's experience commercial superglues are just as effective and do not cause intoxication. Superglue gels are not effective. When using cyanoacrylate, several layers should be applied to build a sturdy repair. Even large opisthosoma wounds can be sealed in this way. The spider will often shed normally at the next ecdysis. If ecdysis occurs soon after the trauma, the new cuticle may also be damaged, and this should be sealed similarly with cyanoacrylate. The cuticle will be normal after the next ecdysis. Successful use of fingernail hardeners has been reported, mainly for arresting hemorrhage from damaged legs, where the application of cyanoacrylate glue may be difficult (Breene, 1998). One benefit is there is no risk of legs being glued together. There are numerous reports among hobbyists of alternatives for hemostasis, including talc, cornstarch, tissue paper, and hematinics. None of these appear to be reliable. Pizzi and Ezendam (2002) showed sutures to be ineffective (see the section Anesthesia and Surgery). Fluid administration may be necessary in some cases. This topic is covered under the section Dehydration.

Autotomy

If limbs are severely damaged or crushed and hemostasis is not possible, the affected limb can be removed by inducing autotomy (Pizzi et al., 2002). Unlike an amputation, this is a voluntary action, and should not be attempted with the spider anesthetized (Figure 10.9). See the section Anesthesia and Surgery for a description and explanation of the technique.

Dehydration

Spiders can become dehydrated from a variety of causes. Theraphosids sent by post can arrive dehydrated due to postal delays. Severely dehydrated spiders cannot move, as extension of ap-

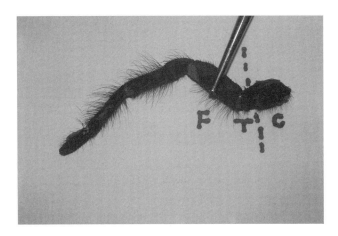

Figure 10.9. Limb autotomy site between the coxa and trochanter on a postmortem specimen.

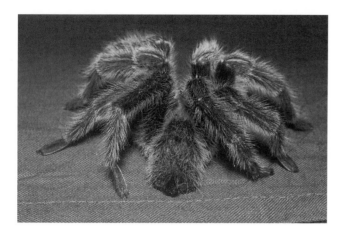

Figure 10.10.   Severe dehydration in a Chilean rose tarantula (*Grammostola rosea*).

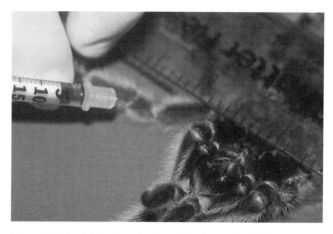

Figure 10.11.   Technique for immobilization and administration of fluids, or hemolymph sampling, using the ventral limb membranes in a theraphosid.

pendages depends on hemolymph pressure (Figure 10.10). In contrast, the limbs are flexed by muscular action. Hemolymph accounts for 20% of a tarantula's body weight. The easiest treatment in most cases of dehydration is placing the front of the spider in a very shallow water dish. Care must be taken not to submerge the book lungs. Most spiders will rehydrate themselves over a few hours, appearing normal after a day.

In severe cases, intrahemolymph injections of sterile physiological fluids may be administered. This author has used physiological saline (sodium chloride, 0.9%), lactated Ringer's solution (LRS), and Hartmann's solution without problems. Physiological saline may have the most similar osmolarity to arachnid hemolymph. A recipe for *spider Ringer's lactate* is listed in Drugs and Therapeutic Agents. This solution is based on analysis of tarantula hemolymph composition (Schartau and Leidescher, 1983).

Fine sterile needles (26 or 27 gauge) are recommended. There are two viable routes of fluid administration. Chitty (2001) quotes Johnson-Delaney as recommending injection into the heart or into the pericardial sac found in the dorsal opisthosoma. Advantages are that a relatively large amount of fluid can be administered rapidly via this route. Another advantage is that placement is not critical, as extracardiac administration is not detrimental due to the open hemolymph system. The main disadvantage of this technique is the risk of any movement by the operator or spider resulting in the needle fatally lacerating the heart or opisthosoma cuticle. This method is best limited to severely dehydrated or to anesthetized spiders.

The second method involves administering fluids into a limb by inserting the needle in the ventral area of the joint membrane (Figure 10.11). The risk of causing a fatal injury is small with this technique, and, even if a limb is crushed, it can be removed by autotomy and the coxal stump wound sealed with cyanoacrylate glue. The spider is usually restrained in dorsal recumbency with a plastic ruler (see Figure 10.11). The disadvantages of this method are that administration is slow and there is a limit to the amount of fluid that can be given.

Intoxication

Like many invertebrates, spiders are extremely sensitive to most insecticides. Certain insects such as *Cyclocephala pasadena* (masked chaffer) are toxic to spiders (Breene, 1998) and their use must be avoided. Numerous other invertebrates can accumulate plant toxins.

Although there is much debate among hobbyists, feeding wild-caught insects does raise the possibility of poisoning captive spiders with pesticides the prey has been exposed to (see the section Feeding). There is no debating that a variety of pesticides, even when used in adjacent dwellings, can kill collections of captive spiders. Proper communication with neighbors can help prevent this situation.

Numerous incidents have been reported of tarantula deaths induced by fipronil (Frontline; Merial, Duluth, GA) (R. Pizzi, unpublished data). One notable case involved a pet shop with enclosures that had previously been used to house snakes that were treated for mites. Although the enclosures had apparently been cleaned well, all spiders placed in the enclosures died acutely (R. Gabriel, personal communication). Other cases have involved handling spiders or invertebrate prey after stroking treated cats and dogs. Some of these incidents did not cause rapid death but gradual deterioration over a period of days. Although these deaths could not be conclusively linked to fipronil, caution should be exercised when there is a risk of its contact with spiders. Similar precautions should be taken when working with acaricides used to control ticks and mites on vertebrate hosts.

There are anecdotal reports of neurological signs in spiders handled by heavy smokers, presumably due to nicotine poisoning. By contrast, smoke itself does not appear irritating, as many hobbyists who smoke in their spider rooms report no problems.

Treating cases of intoxication is difficult and generally unrewarding. Treatment consists of supportive care by hand feeding and assisting the spider to drink. In a small number of cases, spiders have recovered with time and nursing care (Breene, 1998), but owner compliance may be difficult. As with so many environmental conditions, prevention is the best medicine.

Infectious Diseases and Parasites

Microbial Infections

Bacterial Infections

Swabs of the oral cavity, body surface, or any lesions can be taken for microbial culture (Cooper, 1985). Even if a bacterial organism is isolated, determining its pathogenicity may be difficult. There is little knowledge of normal microbial flora of the arachnid body surface and digestive tract. Hemolymph may be sampled for microbiological culture, and the presence of bacteria is likely to be abnormal and significant (Pizzi, 2001b). To prevent contamination of a hemolymph sample with digestive-tract flora, a leg joint should be used. This has the additional benefit of being easier to repair should a spider move and the needle cause a laceration. When collecting hemolymph post mortem for culture, use the most distal leg joints because these areas will be least affected by postmortem invasion of intestinal flora (A.A. Cunningham, personal communication).

Bacillus spp. appear to be normal digestive-tract flora that can act as opportunistic pathogens, especially under poor husbandry conditions. *Bacillus* sp. mortality events have occurred in *Hysterocrates gigas* spiderlings kept under insufficient humidity (R. Pizzi, unpublished data). Antibiotics were not needed, with the number of deaths decreasing rapidly after the substrate moisture level was increased. S. MacGregor (personal communication) reports frequent postmortem isolation of *Bacillus cereus* from older female *Brachypelma smithi*. Mixed secondary or symbiotic bacterial infections, including infection by *Proteus* sp., have been demonstrated on culture and histologically in Panagrolaimidae nematode infections, but their significance is not clear. Attempted treatment of these cases with oral enrofloxacin did not significantly prolong survival. Cooper (1987) reports bacterial infections characterized by discharges from the mouth, genital tract, book lungs, or anus, but the significance of organisms cultured is difficult to access. Very little literature exists on the use, dosages, or efficacy of antimicrobials in the treatment of spiders. Selection should be based on culture and sensitivity results.

Fungal Infections

Fungal infections of the exoskeleton (usually secondary to environmental fungal growth) are common and may be caused by excessive moisture of the substrate and/or waste accumulation (poor hygiene). Fungal infections of the exoskeleton are easily and safely treated by topical application of povidone–iodine with a cotton swab. Infections may recur due to predisposing environmental factors and the persistent nature of fungal spores. Once fungal infections breech the cuticle and become systemic, the prognosis is grave. Systemic infection progresses rapidly, with death occurring within days. Occasionally, a spider is found to have died of a systemic fungal infection with a lack of antemortem clinical signs. These cases appear to develop and progress rapidly (in less than a week).

Adding terrestrial isopods to an enclosure may help reduce decaying matter that would otherwise promote environmental fungal growth in high-humidity enclosures (Schultz and Schultz, 1998).

Fungal Overgrowth of Egg Sacs

Schultz and Schultz (1998) report this as common in captivity. To prevent this, as well as maternal cannibalism of the egg sac, keepers should transfer the egg sac to a slowly rotating artificial incubator where the humidity and temperature are controlled. Most *Brachypelma* spp. egg-sac incubation is advised at 25.5°–28°C (78°–82°F) with a humidity of 60%. If fungal infection of an egg sac is noted, the egg sac should be removed from the mother and placed in a large aquarium and opened, and the infected contents separated from healthy eggs. Although this may not be successful, there is little to lose. If the spiderlings have already hatched, they may be housed normally. Eggs should be kept suspended in a piece of soft cloth over moist substrate to prevent desiccation. Schultz and Schultz (1998) report that once- or twice-daily gentle swirling of the eggs suspended in the cloth may simulate normal maternal movements of the egg sac.

Viruses

Morel (1978) reported the only virus isolated from a spider. This was a baculovirus affecting the hepatopancreas, causing the death of a *Pisaura mirabilis* (nursery web spider). The lack of further reports is likely due to little work in this area.

Parasites

Oral Panagrolaimidae Nematodes

This oral nematode infection of tarantulas has recently been identified from collections in several European countries, including the United Kingdom (Pizzi et al., 2003). There are numerous reports from hobbyists of spiders similarly affected in North America. This is likely an increasingly important disease of captive spiders, posing a risk to collections. The infection initially manifests with anorexia and a gradually increasing lethargy that progresses to a huddled posture. Death occurs after several weeks, or occasionally even months, following the onset of signs. A thick white discharge between the mouth and chelicerae may be noted, especially during the later stages of infection (Figure 10.12). A mass of extremely small, motile nematodes (less than 0.5–3.0 mm long) may be observed microscopically in a drop of saline. In collections with particularly valuable or rare specimens, the area between the chelicera and mouth should be examined with a magnifying lens or stereomicroscopy before the spider leaves quarantine. The nematodes have been classified as belonging to the Panagrolaimidae family (phylum Nemata, order Rhabditida) and are currently undergoing DNA sequencing for accurate phylogenetic placement.

The parasite has been seen in a wide variety of Theraphosidae species from Africa, the Americas, and Asia. It has occurred in

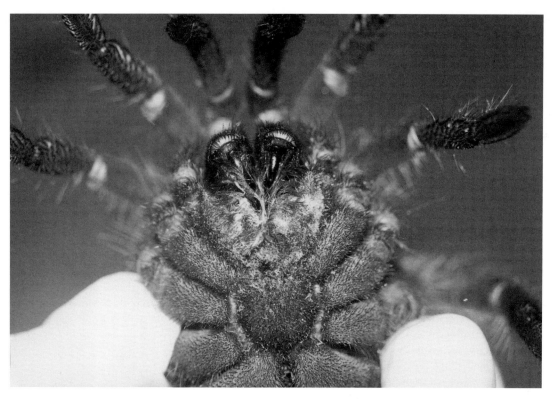

Figure 10.12. Early stage of a Panagrolaimidae nematode infection in a theraphosid. Note the white milky discharge on the chelicerae.

captive and wild-caught arboreal and terrestrial species. Infection has been observed in the most common genera, including *Brachypelma*, *Grammostola*, *Poecilotheria*, and *Theraphosa*. Although the mode of transmission is not yet known, *Phoridae* sp. flies have been suggested as a possible vector (R. Gallon, personal communication). Infections have spread between separate containers that were not adjoining in the same room. The infection also appears more prevalent under conditions of good ventilation and increased humidity. What appears to be a secondary or symbiotic bacterial infection is evident on histopathology, but culture attempts have demonstrated mixed bacteria, including *Proteus* sp. The significance of these bacteria is not clear.

Treatment trials with enrofloxacin, oxfendazole, and fenbendazole were not effective or toxic (R. Pizzi, unpublished data). Topical application of the benzimidazoles appeared initially to irritate the nematodes and decrease the external mass, but similar effects were evident with repeated saline flushing.

One important precaution involves the zoonotic potential of some related nematodes. Human cases have occurred, and deep infections can be difficult to treat. Since large specimens of *Theraphosa blondi* can have fangs longer than 3 cm, secondary infection of bite wounds is possible. Due to this risk, lack of treatment options, and potential spread in a collection, euthanasia of all affected spiders is strongly recommended.

There is a risk that this parasite may adversely affect future captive-breeding plans of rare or endangered species (and thus possible future efforts at reintroduction). Zoological collections

with a spider collection are strongly advised to quarantine all newly arrived spiders (see the section Quarantine). A minimum quarantine period of 30 days in a separate building, or at least a separate room, is advisable. The quarantine period should be prolonged for any anorexic spiders, as these may be approaching ecdysis or are gravid females about to produce an egg sac. Such spiders should leave quarantine only once a return to normal feeding has been observed for 2 weeks.

Nematodes should be preserved in 10% buffered formalin, and not alcohol, which causes distortion and makes identification difficult. In contrast, spiders are best preserved for histopathology in 70% ethanol, as formalin causes marked cuticular hardening that makes sectioning extremely difficult.

Mermithidae Nematodes

Prior to Panagrolaimidae oral infections, only Mermithidae nematodes had been reported from spiders (Poinar, 1985). These uncommon parasites are likely to be of importance only in wild-caught individuals (less than 1% incidence). They have been noted from a large number of spider species worldwide. Mermithid nematodes likely infect spiders via ingestion of a paratenic host. A greatly enlarged opisthosoma is a common sign. Affected spiders may also have an asymmetrical opisthosoma, malformed palps, and shorter legs. These parasites appear to retard host development, whose male secondary sexual characteristics may be poorly developed or absent. Parasites gradually fill the opisthosoma before killing the host, and, in the later stages of infection, the coils may be clearly seen through the cuticle. Foelix (1996) notes that parasitized spiders may show behavior changes and become sluggish and not attempt to escape when approached. Migration toward a water source is often observed. There may be a small risk from feeding wild-caught invertebrate food, but no cases of infection have been reported. Radiography of large adult tarantulas was not helpful in diagnosing this condition (R. Pizzi, unpublished data).

Parasitic and Saprophytic Mites (Acarii)

Mites are a frequently reported problem that usually affects higher-humidity spiders. Many mites are saprophytic and some are parasitic. When mites are observed, it is difficult to evaluate their clinical significance. Breene (1998) proposes that mites may occlude the moist surfaces of the book lungs when present in high numbers. Excessive humidity and accumulated prey remains can contribute to a mite problem. Wood chips and bark substrates have been associated with mites and are best avoided. Many hobbyists routinely microwave nonflammable substrates to prevent mite outbreaks. West (1995) reported using the commercially available predatory mite *Hypoaspis miles* (Laelapidae) that is sold to control fungus gnats (Sciaridae) and pest thrips (Thripidae). These laelapids control mites in tarantula enclosures without irritating the spiders and have been used by many North American keepers. Breene (1998) recommends a half-teaspoon or less per enclosure. The predatory mites will die once no prey mites remain. In the event of a new mite outbreak, more predatory mites will be required. As an alternative, isopods can minimize prey remains that would otherwise provide a food source for mites (Schultz and Schultz, 1998). Other techniques reported by hobbyists include removing mites with an artist's fine paintbrush and immersing spiders in water for a few seconds. A small amount of petroleum jelly on a cotton swab can be used to remove fast-moving mites, but the success rate is variable. Acaricides cannot be used because these compounds are toxic to spiders.

Pompilidae Wasps

These are unlikely to be a problem in captive collections but may occur in areas where captive North American species are native. Spiders are paralyzed by the wasp's sting, and an egg is laid on the spider. The developing larva feeds on the live spider. Paralysis may be temporary or permanent, depending on the wasp species. Most Pompilidae are not species specific but do show host preferences. Paralyzed wild tarantulas are occasionally rescued from parasitic wasps by keepers. Breene (1998) reports some success with intensive nursing and hand feeding of paralyzed spiders.

Ichneumonidae Wasps

These lay their eggs on the spider's legs or abdomen but do not paralyze the spider as do Pompilidae wasps. The larva develops as an ectoparasite, ingesting the spider's hemolymph. This condition is rare in captivity. Treatment involves carefully removing the single parasitic larva. Some ichneumonid larvae also parasitize egg sacs.

Sphecidae Mud Daubers

There are over 1000 species of these solitary wasps in North America and approximately 8000 worldwide (Breene, 1998). The two most common species in North America are *Sceliphron caementarium* and *Chalybion californicum*, which occur under the eaves of buildings. Similar to pompilid wasps, they paralyze spiders for the larvae to feed on. Web spiders belonging to Theridiidae and Araneidae are most commonly parasitized. Mud daubers can impact wild spider populations, since one female may catch up to 300 spiders in a season. This untreatable condition is rare in captivity.

Acroceridae Spider Flies

These are true endoparasites. Larvae slowly crawl from where they are deposited on the spider's body to the book lungs, penetrating the opisthosoma between the lamellae. The larva may be present for several months or even years in tarantulas. The mature fourth instar is the destructive feeding stage, which may last only a few days but is fatal for the spider. The larva consumes opisthosoma tissues before bursting through the dorsal opisthosoma to pupate. Up to 14 larvae have been found in the opisthosoma of one tarantula (Foelix, 1996), but one larva is most common. This condition occurs primarily in wild-caught spiders.

Phoridae: Humpback Flies

These tiny fruit-fly-sized flies lay eggs on prey remains in enclosures and can be abundant in some areas. Schultz and Schultz (1998) report death among adult tarantulas that appears to be caused by the parasitic larvae infecting the book lungs before penetrating the opisthosoma and internal organs. Spiderlings are most susceptible, and Phoridae larvae may kill a large number of spiderlings rapidly before the problem is noticed. The higher humidity requirement of spiderlings is the main contributing factor. The most common species found in North America is *Megaselia scalaris*. Some experienced keepers suspect that phorids may be responsible for the spread of Panagrolaimidae oral nematode infections within a collection. Phorids are controlled by limiting enclosure humidity and frequently removing prey remains. Quarantine of newly introduced spiders is important, as many spider shipments may be affected. New shipments of spiders should be examined closely for the presence of any small flies or larvae.

Ants

Although ants are not parasites, a few species have been reported to injure or even kill captive tarantulas. In some areas, this may be a severe, recurring problem. The main problem species in North America are *Solenopsis* spp. (fire ants), *Iridomyrmex humilis* (the Argentine ant), and *Monomorium pharaonis* (the pharaoh ant). Baits or barriers are the usual methods of control. In severe cases, enclosures may require water moats.

Neoplasia

There are no confirmed reports of neoplasia in the Araneae. What Frye (1992) includes as an illustration of a possible neoplasm may be a melanization reaction to an injury or infection. The Registry of Tumors in Lower Animals has no cases of neoplasia in spiders (Williams, 1992; E.C. Peters, personal communication, 2004)

Miscellaneous Disorders

Opisthosoma Alopecia

Bald patches may be seen on the dorsal opisthosoma of New World theraphosids (Figures 10.13 and 10.14). This condition normally results from the spider projecting urticating hairs when disturbed. Following ecdysis, the opisthosoma will appear normal. This is one of the most commonly reported problems in captive tarantulas and is not biologically similar to true alopecia in mammals.

Another cause of normal alopecia is pending ecdysis. In this case, the cuticle will tend to appear dark (underlying new cuticle and hair), and the opisthosoma will have the typical full or bloated appearance. This is in contrast to the often pale or sometimes pink appearance of the cuticle in a spider that has kicked off its urticating hairs.

Anorexia

This is a frequently reported problem in captive tarantulas. In many cases it is normal. Spiders will become anorexic for weeks

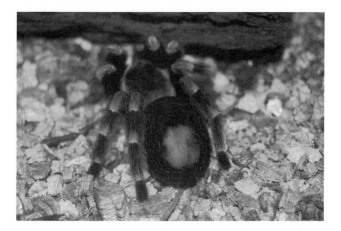

Figure 10.13. Opisthosoma alopecia in a Mexican redknee tarantula (*Brachypelma smithi*) on display in a zoological collection. This was caused by the stress of visitors banging on the glass.

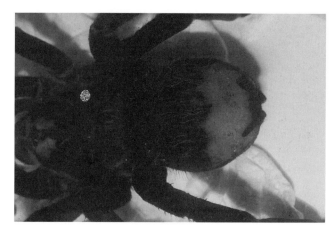

Figure 10.14. Opisthosoma alopecia in the largest spider species, a goliath bird eater (*Theraphosa blondi*).

or months when approaching ecdysis. Gravid females will also often have a period of anorexia before producing an egg sac. Adult male tarantulas are terminal instars and may stop eating, instead spending their time on efforts to escape and find females.

Species such as *Aphonopelma chalcodes* and *Grammostola rosea* often have prolonged periods of anorexia for no apparent reason. Breene (1998) reported anorexia of 3 years in three *Aphonopelma chalcodes*. These spiders died, so a disease condition may have been involved.

In the absence of any clinical signs, the husbandry and captive environment should be reviewed. Increasing the temperature of the enclosure may start some spiders feeding again. If this does not help, Breene (1998) advises increasing the humidity. Waxworms (*Galleria mellonella*) will occasionally be taken by tarantulas that refuse other prey items.

Adult Male Deaths

Adult male theraphosids have a terminal ecdysis and live only for a limited period after this (6–18 months, on average). Adult males are identified post mortem by the palpal organ that is present only in the terminal instar of tarantulas. Some juvenile araneomorphs will also have palpal organs (see the section Reproduction). Histology or cytology will demonstrate spermatozoa in the testicular tissue and palpal organ. When performing cytology on the palpal organ contents, crush the tissue between two glass slides.

Spiders on Their Back

Spiders are normally found dead in an upright position with their legs flexed beneath them. Inverted theraphosids are normally undergoing ecdysis and should not be handled, because they are susceptible to trauma at this time (Figure 10.5). Occasionally, tarantulas will undergo ecdysis on their sides and very rarely while upright. Most araneomorph spiders will undergo ecdysis while upright or suspended from a molting thread.

Dysecdysis

With regard to normal ecdysis, the spider's hydration status is the most important consideration (for details, see the section Natural History and Captive Care). Dysecdysis has been successfully treated by administration of intracardiac fluids. Attempts at aiding dysecdysis by manipulation and removal of the excuvium invariably result in the spider's serious injury or death. Some hobbyists report success with application of detergent solutions or glycerin (carefully avoiding the book lungs). Spiders are most susceptible to injury shortly after a molt, when their exoskeleton is still soft and pliable. If dysecdysis occurs, legs, pedipalps, and/or chelicerae usually become trapped in the excuvium. Limbs can become twisted and deformed, and if the chelicerae are affected, the spider may be unable to catch prey (spiders with autotomized chelicerae have been hand-fed killed, pulverized crickets until the next ecdysis). Any intervention in the molting process should be considered as a last resort. The best results have been in cases where only small sections of leg are trapped in the excuvium. All remaining loose excuvium is trimmed away. In some cases, the spider is severely deformed but can survive until the next ecdysis when it may again have normal limbs. In severe cases, the spider may later need to be induced to autotomize the affected limbs (see the section Anesthesia and Surgery), but this is not without risk. If only a single limb is trapped, autotomy of the limb can be considered but may not be essential for a spider to survive until its next ecdysis. If autotomy is chosen, the cuticle should be allowed to harden for a few days.

Anesthesia and Surgery

Anesthesia

This author has anesthetized many tarantula species with both halothane and isoflurane without any losses. Standard small animal vaporizers set to their maximum vapor concentration (4%–5%) can be used in conjunction with a clear plastic anesthetic chamber designed to hold the spider comfortably (Figure 10.15). A second approach does not use a vaporizer and requires two small, flat, airtight, plastic containers. The inner smaller container has fine perforations at each end to allow diffusion of the anesthetic agent without direct spider/anesthetic contact. The small container (holding the spider) is placed inside the larger plastic container that has a cotton-wool swab soaked with a small amount of the anesthetic agent. Induction usually takes 10–15 min at room temperature. The primary disadvantage of this method is exposure of personnel to the anesthetic gas. The spider's recovery from anesthesia is gradual. Slow leg movements and then righting attempts increase. Slow leg movements may resume 3–20 min after removal from the anesthetic chamber. While spiders may slowly ambulate 30–120 min after anesthesia, prey items should not be offered for at least 48 h. Carbon dioxide gas is commonly used by entomologists for invertebrate anesthesia, but spiders might die (R. Pizzi, unpublished data). Hobbyists commonly use hypothermia to immobilize spiders for shipping. Hypothermia in vertebrates does not

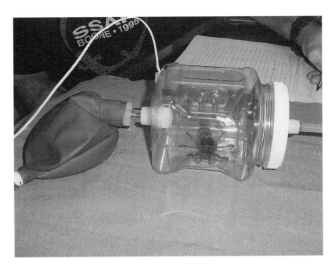

Figure 10.15.   Clear plastic anesthetic chamber with 5% isoflurane and oxygen being used to anesthetize a Chilean rose tarantula (*Grammostola rosea*). Spiders are usually anesthetized in about 5 min by this method.

provide analgesia and is not an anesthetic. While the question of invertebrate pain is a topic for debate, it seems wise to err on the cautious side. If hypothermia is used, it should only be for procedures that would be judged nonpainful in vertebrates. Anesthesia is useful for procedures such as sampling of hemolymph, taking oral swabs for microbiological culture, and saline flushing of the oral area to check for Panagrolaimidae nematode infections. Spiders should not be anesthetized when limb autotomy is to be performed, as this is normally a voluntary action by spiders.

Euthanasia

General anesthesia followed by immersion in 70% ethanol (for histopathology) is the best technique for spider euthanasia (Pizzi et al., 2002). Euthanasia by direct immersion in alcohol is not humane; spider motility may persist for several minutes. Some hobbyist literature recommends rapid freezing for euthanasia, but this will compromise tissues for histopathological examination. Some older texts advise crushing the spider, but this is a crude method unsuitable for most reasonably sized tarantulas.

Limb Autotomy as an Amputation Technique

Autotomy is a natural adaptation used by spiders to escape from an aggressor. Spiders also drop their legs when grasped or stung by scorpions, or when stung in a joint by wasps. Limbs may be autotomized if they are trapped in the shed excuvium during ecdysis. Theraphosids do not autotomize their legs as readily as some other spiders. In captivity, the technique is useful for removing severely damaged legs or pedipalps. It may be needed when an appendage is crushed and hemostasis cannot be achieved. In some cases of dysecdysis, inducing autotomy of a limb may be necessary for the spider's survival.

Autotomy is induced by firmly grasping the femur segment of the limb. Grasping more distal limb segments does not usually lead to autotomy. Autotomy is a voluntary act and cannot be performed with an anesthetized spider (Bonnet, 1930). The usual autotomy site is between the coxa and trochanter. A site between the patella and tibia has been reported in nontheraphosid spiders. The pedipalps may be autotomized, but this can affect feeding. Rarely, the spider may autotomize the limb by rapidly jerking the coxa dorsally while the grasped femur retains its position. Normally, one has to snap the femur rapidly upward.

During limb autotomy, the coxal apodeme fractures, and the joint membrane ruptures dorsally under the tension. Only the gracilis muscle traverses the autotomy site, inserting on the trochanter. This generally detaches easily and retracts into the coxa. The remaining muscles insert on thickenings of the joint capsule (*sclerites*). Contraction of these muscles functions to pull the wound edges closed, limiting hemolymph loss.

Should the site continue to hemorrhage, cyanoacrylate tissue adhesive or commercial superglue may be applied. Application of a cyanoacrylate adhesive is recommended to minimize hemolymph loss in all cases of autotomy.

The autotomized limb will usually regenerate during the next ecdysis and return to normal size and appearance after a further two or three ecdyses. The regenerating limb forms in the coxal stump in a highly folded form and is inflated with hemolymph after ecdysis. Lost chelicerae, labia, and spinnerets can also be regenerated. Some species of araneomorph spiders such as *Latrodectus variolus* (northern black widow spider) seem unable to regenerate a completely autotomized leg (Foelix, 1996). Regeneration will not occur in terminal instar males.

Sutures

The data on the use of surgical sutures in spiders are limited. Schultz and Schultz (1998) report some success, but Pizzi and Ezendam (2002) determined sutures to be ineffective in repairing experimental opisthosoma wounds in tarantulas.

Microchipping

Reichling and Tabaka (2001) describe the implantation of passive integrated transponders (microchips) in the opisthosomas of 12 theraphosids. *Aphonopelma baergi*, *Brachypelma albopilosum*, and *Grammostola pulchra* were used in the study. Four spiders were anesthetized with isoflurane before implantation, and eight were not. All appeared unaffected and accepted food within several hours of the procedure. Setae were scraped from the surface of the dorsolateral opisthosoma, and the cuticle was disinfected with 10% povidone–iodine solution. A 20-gauge needle was used to make a small incision rather than a puncture, and the transponder was inserted with sterile mosquito forceps. The wound was closed using *n*-butyl cyanoacrylate tissue adhesive. The authors describe the technique as providing a permanent identification without interfering with ecdysis. The transponder was successfully read up to a depth of 16 cm

in a simulated burrow environment. This is a potentially useful tool in long-term studies of theraphosids under suitable field conditions.

Radiotelemetry

This has been used in studies of male *Aphonopelma hentzi* movement patterns (Janowski-Bell and Horner, 1999). Transmitters were attached to the carapace of adult males with contact adhesive after removal of surface setae. Several transmitters or spiders were lost in the first few days; the method appears suitable only for very brief study periods. The transmitters seemed to affect movement and survival adversely, probably because of the transmitter size.

Examination and Treatment

Clinical Examination

This should be thorough and systematic. Recording a complete history will also assist in reaching a diagnosis. Helpful points include the spider's gender, when ecdysis last occurred, diet and captive care, and duration of captivity.

The initial external examination may be in a clear plastic container or glass jar. A good-quality magnifying glass is essential. In many cases, anesthesia is needed for a thorough examination, as it will help prevent inadvertent trauma to the spider.

The mouth and the area between the chelicerae should be checked for any signs of discharge or Panagrolaimidae infection.

The joint membranes of the legs should be examined for signs of trauma or hemolymph leakage. Special attention should be paid to the base of the limbs, as mites may also be evident. The book-lung openings should be checked for mites or any signs of Acroceridae or Phoridae larvae. The epigyne area in the ventral midline, just caudal to the book lungs, should be examined, as this may help give an indication of gender in adults. The distal pedipalps should be examined for the presence of the palpal organ in adult terminal instar males. Dried excreta around the anal opening may indicate ill-health. The opisthosoma surface should be examined for signs of cuticular abrasion or trauma and loss of symmetry or swelling. The entire cuticle should be checked for signs of fungal growth. This is especially important if fungal growth in the enclosure is reported. Hemolymph may be collected and examined as detailed under postmortem technique in this chapter (Figure 10.16).

Radiography is generally unrewarding because there is very little soft tissue differentiation (Figure 10.17).

Postmortem Examination

Postmortem examination of ill spiders from a collection may be more rewarding than clinical examination of a live spider. Due to rapid autolysis, dead spiders need to be examined immediately. It may be necessary to sacrifice one or more moribund specimens, especially when a number of spiders in a collection are affected.

(1995). This source also includes appendices on husbandry of shrimp, blue crabs, and hermit crabs. Howard et al. (2004) is another good resource.

Diseases of Special Concern

Some crustacean diseases are of special international significance because of their potential effects on susceptible populations and their potential to spread to uninfected areas. The Office International des Epizooties (OIE) ranks several crustacean diseases in one of two categories (OIE, 2003):

Diseases Notifiable to the OIE are of socioeconomic and/or public health importance and are significant in the international trade in aquatic animals and aquatic animal products. Notifiable crustacean diseases, the type of microbe, and their hosts include Taura syndrome (viral/penaeid shrimp), white spot disease (viral/penaeid shrimp and other decapod crustaceans), and yellowhead disease (viral/penaeid shrimp).

Other Significant Diseases are diseases that have not been included on the notifiable list for one of several possible reasons but still are of current or potential international significance in aquaculture. These include tetrahedral baculovirosis (*Baculovirus penaei*) (viral/penaeid shrimp), spherical baculovirosis (monodon baculovirus) (viral/penaeid shrimp), infectious hypodermal and hematopoietic necrosis (viral/penaeid shrimp), spawner-isolated mortality virus disease (viral/penaeid shrimp), and crayfish plague (*Aphanomyces astaci*) (water mold/freshwater crayfish).

Management of Crustacean Diseases

The great majority of research into managing crustacean diseases has focused on shrimp. Proper management is a critical key to successful control of crustacean diseases in aquaculture. This includes all of the standard methods that would be used in a well-managed farm operation, such as reducing potential sources of contamination by controlling the movement of stock onto the farm with quarantine and testing for specific path-

ogens. Maintaining proper sanitation, such as by disinfection of utensils, footwear, and so on, is advisable. Potential fecal contamination of eggs should be avoided to prevent vertical transmission of pathogens. Segregating various life stages (larvae, juveniles, and broodstock) is advisable.

Other measures to control disease are focused on the reduction or mitigation of stress and include reducing stocking density. There is also considerable ongoing work in the development of specific pathogen-resistant (SPR) stocks. A number of immunostimulants, such as beta-glucans, are used widely to attempt to enhance disease resistance. Probiotics (use of beneficial bacteria to exclude potential pathogens) are also used, especially in hatcheries, where bacterial infections can be especially serious.

Also important is avoidance and quarantine. Unfortunately, failure to adhere to this policy has led to the inadvertent spread of a number of important diseases that have caused major losses in crustacean populations around the world. Disease control is also hampered by a lack of understanding of even the most basic epidemiology (e.g., transmission, hosts, and life cycle) of many diseases.

Analgesia, Anesthesia, and Surgery

The presence of a hard exoskeleton and an open circulatory system makes crustacean survival of major surgery difficult. However, it may be desirable to anesthetize crustaceans for other reasons, for example, for experimental procedures that the animals will not survive, for minor surgical procedures, to prevent stress during shipping or handling, or for sedation prior to euthanasia. Examples of anesthetic agents used in crustaceans are listed in Table 12.2.

Analgesia has not been widely used or investigated in crustaceans. However, since crustaceans can and do respond to noxious stimuli (e.g., by dropping appendages), they should be given the benefit of the doubt when considering anesthesia or analgesia for potentially painful procedures. Anesthetized or sedated crustaceans should never be placed back into their holding tank with unanesthetized tank mates.

Table 12.2. Anesthetics used in crustaceans

Agent	Dose	Comments
Aqui-S[a]	0.125–1.0 mL/L	Bath, induction time 20–70 min in *Pseudocarcinus* (Gardner, 1997)
Chloroform	1.25–2.5 mL/L	Bath, duration 60 min in *Pseudocarcinus* (Gardner, 1997)
Clove oil	0.03–1 mL/L	Bath, long induction time (>85 min) in *Pseudocarcinus* (Gardner, 1997)
Halothane	0.5% by volume	Anesthetizes freshwater crayfish within 15 min (Ingle, 1995)
Isobutanol (100%)	0.5–0.2 μL/10 g	Injected into abdominal sinus in *Homarus*, mortality seen at the higher doses (Gilgan and Burns, 1976)
Ketamine HCl	0.025–0.1 mg/kg	Anesthesia within 15–45 s in *Pseudocarcinus*, can cause rigidity (Gardner, 1997)
	90 μg/g IM[b]	Duration 1 h or less in *Orconectes* (Brown et al., 1996)
Lidocaine HCl	30 μg/g IM	Injected intrathoracically in *Orconectes*, duration 25 min (Brown et al., 1996)
Procaine HCl	25 mg/kg	Anesthesia within 20–30 s, duration 2–3 h, short phase (10 s) of excitement in *Cancer* and *Carcinus* (Oswald, 1977)
Xylazine HCl	70 mg/kg	Anesthesia within 5–6 min in *Cancer* and *Carcinus*, duration 45 min (Oswald, 1977)
	16–22 mg/kg	Anesthesia within 2–3 min in *Pseudocarcinus* (Gardner, 1997)

[a]The active ingredient is iso-eugenol.
[b]IM, intramuscular.

Table 12.3. Drugs used to treat disease in penaeid shrimps

Drug	Dosage[a]	Comments
Benzalkonium chloride	0.6–1.0 ppm, 1 day	Antimicrobial
Chloramphenicol	1–10 ppm, 1 day	Antibiotic[b]
Copper sulfate	0.5–1.0 ppm, 10–12 h	Protozoicide
Formalin	25–30 ppm, 1 day	External parasiticide
Furacin[c]	1–2 ppm	Antibiotic
Furanace[d]	1–2 ppm	Antibiotic
Furazolidone	10–20 ppm, 1 day	Antibiotic
Malachite green	0.5–0.8 ppm, 1 day	Antifungal[b]
Methylene blue	8–10 ppm, 1 day	Antifungal
Oxytetracycline	40–60 ppm, 1 day	Antibiotic
Potassium permanganate	25–30 ppm, 30–60 min	External parasiticide
Romet-30[e]	50–100 mg/kg, 14 days	Antibiotic, administered in feed
Treflan[f]	0.01–0.1 ppm	To treat larval mycosis
Zeolite	100–120 kg/m^2	Applied to environment to inhibit the growth of protozoans

[a]ppm, parts per million.
[b]Not legal for use in U.S. food animals, nor for imports into the U.S.
[c]Nitrofurazone
[d]Nifurpirinol
[e]Ormetoprim–sulfamethoxazole.
[f]Trifluralin

The anesthetic tricaine methanesulfonate (Finquel [Argent, Redmond, WA)] and Tricaine-S [Western Chemical, Ferndale, WA]), is approved for use in aquatic animals not intended for food but is not particularly effective in many crustaceans (Oswald, 1977; Brown et al., 1996; Gardner, 1997). The following agents have also been shown to be ineffective or detrimental to various crustacean species: benzocaine, tubocurarine, gallamine, and chlorpromazine (Oswald, 1977); and carbon dioxide, 2-phenoxy ethanol, and magnesium chloride (Gardner, 1997). In addition, chilling may be effective for immobilizing warm-water species but should be used only for handling, not for painful procedures.

Treatments and Formulary

Drugs used in aquaculture species in the United States are highly regulated by the Food and Drug Administration (FDA). Currently, the only drug that is approved for use in a crustacean species intended for food is oxytetracycline for use in lobsters with gaffkemia (1 g/lb of medicated feed for 5 days). Use of chemotherapeutics in crustaceans not intended for food can be prescribed for extra-label usage by licensed veterinarians, but the user must be absolutely certain that the animals will not end up in the food chain. Table 12.3 is a compilation of drugs used in penaeid shrimp taken from publications by Brock and Main (1994) and Fulks and Main (1992).

References

Anderson DT. 1985. Embryology. In: Bliss DE, ed. The Biology of the Crustacea, volume 2: Embryology, Morphology, and Genetics. Academic, New York, pp 1–36.

Austin B and Austin DA, eds. 1989. Methods for the Microbiological Examination of Fish and Shellfish. Ellis Horwood, Chichester, England, 317 pp.

Battison A, MacMillan R, MacKenzie A, Rose P, Cawthorn R, and Horney B. 2000. Use of injectable potassium chloride for euthanasia of American lobsters (Homarus americanus). Comp Med 50:545–550.

Brock JA and Lightner DV. 1990. Diseases of crustaceans: Diseases caused by microorganisms. In: Kinne O, ed. Diseases of Marine Animals, volume 3: Cephalopoda, Annelida, Crustacea, Chaetognatha, Echinodermata, Urochordata. Biologische Anstalt Helgoland, Hamburg, Germany, pp 245–349.

Brock JA and Main KL. 1994. A Guide to the Common Problems and Diseases of Cultured Penaeus vannamei. Oceanic Institute, Honolulu.

Brown PH, White MR, Chaille J, Russel M, and Oseto C. 1996. Evaluation of three anesthetic agents for crayfish (Orconectes virilis). J Shellfish Res 15:433–435.

De Vosjoli P. 1999. Care of Land Hermit Crabs. BowTie, Irvine, CA, 32 pp.

Edgerton BF, Evans LH, Stephens FJ, and Overstreet RM. 2002. Synopsis of freshwater crayfish diseases and commensal organisms. Aquaculture 206:57–135.

FAO (Food and Agricultural Organization of the United Nations). 2000. http://www.fao.org/waicent/faoinfo/fishery/statist/fisoft/fish-plus.htm.

FAO (Food and Agricultural Organization of the United Nations). 2004. Aquaculture Production: Quantities 1950–2002, version 2.30. (Fishstat Plus: Universal Software for Fishery Statistical Time Series.) FAO Fisheries Department, Fishery Information, Data and Statistics Unit.

Fox S. 2000. Hermit Crabs. Barron's Educational Series, Hauppauge, NY, 64 pp.

Fulks W and Main KL, eds. 1992. Diseases of Cultured Penaeid Shrimp in Asia and the United States. Oceanic Institute, Honolulu.

Gardner C. 1997. Options for humanely immobilizing and killing crabs. J Shellfish Res 16:19–224.

Gilgan MW and Burns BG. 1976. The anesthesia of the lobster (*Homarus americanus*) by isobutanol injection. Can J Zool 54:1231–1234.

Howard DW, Lewis EJ, Keller BJ, and Smith CS. 2004. Histological Techniques for Marine Bivalves and Crustaceans. NOAA Tech Memo NOS NCCOS5, 218 pp.

Ingle RW. 1995. The UFAW Handbook on the Care and Management of Decapod Crustaceans in Captivity. Universities Federation for Animal Welfare, Potters Bar, England.

Lightner DV. 1983. Diseases of cultured penaeid shrimp. In: Moore JR, ed. Handbook of Mariculture, volume 1: Crustacean Aquaculture. CRC, Boca Raton, FL, pp 289–371.

Lightner DV, ed. 1996. A Handbook of Shrimp Pathology and Diagnostic Procedures for Diseases of Cultured Penaeid Shrimp [looseleaf]. World Aquaculture Society, Baton Rouge, LA.

Lightner DV. 2000. DNA-based diagnostic and detection methods for penaeid shrimp viral diseases. FAO Fisheries Technical Paper no. 395, pp 38–44.

Lightner DV and Redman RM. 1998. Shrimp diseases and current diagnostic methods. Aquaculture 164:201–220.

Meyers TR. 1990. Diseases of crustaceans: Diseases caused by protistans and metazoans. In: Kinne O, ed. Diseases of Marine Animals, volume 3: Cephalopoda, Annelida, Crustacea, Chaetognatha, Echinodermata, Urochordata. Biologische Anstalt Helgoland, Hamburg, pp 350–389.

Messick GA and Shields JD. 2000. Epizootiology of the parasitic dinoflagellate *Hematodinium* sp. in the American blue crab *Callinectes sapidus*. Dis Aquat Org 43:139–152.

Murthy HS. 1998. Freshwater prawn culture in India. Inofish Int 5:30–36.

New MB. 2000. History and global status of freshwater prawn farming. In: New MB and Valenti WC, eds. Freshwater Prawn Culture: The Farming of *Macrobrachium rosenbergii*. Blackwell Science, Oxford, UK, pp 1–11.

New MB, Singholka S, and Kutty MN. 2000. Prawn capture fisheries and enhancement. In: New MB and Valenti WC, eds. Freshwater Prawn Culture: The Farming of *Macrobrachium rosenbergii*. Blackwell Science, Oxford, UK, pp 411–428.

Noga EJ. 2000a. Fish Disease. Iowa State University Press, Ames.

Noga EJ. 2000b. Fungal diseases. In: Stickney R, ed. Encyclopedia of Aquaculture. John Wiley and Sons, New York, pp 397–401.

Noga EJ. 2000c. Hemolymph biomarkers of crustacean health. In: Fingerman M and Nagabhushanam R, eds. Recent Advances in Marine Biotechnology, volume 5: Immunobiology and Pathology. Science, Enfield, NH, pp 125–163.

Noga EJ, Sawyer TK, and Rodon-Naveira M. 1998. Disease processes and health assessment in blue crab fishery management. J Shellfish Res 17:567–577.

Noga EJ, Smolowitz R, and Khoo L. 2000. Pathology of shell disease in the blue crab, *Callinectes sapidus*. J Fish Dis 23:389–399.

Office International des Epizooties (OIE). 2003. Manual of Diagnostic Tests for Aquatic Animals, 4th edition. OIE, Paris.

Oswald RL. 1977. Immobilization of decapod crustacea for experimental procedures. J Mar Biol Assoc UK 57:715–721.

Prosser CL, ed. 1991. Comparative Animal Physiology, volume 1: Environmental and Metabolic Animal Physiology, 4th edition. Wiley-Liss, New York, 578 pp.

Rosenberry R. 1999. World Shrimp Farming 1999. Shrimp News International [San Diego] 12:320 pp.

Rosemark R and Conklin DE. 1983. Lobster pathology and treatments. In: Moore JR, ed. Handbook of Mariculture, volume 1: Crustacean Aquaculture. CRC, Boca Raton, FL, pp 289–371.

Ruppert EE, Fox RS, and Barnes RD. 2004. Invertebrate Zoology: A Functional Evolutionary Approach, 7th edition. Thompson-Brooks/Cole, Belmont, CA, 963 pp.

Shields JD. 1994. The parasitic dinoflagellates of marine crustaceans. In: Faisal M and Hetrick FM, eds. Annual Review of Fish Diseases. Elsevier Science, New York, pp 241–271.

Sindermann CJ. 1989. The shell disease syndrome in marine crustaceans. NOAA Tech Memo no. NMFS/NEC-64, 43 pp.

Smolowitz RM, Bullis RA, and Abt DA. 1992a. Mycotic branchitis in laboratory-maintained hermit crabs *Pagurus* spp. J Crustacean Biol 12:161–168.

Smolowitz RM, Bullis RA, and Abt DA. 1992b. Pathologic cuticular changes of winter impoundment shell disease preceding and during intermolt in the American lobster, *Homarus americanus*. Biol Bull 183:99–112.

Smolowitz RM, Bullis RA, Abt DA, and Leibovitz L. 1993. Pathologic observations on the infection of *Pagurus* spp. by plerocercoids of *Calliobothrium verticillatum* (Rudolphi, 1819; Van Benden, 1850). J Invertebr Pathol 62:185–190.

Sparks AK. 1985. Synopsis of Invertebrate Pathology. Elsevier, New York, 423 pp.

Stolen JS, Fletcher TC, Smith, SA, Zelikoff JT, Kaattari SL, Anderson RS, Soderhall K, and Weeks-Perkins BA. 1995. Techniques in Fish Immunology. (Fish Immunology Communications 4 [FITC 4].) SOS, Fair Haven, NJ, 258 pp plus appendices.

TFH Publications. 2003. Quick and Easy Hermit Crab Care. TFH, Neptune, NJ, 64 pp.

Waterman TH and Chase FA. 1960. General crustacean biology. In: Waterman TH, ed. The Physiology of Crustacea, volume 1: Metabolism and Growth. Academic, New York, pp 1–30.

Wickins JF and Lee DO. 2002. Crustacean Farming Ranching and Culture, 2nd edition. Blackwell Science, Oxford, UK, 446 pp.

Chapter 13

MYRIAPODS (CENTIPEDES AND MILLIPEDES)

John R. Chitty

Natural History and Taxonomy

As suggested by the name, myriapods are distinguished from other arthropods by having many legs attached to multiple body segments.

The group is divided into four classes (Buchsbaum et al., 1987; Read and Lewis, 2002):

A. Chilopoda: The centipedes, which have one pair of legs per segment. Over 3000 species are described in five orders (Read and Lewis, 2002):

1. Geophilomorpha: Long, threadlike soil-dwelling burrowers with 27–191 leg pairs.
2. Scolopendromorpha: Flattened burrowers/crevice dwellers that can be extremely large (16–20 cm), with 21–23 leg pairs.
3. Craterostigmomorpha: Flattened crevice dwellers with 15 leg pairs.
4. Lithobiomorpha: Flattened crevice dwellers with 15 leg pairs.
5. Scutigeromorpha: Found in varied habitats, have 15 pairs of long legs and jointed antennae, and can move very fast.

These are found worldwide, with the exception of the craterostigmomorphids (restricted to New Zealand and Tasmania) and the scolopendrids (tropics). Many (typically scolopendrids and lithobiomorphs) are maintained in captivity. Speciation is rarely accurate, although examples include

Scutigera coleopteran: scutigerid
Scolopendra heros (the giant desert centipede): scolopendrid
Copris texanum: scolopendrid

B. Diplopoda: The millipedes, which have two pairs of legs per segment. There are two subclasses of millipedes (Mazer, 1996):

1. Chilognatha: These have a calcified cuticle. Most genera are included in this subclass, including the most common species kept in captivity.
2. Penicillata: These bristly millipedes are characterized by an uncalcified cuticle.

Although over 8000 millipede species have been described, relatively few are regularly maintained in captivity. These tend to be the larger species that are found in tropical rain forest in South America, Asia, and Africa. Most are classified within the orders Spirostreptida and Spirobolida (Murphy, 1985). It is extremely difficult to speciate many of these millipedes accurately, so the identities of many are unknown. This may be a factor in mortality rates, although it is fair to presume that the husbandry needs of these species are very similar. Some examples of captive species are

Isulus spp.: African banded millipede
Aphistogoniulus spp.: Madagascar fire millipede
Spirostreptida spp.: Giant train millipedes
Unknown species: Many unidentified species are commonly advertised and are generally referred to by their common names (e.g., giant train millipede, giant chocolate millipede, African red-legged millipede, and African olive millipede).

C. Symphala: Small eyeless herbivores
D. Pauropoda: Small scavengers

The latter two classes are characterized by one pair of legs per body segment and are rarely kept in captivity.

Anatomy and Physiology

Millipedes

Millipedes live in and burrow in leaf litter and rotting organic matter; most are herbivorous. They generally feed on rotting matter as the action of bacteria and fungi may make nutrients more available. In this role they are very important recyclers of nutrients. Some species will eat live shoots/roots, whereas others have sucking mouthparts that can be inserted into plants. These species may be important agricultural pests. Some species are carnivorous or feed on carrion.

Despite the name, millipedes belonging to the orders Spirostreptida and Spirobolida do not have a thousand legs. The highest number recorded is 752. Most actually have around a hundred (Buchsbaum et al., 1987).

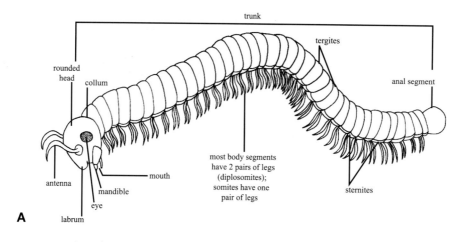

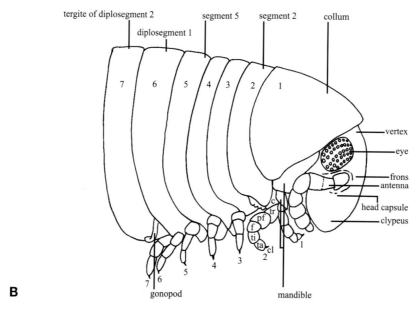

Figure 13.1.   Millipede external anatomy. **A.** Schematic body plan. Reproduced from EnchangedLearning.com by Alison Schroeer. **B.** Head and anterior trunk of a male *Narceus americanus* from North Carolina. *c,* coax; *cl,* claw; *f,* femur, *pf,* prefemur; *ta,* tarsus; *ti,* tibia; and *tr,* trochanter. Reproduced from Richard Fox, Lander University, by Alison Schroeer.

Like the centipedes, each leg represents a body segment. However, during development, the segments fuse in pairs, resulting in two pairs of legs per body ring or *diplosegment*. The fusion of these segments into narrow rings shortens the body and strengthens it for burrowing (Buchsbaum et al., 1987). Not all body rings have two pairs of legs. The first three have only one pair, and the last few pairs lack legs (Figure 13.1). These latter body rings, located between the last leg-bearing segment and the pre-anal ring, are termed *apodous* and are formed at successive molts. The age of an individual can be approximated by counting the apodous segments.

The multiple pairs of legs enable a high power output for burrowing, and the power output is directly linked to the number of legs involved. Their locomotion requires a high degree of coordination resulting in a metachronal wave of movement; each pair is in phase, but consecutive legs on the same side are slightly out of phase. The result is an interesting ripple effect.

Millipedes have two pairs of mouthparts: mandibles and first maxillae. The gnathal lobe of the mandible is responsible for biting and grinding (Enghoff, 1979). The body is strengthened by a calcified exoskeleton (Mazer, 1996), which is formed in three layers: epicuticle, exocuticle, and endocuticle.

Millipedes are sexually dimorphic. In males, the legs on the seventh body ring are replaced by a pair of sperm-transfer organs named *goniopods*. Thus, the presence of legs on the seventh body ring denotes a female or immature male.

Reproduction occurs with the male and female coiled round each other. This enables males to pass sperm into the vulva of the female via the gonopods. The female will lay clutches of eggs a few weeks later, at which time the eggs are fertilized by the stored spermatozoa. The eggs are generally laid just under the substrate surface and hatch within 3 months (Mazer, 1996).

Growth occurs via a succession of molts. The first few stages (stadia) are equivalent to the instar stages of insects. During the first two stadia the millipede is blind and does not eat. With each molt the number of segments increases as does the number of defense glands (Hopkin and Read, 1992). Millipedes molt throughout their lives until reaching sexual maturity, which may take several years in the larger species. Prior to molting the exoskeleton will become dull, and the millipede may lay coiled on its side for a couple of days. After molting the millipede will eat the shed excuvia (Mazer, 1996).

Centipedes

Most centipedes are similarly adapted to burrowing and living in leaf litter. Many dwell in rock crevices. The scutigerids live in a wide variety of habitats and move quickly over substrates. Unlike the other myriapods, centipedes are primarily carnivorous but may consume carrion. They generally feed on invertebrate prey, but the scolopendrids can take small vertebrates. Most ingest by chewing prey, though some geophilomorphs are suctorial feeders.

Although there are similarities in basic body shape to millipedes, there are also many important differences (Figure 13.2):

1. The body is flattened dorsoventrally and considerably more flexible than the millipede's. There is only one pair of legs

per body segment; this enables fast movement as opposed to power. The centipede's gait reflects this speedy locomotion; relatively few of the legs are in contact with the ground at any given moment. The leg movements are out of phase on each side resulting in side-to-side undulations of the body. In scutigerids, the last pair of legs is long (often double the length of the first pair), and these will step over the more cranial limbs as they move.

2. The front pair of legs is adapted to form hollow poison claws or *forcipules*, which are used to seize and perforate prey. Venom is then injected into the prey from attached glands.

3. Centipedes lack a waxy cuticle and calcified exoskeleton.

4. Like millipedes, most centipedes lack or have only simple eyes (ocelli). These (or the cuticle when eyes are not present) detect only light and shade, facilitating the photophobic response (Read and Lewis, 2002). In these species food is located via chemical and tactile receptors on the mouthparts. The surface-dwelling scutigerids, by contrast, have complex eyes.

5. Courtship rituals tend to be more complex in centipedes but there is less contact between the sexes. Courtship often involves tapping with the antennae. A spermatophore is then deposited on a web (except for scutigerids) and is picked up by the female. Some species (lithobiomorphs and scutigerids) lay single eggs in the soil. These contain a rich yolk to nutrify the juvenile

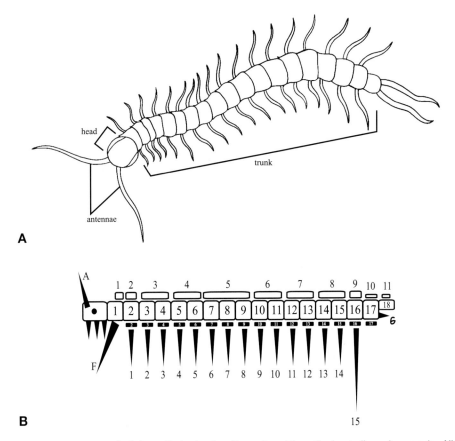

Figure 13.2.   Centipede external anatomy. **A.** Schematic body plan. Reproduced from EnchantedLearning.com by Alison Schroeer. **B.** Side-view diagram of the house centipede, *Scutigera* sp., showing correspondence of appendages, segments, and sclerites. Appendages, *solid triangles*; segments, *heavy-walled rectangles*; tergites, *thin-walled rectangles*; and sternites, *solid rectangles*. *A*, antenna; *F*, forcipule; and *G*, gonopod. Segments, tergites, sternites, and appendages are *numbered*. Reproduced from Richard Fox, Lander University, by Alison Schroeer.

until it can fend for itself. Other species may brood the eggs and guard the young until they are capable of hunting. Scolopendrids have been observed licking eggs to remove mold growths (Murphy, 1985). There is evidence that scolopendrids can reproduce via parthenogenesis (McCowan and Fanney, 1999).

6. There are also differences in growth and development. Lithobiomorphs and scutigerids hatch with less than the full number of legs. The number of legs increases with each molt up to full size. There may be further molts once full size has been attained. Geophilomorph and scolopendrid larvae hatch with the full number of legs but are immobile until after several molts. These continue until they reach maturity after a year or two. The immature stages cannot hunt and fend for themselves; the mother may guard the brood during this period. It has been suggested that the female *Scolopendra gigantea* may sacrifice herself to act as food for her brood (Spencer et al., 1999).

7. Centipedes are not sexually dimorphic; it is nearly impossible to differentiate the sexes safely as they must be persuaded to extend the genital region to do so. The adult female scolopendrid is probably larger than the male (Spencer et al., 1999).

Environmental Disorders and Preventive Medicine

As with most invertebrates, the majority of clinical conditions seen will be due to husbandry problems. It follows that the best preventive medicine is to provide a good environment with proper husbandry. Preventive medicine also involves stock selection and introduction. An overtly unhealthy animal should not be purchased and certainly should not be added to existing stock.

A 4-week quarantine period is advised, even when the new animal is considered to be healthy. During quarantine the animal(s) can be checked for parasites, weighed weekly, and observed for normal feeding behavior. Several other important points regarding mixing of animals include

1. Do not mix stocks of greatly differing ages/life stages. There may be different age-related disease susceptibilities/immunity. Similarly, there may be physical incompatibilities.

2. Do not mix different species unless they are known to be compatible. This can be difficult as many of the myriapods are not accurately identified in the first place. There may also be differences in husbandry needs between different species, but these are likely to be minor.

3. Keep centipedes alone unless uniting individuals for breeding (and even this may end in failure). Centipedes are solitary hunters, and, no matter how many are kept together, the eventual confined population will number one animal.

Husbandry

Millipedes

As mentioned earlier, these are burrowing creatures adapted to living in soil and leaf litter. A plastic or glass tank is ideal, and

heat is essential as the species kept are generally tropical. Heat is best provided by using a heating source placed at one end of the tank to create a thermal gradient. Heating pads may be buried in the substrate or taped to the side of the tank (animals will spend most of their time beneath the surface of the substrate, so heating above the substrate is unnecessary). An ideal temperature range is 20°–25°C. Heating via a bulb is not recommended as these species are photophobic. A light source is not required, and the enclosure is best kept in a dimly lit area. Terraria should have a tight-fitting lid. Millipedes are not climbers but are immensely strong (hence the alternative name of *rammers*). They are quite capable of pushing off a loose-fitting cover if the tank is knocked over or the litter is high enough for the animal to reach the top. A solid lid is also required in order to maintain humidity.

The substrate should consist of 8–10 cm of soil or peat moss with a 3–4 cm of leaf litter above this. Leaf litter may be collected from the garden, but it is important to examine for potential predators (e.g., spiders or centipedes). Litter should be changed every 2–3 months to reduce buildup of microorganisms and fungi. This should be done with great care in case the millipedes have bred. The level of humidity should be maintained so the soil and litter are damp but there are no pools of water.

Millipedes are often kept in zoos as part of a mixed invertebrate exhibit (e.g., with certain beetles) since they are herbivorous, nonaggressive creatures (Murphy, 1985; Mazer, 1996; Cheeseman, 2000).

Centipedes

Centipedes are more difficult to maintain than millipedes. They move extremely fast and, being flat dorsoventrally, can escape from all but the most secure units. They are prone to dehydration as they lack protective layers in the cuticle; their breathing spiracles cannot be closed. They also have the typical wet feces of a carnivore. These factors lead to difficulty in controlling water loss; they must be kept in very humid surroundings. A humidity level of 80%–90% is typically required (Murphy, 1985; Wismann, 1997; Spencer et al., 1999). This should be provided throughout the vivarium for jungle species. Species from arid areas may require a humidity gradient, though part of the vivarium must be at 80%–90% humidity (Murphy, 1985; Frye, 1992). If in doubt, keep it damp! They should therefore be kept in large glass or plastic tanks with tight-fitting lids. Small air holes should be made but care must be taken to maintain humidity levels. A layer of soil or peat should be placed on the base and covered with either damp forest mulch, vermiculite, or ample leaf litter. Sand should not be used as it may result in scoring of the delicate epicuticle (Wismann, 1997). Soil must be carefully sieved to remove abrasive elements. Some species will climb but this should not be encouraged as it may facilitate escape. Most species prefer to burrow. For the surface-living Scutigerids or for crevice dwelling species, bark may be provided. Rocks, though aesthetically pleasing, may cause damage (through blunt trauma or rough contact) to centipedes. Disturbed centipedes may thrash against rocks or stones (Wismann, 1997).

Most species are photophobic and so should be kept in dimly lit surroundings. However, scutigerids do not resent light and have complex eyes, so a light source should be provided with a 12-h light/12-h dark cycle. Humidity is provided by spraying the substrate daily and giving a thorough soaking weekly (Spencer et al., 1999).

Temperature is important, with temperate species being kept at 20°–25°C. Tropical species should be kept at 25°–28°C. Substrate temperature should be maintained at approximately 20°–23°C. Heat should be provided by means of a heating pad, which may be placed under the surface for burrowers or taped to the outside of tank for the surface-living species. The use of heat lamps should be avoided.

Some temperate species may hibernate. Wismann (1997) hibernated a *Scolopendra heros* specimen by using techniques and conditions for snakes. The centipede remained active most of the time but did not feed or lose weight. On rewarming, the centipede resumed feeding within a week.

Scolopendromorphs are extremely hard to maintain in captivity, with few specimens surviving longer than 18 months (though some achieve life spans of up to 5 years [Wismann, 1997]). Beginners should start with the hardier lithobiomorph species before moving on to the scolopendrids (Murphy, 1985).

Nutrition

Millipedes

Most captive species are herbivorous. Although they consume the leaf litter in which they are kept, other fruits and vegetables should be provided. Potatoes appear to be a favorite. Only organically grown foods should be used as many of the commercially used pesticides may harm millipedes and residues may be found in fruit and vegetables. Fish food flakes or tablets and dry poultry mash may also be provided (Frye, 1992). Uneaten food should be removed after a few days.

A calcium source should be provided for growing specimens. This may take the form of high-calcium dark green leaves or a calcium–vitamin D_3 supplement (e.g., Nutrobal; Vetark, Winchester, U.K.). Alternatively, a small piece of sterilized cuttlebone may be buried in the substrate.

A shallow water dish should be provided and care should be taken that the millipede is able to escape should it fall in.

Centipedes

The abiding image of the centipede is that of a voracious hunter, although many of the species maintained in captivity are primarily carrion feeders. Wismann (1997) reports observing wild *Scolopendra heros* feeding on road kill.

Centipedes should be fed a mix of live and dead invertebrates and, if large enough, dead pinky mice, day-old chicks, or adult mice. Wismann (1997) advises that dead prey should be opened or crushed so the internal organs are extruded. This may be necessary to stimulate feeding. Spencer et al. (1999) suggest that *Scolopendra gigantea* is happy to open the skin of a dead mouse by itself.

Both references agree that captive scolopendrids do best if given a varied diet. An *S. gigantea* specimen kept by McCowan

and Fanney (1999) thrived on a simple diet of a dozen live crickets fed weekly with one dead week-old pinky given every 2 weeks.

Most sources recommend feeding on a weekly basis.

Like millipedes, they should be given a shallow dish of water where escape is possible if necessary.

Disinfection

This is an important area for all captive invertebrates. Myriapod enclosures should be completely emptied, cleaned, and disinfected annually. Disinfection using a quaternary ammonium compound appears safe, and F10 (Health & Hygiene, Johannesburg, South Africa) has been used safely in millipede enclosures.

The vivarium should be thoroughly disinfected between batches. A 10% sodium hypochlorite solution is effective; the enclosure should be thoroughly washed out before restocking.

Millipede eggs may be disinfected when transferred between enclosures. The procedure described by Rivers and published in the article by Cooper (1980) is effective:

1. Remove eggs from substrate with 0.1% sodium hypochlorite.
2. Rinse in water.
3. Immerse in 10% formaldehyde for 40 min.
4. Thoroughly wash and ventilate.

Handling

Millipedes

Millipedes are straightforward to handle, as they move slowly and are not aggressive. Their first course of action when threatened is to roll into a tight ball. This makes them easy to pick up and transport but does not facilitate examination. As attempting to unwind the millipede can injure the animal, it is recommended that a thorough clinical examination is performed with the creature under anesthesia (see the section Anesthesia, Analgesia, and Surgery).

Millipedes can, however, exude noxious substances from glands found on each diplosegment. Some species can squirt these compounds 25 cm. Various substances are found in these secretions, including benzoquinones, aldehydes, and hydrocyanic acid. On human skin the effects range from staining to irritation and blistering. The effects can be severe if the substance is squirted into or transferred to the eye. Therapy consists of immediate washing, followed by application of topical antibiotic/steroid ointments (Radford, 1975; Hudson and Parsons, 1997). It is important to wear latex gloves when handling millipedes and to be careful not to transfer secretions to mucous membranes. One should wear goggles if unsure whether a species can squirt.

Centipedes

By contrast, centipedes are extremely hard to handle, and it must be stressed that the larger species, especially the scolopendrids, should never be handled manually. These species are venomous, and some are quite aggressive. Care must be taken not to be bitten. Centipede venom contains many substances, including 5-hydroxytryptamine and cytolysins. Although death from envenomation is rare, there may be severe pain and localized swelling, lymphadenopathy, headaches, palpitations, and nausea. Localized tissue necrosis may occur around the bite. Therapy consists of pain management, systemic analgesics, and local anesthesia around the bite site (Bush et al., 2001; Norris, 2002).

Some species, including *Otostigmus* spp., can exude substances from glands on each segment (Norris, 2002), so even smaller species should be handled with care and only while wearing latex gloves.

When hazardous centipedes are kept in a collection there should be written protocols and risk assessments for dealing with these species.

Centipedes can also be injured by catching and handling. The cuticle is extremely thin, and the cuticle and/or internal organs can be easily injured by handling. Centipedes are inclined to thrash around during capture, thus harming themselves. It is recommended that any detailed examination be performed with the creature under general anesthesia. A reasonable external examination may be performed by capturing the animal within a clear tube as with some venomous snakes (Figure 13.3).

Infectious Diseases

Viruses

There appear to be no descriptions of viral problems in the literature. This is most likely because virology has not been performed in disease outbreaks.

Bacteria and Fungi

There have been extensive studies of the aerobic gut flora of the millipede as this is an important component of its digestive processes and hence important in the biology of leaf-litter decomposition. Gebhart et al. (2002) isolated *Bacillus* spp. from various compartments of the gut, whereas Oravecz et al. (2002) isolated many species from the feces of a healthy African spirostreptid millipede. These isolates included *Arthrobacter, Micrococcus, Leifsonia, Curtobacterium, Cellulomonas, Dietzia, Nocardia, Rhodococcus, Streptomyces,* and *Geodermatophilus* species, and *Promicromonospora enterophila* and *Stenotrophomonas maltophilia.* This is a very wide range of species, many of which are found in the environment. The gut flora of centipedes has not received such attention but is likely to be much simpler as it is a carnivore.

Bacterial and fungal infections occur frequently and are usually opportunistic secondary infections involving environmental organisms. A typical problem is described by Swanson and McCowan (1999). In this report a systemic *Pseudomonas* spp. with involvement of two fungal species, *Rhizomucor* sp. and *Blastoschizomyces capitatus,* resulted in a necrotizing cellulitis and lymphatic thrombosis in a centipede and its death. General symptoms of this type of infection include

Centipedes. Discoloration of the skin, especially head and limbs. Affected areas may eventually turn black. Also occurring are lethargy and a reluctance to feed.

Millipedes. Softening and discoloration of the exoskeleton, lethargy, and reduced feeding.

Causes include inappropriate husbandry (in particular, excessive humidity in centipede vivaria) and cutaneous damage (especially linked to mites in centipedes, although mites may actually reduce the likelihood of these infections in millipedes [see the section Anesthesia, Analgesia, and Surgery).

For a full description of the investigation of bacterial and fungal infections in invertebrates, see Williams (1999).

Parasites

Endoparasites

Frye (1992) reports finding rhabditiform nematodes (morphologically indistinguishable from *Strongyloides stercoralis*) and protozoa in the feces of healthy millipedes. These may be capable of causing disease.

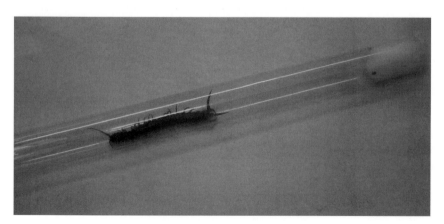

Figure 13.3. Centipede being examined in clear plastic snake-handling tube that is plugged at either end with cotton wool. If required, anesthetic gases may be piped in.

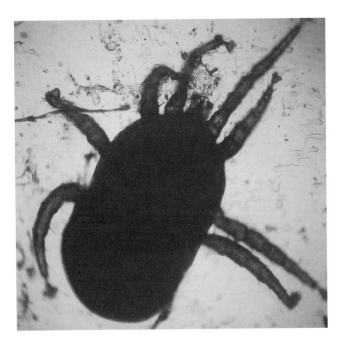

Figure 13.4. Adult mite from a giant train millipede. This is likely to be a commensal mite. Although many were observed on this millipede, there was no associated pathology.

Ectoparasites

These are extremely common in millipedes where many white mobile mites may be seen running over a millipede (Figure 13.4). They do not appear to be a problem, and it has been suggested they may benefit millipedes by consuming organic matter, bacteria, and fungi that accumulate between plates or in leg articulations (Tollefsrud, 1995). Some mites are members of the suborder Astigmata and the form seen may be nonfeeding deutonymphs using the millipede as a dispersal vehicle (Behan-Pelletier, 2001; communication via the Myriapod e-mail discussion group). The likely nonpathogenicity of these mites coupled with the likelihood of harming the millipede by using chemicals contraindicates treatment.

There are reports that these mites may be harmful or irritating (millipedes may be observed rubbing themselves) in excessive numbers and that there may be other, more harmful species (these have been reported as appearing like fixed clusters of grey mites). In these cases therapy may consist of one of the following options that have been developed by millipede keepers:

1. Washing the millipede under a steady stream of warm water.
2. Washing the millipede as above and then coating with flour and placing on a porous screen. Coated mites will fall off and through the screen. After an hour rinse off the millipede.
3. Housing the millipedes with terrestrial isopods that will eat the mites (they can also eat millipede eggs).

Any of the aforementioned methods should be combined with a complete environment change (with all organic material disposed of) in the event of a clinical problem. To reduce the environmental mite load, new substrate may be microwaved before placing in the vivarium (A. Goodwin, 2001; communication via the Myriapod e-mail discussion group).

External parasites appear to be less common in centipedes but often clinically significant. This may be due to their thinner cuticle or because they lack commensal mites that may help control environmental species.

Both mites and nematodes have been described on centipedes and associated with loss of limbs. In these cases the centipede was likely debilitated as they are known to regularly groom and remove parasites.

Therapy is likely to be more difficult than for millipedes as centipedes are more difficult to handle. In these cases a complete environment change and application of flumethrin strips (Bayvarol; Bayer, Newbury, U.K.) may be of use in the environment.

Neoplasia

There appear to be no descriptions of neoplasia in the literature in these species.

Miscellaneous Disorders

Wrinkled Exoskeleton

Discussions in late 2002 on the Inverticap e-mail group mentioned the problem of wrinkled exoskeletons in young, growing millipedes. This may be due to defects in either the

Chitinous part of the exoskeleton. This may be influenced by diet or by external factors (e.g., substrate or organic chemicals that may interfere with chitin production). Alternatively, nonoptimal humidity levels during shedding may affect the chitin.

Exoskeleton calcification. Lack of calcium, excessive protein in the diet, or acidic substrates may interfere with proper calcification.

Young millipedes should receive a calcium supplement but not supplemental protein (e.g., fish flakes) unless the species is known to feed on animal protein. Animals should be kept on an alkaline substrate at appropriate humidity levels.

Dysecdysis

This has been described in both centipedes and millipedes. In the latter, tight bands of retained exoskeleton have been described as cutting into the animal. In both centipedes and millipedes, therapy consists of gentle bathing/softening of the retained shed and supportive care until the animal's next ecdysis. This condition is a significant cause of death, especially in centipedes. Causes include inappropriate environmental humidity, disturbance during shedding, cutaneous irritation, or (in millipedes) overcrowding resulting in the animal being unable to find an appropriate place to shed.

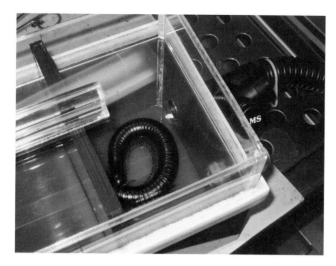

Figure 13.5. Giant train millipede being anesthetized in a scavenged chamber with 5% isoflurane in oxygen.

Anesthesia, Analgesia, and Surgery

The simplest method of anesthesia is to place the animal in an induction chamber (or clear plastic handling tube) and pipe in 5% isoflurane in 100% oxygen (Figure 13.5). Induction may take 15–25 min. It is important to place a piece of open-weave gauze over the end of the anesthetic tubing when dealing with centipedes to prevent escape. It is also useful to humidify the carrier gas, as centipedes are very susceptible to cuticle damage and dehydration in dry conditions. The anesthetized animal can be removed from the chamber and examined/worked on for several minutes. This process can be repeated as necessary.

Anesthetic monitoring is via

1. Loss of voluntary movement
2. Loss of righting and withdrawal (gently stimulate leg/antenna) reflexes

An 8-MHz Doppler ultrasound probe has been used to monitor heart rate under anesthesia in some species (Rees Davies et al., 2000) but appears ineffective in millipedes as good contact on the ventral body surface is difficult to attain; the dorsal body contains a large airspace.

Full recovery from anesthesia may occur in a few hours.

Few, if any surgeries, are described for myriapods. The most likely need to perform surgery is wound repair:

Millipedes. Tissue glue (e.g., Nexaband; Abbott Laboratories, Abbott Park, IL) can be used to repair simple wounds. Major cuticle deficits carry a poor prognosis as repair of the calcified cuticle is unlikely to be successful. Significant loss of hemolymph is unlikely if the injury is to the dorsal part of the body. Prior to closure wounds should be cleansed using a 1:250 dilution of F10 SC (Health & Hygiene) or very dilute povidone iodine. Damaged legs can be removed. If there is loss of hemolymph, the stump can be sealed with tissue glue.

Centipedes. The cuticle is very delicate, so injuries tend to be extensive, severe, and carry a poor prognosis. There is also likely to be significant loss of hemolymph. Again, tissue glue may be useful in repair of injuries. In the larger species it may be possible to place sutures in the soft cuticle (8/0 to 5/0 Vicryl [Ethicon, Somerville, NJ] would be appropriate). Leg injuries can be treated as above.

Diagnostic Techniques

Hemolymph Sampling

This should always be done with the animal under anesthesia. Great care should be taken when sampling centipedes as the cuticle is easily damaged. In both centipedes and millipedes a 25-gauge needle can be inserted between segments. Prior to this, the site should be cleansed with dilute F10 or povidone iodine. In millipedes a site in the ventral third of the body should be selected to avoid the large airspace.

A few drops can be withdrawn for cytology and bacteriology/mycology.

Radiography

Large millipedes are good candidates for radiography because of their calcified cuticle and large dorsal airspace (Figure 13.6). Radiography is best performed with the animal under anesthe-

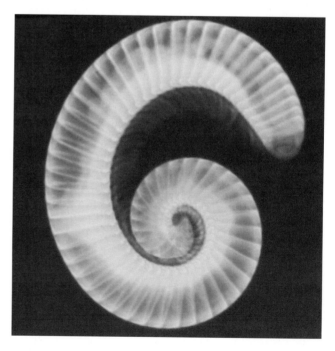

Figure 13.6. Lateral radiograph of a conscious giant train millipede. Barium had been fed the previous day. Note the calcified cuticle, dorsal airspace, and ventrally positioned hemolymph space containing internal organs. The gut is visible in the middle and caudal parts of the viscera as bulges into the airspace. The head is in the center of the coil.

sia as positioning is easier, but productive radiographs can be taken of a conscious, coiled animal. The feeding of barium (e.g., injected into a strawberry) is of great help in outlining the gut.

Centipedes are not obvious candidates as they lack hard structures. However, contrast medium (e.g., barium) can be injected into a cricket that is then fed to the centipede. This will outline the gut and highlight the airspaces seen in some of the cranial segments. Radiography is performed the day after barium administration. Radiographs may be taken by placing the conscious centipede in a clear plastic tube that is positioned over the plate. Alternatively, the centipede may be anesthetized.

Therapeutics

Fluid therapy may be of great importance in sick myriapods. Millipedes may be placed in a shallow bowl of lukewarm water. Centipedes may be placed in a very humid environment surrounded by moistened paper tissue.

Systemic fluid therapy has not been evaluated in myriapods. Oral antimicrobials can be administered:

Millipedes. If still eating, drops may be injected into a small piece of fruit (these animals may refuse treated food).

Centipedes. If eating, these are easier to treat, as drugs may be injected into a small cricket prior to feeding.

In anorexic animals, water-soluble drugs (e.g., trimethoprim–sulfonamide and enrofloxacin) may be injected directly into the hemolymph. The technique is as described earlier for sample taking. Dosing rates are empirical. When using antibiotics, the gut flora of the millipede must be considered. Anderson and Bignell (1980) describe how bacterial populations are amplified as they pass through the gut. These consisted of litter symbionts, so they inferred that fermentation occurs in the gut. Antibiotics (especially per os) should be used judiciously; it may be a good idea to provide probiotics (in the form of fresh feces from a healthy millipede of the same species) to sick millipedes, especially those on antibiotic therapy. It is important not to remove millipedes from a leaf-litter substrate to a more sterile environment when treating as this will have implications for their gut flora and digestion.

References

Anderson JM, Bignell DE. 1980. Bacteria in the food, gut contents and faeces of the litter-feeding millipede, *Glomeris marginata*. Soil Biol Biochem 12:251–254.

Buchsbaum R, Buchsbaum M, Pearse J, Pearse V. 1987. Airborne arthropods: Insects. In: Animals Without Backbones: An Introduction to the Invertebrates, 3rd edition. University of Chicago Press, Chicago.

Bush SP, King BO, Norris RL, Stockwell SA. 2001. Centipede envenomation. Wilderness Environ Med 12:93–99.

Cheeseman V. 2000. Giant millipede care sheet. Vet Invertebr Soc Newsl no. 16, p 20.

Cooper JE. 1980. Invertebrates and invertebrate disease: An introduction for the veterinary surgeon. J Small Anim Pract 21:495–508.

Enghoff H. 1979. Taxonomic significance of the mandibles in the millipede; order Julida. In: Camatini M, ed. Myriapod Biology. Academic, London, pp 27–38.

Frye FL. 1992. Chilopods and diplopods. In: Captive Invertebrates: A Guide to Their Biology and Husbandry. Krieger, Malabar, FL, pp 31–36.

Gebhart K, Schimana J, Müller J, Fiedler HP, Kallenborn HG, Holzenkämpfer M, Krastel P, Zeeck A, Vater J, Höltzel A, Schmid DG, Rheinheimer J, Dettner K. 2002. Screening for biologically active metabolites with endosymbiotic bacilli isolated from arthropods. FEMS Microbiol Lett 217:199–205.

Hopkin SP, Read H. 1992. The Biology of Millipedes. Oxford University Press, New York.

Hudson BJ, Parsons GA. 1997. Giant millipede "burns" and the eye. Trans R Soc Trop Med Hyg 91:183–185.

Mazer C. 1996. Biology, captive propagation and display of an African millipede (Spirostreptida: Spirostreptidae). In: Proceedings of the Sonoran Arthropods Studies Institute Invertebrates in Captivity Conference, 1–4 August, Tucson, Arizona.

McCowan DK, Fanney TE. 1999. The immaculate conception in *Scolopendra gigantea*? In: Proceedings of the Sonoran Arthropod Studies Institute Invertebrates in Captivity Conference, 29 July to 1 August, Rio Rico, Arizona.

Murphy F. 1985. Keeping Spiders, Insects and Other Land Invertebrates in Captivity. Fitzgerald, London.

Norris R. 2002. Centipede envenomation. eMedicine: www.emedicine.com/emerg/topic89.htm.

Oravecz O, Nyir G, Marialigeti K. 2002. A molecular approach in the analysis of the faecal bacterial community in an African millipede belonging to the family Spirostreptidae. Eur J Soil Biol 38:67–70.

Radford AJ. 1975. Millipede burns in man. Trop Geogr Med 27:279–287.

Read HJ, Lewis J. 2002. Millipedes and centipedes. In: O'Toole C, ed. The New Encyclopedia of Insects and Their Allies. Oxford University Press, Oxford, pp 16–21.

Rees Davies R, Chitty JR, Saunders R. 2000. Cardiovascular monitoring of an *Achatina* snail using a Doppler ultrasound unit. In: Proceedings of the British Veterinary Zoological Society Autumn Meeting, 18–19 November, Royal Veterinary College, London, p 101.

Spencer W, Tainton D, Rossiter S. 1999. The general husbandry, display techniques, and breeding of the giant red centipede (*Scolopendra gigantea* Linnaeus 1758) at Bristol Zoo Gardens. In: Proceedings of the Sonoran Arthropods Studies Institute Invertebrates in Captivity Conference, 29 July to 1 August, Rio Rico, Arizona.

Swanson P, McCowan D. 1999. Mortality in captive bred Peruvian centipedes (*Scolopendra gigantea*). In: Proceedings of the Sonoran Arthropods Studies Institute Invertebrates in Captivity Conference, 29 July to 1 August, Rio Rico, Arizona.

Tollefsrud D. 1995. Of mites and men (and millipedes). In: Proceedings of the Sonoran Arthropod Studies Institute Invertebrates in Captivity Conference, 17–20 August, Tucson, Arizona.

Williams DL. 1999. Sample taking in invertebrate veterinary medicine. Vet Clin North Am Exotic Anim Pract 2:777–802.

Wismann K. 1997. Don't let your *Scolopendra* croak: Captive care and exhibit of the giant desert centipede, *Scolopendra heros*. In: Proceedings of the Sonoran Arthropod Studies Institute Invertebrates in Captivity Conference, 31 July to 3 August, Tucson, Arizona.

Chapter 14

INSECTS

John E. Cooper*

Introduction

Interest in the anatomy, physiology, and diseases of insects is not new (Figure 14.1). The economic and social importance of some insects, such as the honeybee (*Apis mellifera*) and the silkworm (*Bombyx mori*) (Mason, 1984), means that awareness of disease in these and certain other species dates back hundreds or even thousands of years. A useful reference in this context is Beavis's book (1988) on *Insects and other Invertebrates in Classical Antiquity*, which recounts the long history of this subject.

Published information on insect diseases is not as rare as many believe. True, relatively little appears to exist in the veterinary literature, but, even there, the fault may lie in assuming that what has been published is in English! The study of diseases of economically important invertebrates is a feature of the veterinary curriculum in many continental European countries, and a surprising amount of information may be found by trawling German, Dutch, French, Polish, and Russian literature. The greatest bulk of relevant data, however, is to be found in nonveterinary journals and books—particularly those that cover invertebrate pathology from the viewpoint of pest control. The objective of those (usually entomologists or invertebrate biologists) who investigate infectious diseases by pests may be different from that of veterinarians, but the techniques used for investigation are very similar. Much useful information about the pathogenesis of infectious diseases in insects is to be found in such publications, together with a certain amount relating to control. A valuable starting point is the *Journal of In-*

vertebrate Pathology and the various books that have appeared over the past few decades, such as those by Boucias and Pendland (1999), Lacey and Kaya (2000), Sparks (1972), Steinhaus (1949, 1963), and Weiser (1977).

A valuable general reference text for those veterinarians and biologists who are concerned with invertebrates in captivity, which includes some articles on health and disease, is the 1990 *International Zoo YearBook* (Olney and Ellis, 1991).

Specific veterinary involvement in the diagnosis and control of insect diseases probably dates back only 2 or 3 decades. A scientific paper on invertebrates was published in 1980 in the *Journal of Small Animal Practice* (Cooper, 1980), and 5 years later a chapter about these animals appeared in Fowler's *Zoo and Wild Animal Medicine* (Frye, 1986). Since then, interest in insects and other invertebrates has burgeoned, with textbooks and chapters (Cooper et al., 1992; Williams, 2002) and articles (Cooper, 1999, 2001; Williams, 1999) on a wide range of relevant topics. A particularly encouraging trend has been the appearance of more specialized articles and reviews—for example, on the dermatology (Cooper, 1993) and stomatology (Williams, 2003) of invertebrate animals.

Natural History and Taxonomy

The Insecta is one of the largest of the classes in the phylum Arthropoda, and three-quarters of the world's animals are insects. Taxonomic nomenclature regarding this group varies. Some consider the insects as a class within the superclass Hexapoda (Ruppert et al., 2004), whereas others list them as a superclass within the phylum Arthropoda (Pearse et al., 1987). For simplicity and consistency, they are referred to as a *class* in this chapter. The class comprises a remarkably diverse group of animals that have been the subject of much study, especially because of the importance of insects in terms of the damage some of them cause to crops and to vertebrate animals (including humans), their use and that of their products as food or other materials, and the widespread study of insects in research laboratories.

Insects are characterized by certain anatomical features (see Table 14.1). Most insects start life as an egg, but subsequent development varies. Some groups undergo a complete metamor-

Acknowledgments. I am grateful to colleagues—entomologists, naturalists, and a very small number of enthusiastic veterinarians—who have encouraged me in my study of invertebrates, especially insects. My interest in these creatures owes much to the encouragement of my parents, Dorothy and Eric Cooper, and to the influence of the Amateur Entomologists' Society (AES), a British organization, which I first joined in 1954 at the age of 10 and of which I am still a member.

I thank John Chitty, MRCVS, for reading and commenting on an early draft, and Terry Hardy, an experienced apiarist, for useful discussions and his advice regarding bees. The typing of this chapter was completed by Ms. Deborah Daniel, to whom I am most grateful for her good-humored support.

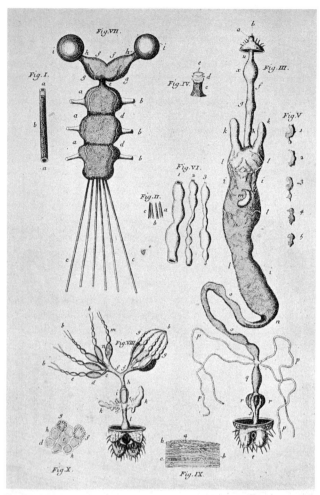

FIG. 112.—Swammerdam. *Pediculus*. Gut, female genitalia, nervous system. In III the oesophagus is much too wide for a blood-sucking animal, and the salivary

Figure 14.1. Interest in insect internal anatomy is not new. Dissections of a *Pediculus* sp. by Jan Swammerdam more than 300 years ago.

Table 14.1.   Important anatomical features

Feature	Comments
Body divided into three parts: head, thorax, and abdomen	A feature of all adult insects: not so well defined in some immature stages
Exoskeleton of chitin, which varies in thickness and extent	Important in defense against physical and infectious insults
Hemolymph present in the body cavity, transports gases, and metabolites	Usually type I: sodium and chloride are main components (Sutcliffe, 1963)
Three pairs of legs attached to thorax	Larval forms may have additional (pseudo) limbs; some adult insects have lost one or more pairs of legs (e.g., certain butterflies)
Usually one or two pairs of wings attached to thorax	Many modifications: some insects (e.g., fleas) appear never to have had wings; Others (e.g., flies) have only one functional pair
Abdomen generally has 11 segments, no limbs	Some variation
Genital apertures near the anus	Some species (and sexes) have appendages associated with courtship, mating, or oviposition

Anatomy and Physiology

The basic anatomy of insects is important and relevant to veterinarians and others who have to examine or treat these animals (Figures 14.2 and 14.3). Traditionally, insects were considered to be arthropods with tracheae in which the body was divided into three distinct regions. The head of an insect usually consists of six segments, and there is a single pair of antenna. The thorax comprises three segments with three pairs of legs and usually two pairs of wings. The main anatomical features and some biochemical features of the class Insecta that should be familiar to veterinarians and others involved with health are listed in Table 14.1.

The anatomy of insects and other invertebrates continues to attract much attention, and in-depth ultrastructural and immunohistochemical studies are reported in the journal *Arthropod Structure and Development*, published by Elsevier.

The physiology of the class Insecta has also been studied in considerable detail over the past 100 years, and there are many standard texts, which provide basic or evolving information. Knowledge and understanding are expanding fast, as is illustrated by the series entitled Advances in Insect Physiology, published for many years by Academic Press. Veterinarians should consider referring to these and other similar state-of-the-art publications. Although some of the papers are complex and relate to basic entomological principles, others include information of practical value. Thus, for example, in volume 18 (edited by Berridge et al. [1985]), there are papers covering such subjects as pheromones, the pattern and control of walking in insects, and the developmental physiology of color patterns in butterflies

phosis, which includes an egg (ovum), larva, pupa, and adult (imago) stage. Well-known examples include the butterflies and moths (Lepidoptera), beetles (Coleoptera), and fleas (Siphonaptera). Others perform an incomplete metamorphosis, whereby the animal that emerges from an egg resembles, to a certain extent, the mature insect. Grasshoppers (Orthoptera) are an example. A series of molts then results in a gradual change to the adult form—for example, the development of wings and genitalia and changes in morphology and color.

Insects are virtually ubiquitous but, in contrast to some other arthropods, such as the Crustacea, are found in only small numbers in the sea and in other environments that are rich in dissolved or suspended chemicals (e.g., alkaline lakes). On the land, however, insects virtually reign supreme; many can fly, and they exploit the vast majority of habitats. In freshwater, also, there is a large insect fauna, and some are important environmental sentinels for the health of such ecosystems.

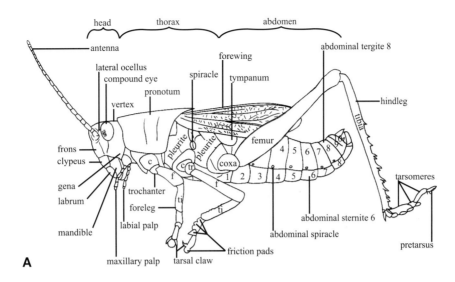

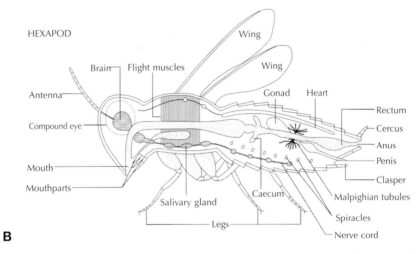

Figure 14.2. **A:** Drawing of a mature grasshopper with major external anatomical features labeled. Reproduced from Richard Fox, Lander University, by Alison Schroeer. **B:** Diagram of a generalized hexapod, indicating the major internal, as well as some external, anatomical features. From Barnes et al. (2001), Figure 8.18.

and moths. The last of these includes discussion of how developmental abnormalities may occur in Lepidoptera as a result of cold or other stressors. Amateur entomologists have long recognized that color aberrations may be induced by exposing pupae to abnormally high or low temperatures, but this and other papers provide an opportunity to consider a scientific explanation.

The *Journal of Insect Physiology*, published by Pergamon, also reports developments in the field and again occasional papers are of relevance to veterinarians and others who work with these animals in captivity.

Some important features of the physiology of insects are listed in Table 14.2.

Environmental Disorders and Preventive Medicine

Insects, being ectothermic and in many cases selected to survive in specific ecosystems, are usually very susceptible to environ-

mental change. High temperatures, low temperatures, the wrong relative humidity, and an unsuitable substrate are all examples of factors that will have an adverse effect on insects and may predispose them to ill-health and/or death (Figures 14.4 and 14.5). Stressors are known to reduce protein and ecdysone values of hemolymph in some species, with corresponding effects on a wide range of body functions. Chemical defenses, including the composition and efficacy of antimicrobial secretions, can also be affected by environmental insults (Blum, 1981). These aspects are all discussed in more detail later.

Preventive medicine for captive insects, therefore, depends largely on providing a suitable environment. In a few cases, often as a result of work by staff of zoological gardens, insectaria, and laboratory animal units, recommended and proven figures for temperature, humidity, etc., are available. For the vast majority of species, however, such data do not yet exist. Extrapolation is then needed—from either (a) the wild or (b) success with allied or similar species. Very frequently it proves necessary to provide a *range* of temperatures, humidity, and

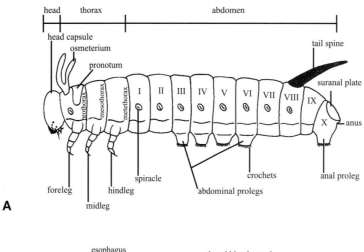

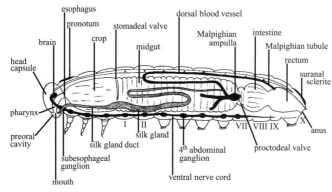

Figure 14.3. Many insects have larval stages that do not resemble the adult form. **A:** A caterpillar's important external anatomical features. **B:** Important internal anatomical features. Reproduced from Richard Fox, Lander University, by Alison Schroeer.

Table 14.2. Important physiological features

Physiological feature	Comments
Ectothermy	The vast majority of insects are ectothermic and thus unable to control their body temperature by internal means. Thermoregulation is achieved by behavioral adaptations, the animal relying on external heat sources.
	A small number of species (e.g., certain autumnal temperate moths) appear able to raise their body temperatures slightly and thus can tolerate a cold climate. Other species are known to produce cryoprotective chemicals.
Metamorphosis	All insects mature by molting their exocuticle (ecdysis). Some species have a complete metamorphosis, with egg (ovum), larva, pupa, and adult (imago) (e.g., Lepidoptera), whereas in others (e.g., Orthoptera) the larval and pupal stages are replaced by gradual differentiation into the adult.

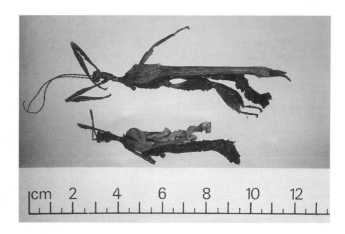

Figure 14.4. Two stick insects (*Phasmidae*) presented for postmortem examination. The *bottom one* shows developmental abnormalities associated with environmental stressors.

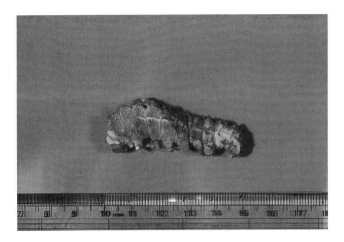

Figure 14.5.   A silkmoth larva (Saturniidae) with dysecdysis. The cause was a low relative humidity in the vivarium.

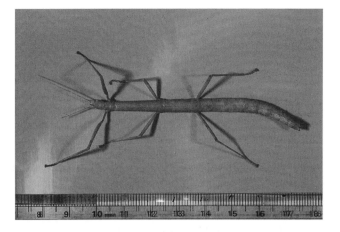

Figure 14.6.   Observation is important. An apparently normal Indian stick insect (*Carausius morosus*). Close examination reveals a damaged antenna.

substrates so that the captive animals can be selective. Keeping batches of captive insects under different conditions and comparing their survival and breeding success will help to elucidate those factors that are important. Such data should be published for the benefit of others.

Other aspects of preventive medicine for insects that should be considered an essential part of good management are

Careful assessment of incoming stock before they are purchased (Figure 14.6)

Quarantining (isolation) of new stock before they join the main collection

Clinical, postmortem, and laboratory health monitoring of stock, both while in quarantine and thereafter

Isolation and or culling (with postmortem examination) of individuals or groups of insects that show signs of disease

Comprehensive record keeping, with regular reviewing of the data, especially analysis of peaks and troughs of morbidity, mortality, or other parameters such as lack of reproductive success or shortened life span

Current interest in the captive breeding of threatened species of invertebrates has resulted in the development of protocols that have proved to be successful in the management, breeding, and propagation of certain invertebrates. An example concerns the endangered wetas (Orthoptera) in New Zealand. Workers in New Zealand and at the Zoological Society of London have successfully bred species of weta, including *Deinacrida fallai*, and in so doing accumulated important information as to how to maintain these animals in good health. Management is all-important and, in the case of *D. fallai*, includes daily temperature and humidity checks, health checks (any dead animals are immediately sent for pathological examination), ascertaining the condition of foliage, removing old feces, and looking out for signs that may indicate imminent problems. The latter includes unusual behavior or the presence of excess amounts of dampness in the cage—which can predispose the animals to disease (P. Pearce-Kelly, personal communication). Similar protocols

are used in many other insect collections, and, as captive breeding of threatened and endangered invertebrates becomes more common, these are likely to prove of increasing value in monitoring and maintaining the health of different species.

Infectious Diseases

A whole range of infectious diseases is now recognized in the class Insecta. The Chinese recorded diseases of the silkworm (*Bombyx mori*) nearly 5000 years ago (Tanada and Kaya, 1993). The brood diseases of the honeybee (*Apis mellifera*) were known to Pliny 2000 years ago, and a few were studied and described scientifically in the 19th century—notably by Agostino Bassi and later by Louis Pasteur in their epic works on the silkworm (*Bombyx mori*) (Bassi, 1835; Pasteur, 1870). For over 150 years, there has been interest in the use of pathogens to control insect pests (see the historical review by Tanada and Kaya [1993]), and organisms used or investigated include fungi, bacteria, viruses, and nematodes. Insect pathology emerged as a bona fide discipline in the mid-20th century, and Edward A. Steinhaus is generally acknowledged as the father of invertebrate pathology.

The epizootiology of insect diseases has been extensively reviewed and discussed by Fuxa and Tanada (1987). Space does not permit detailed discussion here, but important features of any pathogen of insects are its

Virulence

Infectivity

Ability to survive

Some organisms are highly pathogenic (e.g., the bacterium *Bacillus thuringiensis*) but have a low infectivity—in this case, because of its poor powers of dispersal (Gillott, 1980). As a result, natural epizootics caused by the bacterium are rare, but, when used in pest control or when a subspecies gains access to appropriate hosts in captivity, *B. thuringiensis* is a major cause of mortality.

Much work has been carried out on the pathogenesis of certain infectious diseases—notably those caused by bacteria where access to the hemocoel permits rapid multiplication.

Most bacteria, viruses, and protozoa enter the body through the gut, but fungi usually gain access to insects through the integument. A variety of mechanisms enable these various pathogens to damage tissues and to debilitate the host (Gillott, 1980). Bacteria often have their effect on the midgut epithelium or cause a septicemia, whereas viruses disrupt the metabolism of host cells. Fungi physically disrupt tissues and may secrete toxic materials—as may protozoa. Nematodes feed on certain organs and thereby exert specific effects on the host, such as delayed maturity or infertility.

Insects are protected against pathogens in a variety of ways, and an understanding of this helps to explain the different relationships, including symbiosis, that exist between insects and microorganisms.

Our understanding of cellular defense mechanisms in animals dates back to the pioneering research of Metchnikoff (1892), who, in addition to doing research on diseases of Coleoptera, used invertebrates—mainly the crustacean *Daphnia*—in his studies on host responses and coined the term *phagocyte*. Now we have a better understanding of immunity in insects and recognize several types of response, including the following:

1. Cellular responses by hemocytes/plasmacytes (plasmatocytes) that can phagocytose certain pathogens, foreign material, and debris associated with wounds.

2. Coagulocytic responses. The coagulocytes are granular cells that cause the production of a coagulum that surrounds foreign cells.

3. Humoral responses. Some are due to the production of specific antibacterial proteins, such as when live organisms are injected into silkworms (Abraham et al., 1995), whereas others are more basic—for example, in Diptera, whereby melanin can be deposited on the surface of a parasitic worm and thus hamper its growth. One effect of melanin production and deposition is the hardening of the cuticle, and it is suggested that this may have a nonspecific effect on the insect's immune system by making the animal less vulnerable to the attention of mites and, possibly, damage by other parasites. Chemical defenses are important in insects (Blum, 1981).

The role of hemocytes in defense against microorganisms, nematodes, and parasitoids has been well reviewed by Ratcliffe and Rowley (1980).

There is much interest currently in the immune status of insects, and the methods used for research usually involve the investigation of tiny tissue samples, necessitating special techniques (Gilbert and Miller, 1988).

The organisms that can either be the primary cause of disease in insects, or secondary to other infectious or noninfectious insults, include viruses, bacteria (Figure 14.7), mycoplasmas, fungi (Figure 14.8), and various metazoan parasites (Gillott, 1980). Some of the pathogens are familiar to those who work with vertebrates: *Pseudomonas*, for example, can cause morbidity and mortality in a wide range of insect species. The effect of

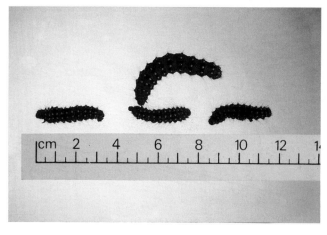

Figure 14.7. Four larvae of the European emperor moth (*Saturnia pavonia*). One has grown normally, whereas the other three are small and stunted, probably as a result of a bacterial infection.

many such infections depends, as it does in other animals, on features of both host and pathogen (Schneider and Dorn, 2001).

Host–parasite relations of insects have attracted considerable interest in recent years and include, for example, substantial work on fungus–insect relationships (Wheeler and Blackwell, 1984). As in other animals, this relationship influences whether a parasite (which might be a macroparasite, such as a metazoan, helminth, or mite [Figure 14.9]; or a microparasite, such as a bacterium or protozoan) causes morbidity or mortality in the insect host. It is important to bear this in mind—and to seek specialist advice, if necessary—when attempting to determine whether organisms identified or isolated from captive insects are likely to be pathogenic. Some specific and frank pathogens of insects are well recognized. Many other organisms, however, may be pathogens if the circumstances are appropriate, but can equally be commensals, symbionts (mutualism in termites, for instance, where the insects, bacteria, and flagellate protozoa coexist), or even environmental contaminants that are of no apparent relevance to the health of the insect. Mites provide many such examples: a few will be mentioned here.

Varroa jacobsoni is considered a scourge of honeybee (*Apis mellifera*) colonies, but, in its natural state, in Asia, it is widespread and infects, without apparent pathogenicity, the local bee *Apis cerana*.

Parasitus fimetorum lives in the nests of bumblebees, *Bombus* spp. It scavenges on debris and, despite its name, is not parasitic.

Symbiosis is illustrated by the life of the mite *Dinogamasus villosior*, which is known only from the bodies and nests of African and Asian carpenter bees (*Xylocopa* spp.). The mites lay their eggs on bee pupae, where the nymphs feed on exudates; in return, the presence of the mite is believed to inhibit fungal infections. The mites live in a special mite pouch (acinarium)—a specific anatomical adaptation on the abdomen of the bee.

Whether or not a parasite causes morbidity or mortality in its insect host depends on many different factors, including the species or strain of both parasite and host and the health status

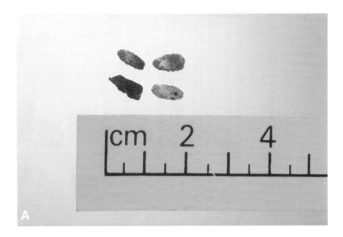

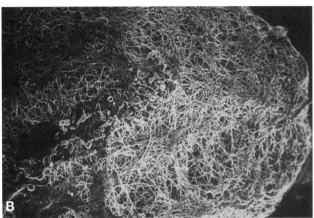

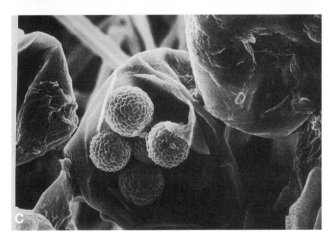

Figure 14.8.   A: A brood disease of bee larvae (*Apis mellifera*). Note the chalky appearance of the larvae in this photograph. **B:** Low-power scanning electron micrography (SEM) reveals filamentous structures. **C:** High-power SEM confirms the presence of fungal hyphae and conidia indicative of an *Aspergillus* infection.

of the latter. Often the numbers of parasites are important; thus, the mite *Acarapsis woodi*, which lives in the tracheae of bees and sucks hemolymph, only usually causes death if present in large numbers. When mites are few, the only observable clinical sign is a reduced life span.

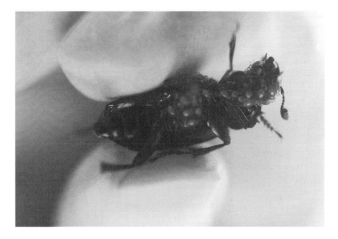

Figure 14.9.   Normal saprophytic mites on the exoskeleton of a carrion beetle.

The association of many insects with nonpathogenic organisms is a complex one—"a fascinating study in itself" (Tanada and Kaya, 1993)—and is relevant to the foregoing examples and many others. Insects may have *exosymbionts* or *endosymbionts*. The latter are perhaps of particular interest because they may live in the hemocoelomic cavity, as well as in various organs. They appear to be protected from the insect's immune system, because most of them are inside *mycetocytes*, protected from phagocytosis (Ermin, 1939; Gupta, 1989).

Some parasites of insects are not only of interest or importance in their own right but are also proving to be useful models for the study of diseases of vertebrates, including humans. A recent example is the study by scientists at King's College, London, of sexually transmitted diseases (STDs) by using a mite (*Coccipolipus hippodamiae*) that is transmitted between ladybirds (ladybugs) during mating.

The implantation of eggs and larvae of various hymenopterans—so-called parasitic wasps or *ichneumons*—into host insects is a well-recognized phenomenon both in the wild and in captivity (Pinches, 2003). Exclusion of such parasites is essential when insects are kept in collections: a suitable size of mesh is often adequate.

Examples of infectious diseases of insects, together with comments on the clinical or postmortem features and on methods of treatment or control, are listed in Table 14.3. This is, of necessity, only a tiny selection. Many organisms cause morbidity and mortality in insects and some, such as *Bacillus thuringiensis*, the most extensively used organism for biological control, have been the subject of countless publications, dissertations and lectures (for example, see Tanada and Kaya [1993]).

A very useful review on the control of diseases in insect cultures is that by Rivers (1991), who described the causes of disease in insects, particularly but not exclusively Lepidoptera, and discussed methods of disease control, including hygiene, surface sterilization, and chemotherapy.

Good record keeping is vital when insects are maintained in captivity and can provide important indicators as to the health of stock. Properly used, it can often serve as an early-warning

Table 14.3. Important insect pathogens

Organism	Disease	Clinical/postmortem features	Treatments/control	Other comments
Various species of bacteria	Bacterial disease of larvae of Lepidoptera and Hymenoptera	Loose feces Dehydration Death	Culling Hygiene	Widespread in captivity and in the wild
Serratia marcescens	Bacterial septicemia	Reddening of body Liquefaction	Isolation Reduce density Antibiotics?	The cage may have a fetid odor (see Callis and Zwart, 1999)
Various species of fungus	Mycotic infections (various)	Blackening of cuticle Rigidity	Hygiene Improved environment	See Hunter-Jones (1966)
Mermis worm	Parasitic helminthiasis of locusts	Weakness and lethargy Weight changes Worms in body cavity	Culling Exclude worm by avoiding infected vegetation	Other Orthoptera can also be affected
Microsporidia	Microsporidiosis	Stiffness of locomotion Colored cysts under skin	Hygiene	
Ophryocystis elektroscirrha	*Oe*	Dark spots under pupae cuticle Incomplete emergence	Hygiene and disinfection	See Figure 14.10
Iridovirus	Iridovirus infection of crickets	Distension of the abdomen	Hygiene	Leong et al. (1992) P. Zwart (personal communication)
Reovirus Fijivirus	Various diseases of silkworms	Loss of condition Loose feces	Hygiene and culling	See Frye (1992)

system enabling a veterinarian/entomologist to take action before an epizootic or other disaster occurs.

Clinical examination is important in work with insects, as it is in other fields of comparative medicine (Figures 14.10–14.12, Color Plate 4.10, Color Plate 4.11). It starts with observation, before any animals are handled. Sometimes, profound behavioral changes are associated with infectious diseases; for example, in the case of polyhedrosis virus infection, affected larvae concentrate in the tops of trees, whereas in *Entomophthora* (fungus) infection the victims are fixed and die on branches, facilitating spread of spores. The apicultural literature abounds with excellent examples of how behavioral signs can be correlated with various diseases and syndromes (for example, see Betts [1934]).

Other clinical signs, some of which are featured in Table 14.3, include

Color changes
Atrophy (shrinkage) of abdomen
Diarrhea
Stiffness of locomotion
Disturbed growth and ecdysis
Behavioral fever

Analysis of records, observation, and clinical examination can be followed by a certain number of investigative procedures. The larger insects can be radiographed (contrast medium may be given per os), and such techniques as ultrasonography and the use of Doppler are beginning to be reported in the study of invertebrates (Davies et al., 2000).

In both diagnostic and research work, accurate sampling and examination of material are essential. Those veterinarians and others who are involved need to be aware of the techniques that

are standard in the study of invertebrates (Weiser, 1977; Cooper and Cunningham, 1991; Lacey, 1997; Williams, 1999).

Certain laboratory investigations need specialized knowledge. Insect hematology—described as "a difficult and controversial subject" by one of its pioneers (Gupta, 1980)—is an ex-

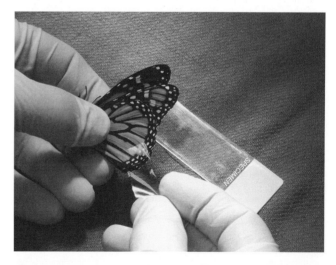

Figure 14.10. A small piece of clean, clear transparent tape is being used on a monarch butterfly (*Danaus plexippus*) to capture the spores of the protozoal parasite *Ophryocystis elektroscirrha*. The ventral abdomen is the ideal place to obtain a sample. The tape is then placed on a clean glass slide and examined under the microscope for the presence of small, brown or gold, football-shaped spores. This parasite is becoming common with the rapid development of butterfly houses (Figures 14.11 and 14.12) and expanding market for butterfly pupae (Dan Dombrowski, personal communication). Photo courtesy of Shane Boylan.

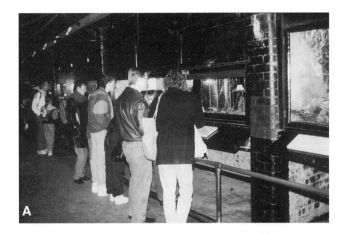

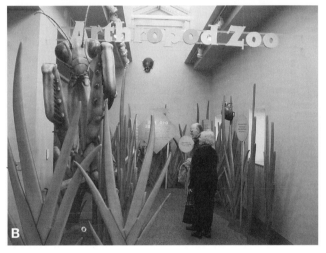

Figure 14.11.   Butterfly houses **(A)** and arthropod zoos **(B)** are becoming very popular in a number of countries.

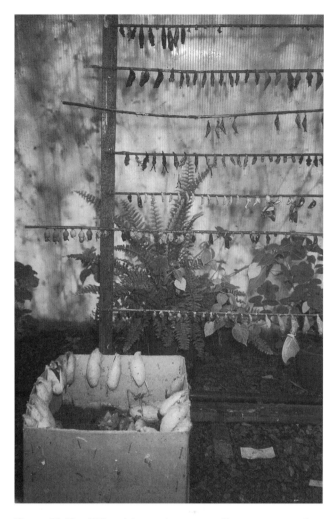

Figure 14.12.   Different types of pupae awaiting emergence of imagines (adults) in a butterfly house. Infections can spread easily under such conditions.

ample. However, the examination of the blood of insects dates back several decades (for example, see information on hemato-cytes of *Tenebrio* in Salt [1970]), and it and other laboratory-based studies are likely to become more important in clinical work with these animals.

Neoplasia

Neoplasms of insects have been increasingly recognized in recent years, to a large extent as a result of the work by the Registry of Tumors in Lower Animals (RTLA) (Harshbarger, 1974) and the research by such authors as Matz (1975, 1996), Gateff (1977), and Tsang and Brooks (1980). Much of the emphasis in such studies has tended to be on oncological research, using these animals as models, rather than on the diagnosis and treatment of neoplasms in individual insects.

Care has to be taken to distinguish true neoplasms from granulomas, which are composed primarily of agglutinated hemocytes (Matz, 1969) and which generally represent a defense reaction to trauma, infectious agents, or hormonal imbalances

(Tanada and Kaya, 1993). In such cases, detailed laboratory examination and accurate differentiation are most important.

Although neoplasms of insects would appear at present to be of relatively little clinical importance, there is a need for veterinarians or others involved with the captive care of these animals to be aware of their existence—as has been emphasized elsewhere (Cooper, 2004). Neoplasms of invertebrates may hold the key to a better understanding of the evolution of oncogenesis, and it is therefore incumbent on those who keep or tend insects to take careful note of tumors and similar lesions. Material that may be neoplastic should always be saved, fixed samples sent to a specialist for histological and/or electron-microscopic investigation, and (where practicable) fresh material frozen for microbiological and other studies.

Miscellaneous Disorders

Morbidity and mortality of captive insects are often due to non-infectious factors. The role of the environment in this respect was emphasized in the section Environmental Disorders and Preventive Medicine.

Nutrition is as important for insects as it is for other animals. Space does not permit more than a brief overview of the nutritional requirements of this large group of animals. Most of the data available are derived from studies on the captive maintenance of economically important species, such as locusts (*Locusta* and *Schistocerca* spp.), silkworms (*Bombyx mori*), tsetse flies (*Glossina* spp.), and various Lepidoptera. A key reference is the two-volume work on insect rearing edited by Singh and Moore (1985), which includes both general chapters (e.g., on artificial diets) and specific sections on different orders. Frye (1992) also provides useful data on culture media and other diets for some of the more commonly kept insects, including prey species.

Nutritional disorders may broadly be divided into those related to (a) quantity and (b) quality. Quantity is mainly relevant in terms of food deprivation or low palatability, whereby the animal does not ingest sufficient nutrients and ultimately succumbs to secondary infection or dies of inanition. In captivity, many factors may combine to cause this; good management and understanding of the dietary requirements of the species are essential. Although most species are fed on natural food (plants or animals), certain insects can be maintained in good health on artificial diets: perhaps the most impressive example is the colony of the aphid *Myzus persicae* that was kept for 26 years on a mixture of amino acids and vitamins (Van Emden, 2003). Pinches (2003) refers to "plant specificity" and points out that some insects eat only one type of food and will refuse to take others, even though they may be edible: this is a well-recognized feature of many phasmids and lepidopterans.

Food deprivation can have multiple effects on insects, and starvation stress is well recognized in some species. Studies on the Colorado (potato) beetle (*Leptinotarsa decemlineata*) by Furlong and Groden (2003) showed that starvation of second-stage instar larvae increased both the duration of the instar and the susceptibility of the larvae to attack by the fungus *Beauveria bassiana*. One reason for the latter may be that a delayed molt enables fungal conidia to accumulate on the surface of the insect, enhancing infection; however, other mechanisms may be involved.

The quality of a diet for insects relates to the nutrients that it contains, not the absolute quantity. Diets for insects, whether natural or artificial, need to contain adequate quantities of protein, carbohydrate, fats, vitamins, and minerals. Requirements vary: growing larvae of, for example, silkworms (*Bombyx mori*) require a high protein intake for them to thrive (Pinches, 2003). Water is all-important. Some insects drink water—a few, such as the European drinker moth (*Philudoria potatoria*), are renowned for this habit—whereas others obtain fluid almost entirely through food or by internal metabolism. Certain groups of insects, such as the tenebrionid beetles that live in arid areas, can either produce water by metabolic means or harvest it by condensing vapor on their exoskeleton.

In any investigation of disease or deaths among insects, the diet must be considered. Not only may it be deficient in quan-

tity or quality, as outlined above, but it may be the source of toxins (e.g., insecticides) or its consistency may be such that it is having an adverse effect on the normal biology and behavior of the animal. Thus, for example, leaves that are too dry and that are ingested by the larvae of Lepidoptera may cause blockage of the intestine, with pathological, sometimes fatal, sequelae (see *laxatives* in Table 14.5).

There are many miscellaneous disorders of insects. The cause of a few is recognized: for others, a syndrome may be familiar to entomologists or hobbyists who manage the species in captivity, but the etiology and pathogenesis are still not known. There is an important role for veterinarians who work with entomologists to elucidate the causes and control of some of these conditions.

Stress is recognized in insects, but its pathogenesis is still poorly understood. Stressors are assumed to include temperature extremes, starvation, and the effects of chemicals. The immune responses of the insect may be affected (Brey, 1994), increasing vulnerability to infectious diseases. Even symbionts may then become pathogenic (Tanada and Kaya, 1993).

Environmental factors play a large part in the health and diseases of insects. An adverse temperature may affect individual animals or influence the behavior of whole colonies. Thus, for example, John Chitty (personal communication) has reported changes in the colonial activity of leaf-cutting ants (*Atta* sp.), characterized by an increased production of winged queens, as a response to high temperatures, and Pinches (2003) has described sterility in the wasp *Dahlbominus* and leaf-cutting ants that is caused by thermal damage to gametocytes. Low temperatures can also affect insects, but it should be noted that some species can produce cryoprotective chemicals (Tanada and Kaya, 1993). The effects of high humidity or low humidity have been discussed by Pinches (2003): often the picture is complicated by secondary infection, possibly the result of reduced host resistance.

Trauma is commonly a cause of ill-health or death. If the chitinous exoskeleton of an insect is breached, hemolymph escapes and, if this is not stemmed, the animal will die. Methods of sealing such defects include the application of tissue glue, talc, or caster sugar (Cooper, 1999) (see this chapter's appendix). Traumatic injuries are particularly common during ecdysis: for example, wetas (*Deinacrida*) may damage their ovipositors, leading to dilatation of Malpighian tubules with eggs and causing death (Pinches, 2003). Predation, including cannibalism, can be considered a form of trauma and is common among insects, both in captivity and in the wild (Pinches, 2003).

A word should be said about genetics and developmental disorders. Much of what we understand of animal genetics is based on long-term studies of insects, especially fruit flies (*Drosophila* species). Genetic disorders may be a feature of such colonies because the aberration is being used in research, but genetic diseases can also occur spontaneously, perhaps as a result of inbreeding from small founder stocks. The latter is an important consideration when dealing with small populations of threatened or endangered species, especially when these have already been through a bottleneck as a result of, for example, environmental catastrophes or human persecution. Lethal or semilethal genes are prevalent, in the heterozygous form, in some butterflies and moths, where they are linked with loci containing genes for beneficial traits, such as camouflage (Benz, 1963).

Developmental abnormalities may be genetic in origin or may be associated with environmental factors. They can take the form of duplication of limbs, asymmetry of organs, transposition of organs, and so on. The frequency of such abnormalities in a colony should be recorded, and, periodically, the prevalence should be studied and analyzed to determine whether there is any association with an extrinsic managemental factor.

Conditions that are congenital are present at birth and might be genetic in origin. Again, although culling is usually the appropriate course of action, the keeping of good records about such occurrences and the retention of material for scientific study is good practice and may contribute to our understanding of insect pathology.

Neoplasms of insects can also be of genetic origin, and these have been extensively studied in, for example, *Drosophila* (Gateff, 1977). Generally speaking, however, neoplasms do not appear to be prevalent in insects, in contrast to the situation in some other invertebrates (Williams, 2002; Pinches, 2003).

Poisoning is an ever-present threat to most insects, even in the wild. Some toxic materials are natural, being produced by plants or by other animals as part of their defense mechanism. There are many instances in which insects have evolved to cope with such toxins—for example, lepidopterous larvae that feed safely on plants that are rich in alkaloids. Other poisons that are produced, accidentally or intentionally, by humans may kill or incapacitate insects in the wild or in captivity.

Pesticides are, by definition, intended to kill pests, which may include insects, and may be used to control wild (free living) populations of, say, locusts or mosquitoes, or they may be employed in a more general way (e.g., in a house or garden) as a safeguard against unwanted invertebrates. Insofar as captive colonies of insects are concerned, both categories of pesticide are potentially dangerous, but the latter are sometimes less easy to detect and control. Thus, insects kept for educational purposes in a classroom or laboratory may be exposed to fly sprays or other insecticides that have been used in the location for other, apparently innocuous, purposes. The same applies to certain inorganic chemicals. A few insects are remarkably resistant to toxic chemicals—the American cockroach (*Periplaneta americana*), for example, will even survive many hours of exposure to formaldehyde vapor—but others can succumb rapidly to even low concentrations of such substances. Therefore, when investigating morbidity or mortality among captive insects, all lines of enquiry should be followed. Fumes from a recently painted fence, disinfectant used to clean table surfaces, or gases liberated from an apparently harmless science lesson in an adjacent school laboratory may be the clue as to why animals have died or failed to perform well.

Likewise, care must be taken with any food that is provided, since the diet may be a source of toxins. Foliage may have been sprayed with a toxic chemical such as an organophosphate or may merely be unpalatable because it has, for example, been treated with soapy water to control aphids in the garden. Genetically modified crops may present a new threat. Losey et al. (1999) have described how maize modified with genetic material from *Bacillus thuringiensis* to protect against the corn borer (*Ostrinia nubilalis*) affected the development of monarch butterfly (*Danaus plexippus*) larvae. Food of animal origin is also a possible source of toxicity. Crickets or mealworms, used as a food source for other insects, can appear to be healthy but may harbor sufficient toxic chemical on their exoskeletons, or sometimes within their bodies, to cause disease in, or the death of, the predator. Health monitoring of food items is part of quality control whenever insects are kept in captivity and should include a check for chemicals as well as pathogens.

Pinches (2003) has discussed in some detail the effect of chemical agents on invertebrates and emphasized the importance of "good display management" as a preventive measure.

Analgesia, Anesthesia, and Surgery

Over the past 15 years, there has been considerable debate about pain in different taxa of animals. Certain species of insect have been investigated scientifically in addressing the question "Do invertebrates feel pain?" Many of the findings are equivocal, but there is a growing recognition among scientists and concerned laypeople, perhaps particularly in Britain and other European countries where animal-welfare issues are of high priority, that insects, like other animals, should be given the benefit of the doubt. In other words, it should be assumed that invertebrates feel pain unless it can be proved to the contrary—and this has led to measures in research laboratories and elsewhere to minimize or to refine traumatic procedures on these creatures. The idea that insects might feel pain is not a new one. William Shakespeare in his play *Measure for Measure* wrote, "[T]he poor beetle that we tread upon . . . feels a pang as great as when a giant dies."

Pain relief for insects is not, therefore, as far-fetched as it might appear. In captivity, where animals depend entirely on their keepers, any lesions or procedures that might cause pain or distress should receive appropriate attention (Cooper, 2001). It is sometimes difficult, however, to distinguish between what are truly pathological events and what are part of an animal's normal physiology; for example, some insects, particularly if they are immature, can regenerate all or part of a lost limb. This is a well-developed and vital strategy for survival, and no veterinary intervention is justified. However, extensive damage or injuries to sensitive areas of the body, where regeneration is not a characteristic, may warrant attention. Usually the only action that can be taken to alleviate presumed pain in insects is either (a) to kill the animal humanely or (b) to apply supportive care. The latter may include, for example, irrigation of a lesion that is dry and causing disturbance to locomotion, feeding, or skin shedding (ecdysis). The days of giving analgesics to insects, though, other than experimentally to study the physiology of endorphins, may still be a long way off.

Table 14.4.   Anesthetic agents

Method of administration	Anesthetic agents	Comments
1. Inhalation (terrestrial insects) by using an anesthetic chamber through which the agents are pumped	Carbon dioxide	Effective and generally safe, but its analgesic properties are unknown
	Diethyl ether	Effective and generally safe, but an irritant to the operator's mucous membranes and inflammable
	Halothane	Effective and generally safe
	Isoflurane	Effective and apparently very safe
	Sevoflurane	Effective and apparently safe
2. Absorption (aquatic insects) by using a measured container of water	Benzocaine	Must first be dissolved in acetone
	Tricaine methanesulfonate	Can be dissolved in water; may prove an irritant
	Carbon dioxide	Bubbled through the water from a cylinder or produced by the addition of soda water

In contrast to the foregoing, anesthesia of insects has long been carried out in certain species for research purposes and, in recent years, has begun to be studied and refined. Decades ago, certain varieties of *Drosophila* were designated *ether sensitive* or *ether resistant*, depending on their susceptibility to the effects of anesthetic ether. In recent years, anesthesia of insects and other arthropods has become commonplace in veterinary practices and zoos that deal with these animals (Cooper, 2001). Some examples of agents that can be used are presented, with comments, in Table 14.4.

Hypothermia (chilling/cooling) can often be of use in temporary immobilization of a specimen—for example, to take photographs or to perform radiography—but should never be employed for surgical treatment or other procedures that may cause pain or be stressful.

Assessing depth of anesthesia is not easy. In many cases, total immobility, absence of a righting reflex, and apparent lack of awareness of stimuli shown by an insect that has been given an anesthetic agent are usually reversible. If the source of the anesthetic agent is removed—for example, if an insect in an anesthetic chamber that has been exposed to isoflurane is placed in fresh air or oxygen—recovery will usually follow. Initially, often within a few minutes, the limbs will twitch slightly, and then the animal gradually recovers fully, but this may take several hours. Sick or debilited insects may succumb to anesthesia, but generally the agents and techniques that are listed prove safe.

The killing (euthanasia) of invertebrates, including insects, has attracted interest and attention in recent years, particularly in Western Europe but also increasingly in North America (Hackendahl and Mashima, 2002). The subject is covered in a publication commissioned by the World Society for the Protection of Animals (WSPA) (1994) and led to the production of guidelines by the National Federation of Zoos in the United Kingdom (National Federation of Zoos, 1990).

Ascertaining whether an insect is dead, whether or not the result of anesthesia or euthanasia, is often far from easy. This was recognized over a century ago when one correspondent felt prompted to write to an entomological journal, in the con-

text of parasite control, "It is as difficult to determine that a flea is dead as it is to tell an Englishman that he is defeated in battle . . . !"

There are important reasons for being able to assess an insect's death. The ability of many species to recover fully from anesthesia and other toxic insults means that there is a danger that a discarded "dead" body may prove still to be alive. The best approach is either (a) to await signs of autolysis or rigor mortis (the animal becomes stiff and brittle) or (b) to destroy the animal physically so that recovery is impossible.

Some minor procedures can be performed on insects without recourse to anesthesia. Ectoparasites can be removed by using cotton buds soaked in either water (to keep the creature alive) or in methanol (to fix the parasite). Chitinous debris can be debrided using a scalpel. Impacted fecal material can sometimes be expressed from, for example, a caterpillar by administering mineral oil (liquid paraffin in Europe) and applying gently rolling pressure to the abdomen with a blunt instrument, such as a round-bodied pencil.

Surgery on insects has also been performed over the years, particularly in research laboratories. A whole range of experimental scientific procedures has been described, including gonadectomy and implantation of various materials. In veterinary clinical medicine, surgical techniques are still used very infrequently. Nevertheless, with appropriate anesthesia, a variety of surgical tasks can be attempted, including limb amputation, lesion removal, and wound suturing or repair. Dehydration is always a threat when the chitinous exoskeleton is breached, and insects should therefore receive fluids (see this chapter's appendix) before and after surgery.

Treatment Protocols and Formulary

Treatment of insects by using medical compounds is possible, but there is very little scientific information on its usefulness or safety. Most of the available data relate to the honeybee (*Apis mellifera*), and such work has resulted in a certain amount of information about the efficacy of treatment with antibiotics, antimycotics, and acaricides. Some examples are presented in the Formulary (Table 14.5). Resistance to standard treatments can be a problem in apicultural medicine—for instance, the resistant *Varroa* mites that are now threatening colonies of bees in Britain (Vidal, 2003)—and has to be borne in mind whenever insects are treated.

Because so few agents are licensed for invertebrates, care must always be taken in their use. Before using a medicine, it is wise to consult the literature, speak to the manufacturer, and discuss the proposed treatment with experienced colleagues. When a colony of insects is involved, it is also sensible to consider first treating a small number of animals, as a pilot study, before embarking on therapy for the whole group.

All findings and results relating to attempted treatment of insects should be recorded and the information published or disseminated to interested parties. Much remains to be learned, and learning more depends on the sharing of experiences.

Although a few of the agents are licensed for use in insects, mainly honeybees, in Europe and elsewhere, the vast majority have no product license. Care must therefore be taken in their use. No liability is taken by the author, the editor, or the publisher for any adverse reactions that may occur as a result of trying the agents listed in this appendix.

The methods of medication and disinfection/fumigation used by apiarists can sometimes be applied to other species. A useful guide is the book by Bailey (1981). It should be noted that beekeepers are not keen to treat their bees unnecessarily, because of the effects that drugs might have on honey and other products. Nevertheless, the experience gained by such people is worthy of note and some methods of therapy show ingenuity (Rendall, 1996).

As an example, the methods of administering medication to honeybees to treat *Varroa* mite infestation are many and varied, and include (in addition to standard treatment with pyrethroids) the following:

1. The use of fine powders, such as talc, which stick to the feet of parasites and cause them to lose their grip from the bee host and fall off. This method, it is claimed, can eliminate up to 90% of the mites (Rendall, 1996).
2. Mixing fat (lard) with sugar that is put out to attract the bees. After feeding, bees groom and, as a result, fat is spread over their bodies. This appears to deter parasitic mites or to make it less easy for them to hold on to their hosts.
3. Spraying of lactic acid (15%) onto combs and bees. This again can kill up to 90% of the mites. In Germany, formic acid has been used with similar success.
4. Mechanical control. *Varroa jacobsoni* selectively enters the drone brood cells rather than the worker cells. If the drone brood cells are killed—usually by removing the comb and freezing it or washing it with cold water—many of the mites are killed.

It will be apparent from the foregoing that *external* application of medicinal agents to insects often presents few problems—so long as it is not toxic if subsequently ingested or if it comes into contact with, for example, thin-skinned larvae. Oral and systemic administration can be more problematic.

Some agents that can be used in insects are listed in Table 14.5.

The Future

Invertebrate medicine is a new discipline that presents a challenge to veterinarians and to others who have a concern for the health, welfare, and conservation of these animals.

The publication of this book is a significant step forward, but the truth is that there remains a paucity of literature in the veterinary press about insects and other invertebrate animals. As a result, access to information remains a barrier to the proper development of invertebrate medicine. Obtaining access to published data on insects is a problem, even for entomologists, and prompted the organization, in October 2000, of the first international conference on the subject, entitled *Insect Information: From Linnaeus to the Internet*. The gathering, hosted by the Royal Entomological Society and the Natural History Museum, London, was convened by the Entomology Libraries and Information Network (ELIN): their and other valuable Web sites are listed under the section on Web Sites Relating to Insects.

The Veterinary Invertebrate Society (VIS), based in Great Britain, possibly the first organization of its kind, has a small but active membership. Articles in its newsletter cover various aspects of the health and disease of invertebrates, and the publication is therefore of great value to those veterinarians and others who deal with these species. Such people should also consider joining entomological societies to learn more about the biology and natural history of these animals. Success in managing and treating invertebrates is facilitated by knowing how they live in the wild.

Jean-Henri Fabre, the 19th-century French entomologist and author of *Souvenirs Entomologiques*, often considered to be the father of entomology, was described by Charles Darwin as the "incomparable observer." This was a fitting description of a man who spent so much of his life studying the world of insects. Fabre's writings illustrate the empathy that he felt with invertebrate animals, and, as a result, he was better able to interpret their biology and lifestyle. A similar approach is needed by those veterinarians and others who work with these fascinating creatures.

Web Sites Relating to Insects

ELIN—http://www.nhm.ac.uk/hosted_sites/elin

The USDA Animal Welfare Center, Care and Use of Invertebrates—http://www. nal.usda.gov/awic/pubs/invertebrates.htm

The Royal Entomological Society—http://www.royensoc.co.uk

The Entomology Department, The Natural History Museum—http://www.nhm.ac.uk/researach-curation/departments/entomology/

Table 14.5.   Formulary

Type	Name	Comment
Fluids	Water Hypotonic saline (0.2%–0.5%)	Administer by mouth, by nebulization or, with caution, intracoelomically. Do not use saline in phasmids, as their body fluids contain potassium, not sodium, ions (Stonehouse, 2003).
Sulfonamides	Sulfadiazine	Sulfonamides have been used orally for some decades, e.g., in bees (Bailey, 1981), in grasshoppers (Henry, 1968) and, more recently, in crickets (Callis and Zwart, 1999). Oral.
Antibiotics	Chlortetracycline Oxytetracycline	Often reported as safe, and possibly efficacious orally and topically. For long, used in bees (Bailey, 1981). Beware of toxicity. Oral or topical.
Laxatives	Mineral oil (liquid paraffin, Europe)	Administer by mouth. Gives feces an oily appearance.
Antimycotics	Povidone–iodine	Paint on surface.
	Ketoconazole or nystatin	Dust or spray (Chitty, 2000).
	Fumagillin	Fed to bees but also used safely in lepidopterous larvae; sprayed on to foliage (Rivers, 1991).
Antiprotozoals	Benomyl	Incorporated into diet of Lepidoptera or used as a spray (Rivers, 1991). Avoid insecticidal overdosage.
Antiseptics/disinfectants	Povidone–iodine, hypochlorite, and others	Apply to surface with care (see Chitty, 2000, and Rivers, 1991). Caution may be needed if there are surface ectosymbionts that are beneficial to the host (antibiosis) (Schabel, 1978).
Repair materials	Cyanoacrylate or Talc Icing sugar Various adhesive tapes	For damaged (split) exoskeleton (Cooper, 1999).

References

Abraham EG, Nagaraju J, Salunke D, Gupta HM, and Datta RK (1995). Purification and partial characterization of an induced antibacterial protein in the silkworm *Bombyx mori*. Journal of Invertebrate Pathology 65:17–24.

Bailey L (1981). Honey Bee Pathology. Academic, New York, 124 pp.

Barnes RSK, Calow P, Olive PJW, Golding DW, and Spicer JI. (2001). The Invertebrates: A Synthesis, 3rd edition. Blackwell Science, Oxford, 497 pp.

Bassi A (1835). Del mal del sengno, calcinaccio o moscardino, malatti ache affigge i bachi de seta e sul modo di liberarne le bigattaie anche le piu infestate. Part 1: Teoria. Orcesi, Lodi, Italy.

Beavis IC (1988). Insects and Other Invertebrates in Classical Antiquity. Exeter University Publications, Exeter, UK.

Benz G (1963). Genetic diseases and aberrations. In: Steinhaus EA, ed. Insect Pathology: An Advanced Treatise, volume 2. Academic, New York.

Betts AD (1934). The Diseases of Bees: Their Signs, Causes and Treatment. Privately published, UK.

Blum MS (1981). Chemical Defenses of Arthropods. Academic, New York, 562 pp.

Boucias DG and Pendland JC (1999). Principles of Insect Pathology. Kluwer, Dordrecht, The Netherlands.

Brey PT (1994). The impact of stress on insect immunity. Bulletin de l'Institut Pasteur 92:110–118.

Callis H and Zwart P (1999). An outbreak of disease in a colony of crickets *Gryllus assimilis*: Case report. Veterinary Invertebrate Society Newsletter 15:17–20.

Chitty J (2000). Therapeutics of pet invertebrates. Veterinary Invertebrate Society Newsletter 2(16):5–7.

Cooper JE (1980). Invertebrates and invertebrate disease: An introduction for the veterinary surgeon. Journal of Small Animal Practice 21:495–508.

Cooper JE (1993). Skin disease in invertebrates. In: Locke PH, Harvey RG, and Mason IS, eds. Manual of Small Animal Dermatology. British Small Animal Veterinary Association, Cheltenham, UK, pp 198–212.

Cooper JE (1999). Emergency care of invertebrates. Veterinary Clinics of North America: Exotic Animal Practice 1:251–264.

Cooper JE (2001). Invertebrate anesthesia. Veterinary Clinics of North America: Exotic Animal Practice 4:57–67.

Cooper JE (2004). Oncology of invertebrates. Veterinary Clinics of North America: Exotic Animal Practice 7:697–703.

Cooper JE and Cunningham AA (1991). Pathological investigation of captive invertebrates. International Zoo Yearbook 30:137–143.

Cooper JE, Pearce-Kelly P, and Williams DL, eds (1992). Arachnida. Chiron, Keighley, UK.

Davies RR, Chitty JR, and Saunders RA (2000). Cardiovascular monitoring of an *Achatina* snail with a Doppler ultrasound probe. In: Proceedings of British Veterinary Zoological Society Conference. BVZS, London.

Ermin R (1939). Uber bau und Funktion der Lymphocyten bei Insekten (*Periplaneta americana* L.). Zeitschrift für Zellforschung und Mikroskopische Anatomie 29:613–669.

Frye FL (1986). Care and feeding of invertebrates as pets or study animals. In: Fowler ME, ed. Zoo and Wild Animal Medicine, 2nd edition. WB Saunders, Philadelphia.

Frye FL (1992). Captive Invertebrates: A Guide to Their Biology and Husbandry. Krieger, Malabar, FL, 136 pp.

Furlong MJ and Groden E (2003). Starvation induced stress and the susceptibility of the Colorado potato beetle, *Leptinotarsa decemlineata* to infection by *Beauveria bassiana*. Journal of Invertebrate Pathology 83:127–138.

Fuxa JR and Tanada Y, eds (1987). Epizootiology of Insect Diseases. John Wiley and Sons, New York, 555 pp.

Gateff E (1977). The genetics and epigenetics of neoplasms in *Drosophila*. Biological Reviews of the Cambridge Philosophical Society 53:123–168.

Gilbert LI and Miller TA, eds (1988). Immunological Techniques in Insect Biology. Springer-Verlag, New York.

Gillott C (1980). Entomology. Plenum, New York, 727 pp.

Gupta AP, ed (1980). Insect Hemocytes. Cambridge University Press, Cambridge, MA.

Gupta AP (1989). Insect host immune system and endocytobionts: Their avoidance strategies. In: Schwemnler W and Gassnre G, eds. Insect Endocytobiosis, Morphology, Physiology, Genetics, Evolution. CRC, Boca Raton, FL.

Hackendahl N and Mashima TY (2002). Considerations in aquatic invertebrate euthanasia. In: Proceedings of the American Association of Zoo Veterinarians, pp 324–329.

Harshbarger JC (1974). Radiation, neoplasms, carcinogenic chemicals and insects. In: Cantwell GE, ed. Insect Diseases. Marcel Dekker, New York.

Henry JE (1968). *Malameba locustae* and its antibiotic control in grasshopper cultures. Journal of Invertebrate Pathology 11:224–233.

Hunter-Jones P (1966). Rearing and Breeding Locusts in the Laboratory. Anti-Locust Research Centre (Ministry of Overseas Development), London.

Lacey LA, ed (1997). Manual of Techniques in Insect Pathology. Academic, San Diego, 409 pp.

Lacey LA and Kaya HK (2000). Field Manual of Techniques in Invertebrate Pathology. Kluwer, Dordrecht, The Netherlands.

Leong KLH, Kaya HK, Yoshimura MA, and Frey DF (1992). The occurrence and effect of a protozoan parasite *Ophryocystis elektroscirrha* (Neogregarinida: Ophryocystidae) on overwintering monarch butterflies *Danaus plexippus* (Lepidoptera: Danaidae) from two California winter sites. Ecological Entomology 17:338–342.

Losey JE, Raynor LS, and Cater ME (1999). Transgenic pollen harms monarch larvae. Nature 399:214.

Mason IL, ed (1984). Evolution of Domesticated Animals. Longman, New York, 452 pp.

Matz G (1969). Manifestations inflammatoires at tumorales chez les orthopteres. Annales de Zoologie Ecologie Animale 1:4–65

Matz G (1975). Les tumeurs chez les Insects. Comptes Rendus des Séances de la Société de Biologie et de ses Filiales 169(Suppl 3):784–787.

Matz G (1996). Cancérologie comparée. La Santé en Pays de la Loire 39:35–37.

Metchnikoff E (1892). Lecons sur la Pathologic Comparée de L. Inflammation. Paris.

National Federation of Zoos (1990). Euthanasia of Invertebrates. Codes of Practice for the Care of Invertebrates in Captivity: 2. National Federation of Zoological Gardens of Great Britain and Ireland, London.

Olney PJS and Ellis P, eds (1991). International Zoo Yearbook, volume 30. Zoological Society of London, London.

Pasteur L (1870). Études sur la Maladie des Vers à Soie, volumes 1 and 2. Gauthier-Villars, Paris.

Pearse V, Pearse J, Buchsbaum M, and Buchsbaum R (1987). Living Invertebrates. Blackwell Scientific, Palo Alto, CA, 848 pp.

Pinches M (2003). Non-infectious diseases of invertebrates. UKVet 8(7):1–4.

Rendall G (1996). The world of the bee. Veterinary Invertebrate Society Newsletter 10:5–6.

Rivers CF (1991). The control of diseases in insect cultures. International Zoo Year Book 30:131–137.

Ruppert EE, Fox RS, and Barnes RD (2004). Invertebrate Zoology: A Functional Evolutionary Approach, 7th edition. Brooks/Cole—Thomson Learning, Belmont, CA, 963 pp.

Salt G (1970). The Cellular Defence Reactions of Insects (Cambridge Monographs in Experimental Biology, volume 16.) Cambridge University Press, Cambridge, MA, 118 pp.

Schabel HG (1978). Percutaneous infection of *Hylobius pales* by *Metarhizium anisopliae*. Journal of Invetebrate Pathology 31:180–187.

Schneider M and Dorn A (2001). Differential infectivity of two *Pseudomonas* species and the immune response in the milkweed bug, *Oncopeltus fasciatus* (Insecta: Hemiptera). Journal of Invertebrate Pathology 78:135–140.

Singh P and Moore RF, eds (1985). Handbook of Insect Rearing, volumes 1 and 2. Elsevier, Amsterdam.

Sparks AK (1972). Invertebrate Pathology: Noncommunicable Diseases. Academic, New York, 387 pp.

Steinhaus EA (1949). Principles of Insect Pathology. McGraw-Hill, New York.

Steinhaus EA, ed (1963). Insect Pathology: An Advanced Treatise. Academic, New York.

Stonehouse J (2003). Hexapod. Antenna 27:341–342.

Sutcliffe DQ (1963). The chemical composition of the haemolymph in insects and some other invertebrates in relation to their phylogeny. Comparative Biochemistry and Physiology 9:121–135.

Tanada Y and Kaya HK (1993). Insect Pathology. Academic, New York, 666 pp.

Tsang KR and Brooks MA (1980). Neoplasias caused by cultured insect cells. In: Kurstak E, Maramorosch K, and Dubendorfer A, eds. Invertebrate Systems In Vitro. Elsevier/North-Holland Biomedical, Amsterdam.

Van Emden H (2003). Twenty-six years without plant food: An aphid still going strong. Antenna 27:95–98.

Vidal J (2003). "Apian Aids" threatens bees. Guardian Weekly, 8–14 May, p 19.

Weiser J (1977). An Atlas of Insect Diseases. Dr W Junk, The Hague.

Wheeler Q and Blackwell M, eds (1984). Fungus–Insect Relationships: Perspectives in Ecology and Evolution. Columbia University Press, New York, 514 pp.

Williams DL (1999). Sample taking in invertebrate veterinary medicine. Veterinary Clinics of North America: Exotic Animal Practice 2:777–801.

Williams DL (2002). Invertebrates. In: Meredith A and Redrobe S, eds. Manual of Exotic Pets. British Small Animal Veterinary Association, Gloucester.

Williams DL (2003). Oral biology and disease in invertebrates. Veterinary Clinics of North America: Exotic Animal Practice 6:459–465.

World Society for the Protection of Animals (WSPA) (1994). Pain Assessment and Euthanasia of Ectotherms. Scientific Advisory Panel Report 09/90, revised 02/94. WSPA, London.

Further Reading

Bellas PE (1982). Insects as a Cause of Inhalant Allergy: A Bibliography. Report no. 25. CSIRO, Hobart, Australia.

Charles J-F, Delécluse A, and Nielsen-Le Roux C, eds (2000). Entomopathogenic Bacteria: From Laboratory to Field Application. Kluwer, Dordrecht, The Netherlands.

Cooper JE (1986a). Veterinary work with invertebrates: A new challenge for the profession. In: Scott PW and Greenwood AG, eds. Exotic Animals in the 80s: Proceedings of the 25th Anniversary Conference of the British Veterinary Zoological Society Conference. BVZS, London.

Cooper JE (1986b). Captive-breeding of invertebrates. International Zoo Yearbook 24/25:74–76.

Chapter 15

NEMATODES

Michael S. Bodri

Natural History and Taxonomy

The most numerous of the multicellular organisms, almost 500,000 species of nematodes are known worldwide (Platt et al., 1984; Giblin-Davis, 2000), with estimates of up to 100 million species (Dorris et al., 1999). The bulk of information about the phylum Nematoda is concerned with the thousands of parasitic species and the free-living *Caenorhabditis elegans*. It is believed that nematodes originated in freshwater and migrated and colonized saltwater and terrestrial habitats. Of the free-living species, they occur in widely differing habitats, including pools of polar ice, hot springs, marine waters, and the bottoms of beer-fermenting vats, as well as soils and detritus of all types. They are the most highly ecologically and physiologically adaptable metazoans.

The typical nematode is bilaterally symmetrical, elongated, and tapered at both ends, although the head is somewhat bluntly rounded or truncate and has a terminal mouth (Figures 15.1–15.3). A slitlike anus is subterminal at the posterior tip, which generally tapers to a point. Nematodes are more or less circular in cross section. Coloration may range from colorless to blackish, with most species translucent, their color imparted by the gut contents and intestinal cell inclusions. The cuticle is variously marked, sculptured, or scaly, usually in a transverse pattern that may be difficult to detect. Markings and ornamentations include shallow punctuations, deeper pores, and spines (*setae*). Transverse striations may consist of fine lines or rows of dots to prominent grooves, rows of dots, or scalelike folds. In some species, both sexes possess longitudinal striations or long, low, keel-like wings (*alae*) that extend the entire length of the worm and may assist in its stiffening. Longitudinal ridges, whose pattern is called the *synlophe*, may aid in locomotion. Cervical alae, if present, are found on the anterior end of the animal. Some males may have a caudal bursa, composed of two or more alae, on the end of the tail. Setae, sometimes present on the anterior end, are elongated projections of the cuticle.

Nematodes have both males and females known for most species, with syngamic reproduction. In many species, though, males are rare or unknown, and reproduction is usually parthenogenic. In dioecious forms, females are generally larger; in addition, the sexes can generally be distinguished by male sexual characteristics. The males tend to have a more coiled tail than do females, as well as bursae, alae, or papillae.

The different sexes find each other by chemotactic and thigmotactic means. Pheromones have been shown for 40 species (MacKinnon, 1987; Haseeb and Fried, 1988). Thigmotaxis, assisted by papillae, facilitates copulation. Females often seek the more coiled posterior of the male. The vulva is detected by the caudal papillae of the male, who then extrudes a pair of sclerotized copulatory spicules from the cloaca through the anus. The spicules are innervated, and the sensory nature likely enables entry into the female reproductive system without damage to the tissues. Once inserted into the vulva, the spicules hold the vulva open so that sperm are more easily propelled into the vagina against the high hydrostatic pressure present in the female.

Reproduction is by the production of eggs that are often highly resistant to desiccation (for periods of up to 20 years) and temperature extremes. Eggs can be transported by animals or carried on air currents. Larvae and adults of many soil-dwelling species may also survive times of desiccation by entering a state of developmental arrest, or *hypobiosis*. If conditions are unfavorable, special third-stage juveniles called *dauer juveniles* are produced that require a more or less specific stimulus for resumption of development.

Most nematodes reproduce by means of eggs, but there are viviparous and ovoviviparous species. Eggs are laid following fertilization in the upper end of the uterus. The shell, which is formed in the lower uterus, consists of an outer vitelline layer, a chitinous layer, and an inner lipid layer. The chitinous layer provides structural support while the lipid layer confers resistance to desiccation and penetration of water-soluble substances. Embryonation and hatching occur in as little as a few hours to a few weeks. Newly hatched young are miniature adults, with the exception of the reproductive system and specializations, such as the lips surrounding the mouth, the pharynx, and the esophagus. With the exception of germinal cells, the nuclei of all other cells cease to divide. Termed *nuclear constancy* or *eutely*, all adult cells are present at hatching, and growth, with few exceptions, occurs by cell enlargement rather than cell division. Cellular numbers within a species are fairly constant, and this constancy has been exploited in *C. elegans*, where all the cells have been identified and mapped.

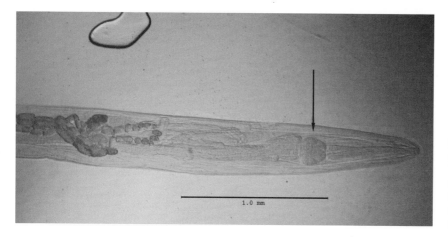

Figure 15.1. Photomicrograph of the anterior end of *Enterobius* sp., a typical nematode. The *arrow* indicates the spherical bulb of the esophagus immediately anterior to its junction with the intestine. The nerve ring, or circumesophageal commissure, is evident as a constriction anterior to the bulb.

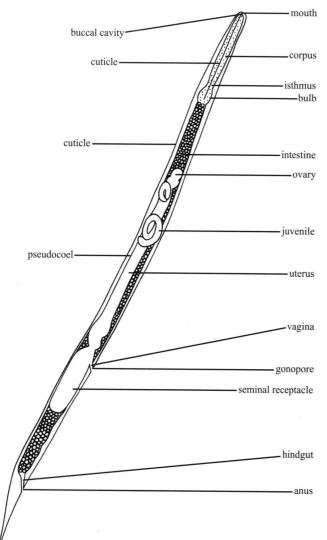

Figure 15.2. This drawing indicates the key anatomical features of a female *Cephalobus* sp. Reproduced from Richard Fox, Lander University, by Alison Schroeer.

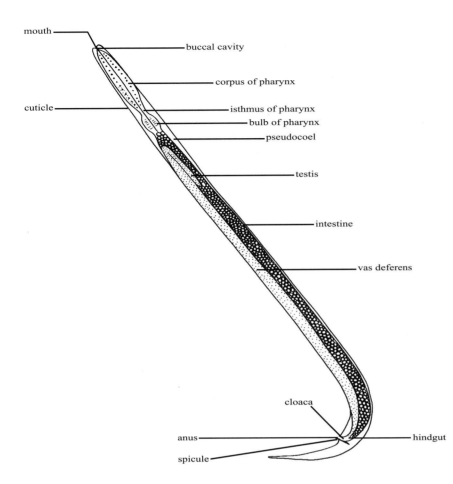

mouth

buccal cavity

corpus of pharynx

cuticle

isthmus of pharynx

bulb of pharynx

pseudocoel

testis

intestine

vas deferens

cloaca

anus

hindgut

spicule

Figure 15.3. This drawing indicates the key anatomical features of a male *Cephalobus* sp. Reproduced from Richard Fox, Lander University, by Alison Schroeer.

The developmental cycle of nematodes is punctuated by a series of four molts (five instars) of the cuticle. Molting involves the loss of the external cuticle and the cuticular lining of the pharynx, esophagus, vulva, and rectum. Molting is critical in parasitic nematodes because it provides the opportunity for the worms to alter the characteristics of the cuticle and thus interact more appropriately with a new or changing environment and to accommodate growth (Davey, 1982). *Molting* involves two physiologically distinct processes: *cuticle formation*, during which new cuticle is laid down beneath the existing cuticle, and *ecdysis*, where the old cuticle is shed and the new cuticle exposed to the environment. Synthesis, transport, secretion, and organization of precursors into a new cuticle and loss of the old cuticle constitute a *molt* (Bonner et al., 1976).

Because of the similar punctuated development of insects and nematodes through a series of molts to the adult stage, it has been postulated that molting in nematodes may also be influenced or even controlled by insect juvenile hormone (JH) and α-ecdysone, the insect molting hormone (Rogers, 1973; M.S.B., unpublished doctoral dissertation). Rodgers (1973) demonstrated that extracts from nematodes showed the activity of JH and had molt-promoting activity in insects. Ecdysteroids have been detected and characterized in nematodes (Dennis, 1977; Mendis et al., 1983; Bottjer et al., 1984; Fleming, 1985; Cleator et al., 1987). Both free and conjugated ecdysteroids occur in nematodes. Davey (1971) showed that farnesyl methyl

ether and synthetic JH inhibit ecdysis but leave cuticle formation unaffected in vitro in *Pseudoterranova (Phocanema) decipiens*. Similarly, under in vitro conditions not conducive to molting for *P. decipiens* (i.e., 0.9% NaCl), addition of either compound stimulated ecdysis. Examination of neurosecretory activity indicated a stimulatory effect on the presumptive neuroendocrine system by the two compounds.

Secondary sex characters become apparent after the penultimate or last molt. Longevity information about free-living nematodes is lacking, but males are believed to be much shorter-lived than females. In *C. elegans*, reduction of male life span is caused by additional sperm production, contradicting the biological assumption that large oocytes are much costlier to produce than are small sperm (Van Voorhies, 1992). Extension of life span in *C. elegans* (by mutation of a single gene) has been shown to reduce fitness, validating the pleiotropy theory of aging (Walker et al., 2000).

Feeding by free-living nematodes exploits many different food habits. Some species feed only on dead plant material, whereas others feed only on dead animal material. Detritus feeders will consume both dead plant and dead animal material. Herbivores have modifications that enable biting and chewing of living plant tissues or possess a rigid hollow stylet that pierces plant cells. Cytoplasm is sucked into the intestine by the pumping action of the muscular pharynx. Predaceous and carnivorous species also have anatomical modifications that assist in feeding. The lips may be modified for seizing or tearing of prey. The pharynx, often equipped with onchia or rasps for crushing, rasping, or macerating, may be partially eversible. Many carnivorous nematodes have a hollow stylet that is used to feed upon protozoa, metazoa, and other nematodes.

The phylogeny of nematodes is unclear because they lack clearly homologous characters, convergent morphological evolution is extensive, and there is no fossil record. The phylum Nematoda is a modification of Rudolphi's Nematoidea and was originally used to categorize worms within the class Nemathelminthes, phylum Vermes (Roberts and Janovy, 2000). The Nematoda can be distinguished from other pseudocoelomate groups by their spicules and a ventral excretory pore.

Classification has been based on morphological and ecological traits. A framework based on analysis of full-length small subunit rDNA sequences has elucidated the relationships between major taxa (Aboobaker and Blaxter, 2000). Nematodes and arthropods are considered sister taxa in a clade of molting animals: the Ecdysoxoa (Aguinaldo et al., 1997). Traditionally, taxonomists have divided the group into two classes: The Secernentea are predominantly terrestrial parasitic and free-living groups containing nine orders, five of which are exclusively animal parasites; whereas the Adenophorea include a wide range of marine, freshwater, and soil nematodes, relatively few of which are parasites of animals and plants, and contain eight orders. The adenophoreans traditionally included the following orders: Chromadorida (including Plectidae), Monohysterida, Enoplida, Monochida, Triplonchida, Dorylaimida, Trichocephalida, and Mermithida. The secernentean orders were postulated to be derived from the adenophoreans, but now, based on the molecular data, it is likely that the Adenophorea is monophyletic, and the secernentean Rhabditida paraphyletic. The secernenteans traditionally included the orders Tylenchida, Aphelenchida, Diplogasterida, Rhabditida, Oxyurida, Rhigonematida, Ascaridida, Spirurida, and Strongylida. The taxonomic traits used for classification are the buccal and pharyngeal structure, cuticle, lip region, intestine, reproductive system, sense organs, and tail. Life-history traits have also been used.

Based on small subunit ribosomal DNA analysis (SSU rDNA) (Blaxter et al., 1998; Dorris et al., 1999), it is obvious that the Nematoda will be in a taxonomic state of flux for quite some time. It is likely that groups will need to be reexamined in light of the molecular evidence for convergence, with the probability of five major clades, with animal parasitism arising independently at least six times and plant parasitism three times (Dorris et al., 1999). The likely framework recognizes two purely adenophorean clades, clade I including the Monochida (free living), Mermithida (insect parasites), Dorylaimida (Longidoridae) (plant parasites), and Trichocephalida (vertebrate parasites). Clade II includes the Triplonchida (plant parasites) and Enoplida (free living). In standard taxonomic works, the Triplonchida was linked with the Dorylaimida as sister taxa.

Clade III recognizes the Ascaridida (large gut roundworms), Rhigonematida (millipede gut parasites), Spirurida (filarial nematodes), and Oxyurida (pinworms). Between clade II and III are the Monohysterida and Chromadorida. The Chromadorida are a large and diverse group of microbivorous nematodes, a

family of which, the Plectidae, may be the group from which the secernentean radiation began.

Clade IV includes the plant parasitic tylenechidans, the Aphelenchida (vertebrate and insect parasites), and four subgroupings of the Rhabditida: the Cephalobidae (bacterivores), Steinernematidae, Panagrolaimidae (bacterivores), and Strongyloidae. The Rhabditida are again represented in clade V by the Rhabditoidea, which include *C. elegans*, the Diplogasteridae, and the Strongylida (small gut and insect parasites):

Order Chromadorida: These nematodes are found in marine and brackish water and freshwater, and are also encountered in marshy and moist soils.

Order Monohysterida: These marine nematodes are found in freshwater and brackish water and wet soil.

Order Enoplida: These marine nematodes are found in freshwater and brackish water and wet to dry soils.

Order Monochida: These soil nematodes are well adapted as predators, with large buccal cavities armed with a large tooth and, sometimes, a subventral denticulate ridge.

Order Triplonchida: These plant-feeding nematodes are important because they are vectors of viral diseases. They possess a movable tooth (onchiostyle) important in their classification.

Order Dorylaimida: Some are plant parasites, whereas others are animal parasites, predatory, or free living.

Order Trichocephalida: This order contains the well-known vertebrate parasitic genera *Trichinella* and *Trichuris*.

Order Mermithida: The juvenile stages are infective to a variety of invertebrates, where they are parasites of the body cavities.

Order Tylenchida: These nematodes are primarily plant and, to a lesser extent, insect parasites. Insects are often used as phoretic hosts. Others are fungus feeders, predatory, and free living. These nematodes have a buccal stylet.

Order Aphelenchida: These nematodes are plant parasites, fungus feeders, insect parasites, predatory, and free living.

Order Diplogasterida: These nematodes are characterized by movable teeth in the stoma. They are predatory, omnivores, bacterivores, and fungus feeders. They are also insect associates.

Order Rhabditida: These small nematodes possess six lips. Many are free living, with some group members parasitic in the lungs of amphibians and reptiles, or the intestinal tract of amphibians, reptiles, birds, and mammals.

Order Oxyurida: As the common name pinworm implies, these parasites are sharply pointed at the posterior end. They parasitize the colon or rectum of invertebrates and vertebrates.

Order Rhigonematida: These millipede gut parasites infect the posterior gut.

Order Ascaridida: These parasitic nematodes have a variable life cycle, with direct or indirect development and invertebrate or vertebrate intermediate hosts. These nematodes usually have three prominent lips.

Order Spirurida: These parasitic nematodes require an invertebrate for development from the L1 to L3. Adults parasitize the intestine or blood and cutaneous and subcutaneous tissues, and lymphatic system, of all vertebrate classes.

Order Strongylida: Long and slender, these worms have free-living larvae, or the L1, L2, and L3 stages are parasitic in invertebrates. The adults are parasitic in all classes of vertebrates.

Anatomy and Physiology

Much of our discussion of nematode anatomy in this chapter is based on *C. elegans*. The anatomy of *C. elegans* is well known, consisting of 959 somatic cells in hermaphrodites (1031 in males), including neuronal cells (302, representing 118 different subtypes), 111 muscle cells, 213 epidermal cells, and 34 intestinal cells (Aboobaker and Blaxter, 2000). Molecular techniques, as well as forward and reverse genetics enabling investigation of gene function, coupled with the intimate understanding of the animal's cell cycle, have contributed greatly to the understanding of nematode molecular, physiological, and developmental mechanisms.

Two concentric tubes separated by a fluid-filled space, the pseudocoelom, constitute the basic nematode body plan. The body shape is maintained by internal hydrostatic pressure. The body cavity, which is derived from the embryonic blastocoel, is termed the pseudocoel. The inner tube is composed of a muscular pharynx with a reradiate lumen, its autonomous nervous system, and the intestine. In males, the digestive system opens into a cloaca, as does the reproductive system. Females have a ventral genital pore as the termination of their reproductive system. The secretory–excretory system varies throughout the phylum and may be lacking entirely in some genera. All the muscles are longitudinally arranged and are a single layer in thickness. A noncellular collagenous cuticle, secreted by the underlying hypodermis, covers the body.

Body Wall

A barrier between the environment and the nematode, the cuticle is a multilayered extracellular structure secreted by the underlying hypodermis. Most nematodes have a surface coat, external to the cuticle, that may act as its protective layer (Nowell et al., 1997). This epicuticle is an electron-dense multilaminate layer whose lipid-rich structure is environmentally dependent.

Three regions may be distinguished within the cuticle: the cortical, median, and basal zones. The individual zones, however, are difficult to distinguish. Cuticlin, a highly resistant protein, is the primary component of the cortical zone. The median zone is primarily composed of collagen, as is the basal zone. Within the basal zone, the collagen is arranged in 2–3 layers of parallel strands that run at an angle of 75° to the longitudinal axis of the worm. A latticelike arrangement of the collagen is the result of the middle layer lying at an angle of 135° to those of the first layer. The collagen is the primary component of the hydrostatic skeleton. A basement membrane merges the cuticle with the underlying hypodermis. The cuticle lines the mouth, esophagus, posterior intestinal tract, and vulva.

The hypodermis is a syncytial tissue responsible for the secretion of the cuticle. In *C. elegans*, the hypodermis (subcuticle) consists of four longitudinal ridges (dorsal, ventral, and left and right lateral), the hypodermal cords, joined circumferentially by thin sheets of cytoplasm that separate the muscle cells from the cuticle (Nelson and Riddle, 1984). In other species, there may be 6–8 thickened portions. These cords protrude inward and divide the musculature into quadrants. Longitudinal nerve trunks lie within the dorsal and ventral cords, whereas the lateral cords contain excretory canals.

Muscles

The body musculature is arranged in four longitudinal strips. *Muscle cells* are usually long and spindle shaped with a contractile portion and a noncontractile cell body, or *myocyton*. They contain numerous ribbon-shaped muscle fibrils that either lie at the base of the cell, adjacent to the hypodermis, or extend up the sides of the cells, partially enclosing the sarcoplasm (Pennak, 1978). *Platymyarian cells* are wide and shallow with the contractile portion close to the hypodermis. *Coelomyarian cells* are the typical spindle shape with the contractile portion in the form of a U and the distal end of the U placed against the hypodermis. These cells are important in glycogen storage. Other body-wall muscles include *circomyarian cells*. In these, the sarcomeres form a system of continuous peripheral helices and resemble striated muscle (Restelli et al., 2002). The contractile fibrils at the periphery completely encircle the myocyton in circomyarian cells (Roberts and Janovy, 2000).

The hydrostatic skeleton is a result of the nematode pseudocoel. The body wall and muscles enclose the fluid-filled pseudocoel, which is derived from the blastocoel. Because it lacks a mesodermal lining, as in cavities formed within the endomesoderm, the pseudocoel is not a true coelom. Hydrostatic pressure within the pseudocoel is high. The incompressibility of the fluid (*hemolymph*) within this space, the ability of the muscles to apply pressure to the fluid, and the transmission of the pressure in all directions as a result of compression create a hydrostatic skeleton. Hemolymph, in addition to being structurally important, is also involved in transport of solutes. Nematode muscles act against the stretching and compression of the cuticle and do not change in length or diameter.

The muscle strips are attached to the cuticle by means of a thin layer of hypodermis. Sinusoidal movements in the dorsoventral plane are generated by contraction of the two subventral muscle strips with relaxation of the subdorsal strips. Contraction of the muscles compresses the cuticle on that side, with transmission of the force through the fluid of the pseudocoel to the other side of the nematode, where the cuticle stretches. Movement is achieved by alternate relaxation and contraction of these muscle strips, with forward propulsion of the animal lying on its side. Coordination of contraction is influenced by the unique innervation of the muscle cells. Processes run from the myocytons to the nerves, and the muscle cells themselves may have numerous muscle–muscle connections between the innervation processes.

Digestive System

The primitive form of nematode lips is six, surrounding the mouth. Each lip has a small papilla on its summit. Fusion of the lips in pairs is common, but some species lack lips entirely. Two lateral lips may develop as new structures derived from the inner margin of the mouth. The lips may be variously modified for sucking, gripping, or ripping or form toothlike odontia.

The mouth is circular or triangular and may be capable of great distension. It opens into the buccal cavity, which is lined with cuticle that may be quite thick, forming a rigid structure termed the *buccal capsule*. The buccal cavity may be cylindrical, subglobular, cup shaped, conoid, inconspicuous, or even absent. The walls are often supplied with stiffening rods or plates, and rasps and teeth (*onchia*) are common.

Food moves from the buccal cavity into the esophagus or pharynx. The esophagus is circular in cross section, lined with cuticle, composed primarily of radial muscle fibers, and has a small triquetrous cavity (Pennak, 1978). In some species, it is supplied with a solid or hollow protrusable stylet. The muscular pharynx may be elongated, plain, and cylindrical, but more commonly has one or two ellipsoid or spherical bulbar swellings. Placement of a single bulb is at the posterior end of the esophagus and is termed *cardiac*. If present, the second, or middle bulb is located near midlength.

The pharynx is both suctorial and peristaltic and functions in pumping food into the intestine. The pumping action is necessary to overcome the high pressure in the surrounding pseudocoel. Suspended bacteria and organic molecules are drawn into the esophagus of bacteria-feeding nematodes by pharyngeal pumping. Hydrostatic pressure closes the mouth and esophageal lumen when the muscles relax. Esophageal valves may be present in the posterior bulb to prevent regurgitation. The structure of the alimentary system suggests that rhabditids feed nonselectively, whereas members of the cephalobids may use probolae to restrict the size of food entering the buccal cavity. The second bulb has the additional function of grinding food. Once ingested, bacteria are crushed by cuticularized plates in the posterior pharyngeal bulb.

Three unicellular salivary glands, whose ducts open into the lumen of the esophagus or buccal cavity, are embedded in the esophageal wall. Digestive enzymes secreted in the pharynx and intestine assist in the digestion of lipids, carbohydrates, and fats (Venette and Ferris, 1998).

The pharynx, which contains its own nervous system of 20 neurons (in *C. elegans*), is isolated from the rest of the worm by a basal lamina. A pair of extrapharyngeal neurons form the only anatomical connection between the pharyngeal nervous system and extrapharyngeal nervous system (Avery and Horvitz, 1990).

Consisting of a single layer of simple columnar epithelial cells, the intestine extends from the esophagus to rectum. There may be an obscure valvular apparatus at the junction of esophagus and intestine, as well as a comparable structure between the intestine and rectum. It is a simple tubelike structure that may have a flimsy covering of connective tissue or muscle fibers. In males, the rectum terminates in a cloaca, as it also receives the products of the reproductive system. The dorsal wall is invaginated into two spicule sheaths containing the copulatory spicules. Females have a short cuticle-lined rectum that terminates in the anus.

The central lumen of the intestine is surrounded by intestinal cells. Ingesta are moved by the pumping action of the esophagus as it adds more food to the front end of the system. The inner surface is lined with a layer of rodlike outgrowths or microvilli, constituting the brush border (Pennak, 1978). The cells sit on a basement membrane that randomly attaches to extensions of the body-wall musculature. Some digestion takes place in the anterior portion, but the primary function of the intestine is absorption and excretion of nitrogenous and water-soluble wastes. The thin-walled intestine with its brush border makes up in efficiency of absorption what it lacks in digestive capability.

Nervous System

The nervous system of nematodes is quite simple and consists of only a few hundred neurons, allowing for at least three sensory responses: chemical, mechanical, and thermal (Ward et al., 1975). Consisting almost entirely of fibers from associated ganglia, the circumpharyngeal or circumesophageal nerve ring is the most prominent feature of the nematode nervous system. The ring contains 2–4 large associative cells and paired lateral ganglia, paired ventral ganglia, and the unpaired dorsal ganglion (Davey, 1966). Two amphidial nerves leave the lateral ganglia to innervate the *amphids*. Cell bodies of most neurons are positioned around the pharynx, with their cell processes forming a ring around the basement membrane that surrounds the pharynx. Chemosensory and mechanosensory neurons extend afferent processes as six small papillary nerves from the region of the nerve ring to the cephalic sensory papillae surrounding the mouth. Nerve processes, four or more longitudinal nerves, may also be extended along the body within the hypodermal cords to the tail. Numerous ganglia, particularly of the ventral nerve trunk, and branch nerves connecting the longitudinal nerves with one another are found posterior to the nerve ring. Reception and integration of sensory input occur within the nerve ring, with subsequent relay of signals to motor neurons in the head or along the nerve cords. Those that are not involved in the ring formation join the dorsal or ventral nerve cords. The ventral nerve trunk terminates in the pre-anal ganglion. Two branches from the pre-anal ganglion encircle the rectum as the posterior nerve ring, or *rectal commissure*. Other cell bodies are positioned along the ventral midline and in the tail.

Paired ocelli—small clumps of reddish, violet, or blackish granules embedded in the esophagus or between the esophagus and body wall—are present in some species (Pennak, 1978). A lenslike device might be present in front of the pigment clumps. There is some controversy regarding the innervation, or lack thereof, between the eyespots and the nervous system.

The innervation of nematode *sensilla* is similar within the phylum, with the number of neurons in each type of sensillum varying by species. The six inner labial sensilla, each associated with a lip, contain nerve endings from two neurons, one of which is exposed to the exterior (Davis et al., 1986). The cephalic papillae and setae, as well as the caudal setae, are considered tactile receptors. Somatic setae, present between the anterior and posterior ends, are also tactile.

Containing nine sensory neurons, the amphids are blind, pouchlike invaginations in the cuticle located in the head region, whose sensory receptors connect to the circumpharyngeal nerve ring via their axons (McLaren, 1972; Albert and Riddle, 1983; Haseeb and Fried, 1988). An amphid is located on each of the two lateral lips. The amphidial openings may have the shape of a narrow slit, an oval, a circle, or spiral ridges and grooves and are in direct contact with the environment. At the base of the pouch is a nerve bulb with several nerve processes. In *C. elegans*, the two amphids each contain the endings of 12 neurons, eight appearing to be exposed to the external environment (Davis et al., 1986). The sensory endings are modified cilia that extend into the amphidial channel; one is very short. The supporting or sheath cell is highly vacuolated (McLaren, 1972). The amphidial sheath cell in *C. elegans* contains a large Golgi apparatus that presumably produces and stores secretions in vesicles within these cells (Ward et al., 1975). Although amphids are considered chemoreceptors, these neurons stain prominently with paraldehyde fuchsin or chrome–hematoxylin, the histological basis for their classification as neurosecretory in nature (Ewen, 1962; Davey, 1988).

Deirids (cervical papillae), which are located at the level of the nerve ring, are cuticular modifications that are sensory in nature. Other sensory papillae occur at various levels along the body of many species. Caudal papillae, particularly elaborate in males, assist in proper alignment during copulation.

At the posterior end of many nematodes are a pair of cuticle-lined organs: the *phasmids*. Phasmids, similar to the amphids, contain the nerve endings from two neurons, both of which are exposed to the external environment (Davis et al., 1986). The sensory nerve endings are a modified cilium extending into a receptor cavity that opens to the outside at the ampulla. They are considered chemoreceptors.

Dendritic nerve endings are also located within body pores, which are filled with glycoprotein exudates produced in gland cells (Aumann, 1993).

Secretory–Excretory System

There is little evidence to support the role of the excretory system in the elimination of wastes. In some species, there is a complete lack of an excretory system, with waste products being eliminated through the digestive system. At its simplest, there is a single ventral excretory cell, the *renette*, which opens through the excretory pore on the midventral line at the level of the esophagus by way of a short to long duct (Pennak, 1978). In most nematodes, the excretory system is composed of only a few cells. The form of the excretory system is typically that of long excretory canals joined to a sinus located at the origin of the duct, which leads to the exterior of the body. A gland may be associated with the duct. Studies in a number of species, including parasitic worms, have demonstrated its involvement in

excretion of waste products, osmoregulation, and release of molting enzymes (Nelson and Riddle, 1984). In *C. elegans*, the secretory–excretory system is comprised of four cells. The cell bodies are located near the ventral side of the pharynx. The excretory canals are formed from bilateral processes from large, H-shaped excretory cells, extend anteriorly and posteriorly the length of the worm, and are connected to an excretory pore on the ventral side of the head. Extensive gap junctions form with the hypodermis, and the excretory canals are exposed to the pseudocoelom for much of their length. An *excretory sinus*, a system of small channels joining the lumena of the four excretory canals with the origin of the excretory duct, is contained within the cell body. A duct cell surrounds the duct. The plasma membrane of the duct cell and a collagenous cuticular wall line the excretory duct, becoming continuous with the cuticle at the excretory pore. At the terminus of the duct cell is a pore cell, enclosing the terminal one-third of the duct. Synaptic input occurs via an A-shaped, excretory gland cell, which has the appearance of two lateral, nucleated cell bodies just below the level of the pharynx that forms anterior processes that join at the level of the circumpharyngeal nerve ring. The processes also join across the anterior edge of the excretory cell body. A tight junction surrounds the origin of the excretory duct, involving the gland cell, duct cell, and excretory cell. Destruction of the pore cell, duct cell, or excretory cell will cause *C. elegans* to die due to water accumulation. Osmoregulation and secretion of glycoproteins occur through the action of the excretory cell, the largest cell in the body.

Reproductive System

Nematodes may be monoecious or dioecious, with the majority dioecious. Parthenogenesis can also occur in a number of species. The reproductive systems of free-living nematodes tend to be simpler and less extensive than those of parasitic species.

The gonads are solid cords of cells continuous with the ducts. *Telogonic* gonads have germ cell proliferation at the inner end of the gonad only. Germ cell proliferation along the entire length of the gonad is termed *hologonic*. Telogonic testes are divided into three zones. Spermatogonial divisions take place within the germinal zone at the terminal end. A maturation or growth zone occupies the middle region, whereas the seminal vesicle or storage zone terminates at the vas deferens. The female reproductive tracts of most nematodes are telogonic. The proximal end is the germinal zone, which produces oogonia, which become oocytes and move into the growth zone of the ovary. Oocytes leave the ovary to enter the oviduct, where fertilization occurs.

The genital pore or vulva of the female is a transverse slit on the ventral midline located anywhere from the mouth to immediately in front of the anus, but most commonly near the middle of the body. A short muscular vagina may connect with a single thin-walled, tapering reproductive tubule or, more typically, to a branched system with one anterior and one posterior tubule (Pennak, 1978). Each tubule consists of a uterus, an oviduct, and an ovary containing small oocytes. Depending on the species, some females have up to six ovaries. The uterus may have an associated seminal receptacle. Tubules may be reflexed or outstretched, presenting four possible configurations: double and outstretched, double and reflexed, single and outstretched, or single and reflexed (Pennak, 1978). The reproductive tract is divided roughly into developmental, storage, and ejective areas. Eggs move down the ovary to the proximal end of the oviduct, the *spermatheca*, where fertilization takes place. Shell formation commences after fertilization and meiosis. Eggs are moved through the uterus by contraction of well-developed circular and diagonal muscles. Egg shape is influenced by the uterus, and additional materials may be added to the shells by uterine secretory cells. The distal end of the uterus is muscular and constitutes an ovijector (Roberts and Janovy, 2000). The ovijectors fuse to form the vagina, which opens into the vulva. The vagina and vulva control egg release. When the muscles of the vulva dilate the opening, constriction of the circular muscles of the ovijectors expels the eggs while retaining more proximal, undeveloped eggs.

A single tapering tubule is typical of males, with the paired condition likely plesiomorphic. From the ventral opening in the cloaca, the tubule consists of a long vas deferens, short seminal vesicle, and thin testis. The vas deferens is divided into an anterior glandular region and a posterior muscular region, the *ejaculatory duct*. The testis may be bifurcated or reflexed. Ejaculatory glands may open into the basal part of the vas deferens. These glands secrete a hard brown material that plugs the vulva after copulation. Some males may have a copulatory bursa. This clasping device consists of two thin transparent longitudinal flaps of cuticle near the posterior end. Widest opposite the anus, it may be long enough to encompass the posterior tip of the worm (Pennak, 1978).

Hermaphroditic nematodes have functionally independent anterior and posterior arms of the reproductive system.

Environmental Disorders and Preventive Medicine

Temperature fundamentally affects the physiological processes and population dynamics of most nematodes (Venette and Ferris, 1997). Thermal optima exist for metabolism, embryogenesis, egg hatching, growth, and activity. Population growth rates of bacterial-feeding nematodes change in a species-specific manner with changes in temperature.

Temperature can affect nematodes directly or indirectly. Indirect effects are generally by the action of temperature on food source, decreasing food supply and increasing numbers of males. Increased temperatures may directly affect worms by interfering with sexual differentiation (Hansen and Hansen, 1988).

The life span of *C. elegans* is rigidly determined by somatic cells and markedly influenced by the effects of temperature on the cells during the postmitotic state (Hosono et al., 1982). High temperatures during the growing phase or shortly after the adult phase cause an earlier start to the dying phase, whereas an increase in population half-life results with downward temperatures during the adult phase.

Microwave radiation (750 MHz, 0.5 W) can induce both a heat-shock response and enhanced growth in *C. elegans* through one or more nonthermal routes (De Pomerai et al., 2000).

Most free-living nematodes can attenuate the ultraviolet (UV) effects of sunlight by avoidance behaviors, including burrowing into the ground or moving into the shade. Solar UV radiation induces a fluence-dependent reduction in fertility in *C. elegans* (Mills and Hartman, 1998). Longer wavelengths (in the UVA region) interact to promote lethality.

Caenorhabditis elegans have a wide tolerance range for pH, salinity, and hardness in aquatic media (Khanna et al., 1997). With changes in pH, the chemical form of compounds can change, resulting in toxicants. *Caenorhabditis elegans* can withstand a pH range of 3.2–11.8, depending on the media. Toxicity is attributed to H^+ and OH^-. Osmotic stress induced by NaCl and KCl at greater than 20 ppt causes mortality in *C. elegans*. Alkalinity, induced into culture systems with $NaHCO_3$, is tolerated up to 0.236–0.241 g/L.

All nematodes require periods of aerobic respiration to complete their life cycle (Van Voorhies and Ward, 2000). *Caenorhabditis elegans* maintains a constant metabolic rate until a lower critical oxygen tension is reached. At that time, it reduces its metabolic rate. Under hypoxic conditions, a relatively high metabolic rate may be maintained by the location of metabolically active tissue closer to the cuticular surface, by movement of air through the digestive tract, or by the increase of mixing rates in the pseudocoelomic fluid by use of locomotory movements. Many nematodes contain oxygen-transport pigments, although these pigments may have evolved to prevent oxygen from reaching cells rather than as a mechanism to supply oxygen to cells. Prolonged anaerobic conditions will cause death.

Many stressors—including alcohols (methanol and ethanol), heavy metals (cadmium and mercury), sulfhydryl-reactive compounds (the phthalimide fungicide captan and diamide), and salicylate—inhibit *C. elegans* feeding, as determined by a decrease in pharyngeal pumping. This response may be an important survival mechanism that limits the intake of toxic solutes (Jones and Candido, 1999). Heavy metals interfere with nutrient uptake and assimilation in *C. elegans*.

Volatile fatty acids produced by soil bacteria are toxic for nematodes. Formic, acetic, propionic, and butyric acids readily immobilize nematodes in their undissociated states (Sayre and Starr, 1988). Hydrogen sulfide is also a potent nematicide. Ammonifying bacteria active in decomposition of plant residues can also influence soil nematode populations.

Secondary metabolites from the soil-inhabiting fungi *Arthrobotrys conoides*, *Nematoctonus robustus*, *Hohenbuehelia* sp., *Chlorosplenium* sp., *Neobulgaria pura*, *Daldinia concentrica*, and *Lachnum papyraceum* have nematicidal activity (Anke et al., 1995).

Streptomyces griseus-derived faeriefungin, a polyol polyene macrolide lactone antibiotic, has nematicidal properties. Fractionation and purification enable isolation of aromatic nitro compounds and griseulin, with concentrations of 0.1–1.0 μg/mL fatal within 24 h (Nair et al., 1995).

Pleurotus ostreatus and *P. pulmonarius* are nematode-feeding fungi that produce tiny droplets of toxin—*trans*-2-decenedioic acid in *P. ostreatus* and lineolic and *S*-corioloc acid in *P. pulmonarius*—from minute spatulate secretory cells, immobilizing 95% of *Panagrellus redivivus* within 1 h at 300 ppm. Death is likely due to increased membrane permeability, with leakage of the cytoplasm (Kwok et al., 1992). *Hericium coralloides, H. abietis,* and *H. ramosum* also produce fatty-acid mixtures (Anke et al., 1995). *Irpex lacteus* forms three nematicidal metabolites (Anke et al., 1995).

Infectious Diseases

Viruses

Hess and Poinar (1988) report a single case of a biochemically characterized virus (iridovirus) in the mermithid nematode *Thaumamermis cosgroveri*, a parasite of terrestrial isopods. The virus was found to infect the host, as well as the nematode. Nematodes, particularly plant parasitic species, are well-known vectors of virus, with associations that are transient to persistent. Plant viruses are not found within the tissues of nematode vectors. Free-living nematodes have been found harboring replicating virus within their intestinal lumen but not within their tissues (Hess and Poinar, 1988). The nematode cuticle likely acts as an effective barrier against viral infection.

Bacteria

The association of bacteria and nematodes is frequently a coincidental observation or an intentional exposure in an attempt to model infectious mechanisms. *Caenorhabditis elegans* is not known to be infected naturally by bacterial pathogens (Finlay, 1999). It does, however, have both amoebapore-like and defensin-like antimicrobial peptides (Mallo et al., 2002). A slow-growing Gram-positive rod bacterium of the coryneform genus, *Microbacterium nematophilum*, adheres to the surface of the rectum and post-anal region of *C. elegans*. It induces swelling of the hypodermal tissue but does not invade across the cuticle. The swelling interferes with defecation, causing constipation and a slower growth rate. The infection is likely responsible for the Dar phenotype in some isolates (Hodgkin et al., 2000). This may be the only case of naturally occurring infection in a free-living nematode.

Pseudomonas strains may be highly nematicidal (Sayre and Starr, 1988). *Pseudomonas aeruginosa* fed to *C. elegans* is fatal (Dvorak, 1994; Strauss, 2000; Hendrickson et al., 2001). Pyocyanin, the blue redox-active phenazine pigment, is an important toxin mediating the killing process and may kill through the generation of active oxygen species (Hendrickson et al., 2001; O'Quinn et al., 2001). Hydrogen cyanide may be the sole or primary toxic factor that is responsible for the killing via the inhibition of mitochondrial cytochrome oxidase (Gallagher and Manoil, 2001). Specific virulence factors produced by the bacterium include adhesions (e.g., pili and filamentous hemagglutinin), protein toxins (e.g., phospholipase, proteases, and ADP-ribosylating enzymes), and small-molecule poisons (e.g., phenazines, rhamnolipid biosurfactant, and cyanide) (Gallagher and Manoil, 2001). Worms fed toxic strains lose pharyngeal pumping ability within minutes after placement on dense lawns; defecation and egg laying cease. Locomotion becomes sluggish and is sometimes accompanied by spasmodic twitching. Almost all worms are paralyzed within 4 h of exposure and exhibit a kinked tail and blunted nose indicating a hypercontraction of the body-wall muscles. The speed of the lethal effect suggests a diffusible chemical (Darby et al., 1999).

Serratia marcescens is also toxic to *C. elegans* (Dvorak, 1994). *Serratia marcescens* are found intact in the intestinal lumen within 6 h after feeding, resulting in a progressive outward distension of the lumen. This is followed by a progressive destruction of the intestinal epithelium and of the germ line, accompanied by a decrease in egg production. Death begins in 72 h (Mallo et al., 2002).

An intoxication mechanism, possibly a disruption of normal Ca^{2-} signal transduction by *Burkholderia thailandensis* and some strains of *B. cepacia*, kills *C. elegans* (O'Quinn et al., 2001). Both the body-wall muscles and neuromuscular junction are targeted with a toxin-mediated inability to restore Ca^{2+} membrane potentials. The condition is characterized by rapid onset of lethargy with decreased locomotion, cessation of pharyngeal pumping, and inhibition of egg laying.

Salmonella typhimurium, and *S. enterica* serovars including *S. enteritidis* and *S. dublin,* when fed to *C. elegans* accumulate in the intestinal lumen, with death occurring over several days. The motility of the worms and rate of pharyngeal pumping decline until the worms become immobile and die. The lumen of the intestine distends within 2 days of feeding. Worms ingesting a low initial dose become chronically infected due to proliferation of the bacterium in the intestine until it reaches a high enough titer to be fatal (Aballay et al., 2000). Few bacteria pass the terminal bulb of the pharynx during the first day of contact. Marked decrease in the volume of the intestinal cells is coincident with an increase in the number of bacteria seen in the intestinal lumen. The cells of the terminal bulb of the pharynx are progressively destroyed at the same time. As little as 8 h of contact with the bacteria is sufficient for reduced survival (Labrousse et al., 2000).

Bacillus thuringiensis have nematicidal strains. The toxicity is temperature dependent, with no toxicity below 16°C (maximal, 25°C). Toxicity is also pH sensitive. The nematicidal factor is internalized into the intestinal cells (Borgonie et al., 1996).

Aeromonas hydrophila is also reportedly toxic to *C. elegans* (Dvorak, 1994).

Protozoa

Most protozoan parasites of nematodes are associated with animal or plant parasitic species (Poinar and Hess, 1988). Most reports are descriptive and preclude the identification or placement in a systematic category. Several sporozoans in the genus *Dubosqia* have been identified from various free-living freshwater species of nematode. Sporozoans may kill their host or, at low infection rates, castrate the worm. A *Pleistophora* sp. has been presumptively identified from the free-living marine nematode *Metoncholaimus scissus* (Hopper et al., 1970).

A *Mononchus composticola* female isolated from leaf litter in New Zealand was found to be infected by the coccidian *Legerella helminthorum*. This parasite was restricted to invasion of the intestinal cells, where schizogony was observed. *Adelea* spp. are also reported from a number of nematode genera, including *Actinolaimus*, *Cephalobus*, *Dorylaimus*, *Trilobus*, and *Tripyla*, primarily within the body cavity (Poinar and Hess, 1988). Stylet-feeding nematodes would be immune to infection if ingestion were required for infection. Most infections by protozoa are associated with relatively long-lived nematode species in freshwater and moist soil habitats. Amoebic infections of the gut wall or body cavity have been recorded for *Archromadora* sp., *Chromadora* sp., *Dorylaimus* spp., *Monhystera* spp., *Paraphanolaimus* sp., *Trilobus* spp., *Tripyla* sp., and *Tylenchus* spp. Flagellates are also reported from a number of genera, including *Chromadora* sp., *Diplogaster* spp., and *Trilobus* sp. (Poinar and Hess, 1988).

Neoplasia

There are no reports of neoplasia in nematodes.

Miscellaneous Disorders

Nutritional Disorders

Nutritional diseases are observed in free-living nematodes as a retardation of the normal life cycle. This is complicated by the production of dauer juveniles, which are normally produced under adverse environmental conditions (e.g., food deficiency and dense populations). If nutritionally deficient, worms may be less robust. Failure to reach sexual maturity is the most sensitive aspect of the life cycle, due to nutritional deprivation (Hansen and Hansen, 1988). This is most easily recognized by an absence of progeny. The decrease in progeny is due to individual fitness changes, as well as a decrease in the number of females producing progeny. Males often become more predominant in populations under restricted nutritional conditions.

Metabolic Disorders

Metabolic diseases or disease conditions have been observed by the incorporation of inhibitors into culture media. Many inhibitors have been tested, are dose dependent, and generally act to inhibit growth and inhibit sexual maturity, as well as decrease fecundity. Compounds tested include actidione, actinomycin D, acriflavin, aminopterin, azaserine, azasteroid, 5-bromouracil, hydroxyurea, γ-glutamyl hydrazone, mitomycin, and puromycin (Hansen and Hansen, 1988). The worms themselves may produce inhibitory materials as waste products, in particular, ammonia. Dense populations may become sluggish with decreased motility. Bacterial products including organic acids, phenols, methane, and hydrogen sulfide may be inhibitory to nematodes.

Genetic Disorders

Genetic diseases are primarily caused by recessive mutations in genes coding for proteins essential for normal growth and development. The genome of *C. elegans* has been sequenced, and ongoing work with this animal has resulted in a plethora of aberrant phenotypes that can be considered genetic disorders (a discussion of the many forms is beyond the scope of this review). Many of these mutations are the direct result of chemical mutagenesis, most commonly the DNA-alkylating agent ethylmethane sulfonate (Edgar, 1988). Naturally occurring mutants in *C. elegans* are infrequent because of facultative hermaphroditism encouraging homozygosity. The mutant phenotypes of *C. elegans* have been classified by Edgar (1988) as aberrant morphology, aberrant behavior, aberrant development, and others.

Predation

In soil, the largest group of natural enemies of nematodes are nematophagous fungi, with over 24 species observed to subsist on free-living species (Drechsler, 1940). Fungi are classified as either endoparasitic or predatory. Endoparasites exist in the environment as small infective conidia or zoospores, which infect nematodes by adhering to the surface of the worm. Zoospores are free-swimming flagellate spores that swim toward nematodes and encyst on their surface near an orifice, followed by penetration. Zoospores find their host by following the chemical gradient formed by nematode exudates. Predatory fungi produce hyphal systems that produce trapping devices along the hyphae. In both instances, fungal hyphae develop within the nematode, and the body contents are assimilated by the fungus.

The endoparasitic fungus *Verticillium balanoides* infects nematodes (*Panagrellus redivivus*) by means of adhesive conidia, which stick by means of a trilayered adhesive pad located at the apical end of the conidia. Adhesion is random on the surface of the nematode, with subsequent growth of an appressorium through the adhesive pad, establishing firm contact between the fungal cell wall and nematode cuticle. Hyphal outgrowth on the appressorium is followed by the formation of an infection bulb. Trophic hyphae develop from this bulb and invade the nematode. Numerous conidia are produced by externally developing conidiophores (Sjollema et al., 1993).

Drechmeria coniospora infects by means of clavate conidia, which adhere by means of sticky knobs at their apical end. Adherence is preferential for the chemosensory structures of the head of males, females, and juveniles and the tail of male *P. redivivus*. An appressorium is formed on the adhesive knob, from which a penetrating germ tube emerges. Trophic hyphae colonize the nematode body, and conidiophores are formed outside the body that produce conidia (Jansson, 1993; Sjollema et al., 1993). Invasion is by means of the pseudocoel, with no penetration of the internal organs (Dijksterhuis et al., 1991).

Harposporium microsporum infects *Rhabditis* spp. The method of infection is unknown but is attributed to microconidia rather than macroconidia (Glockling and Dick, 1994). Assimilative hyphae fill the body and then produce protruding conidiophores, which bear microconidia or narrow, curved conidia.

Nematode-destroying fungi may form traps that ensnare nematodes. Capture is followed by paralysis caused by toxins. *Arthrobotrys oligospora* (penetration due to enzymatic weakening and exertion of mechanical force), *Dactylaria pyriformis*, and *D. thaumasia*, *Monacrosporium* sp., *Nematoctonus haptocladus*, and *N. concurrens* all produce traps and toxins (Kwok et al., 1992).

Arthrobotrys oligospora and *A. superba* form adhesive network traps, whereas *A. dactyloides* forms constrictive ring traps (Jansson et al., 2000). *Arthrobotrys dactyloides* captures nematodes when they enter the constricting ring and, by touching the inner surface, trigger the trap cells to swell. Nematophagous fungi tend to be nonselective in regard to prey preference; the work by Jansson et al. (2000) used laboratory cultures of *P. redivivus* and *Meloidogyne* spp.

Fungivorous Collembola (sprintails), in particular *Folsomia candida*, may preferentially feed on free-living nematodes, as demonstrated by Lee and Widden (1996), who used a wild strain of bacterivorous nematode isolated from Norway spruce litter and *C. elegans*. *Isotoma* sp. have also been observed ingesting nematodes of an unidentified species (Brown, 1954).

Some species of soil mites feed on nematodes. Protonymphs and deuteronymphs of *Macrocheles muscaeidomesticae* feed preferentially on nematodes, as does the oribatid mite *Pergalumna* sp., feeding on *Pelodera lambdiensis* and *Tylenchorhynchus martini*. The neostigmatid mite *Lasioseius scapulatus* feeds on *Aphelenchus avenae* and *Cephalobus* sp. The sarcoptiform mite *Tyrophagus putrescentiae* has been observed feeding on *Rhabditis* sp., *Cephalobus* sp., *Hirschmanniella oryzae*, and *Tylenchorhynchus mashhoodi* (Bilgrami and Tahseen, 1992).

Anesthesia, Analgesia, and Surgery

Nematodes have determinate cleavage, precluding any possibility of epimorphic regeneration. Coupled with the hydrostatic skeleton, surgery is risky and limited to microinjection techniques.

A great number of anesthetic protocols have been developed for working with nematodes, as an adjunct to surgical manipulation or simply to assist in observation and sorting of material. The worms can be straightened when chilled at 4°C for 30–60 min (Nelson and Riddle, 1984). A stream of carbon dioxide (CO_2) blown over *C. elegans*, a technique widely used for invertebrates such as insects, has an anesthetic effect, with worms ceasing movement almost immediately and recovering within a few seconds after removal from the CO_2 source.

Caenorhabditis elegans can also be anesthetized in 0.1% tricaine and 0.01% tetramisole in N buffer (100 mM NaCl, 25 mM potassium phosphate, pH 6.0) or with sodium azide at 100 μg/mL in N buffer or cold N buffer saturated with CO_2. Sodium azide and CO_2-treated nematodes recover within 30–90 min (Davis et al., 1986).

Homologous series of n-alkanes (C5–C9) and primary alcohols (C1–C9) have anesthetic potencies in *C. elegans* directly related to their relative lipid solubility, with alcohols much more potent than alkanes, even though the alkanes are much more lipid soluble (Anton et al., 1992). Ethanol at a concentration of 4.5% causes a reversible cessation of movement in *C. elegans* (Jones and Candido, 1999).

Caenorhabditis elegans is a good model for the study of volatile anesthetics because it responds to them in a manner similar to all other species, including humans. A typical anesthetic chamber consists of a flat glass Pyrex dish, covered with a ground-glass lid and sealed with C-clamps. Steel needles are fitted through a hole in the side of the dish—one for injection of anesthetic and the second for sampling atmospheric concentrations of anesthetic, if necessary (Morgan and Cascorbi, 1985). Volatile anesthetic-induced immobility in *C. elegans* is totally reversible and correlates closely with loss of response to a noxious stimulus. At low doses, the worms become excited, moving more than animals not similarly exposed. As the concentration increases, the worms become uncoordinated and, at the highest concentrations, are immobilized. When removed from the anesthetic, they quickly resume normal behavior. ED_{50} values (effective dose where the concentration of anesthetic is expressed as % volume [vol %] at standard temperature and pressure in air and 50% of the animals were immobile for longer than 10 s) for nine agents are as follows: trimethoxyflurane, 0.10–0.11; methoxyflurane, 0.45–0.58; chloroform, 1.25–1.63; halothane, 2.7–3.28; enflurane, 4.2–6.05; isoflurane, 5.6–7.18; diethyl ether, 4.8–7.5; fluroxene, 8.8–10.8; and flurothyl, 8.1–15.0 (Morgan and Cascorbi, 1985; Morgan et al., 1990). Sensitivity is influenced by a neuronal protein capable of controlling ion flux through a sodium channel crucial in mediating the response of volatile anesthetics (Rajaram et al., 1999). Although it has been postulated that γ-aminobutyric acid (GABA) may contribute to the action of volatile anesthetics because it is a central inhibitory neurotransmitter, GABA by itself does not mediate sensitivity to halothane or enflurane in *C. elegans* (Boswell et al., 1990). Worms typically recover within 3–5 min after removal from the anesthetics. At 2–3 times ED50, exposure to volatile anesthetics is lethal.

Aqueous 1-phenoxy-2-propanol (propylene phenoxetol) has been used as an anesthetic agent and studied in the plant pathogenic nematodes *Panagrellus redivivus*, *P. penetrans*, *Heterodera rostochiensis*, *H. schachtii*, and *H. trifolii*, with specific evaluation of the effect of concentration on anesthesia and revival time, as well as infectivity after anesthesia (Townshend, 1983). Also using a plant parasitic nematode, Riddle and Bird (1985) suspended worms in a 1% aqueous solution and determined that 70–105 min of exposure was necessary for complete anesthesia. Fewer nematodes in Townshend's study (1983) survived the highest concentrations (0.5%), and infective capacity of worms thus exposed was reduced. The ideal concentration was found to be between 0.25% and 0.5%, with immediate removal from the agent once the nematode is anesthetized.

Propylene phenoxetol incorporated into a 5% agar pad at 0.5 μL/mL (for first-stage larvae), 1.5 μL/mL (second-stage larvae), 2.0 μL/mL (third-stage larvae), 4.0 μL/mL (dauer larvae), 2.5 μL/mL (fourth-stage larvae), and 3.0 μL/mL (adult) is effective for the immobilization and anesthesia of *C. elegans* (Nelson and Riddle, 1984). This agent makes the worms permeable to dyes and other chemical agents, possibly due to altered permeability of the body wall.

Microinjection is typically used to transfer foreign DNA into the worm. Injection directly into the gonad cytoplasm with subsequent transformation was first performed by Stinchcomb et al. (1985). For microinjection, an inverted microscope with differential interference contrast (DIC) optics or Hoffman modulation contrast (HMC) optics, coupled with a microinjection controller, are essential. A micropipette puller producing needles with a tip of 1-μm diameter is also essential. A pressure source, typically nitrogen gas, must maintain 30 psi during the injection (Hashmi et al., 1995).

Caenorhabditis elegans are immobilized on dried (2%) agarose pads. Prior to injection, the agarose pads should be spread with halocarbon oil. Injections are typically into the distal arm of each half of the gonad. Rehydration of the animals with a high-viscosity recovery buffer and M9 salts (3 g KH_2PO_4, 6 g Na_2HPO_4, 5 g NaCl, and 0.25 g $MgSO_4$ per liter of water, pH 7.2) is necessary (McCoubrey et al., 1988). After injection, osmotic strength can be reduced by placing a drop of M9 buffer on the nematode.

Cells are ablated via laser microbeam. Laser ablation is performed with a tunable or flashlamp-pumped dye laser system, with the laser light entering a microscope through the optics via an epifluorescence condenser fitted with a dichroic reflector. Output typically requires about 0.06–0.10 J/pulse at 15–18 kV. Coumarin 2 dye with a 480-nm emission maximum is used at a concentration of 0.23 mM (Nelson and Riddle, 1984). Extreme intensity, leading to a linear, multiphoton process, means no absorbing pigment is necessary (Davis et al., 1986).

Treatment Protocols and Formulary

Anesthetics

Chloroform: 1.25%–1.63% (Morgan and Cascorbi, 1985; Morgan et al., 1990)

Diethyl ether: 4.8%–7.5% (Morgan and Cascorbi, 1985; Morgan et al., 1990)

Enflurane: 4.2%–6.05% (Morgan and Cascorbi, 1985; Morgan et al., 1990)

Ethanol: 4.5% ethanol causes a reversible cessation of movement (Jones and Candido, 1999)

Flurothyl: 8.1%–15.0% (Morgan and Cascorbi, 1985; Morgan et al., 1990)

Fluroxene: 8.8%–10.8% (Morgan and Cascorbi, 1985; Morgan et al., 1990)

Halothane: 2.7%–3.28% (Morgan and Cascorbi, 1985; Morgan et al., 1990)

Isoflurane: 5.6%–7.18% (Morgan and Cascorbi, 1985; Morgan et al., 1990)

Methoxyflurane: 0.45%–0.58% (Morgan and Cascorbi, 1985; Morgan et al., 1990)

Propylene phenoxetol: 0.25%–1.0% aqueous solution (Townshend, 1983; Riddle and Bird, 1985); 0.5–4.0 μL/mL in a 5% agar pad (Nelson and Riddle, 1984)

Sodium azide: Anesthetize with sodium azide 100 mM (Avery and Horvitz, 1990). Larvae and adults can remain in the azide for 2 h without ill-effect. Sodium azide is a mutagen in bacterial, plant, and mammalian cell culture systems.

Tricaine and tetramisole: A 0.1% tricaine and 0.01% tetramisole solution in an appropriate buffer (Davis et al., 1986)

Trimethoxyflurane: 0.10%–0.11% (Morgan and Cascorbi, 1985; Morgan et al., 1990)

Neuroactive Drugs

Gramine: This serotonin antagonist inhibits pumping at 0.01 mg/mL (Avery and Horvitz, 1990).

Imipramine: This stimulates pumping at 20 μg/mL. High concentrations have an anesthetic effect (Avery and Horvitz, 1990).

Ivermectin: This inhibits pumping at 0.05 ng/mL (Avery and Horvitz, 1990).

Muscimol: This GABA agonist inhibits pumping at 2 μg/mL (Avery and Horvitz, 1990).

Serotonin: This stimulates pumping at 1 mg/mL (Avery and Horvitz, 1990).

Miscellaneous

Alkaline bleach: To obtain large quantities of age synchronous adults, dissolve gravid worms with alkaline bleach. Eggs released are allowed to hatch overnight, and in the absence of food all larvae will arrest at the first stage (Braeckman et al., 2000).

5-Fluorodeoxyuridine (FudR): Immature *C. elegans* and *Turbatrix aceti* have been treated with this to preserve the age synchrony of adult populations. Treatment of larvae with this DNA inhibitor causes stunted development and morphological abnormalities. A low level (25 μM) added just before the larvae reach maturity stops reproduction by blocking embryogenesis (Ghandi et al., 1980).

M9 salts buffer: This is 3 g KH_2PO_4, 6 g Na_2HPO_4, 5 g NaCl, and 0.25 g $MgSO_4$ per liter of water, at pH 7.2 (McCoubrey et al., 1988).

N buffer: This is 100 mM NaCl and 25 mM potassium phosphate, at pH 6.0 (Davis et al., 1986).

Vitamin E: At 200 μg/mL, this significantly prolongs the life span of *C. elegans*, *Turbatrix aceti*, and *C. briggsae* when added from hatching to day 3 but reduces fecundity and increases the mean day of reproduction. Although the mechanism of action is not known, life span may increase in part by slowing development (Harrington and Harley, 1988).

References

Aballay A, P Yorgey, and FM Ausubel. 2000. *Salmonella typhimurium* proliferates and establishes a persistent infection in the intestine of *Caenorhabditis elegans*. Curr Biol 10:1539–1542.

Aboobaker AA and MI Blaxter. 2000. Medical significance of *Caenorhabditis elegans*. Ann Med 32:23–30.

Aguinaldo AAM, JM Turbeville, LS Linford, MC Rivera, JR Garey, RA Raff, and JA Lake. 1997. Evidence for a clade of nematodes, arthropods, and other moulting animals. Nature 387:489–493.

Albert PS and DL Riddle. 1983. Developmental alterations in sensory neuroanatomy of the *Caenorhabditis elegans* dauer larva. J Comp Neurol 219:461–481.

Anke H, M Stadler, A Mayer, and O Sterner. 1995. Secondary metabolites with nematicidal and antimicrobial activity from nematophagous fungi and Ascomycetes. Can J Bot 73(Suppl 1):S932–S939.

Anton AH, AI Berk, and CH Nicholls. 1992. The "anesthetic" effect of alcohols and alkanes in *Caenorhabditis elegans* (C.e.). Res Commun Chem Pathol Pharmacol 78:69–83.

Aumann J. 1993. Permeability of chemosensillum-associated exudates for lectins in a plant-parasitic and in a free-living nematode. Fundam Appl Nematol 16:381–384.

Avery L and HR Horvitz. 1990. Effects of starvation and neuroactive drugs on feeding in *Caenorhabditis elegans*. J Exp Zool 253:263–270.

Bilgrami AL and Q Tahseen. 1992. A nematode feeding mite, *Tyrophagus putrescentiae* (Sarcoptiformis: Acaridae). Fundam Appl Nematol 15:477–478.

Blaxter ML, P DeLey, JR Garey, LX Liu, P Scheldeman, A Vierstraete, JR Vanfleteren, LY Mackey, M Dorris, and LM Frisse. 1998. A molecular evolutionary framework for the phylum Nematoda. Nature 392:71–75.

Bonner TP, K Evans, and L Kline. 1976. Cuticle formation in parasitic nematodes: RNA biosynthesis and control of molting. Int J Parasitol 6:473–477.

Borgonie G, M Claeys, F Leyns, G Arnaut, D de Waele, and A Coomans. 1996. Effect of a nematicidal *Bacillus thuringiensis* strain on free-living nematodes. 3. Characterization of the intoxication process. Fundam Appl Nematol 19:523–528.

Boswell MV, PG Morgan, and MM Sedensky. 1990. Interaction of GABA and volatile anesthetics in the nematode *Caenorhabditis elegans*. FASEB J 4:2506–2510.

Bottjer KP, LR Whisenton, and PP Weinstein. 1984. Ecdysteroid-like substances in *Nippostrongylus brasiliensis*. J Parasitol 70:986–987.

Braeckman BP, K Houthoofd, and JR Vanfleteren. 2000. Patterns of metabolic activity during aging of the wild type and longevity mutants of *Caenorhabditis elegans*. Age 23:55–73.

Brown WL. 1954. Collembola feeding upon nematodes. Ecology 35:421.

Cleator M, CJ Delves, RE Howles, and HH Rees. 1987. Identity and tissue localization of free and conjugated ecdysteroids in adults of *Dirofilaria immitis* and *Ascaris suum*. Mol Biochem Parasitol 25:93–105.

Darby C, CL Cosma, JH Thomas, and C Manoil. 1999. Lethal paralysis of *Caenorhabditis elegans* by *Pseudomonas aeruginosa*. Proc Natl Acad Sci USA 96:15202–15207.

Davey KG. 1966. Neurosecretion and molting in some parasitic nematodes. Am Zool 6:243–249.

Davey KG. 1971. Molting in a parasitic nematode, *Phocanema decipiens*. VI. The mode of action of insect juvenile hormone and farnesyl methyl ether. Int J Parasitol 1:61–66.

Davey KG. 1982. Growth and molting in nematodes. In: E Meerovitch, ed. Aspects of Parasitology. McGill University, Montreal, pp 58–70.

Davey KG. 1988. Endocrinology of nematodes. In: H Laufer and RGH Downer, eds. Endocrinology of Selected Invertebrate Types. Alan R Liss, New York, pp 63–86.

Davis BO, M Goode, and DB Dusenbery. 1986. Laser microbeam studies of role of amphid receptors in chemosensory behavior of nematode *Caenorhabditis elegans*. J Chem Ecol 12:1339–1347.

Dennis RDW. 1977. On ecdysone-binding proteins and ecdysone-like material in nematodes. Int J Parasitol 7:181–188.

De Pomerai, C Daniells, H David, J Allan, I Duce, M Mutwakil, D Thomas, P Sewell, J Tattersall, D Jones, and P Candido. 2000. Microwave radiation induces a heat-shock response and enhances growth in the nematode *Caenorhabditis elegans*. IEEE Trans Microwave Theory Tech 48:2076–2081.

Dijksterhuis J, W Hrder, U Wyss, and M Veenhuis. 1991. Colonization and digestion of nematodes by the endoparasitic nematophagous fungus *Drechmeria coniospora*. Mycol Res 95:873–878.

Dorris M, P DeLey, and ML Blaxter. 1999. Molecular analysis of nematode diversity and the evolution of parasitism. Parasitol Today 15:188–193.

Drechsler C. 1940. Three fungi destructive to free-living terricolous nematodes. J Wash Acad Sci 30:240–254.

Dvorak TJ. 1994. Bioassay and studies of bacterial pathogens to the free-living nematode *Caenorhabditis elegans*. Unpublished thesis, Graduate College of the University of Nebraska.

Edgar RS. 1988. Genetic diseases. In: GO Poinar Jr and H-H Jansson, eds. Diseases of Nematodes, volume 1. CRC, Boca Raton, FL, pp 35–47.

Ewen AB. 1962. An improved aldehyde fuchsin staining technique for neurosecretory products in insects. Trans Am Microsc Soc 81:94–96.

Finlay BB. 1999. Bacterial disease in diverse hosts. Cell 96:315–318.

Fleming MW. 1985. *Ascaris suum*: Role of ecdysteroids in molting. Exp Parasitol 60:207–210.

Gallagher LA and C Manoil. 2001. *Peudomonas aeruginosa* PAO1 kills *Caenorhabditis elegans* by cyanide poisoning. J Bacteriol 183:6207–6214.

Ghandi S, J Santelli, DH Mitchell, JW Stiles, and DR Sanadi. 1980. A simple method for maintaining large, aging populations of *Caenorhabditis elegans*. Mech Ageing Dev 12:137–150.

Giblin-Davis RM. 2000. Pasteuria sp. for biological control of the sting nematode, *Belonolaimus longicaudatus*, in turfgrass. In: JM Clark and MP Kenna, eds. Fate and Management of Turfgrass Chemicals. (ACS Symposium series 743.) American Chemical Society, Washington, DC, pp 408–442.

Glockling SL and MW Dick. 1994. A new species of *Harposporium* infecting *Rhabditis* nematodes with microspores. Mycol Res 98:854–856.

Hansen EL and JW Hansen. 1988. Nutritional and metabolic diseases. In: GO Poinar Jr and H-H Jansson, eds. Diseases of Nematodes, volume 1. CRC, Boca Raton, FL, pp 23–33.

Harrington LA and CB Harley. 1988. Effect of vitamin E on lifespan and reproduction in *Caenorhabditis elegans*. Mech Ageing Dev 43:71–78.

Haseeb MA and B Fried. 1988. Chemical communication in helminthes. Adv Parasitol 27:169–207.

Hashmi S, G Hashmi, and R Gaugler. 1995. Genetic transformation of an entomopathogenic nematode by microinjection. J Invertebr Pathol 66:293–296.

Hendrickson EL, J Plotnikova, S Mahajan-Miklos, LG Rahme, and FM Ausubel. 2001. Differential roles of the *Pseudomonas aeruginosa* PA14 *rpoN* gene in pathogenicity in plants, nematodes, insects, and mice. J Bacteriol 183:7126–7134.

Hess R and GO Poinar Jr. 1988. Viral diseases. In: GO Poinar Jr and H-H Jansson, eds. Diseases of Nematodes, volume 1. CRC, Boca Raton, FL, pp 51–67.

Hodgkin J, PE Kuwabara, and B Corneliussen. 2000. A novel bacterial pathogen, *Microbacterium nematophilum*, induces morphological change in the nematode *C. elegans*. Curr Biol 10:1615–1618.

Hopper BE, SP Meyers, and R Cefalu. 1970. Microsporidian infection of a marine nematode, *Metoncholaimus scissus*. J Invertebr Pathol 16:371–377.

Hosono R, Y Mitsui, Y Sato, S Aizawa, and J Miwa. 1982. Life span of the wild and mutant nematode *Caenorhabditis elegans*. Exp Gerontol 17:163–172.

Jansson H-B. 1993. Adhesion to nematodes of conidia from the nematophagous fungus *Drechmeria coniospora*. J Gen Microbiol 139:1899–1906.

Jansson H-B, C Persson, and R Odeslius. 2000. Growth and capture of nematophagous fungi in soil visualized by low temperature scanning electron microscopy. Mycologia 92:10–15.

Jones D and EPM Candido. 1999. Feeding is inhibited by sublethal concentrations of toxicants and by heat stress in the nematode *Caenorhabditis elegans*: Relationship to the cellular stress response. J Exp Zool 284:147–157.

Khanna N, CP Cressman III, CP Tatara, and PL Williams. 1997. Tolerance of the nematode *Caenorhabditis elegans* to pH, salinity, and hardness in aquatic media. Arch Environ Contam Toxicol 32:110–114.

Kwok OCH, R Plattner, D Weisleder, and DT Wicklow. 1992. A nematicidal toxin from *Pleurotus ostreatus* NRRL 3526. J Chem Ecol 18:127–136.

Labrousse A, S Chauvet, C Couillault, CL Kurz, and JJ Ewbank. 2000. *Caenorhabditis elegans* is a model host for *Salmonella typhimurium*. Curr Biol 10:1543–1545.

Lee Q and P Widden. 1996. *Folsomia candida*, a "fungivorous" collembolan, feeds preferentially on nematodes rather than soil fungi. Soil Biol Biochem 28:689–690.

MacKinnon BM. 1987. Sex attractants in nematodes. Parasitol Today 3:156–158.

Mallo GV, CL Kurz, C Couillault, N Pujol, S Granjeaud, Y Kohara, and JJ Ewbank. 2002. Inducible antibacterial defense system in *C. elegans*. Curr Biol 12:1209–1214.

McCoubrey WK, KD Nordstrom, and PM Meneely. 1988. Microinjected DNA from the X chromosome affects sex determination in *Caenorhabditis elegans*. Science 242:1146–1151.

McLaren DJ. 1972. Ultrastructural and cytochemical studies on the sensory organelles and nervous system of *Dipetalonema vitae* (Nematoda: Filaroidea). Parasitology 65:507–524.

Mendis AHW, ME Rose, HH Rees, and TW Goodwin. 1983. Ecdysteroids in adults of the nematode, *Dirofilaria immitis*. Mol Biochem Parasitol 9:209–226.

Mills DK and PS Hartman. 1998. Lethal consequences of simulated solar radiation on the nematode *Caenorhabditis elegans* in the presence and absence of photosensitizers. Photochem Photobiol 68:816–823.

Morgan PG and HF Cascorbi. 1985. Effect of anesthetics and a convulsant on normal and mutant *Caenorhabditis elegans*. Anesthesiology 62:738–744.

Morgan PG, M Sedensky and PM Meneely. 1990. Multiple sites of action of volatile anesthetics in *Caenorhabditis elegans*. Proc Natl Acad Sci USA 87:2965–2969.

Nair MG, A Chandra, DL Thorogod, and RMG Davis. 1995. Nematicidal and mosquitocidal aromatic nitro compounds produced by *Streptomyces* spp. Pestic Sci 43:361–365.

Nelson FK and DL Riddle. 1984. Functional study of the *Caenorhabditis elegans* secretory–excretory system using laser microsurgery. J Exp Zool 231:45–56.

Nowell M, A Wardlaw, D de Pomerai, and D Pritchard. 1997. The measurement of immunological stress in nematodes. J Helminthol 71:119–123.

O'Quinn AL, EM Wiegand, and JA Jeddeloh. 2001. *Burkholderia pseudomallei* kills the nematode *Caenorhabditis elegans* using an endotoxin-mediated paralysis. Cell Microbiol 3:381–393.

Pennak RW. 1978. Nematoda (roundworms). In: Freshwater Invertebrates of the United States. John Wiley and Sons, New York, pp 211–230.

Platt H, K Shaw, and P Lambshead. 1984. Nematode species abundance patterns and their use in the detection of environmental perturbations. Hydrobiologia 118:59–66.

Poinar GO Jr and R Hess. 1988. Protozoan diseases. In: GO Poinar Jr and H-H Jansson, eds. Diseases of Nematodes, volume 1. CRC, Boca Raton, FL, pp 103–131.

Rajaram S, TL Spangler, MM Sedensky, and PG Morgan. 1999. A stomatin and a degenerin interact to control anesthetic sensitivity in *Caenorhabditis elegans*. Genetics 153:1673–1682.

Restelli MA, CL de Villalobos, and Z Fernanda. 2002. Ultrastructural description of the musculature, the intraepidermal nervous system, and their interrelation in *Pseudochordodes bedriagae* (Nematomorpha). Cell Tissue Res 308:299–306.

Riddle DL and AF Bird. 1985. Response of *Anguina agrostis* to detergent and anesthetic treatment. J Nematol 17:165–168.

Roberts LS and J Janovy Jr. 2000. Phylum Nematoda: Form, function, and classification. In: Gerald D. Schmidt and Larry S. Roberts' Foundations of Parasitology, 6th edition. McGraw-Hill, New York, pp 355–384.

Rogers WP. 1973. Juvenile and molting hormones from nematodes. Parasitology 67:105–113.

Sayre RM and MP Starr. 1988. Bacterial diseases and antagonisms of nematodes. In: GO Poinar Jr and H-H Jansson, eds. Diseases of Nematodes, volume 1. CRC, Boca Raton, FL, pp 69–101.

Sjollema KA, J Dijksterhuis, M Veenhuis, and W Harder. 1993. An electron microscopical study of the infection of the nematode *Panagrellus redivivus* by the endoparasitic fungus *Verticillium balanoides*. Mycol Res 97:479–484.

Stinchcomb DT, JE Shaw, SH Carr, and D Hirsh. 1985. Extrachromosomal DNA transformation of *Caenorhabditis elegans*. Mol Cell Biol 5:3483–3496.

Strauss E. 2000. Simple hosts may reveal how bacteria infect cells. Science 290:2245–2247.

Townshend JL. 1983. Anesthesia of 3 nematodes species with propylene phenoxetol. Nematologica 29:357–360.

Van Voorhies WA. 1992. Production of sperm reduces nematode lifespan. Nature 360:456–458.

Van Voorhies WA and S Ward. 2000. Broad oxygen tolerances in the nematode *Caenorhabditis elegans*. J Exp Biol 303:2467–2478.

Venette RC and H Ferris. 1997. Thermal constraints to population growth of bacterial-feeding nematodes. Soil Biol Biochem 29:63–74.

Venette RC and H Ferris. 1998. Influence of bacterial type and density on population growth of bacterial-feeding nematodes. Soil Biol Biochem 30:949–960.

Walker DW, G McColl, NL Jenkins, J Harris, and GJ Lithgow. 2000. Evolution of lifespan in *C. elegans*. Nature 405:296–297.

Ward S, N Thomson, JG White, and S Brenner. 1975. Electron microscopical reconstruction of the anterior sensory anatomy of the nematode *Caenorhabditis elegans*. J Comp Neurol 160:313–337.

Chapter 16

CHAETOGNATHS (ARROWWORMS)

Laura Foster

Natural History and Taxonomy

The Arrowworms (phylum Chaetognatha), are an abundant and important component of the zooplankton community. They occupy benthic and planktonic habitats in every ocean. There is even a fully troglobitic species, *Paraspadella anops* (Bowman and Bieri, 1989), as well as a luminescent species, *Caecosagitta macrocephala* (Haddock and Case, 1994). Chaetognaths are ecologically important as carnivorous predators feeding primarily on zooplankton (copepods, crustaceans, appendicularians, fish larvae and even other chaetognaths) (Nagasawa and Marumo, 1976). They, in turn, contribute to the marine food web as valuable prey for fish.

Chaetognaths are hermaphrodites with the male and female gonads located in different regions of the body. Species range in size from about 2 to 120 mm. The majority of chaetognaths are transparent, but some deeper-water species are pigmented blue, brown, orange, or red (Kapp, 1991).

There are about 23 genera and 115 species of chaetognaths recorded, with many more in an unresolved status (Bieri, 1991). There is much debate about their taxonomy as well as their origin and evolutionary development. Future research is needed to resolve some of the taxonomy questions. For now, they are roughly divided into benthic and planktonic groups that are not entirely accurate. The genera *Spadella*, *Paraspadella*, *Bathyspadella*, *Xenokrohnia*, and *Krohnittella* are considered benthic whereas the rest are planktonic (Bieri, 1991; Casanova, 1993a). Some planktonic genera mentioned in this chapter are *Eukrohnia*, *Bathybelos*, *Krohnitta*, *Pterosagitta*, *Sagitta*, *Ferosagitta*, and *Parasagitta*.

Anatomy

Chaetognaths are streamlined and bilaterally symmetrical, with bodies divided into the head, trunk, and tail segments. Chaetognaths are probably best known for their grasping spines (hooks) from which they are named (*chaete*, "spine," and *gnathos*, "jaw") (Kapp, 1991) (Figure 16.1). Other structures at their anterior end include teeth, vestibular organs, and eyes (most species), as well as a ventral mouth. Posteriorly are one or two pairs of lateral fins, as well as a caudal fin (Figure 16.1). Many of these external features are used for taxonomy (e.g., number of hooks or teeth, number of lateral fins, and presence of an eye, as well as the shape and size of the pigment cell in the eye). The internal organs primarily consist of a gut that stretches the length of the body, as well as gonads.

The epidermis is delicate and easily damaged. The epidermis overlying the dorsal head, trunk, tail, and fins is composed of a stratified squamous epithelium unique to invertebrates. The outer layer has a secretory function and continuously produces a coating over the surface of the chaetognath. The function and chemical composition of this secretion have not been explored (Shinn, 1997). The inner layer is separated from the underlying muscles by a basement membrane that prevents physical contact but is permeable to diffusion (Kapp, 1991).

The head contains a set of chitinous lateral and ventral plates that serve as a site for head-muscle attachment (Figure 16.2). The larger lateral plates are positioned dorsolaterally and are bordered by the teeth on their anterior end and the base of the spines on their posterior end. The ventral plates are smaller and more triangular and are located ventral to the base of the spines (Hyman, 1959).

There are pairs of anterior and posterior teeth but not all species have all sets. All known chaetognaths have grasping spines, which are much longer and larger than the teeth, though structurally they are very similar. The core of each is composed of chitin crystallite tubes that contain zinc, whereas the tips are coated in silicon that gives them their hardness (Bone et al., 1983). The spines are used mainly for grasping prey and working it into the mouth, whereas the teeth are possibly used to puncture the prey and allow for tetrodotoxin penetration (Bieri et al., 1983).

A hood with retractor and extensor muscles covers the teeth and spines. The hood covers the head completely, except for a hole located by the mouth, streamlining the body (Kapp, 1991) (Figure 16.3). The hood is an extension of the epidermis on the head and, as such, is composed of stratified squamous epithelium on the dorsal surface, whereas the ventral surface is a simple epidermis. Glandular cells are located on the inner wall of the hood as well as on the head, where the hood attaches. Kapp (1991) presumes that they secrete a lubricant that facilitates the quick retracting of the hood during prey capture.

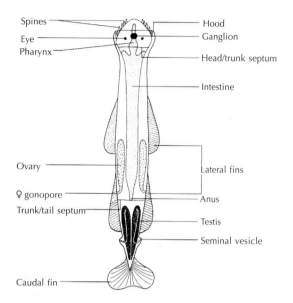

Figure 16.1. Diagram of a representative chaetognath from the dorsal surface illustrating the important anatomical features. From Barnes et al. (2001), Figure 7.1 (p. 147).

Vestibular ridges are located in close proximity to the posterior teeth on the head (Figure 16.3). They contain a row of papillary pores that appear to contain cilia, suggesting a possible chemosensory function (Bone and Pulsford, 1984). Another function suggested by Bieri et al. (1983) and Thuesen and Bieri (1987) is that this is the possible area where toxin is stored or produced to aid in prey capture. Located near the vestibular ridges are vestibular pits comprised of a circular ring of columnar secretory cells whose function is not known (Figure 16.3).

Transvestibular pores that are located on the head of some chaetognaths parallel the vestibular ridge and then spread out laterally toward the base of the grasping spines. Thuesen et al. (1988b) studied 17 species and identified transvestibular pores on 15 of them. The exact pattern of the pores varied not only within the species but also from the right side to the left side of the same individual. Bone and Pulsford (1984) noticed a material located in each and concluded that they contain cilia. The exact function is not clear, though speculation is that they are used as a chemosensory device or possibly to release pheromones used during the mating process (Thuesen et al., 1988b).

Xenokrohnia sorbei, described by Casanova (1993a), was found to have a ventral secretory gland—a new structure not previously seen in chaetognaths (Figure 16.4). This ventral secretory gland is located in the neck region along the gut. Cytological studies show that it is a serous gland rather than a mucous gland and is therefore believed to have a role in feeding.

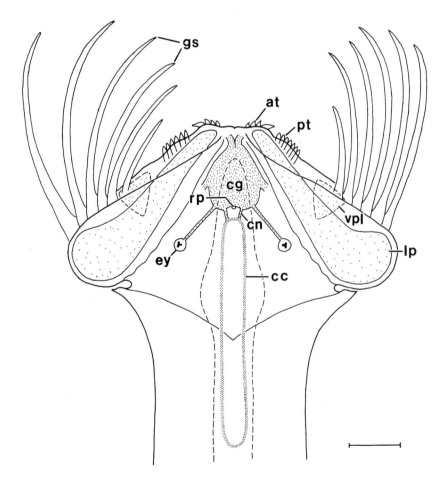

Figure 16.2. Diagram of dorsal head structures with grasping spines open. *at*, anterior teeth; *cg*, cerebral ganglion; *cc*, corona ciliata; *cn*, coronal nerve; *ey*, eye; *gs*, grasping spines; *lp*, lateral plate; *pt*, posterior teeth; *rp*, retrocerebral pore; and *vpl*, ventral plate. Scale bar = 100 μm. From Shinn (1997), after Beauchamp (1960).

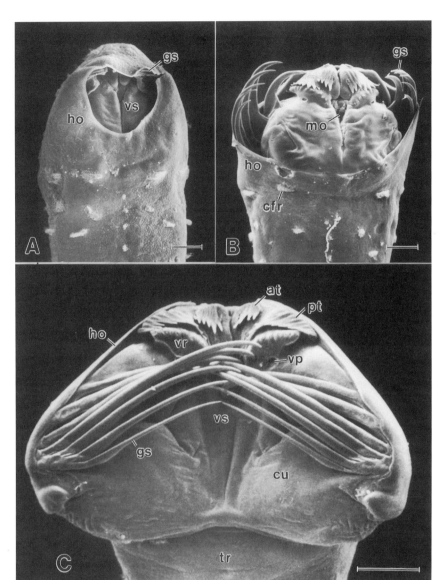

Figure 16.3. Scanning electron micrograph of *Adhesisagitta hispida*. Ventral view of head. **A:** Hood extended over head. **B:** Hood partially retracted. **C:** Hood fully retracted. *at*, anterior teeth; *cfr*, ciliary fence receptor; *cu*, cuticle of ventral epidermis; *gs*, grasping spines; *ho*, hood; *mo*, mouth; *pt*, posterior teeth; *tr*, trunk; *vp*, vestibular pit; *vr*, vestibular ridge; and *vs*, vestibular stoma. All scale bars = 100 μm. From Shinn (1997).

There is no evidence that it opens into the gut. Therefore, it is postulated that it helps to predigest the food outside of the body to make the prey easier to swallow. If this mechanism were correct, it could also enable chaetognaths to scavenge dead animals. Another suggestion is that it may enable chaetognaths to attach to a host and act as an external parasite (Casanova, 1993a).

The fins of chaetognaths are epidermal folds with several possible functions. Shinn (1997) found that *Sagitta hispida* has a transverse body-wall musculature that can deflect the fins, and therefore the fins may function in directional control of locomotion. Jordan (1992) used a mathematical model to show that they may be used to stop any rotational forces of the body induced from opposing muscle contractions. This rotational stability would come at the expense of performance, since the fins would add to the drag and mass of the streamlined body (Jordan, 1992). A study using *Eukrohnia hamata* shows they use their fins as a brood pouch to cover their eggs (Terazaki and Miller, 1982). It is also known that, as some chaetognaths ma-

ture, the fins fill up with a gel-like substance, which may increase buoyancy to counteract the weight of their gonads (Kapp, 1991).

The ovaries are located in the posterior portion of the trunk between the body wall and the gut (Figure 16.1). They contain an oviducal complex that has a syncytium where the sperm are stored until fertilization. The ovaries also contain developing oocytes. Each oocyte has its own pair of accessory fertilization cells (AFCs) that help with the fertilization process. Each AFC of the pair is different: AFC1 forms the tunnel between the oocyte and the sperm stored in the syncytium of the oviducal complex, and AFC2 forms a plug to this tunnel. After fertilization, AFC2 disappears, and the sperm are able to travel through the tunnel to fertilize the oocyte (Shinn, 1994). Contractions of the ovarian wall then occur that force the eggs into the oviducal complex, through the vagina, and out through the gonopore on the external surface of the body (Shinn, 1997).

The male reproductive system is contained within the tail coelom (Figure 16.1). The testes of chaetognaths contain sper-

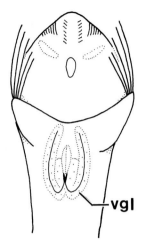

Figure 16.4. *Xenokrohnia sorbei*. Diagram showing position of ventral gland (*Vgl*). From Shinn (1997), after Casanova (1993a).

matogonia that are released into the coelom, where they are continuously in motion during maturation. The sperm ducts conduct the mature spermatozoa to the seminal vesicles that have no area for exit. The seminal vesicles have a line of suture cells where a temporary hole is made when the sperm exit (Shinn, 1997).

Physiology

Feeding

As previously mentioned, chaetognaths are voracious carnivores. Many of the *Sagitta* species appear to feed both during the day and at night, with more feeding occurring at night (Reeve et al., 1975; Feigenbaum and Reeve, 1977; Nagasawa, 1985). They are ambush predators that detect prey by sensing movement. Chaetognaths appear to have a maximal attack distance where they can recognize the vibration of prey. A study using a vibrating probe determined the maximum distance as 3 mm for *Spadella schizoptera* and *Sagitta hispida* (Feigenbaum and Reeve, 1977), whereas a separate study on *Sagitta elegans* that used different prey items showed the distance to be between 0.09 and 1.32 cm, depending on the prey (Saito and Kiørboe, 2001). The prey must be of a certain size and swimming with a certain velocity to elicit the attack response (Saito and Kiørboe, 2001). The mean digestive efficiency for *Sagitta hispida* Conant is about 80%, whereas that for *Sagitta crassa* Tokioka is about 83% (Cosper and Reeve, 1975; Nagasawa, 1985).

Chaetognaths can likely detect the difference between water turbulence and prey. Sensory hairs located over the surface of their body might play a role in this. The movement of many sensory hairs causes an escape action, whereas the movement of a few causes an attack behavior (Saito and Kiørboe, 2001).

Toxin

Once the prey is detected, chaetognaths begin the attack by flexing and flicking their tail very rapidly. The prey is grabbed by the spines and immobilized before consumption (Feigenbaum, 1991). The toxin used by chaetognaths is tetrodotoxin (TTX) and appears to be located in the head of the chaetognath. TTX works as a very potent neurotoxin that blocks sodium channels. The bacteria *Vibrio alginolyticus* is the likely source of the TTX in chaetognaths (Thuesen et al., 1988b; Thuesen, 1991). The exact location of the bacteria or the mechanisms for TTX storage is unknown, but the most likely location according to Bieri et al. (1983) is the vestibular papillae on the vestibular ridge. They suggest that the spines hold the prey while the posterior teeth (located next to the vestibular ridge) facilitate envenomation. Neither the teeth nor the grasping spines are hollow and so cannot be used to inject prey directly (Bone et al., 1983). The susceptibility of the chaetognath nervous system to the TTX is unknown.

Digestive System

The digestive system consists of a simple tube running from one end of the animal to the other. At the anterior end is the mouth, a slitlike opening on the ventral surface. It is thought that the dilator vestibuli externus and dilator vestibuli internus muscles open the mouth during feeding (Shinn, 1997). Intrabuccal pores have been located just inside the mouth of *Parasagitta hispida* but have not been well studied (Thuesen et al., 1988b). The mouth is contiguous with the esophagus that is located in the head region and contains an esophageal bulb (pharynx) at the posterior end.

The esophagus is continuous with the intestine that travels the length of the trunk and is collapsed laterally when empty. It is a straight tube with the exception of an intestinal diverticula (function not understood) (Figure 16.1). Longitudinal mesenteries attach the intestines to the body wall along its dorsal and ventral surfaces (Kapp, 1991). The entire esophagus contains both absorptive and glandular cells, but the glandular cells appear to be more concentrated at the anterior end and the absorptive cells at the posterior end (Parry, 1944). A study by Perez et al. (2000) showed that after about 20 days of starvation the absorptive cells, as well as some longitudinal muscle, will show signs of necrosis. The animal may live up to 35 days during starvation while the reproductive behavior is still functioning.

The intestine connects to the short rectum that is lined with ciliated columnar cells and is surrounded by a rectal sphincter composed of circular muscle that controls the movement of feces. There is debate as to whether chaetognaths have anal sphincters. Most literature states that they do not, but Cosper and Reeve (1975) found a well-developed anal sphincter in *Adhesisagitta hispida*. Ultrastructural studies by Duvert and Salat (1995) also found the presence of an anal sphincter in several species of *Sagitta* (Shinn, 1997).

Filling up much of the coelomic cavity in some species, like *Sagitta elegans*, are vacuolated gut cells that replace Na^+ with NH_4^+. For species without these specialized cells, like *Sagitta se-*

tosa, their coelomic cavity is very similar in composition to seawater. Because NH_4^+ is less dense than seawater, the species containing NH_4^+ are less dense and can attain neutral buoyancy (Bone et al., 1987). This plays an important role in the amount of energy the animal must expend and may dictate hunting techniques.

Hemal System

For many years, there was no evidence of a hemal system, and the transport of important nutrients from the intestine during digestion was a mystery. Shinn (1997) reports that *Adhesisagitta hispida* and *Parasagitta elegans* do actually have a peri-intestinal sinus that is similar in some ways to the hemal system of other invertebrates. In these two species, it is located between the basal laminae of the intestinal epithelium and the overlying gut musculature. On the dorsal side, it extends into the mesentery, but there is no evidence of this in the ventral mesentery. Shinn (1997) postulates that the sinus functions by alternating posteriorly directed peristalsis with reverse peristalsis. Much research is still needed in this area to determine whether other species have a similar system and to define the exact mechanism.

Metabolism

Duvert et al. (2000a) have shown that the chaetognath *Sagitta friderici* uses the Krebs cycle to break down glucose rather than using the pentose cycle that is more commonly used in other invertebrates like insects. Glucose and leucine can freely diffuse through the body wall, and carbon dioxide can diffuse out. Although diffusion is possible, Duvert et al. (2000a) believe that energy obtained from food is more important than diffusion. Their study also was the first to show that glycogen is stored in tissues other than muscle or intestine. It is believed the gap junctions found between all of the cells may play a role in glycogen transport for energy (Duvert et al., 2000a).

Reproductive System

The first record of mating for planktonic chaetognaths was with *Sagitta hispida*. They grasp each other by the spines, which is followed by a series of violent positions that result in the transfer of sperm masses (Reeve and Walter, 1972). It is thought that these maneuverings cause the force needed to split open a seminal vesicle for sperm transfer. Experiments showed the sperm were always deposited on the body surface between the anterior and posterior fins of the other chaetognath (Reeve and Walter, 1972). Usually, mating results in both chaetognaths attaching their sperm masses to the other. Once attached to the body, the sperm mass divides, and some sperm enter the attachment-side gonopore while the rest travel around to the opposite gonopore (Reeve and Walter, 1972).

Fertilization occurs internally at the ovary. Once fertilized, the eggs of some genera (e.g., *Sagitta*) are released free into the water. Other genera, such as *Pterosagitta*, release the fertilized eggs bound together in a jellylike sac. Species of the genus *Eukrohnia* will release fertilized eggs into a marsupial sac for brooding up to and after hatch for a short period (Terazaki and Miller, 1982).

Instances of self-fertilization have been recorded. Experimentally, Reeve and Walter (1972) observed what looked like a leak of small amounts of sperm leaving the seminal vesicles and traveling to the gonopore of the same animal. In each case, the animal died before the outcome could be observed. In this same experiment, they split open the seminal vesicles and induced self-fertilization. In each case, fertile eggs were produced. This shows that self-fertilization as well as cross-fertilization can occur in *S. hispida*, but the frequency of each in nature is not known.

Nervous System

The main part of the nervous system includes six ganglia on the head and a large ventral trunk ganglion (Figure 16.1). A dorsal cerebral ganglion is located in the head and acts as the control center. It has connecting branches to the ventral ganglion, as well as branches to the paired optic nerves and paired coronal nerves (Figure 16.2). The largest ganglion in the chaetognath is the ventral ganglion that acts to innervate the muscles of the trunk and coordinate swimming (Goto and Yoshida, 1987; Bone and Goto, 1991; Shinn, 1997). Another observation by Shinn (1997) is that the ventral ganglion may also innervate the ciliary fence receptors that aid in detection of prey.

The sensory receptor organs for chaetognaths include the eyes, ciliary tufts along the body, and the ciliary loop (corona). Most, but not all, chaetognaths have eyes that are innervated by the optic nerve. The eye contains a pigment spot that has photoreceptor cells around it (the arrangement and location of both ocular structures vary depending on the species). The eye plays a role in the phototaxis that chaetognaths exhibit (Goto and Yoshida, 1987). The ciliary tufts (ciliary fence receptors) are elongated cilia that are located in different patterns along the head, trunk, and tail, depending on the species. Most are positioned at right angles to the body, but some can be found parallel to it (Bone and Goto, 1991). Ciliary tufts detect motion and are the main means of detecting prey. Located dorsally on the surface of the head is the ciliary loop that forms a ring of glandular and ciliated cells. The ciliary loop is connected to the cerebral ganglion, but there is no information as to whether the loop has a sensory or motor function (Shinn, 1997). Ghirardelli (1968) suggests chemoreception, excretion of metabolic wastes, or even possible use during reproduction for secretion of a substance that helps guide sperm to the gonopores.

Muscular System

There are about 16 muscles of the head, depending on the species, which function to move the grasping spines, as well as the mouth and teeth during feeding (Shinn, 1997). Of the trunk muscles, there are two kinds of longitudinal muscles, primary and secondary. The primary muscles constitute about 80% of the tissue volume in the trunk and have a single sarcomere.

Secondary muscles total less than 1% of the tissue volume in the trunk and are unique among animals in that they have two types of sarcomeres.

Most chaetognaths have primary muscle that contains two types of muscle fibers, A and B, whereas the benthic *Spadella* species have only type A. It is thought that the B-fibers are faster than the A-fibers. The sarcomeres are short with short I-bands and A-bands. The ratio of thin to thick filaments is 3:1. These muscles are thought to act in the normal sliding-filament manner of contraction (Shinn, 1997).

The secondary fibers are located only in small areas around the dorsal and ventral midlines, as well as in the ventral parts of the lateral fields (Shinn, 1997). The s1 sarcomeres are thought to operate much like the regular sarcomeres found in primary muscle. The s2 sarcomeres, which are different and contain no A-bands, are not thought to work by the normal sliding-filament theory (Shinn, 1997).

The other group of muscles that are found in some chaetognath species are the transverse muscles. They have been found in the genera *Eukrohnia*, *Spadella*, *Heterokrohnia*, *Archheterokrohnia*, and *Xenokrohnia* at varying locations in their trunk and tail (Shinn, 1997). The exact function of these muscles is unknown.

There has been much debate about how muscle contraction works in chaetognaths. A study by Tsutsui et al. (2000) showed that, for the locomotor muscle fibers, the action potential is carried by Ca^{2+} and that external Ca^{2+} is required. The action potential for the grasping spine muscles is carried by both Na^+ (rare in invertebrates) and Ca^{2+} (Tsutsui et al., 2000). In *Sagitta* sp., acetylcholine is the only neuromuscular transmitter known to produce a stimulatory effect on the contraction of trunk muscles (Duvert et al., 1997).

Regeneration

There has been much debate on the issue of regeneration in chaetognaths. A study by Duvert et al. (2000b) showed that *Spadella cephaloptera* can survive for 30 days after a major amputation (either the head or the tail) but without regeneration. Although chaetognaths do not appear to regenerate missing parts, they can restore their body cavities in order to continue to reproduce and survive an additional month. *Spadella cephaloptera* can produce seminal vesicles and spermatozoa, lay ripe eggs, attack prey, and even mate after decapitation. They cannot develop immature eggs, because that requires energy that they cannot acquire with the head missing (Duvert et al., 2000b).

Although these studies did not show regeneration, they did enable wound healing to be documented. Within the first 2 h after the wound is made, the surrounding uninjured muscles contract to seal it off while the gut flattens itself against the space to fill in any gaps. This enables the animal to seal off its internal space and restore the mechanical integrity of the body. After 2 h, a clot forms and eventually penetrates the muscular tissue. After 6 h, the wound is closed and the muscles are being rebuilt as the gut is resealed (Duvert et al., 2000b).

Environmental Disorders

Temperature Effects

Different studies have shown that, as the temperatures increase, egg development, sexual maturation, and growth rates all increase. Chaetognaths at lower temperatures reach a larger size at maturity (Pearre, 1991).

Infectious Diseases

Viruses

Shinn (personal communication) has discovered nucleus-inhabiting viruses in *P. elegans*. Further work is needed to determine their impact on chaetognaths.

Bacteria

Bacterial infections may cause deformities. Some bacteria, found in the laboratory and in Suruga Bay (Japan), seem to destroy the head and organs, whereas other bacteria, found in Tokyo Bay, cause chaetognaths to lack body tone and appear sick. An estimated 10% of the chaetognaths in Japanese waters are infected with bacteria (Nagasawa, 1991).

Protozoal Parasites
Dinoflagellates

The only documented account of a dinoflagellate parasite on *Sagitta elegans* was *Oodinium jordani*, which was most commonly found attached to the fin of chaetognaths but also found on the body. Unusual for a dinoflagellate, it was attached by a peduncle (rather than by a sucking disk) that penetrated the epithelium of the chaetognaths, causing considerable damage (McLean and Nielsen, 1989) (Figure 16.5).

Ciliates

Large numbers (average of 100 cells per host) of the ciliate *Metaphrya sagittae* are found in several different chaetognath species, including *S. enflata*, *S. minima*, *S. bipunctata*, *S. nagae*, *S. pacifica*, *S. elegans*, *S. tasmanica*, and *Eukrohnia hamata*. They are typically found in the main coelom and are randomly dispersed but can be found in the tail coelom, as well (Jarling and Kapp, 1985; Nagasawa, 1991). The affected chaetognaths appear to be swollen and not very responsive, and their gonads were also affected (Nagasawa, 1991).

Helminths
Trematodes

Jarling and Kapp (1985) documented the trematode *Ectenurus lepidus*, primarily in the tail coeloms of chaetognaths. The pres-

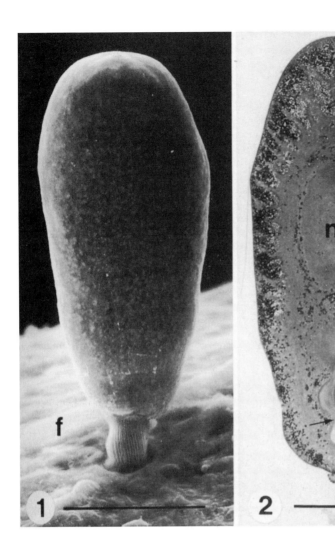

Figure 16.5.   1: Scanning electron micrograph of *Oodinium jordani* attached to the fin (*f*) of *Sagitta elegans* by the peduncle. **2:** Photomicrograph of a sectioned *O. jordani* trophozoite. *a*, aperture; *f*, fin of *S. elegans*; *g*, granular cytoplasm; *p*, peduncular bulb; *area between small arrows*, transverse constriction; *arrowhead*, osmiophilic ring; and *long arrow*, secondary osmiophilic ring. Scale bars = 100 μm.

ence of eggs in some of the trematodes may indicate chaetognaths are true intermediate hosts (Jarling and Kapp, 1985). Many other reports of trematode infestations have been recorded. Most such infestations appear clinically innocuous, though there is a report of a trematode observed while burrowing through the gut wall (Nagasawa, 1991).

Some parasites can affect the growth of the ovaries or testes by occupying space in the body cavity (Pearre, 1991). Other parasites, such as larval trematodes, act to change the color of chaetognaths from transparent to opaque. Larval trematodes may also cause chaetognaths to swim close to the surface. This behavioral change puts them at greater risk for predation (Nagasawa, 1991).

Nematodes

Most nematodes found in chaetognaths are ascarids. The incidence of nematode infestation depends on location. Nematode infestation is rare in some areas but is more common in others. It is reported that 33% of the *Sagitta* species in the Black Sea are infected, and the chaetognath plays an important role in the life cycle of the nematodes (Nagasawa, 1991). Another report found that III-stage larval *Hysterothylacium aduncum* are the most common nematodes found in *Sagitta setosa* and *Sagitta elegans* (Øresland, 1986).

Cestodes

Cestode infections are uncommon. Chaetognaths found to contain cestodes include *Sagitta elegans*, *Eukrohnia hamata*, *Pterosagitta draco*, *Sagitta tasmanica*, and *Sagitta setosa* (Nagasawa, 1991).

In addition to the aforementioned parasites, Shinn (personal communication) recently discovered an amoeboid parasite located in the tail coelom of *Parasagitta elegans*. He speculates that transfer is similar to that of a venereal disease.

Neoplasia

No cases of neoplasia in chaetognaths have been documented.

Miscellaneous Disorders

Chaetognaths may suffer from malnutrition when kept in laboratory conditions. Casanova (1993b) reports that *Artemia salina* nauplii, which are often the main diet of laboratory chaetognaths, are not very good for *Spadella*. He reports that a diet of *A. salina* nauplii can cause the epidermis to become thin and deformed. Perez et al. (2000) noticed that specimens fed *A. salina* nauplii in the laboratory had large amounts of lipids stored in their intestinal absorptive cells.

Nagasawa (1991) reported diseases of unknown origin in captive *Sagitta crassa*. In one case, the head suddenly came off but did not appear damaged. In another incident, the ciliary sense organs stuck together, which may lead to starvation. In the third case, the body turned opaque and the epithelium degenerated. None of the cases appeared to be caused by bacteria or damage that could be detected, so the diagnosis was termed "X disease" (Nagasawa, 1991).

Analgesia, Anesthesia, and Surgery

There are currently no known reports of anesthesia use in chaetognaths or performing surgery.

Treatment Protocols and Formulary

There are currently no known reports of a treatment protocol for chaetognaths.

References

Barnes RSK, Calow P, Olive PJW, Golding DW, and Spicer JI. 2001. The Invertebrates: A Synthesis, 3rd edition. Blackwell Science, Oxford, 497 pp.

Beauchamp P de. 1960. Class des Chétognathes [Chaetognatha]. In: Grassé P-P, ed. Traité de Zoologie, volume 5: Anatomie, Systématique, Biologie. Paris: Masson, pp 1500–1520.

Bieri R. 1991. Systematics of the Chaetognatha. In: Bone Z, Kapp H, and Pierrot-Bults AC, eds. The Biology of Chaetognaths. Oxford University Press, New York, pp 122–136.

Bieri R, Bonilla D, and Arcos F. 1983. Function of the teeth and vestibular ridge in the Chaetognatha as indicated by scanning electron microscope and other observation. Proc Biol Soc Wash 96:110–114.

Bone Q and Goto T. 1991. The nervous system. In: Bone Z, Kapp H, and Pierrot-Bults AC, eds. The Biology of Chaetognaths. Oxford University Press, New York, pp 18–31.

Bone Q and Pulsford AL. 1984. The sense organs and ventral ganglion of *Sagitta* (Chaetognatha). Acta Zool (Stockh) 65:209–220.

Bone Q, Ryan KP, and Pulsford AL. 1983. The structure and composition of the teeth and grasping spines of chaetognaths. J Mar Biol Assoc UK 63:929–939.

Bone Q, Brownlee C, Bryan GW, Burt GR, Dando PR, Liddicoat MI, Pulsford AL, and Ryan KP. 1987. On the differences between the two 'indicator' species of chaetognath, *Sagitta setosa* and *S. elegans*. J Mar Biol Assoc UK 67:545–560.

Bowman TE and Bieri R. 1989. *Paraspadella anops*, new species, from Sagittarius Cave Grand Bahama Island, the second troglobitic chaetognath. Proc Biol Soc Wash 102:586–589.

Casanova JP. 1993a. A new genus and species of deep-sea chaetognath from the Bay of Biscay with a strange ventral secretory gland. J Nat Hist 27:445–455.

Casanova JP. 1993b. *Spadella japonica*, a new coastal benthic chaetognath from Japan. Proc Biol Soc Wash 106:359–365.

Cosper TC and Reeve MR. 1975. Digestive efficiency of the chaetognath *Sagitta hispida* Conant. J Exp Mar Biol Ecol 17:33–38.

Duvert M and Salat C. 1995. Ultrastructural studies of the visceral muscles of chaetognaths. Acta Zool (Stockh) 76:75–87.

Duvert M, Savineau JP, Campistron G, and Onteniente B. 1997. Distribution and role of aspartate in the nervous system of the chaetognath *Sagitta*. J Comp Neurol 380:485–494.

Duvert M, Gourdoux L, and Moreau R. 2000a. Cytochemical and physiological studies of the energetic metabolism and osmotrophy in *Sagitta friderici* (chaetognath). J Mar Biol Assoc UK 80:885–890.

Duvert M, Perez Y, and Casanova JP. 2000b. Wound healing and survival of beheaded chaetognaths. J Mar Biol Assoc UK 80:891–898.

Feigenbaum D. 1991. Food and feeding behaviour. In: Bone Z, Kapp H, and Pierrot-Bults AC, eds. The Biology of Chaetognaths. Oxford University Press, New York, pp 45–54.

Feigenbaum D and Reeve MR. 1977. Prey detection in the Chaetognatha: Response to a vibrating probe and experimental determination of attack distance in large aquaria. Limnol Oceanogr 22:1052–1057.

Ghirardelli E. 1968. Some aspects of the biology of chaetognaths. Adv Mar Biol 6:271–375.

Goto T and Yoshida M. 1987. Nervous system in Chaetognatha. In: Ali MA, ed. Nervous Systems of Invertebrates. (NATO ASI series.) Plenum, New York, pp 461–481.

Haddock S and Case JF. 1994. A bioluminescent chaetognath. Nature 367:225–226.

Hyman LH. 1959. The Invertebrates, volume 5: Smaller Coelomate Groups. McGraw-Hill, New York, pp 1–71.

Jarling C and Kapp H. 1985. Infestation of Atlantic chaetognaths with helminths and ciliates. Dis Aquat Org 1:23–28.

Jordan CE. 1992. A model of rapid-start swimming at intermediate Reynolds number: Undulatory locomotion in the chaetognath *Sagitta elegans*. J Exp Biol 163:119–137.

Kapp H. 1991. Morphology and anatomy. In: Bone Z, Kapp H, and Pierrot-Bults AC, eds. The Biology of Chaetognaths. Oxford University Press, New York, pp 5–17.

McLean N and Nielsen C. 1989. *Oodinium jordani* n. sp., a dinoflagellate (Dinoflagellata: Oodinidae) ectoparasitic on *Sagitta elegans* (Chaetognatha). Dis Aquat Org 7:61–66.

Nagasawa S. 1985. The digestive efficiency of the chaetognath *Sagitta crassa* Tokioka, with observations on the feeding process. J Exp Mar Biol Ecol 87:271–281.

Nagasawa S. 1991. Parasitism and diseases in chaetognaths. In: Bone Z, Kapp H, and Pierrot-Bults AC, eds. The Biology of Chaetognaths. Oxford University Press, New York, pp 76–85.

Nagasawa S and Marumo R. 1976. Further studies on the feeding habits of *Sagitta nagae* Alvarino in Suruga Bay, central Japan. J Oceanogr Soc Jpn 32:209–218.

Øresland V. 1986. Parasites of the chaetognath *Sagitta setosa* in the western English Channel. Mar Biol 92:87–91.

Parry DA. 1944. Structure and function of the gut in *Spadella cephaloptera* and *Sagitta setosa*. J Mar Biol Assoc UK 26:16–36.

Pearre S Jr. 1991. Growth and reproduction. In: Bone Z, Kapp H, and Pierrot-Bults AC, eds. The Biology of Chaetognaths. Oxford University Press, New York, pp 61–75.

Perez Y, Casanova JP, and Mazza J. 2000. Changes in the structure and ultrastructure of the intestine of *Spadella cephaloptera* (Chaetognatha) during feeding and starvation experiments. J Exp Mar Biol Ecol 253:1–15.

Reeve MR and Walter MA. 1972. Observations and experiments on methods of fertilization in the chaetognath *Sagitta hispida*. Biol Bull 143:207–214.

Reeve MR, Cosper TC, and Walter MA. 1975. Visual observations on the process of digestion and the production of faecal pellets in the chaetognath *Sagitta hispida* Conant. J Exp Mar Biol Ecol 17:39–46.

Saito H and Kiørboe T. 2001. Feeding rates in the chaetognath *Sagitta elegans*: Effects of prey size, prey swimming behaviour and small-scale turbulence. J Plankton Res 23:1385–1398.

Shinn GL. 1994. Ultrastructural evidence that somatic "accessory cells" participate in chaetognath fertilization. In: Wilson WH, Stricker SA, and Shinn GL, eds. Reproduction and Development of Marine Invertebrates. Johns Hopkins University Press, Baltimore, pp 95–105.

Shinn GL. 1997. Chaetognatha. In: Harrison FW and Ruppert EE, eds. Microscopic Anatomy of Invertebrates, volume 15: Hemichordata, Chaetognatha, and the Invertebrate Chordates. Wiley-Liss, New York, pp 103–220.

Terazaki M and Miller CB. 1982. Reproduction of meso- and bathy-pelagic chaetognaths in the genus *Eukrohnia*. Mar Biol 71:193–196.

Thuesen EV. 1991. The tetrodotoxin venom of chaetognaths. In: Bone Z, Kapp H, and Pierrot-Bults AC, eds. The Biology of Chaetognaths. Oxford University Press, New York, pp 55–60.

Thuesen EV and Bieri R. 1987. Tooth structure and buccal pores in the chaetognath *Flaccisagitta hexaptera* and their relation to the capture of fish larvae and copepods. Can J Zool 65:181–187.

Thuesen EV, Kogure K, Hashimoto K, and Nemoto T. 1988a. Poison arrowworms: A tetrodotoxin venom in the marine phylum Chaetognatha. J Exp Mar Biol Ecol 116:249–256.

Thuesen EV, Nagasawa S, Bieri R, and Nemoto T. 1988b. Transvestibular pores of chaetognaths with comments on the function and nomenclature of the vestibular anatomy. Bull Plankton Soc Jpn 35:133–141.

Tsutsui I, Inoue I, Bone Q, and Carre C. 2000. Activation of locomotor and grasping spine muscle fibres in chaetognaths: A curious paradox. J Muscle Res Cell Motil 21:91–97.

Chapter 17

ECHINODERMS

Craig A. Harms

Natural History and Taxonomy

Phylum Echinodermata

Class Crinoidea: crinoids, sea lilies, and feather stars, 600 species
Class Asteroidea: sea stars or starfish, 1500 species
Class Ophiuroidea: brittle stars or serpent stars, and basket stars, 2000 species
Class Echinoidea: sea urchins and sand dollars, 950 species
Class Holothuroidia: sea cucumbers, 900 species
Class Concentrocycloidea: two little-known species

The phylum Echinodermata comprises about 6000 species grouped in six rather disparate classes (Ruppert and Barnes, 1994). Characteristics linking the groups include pentamerous radial symmetry (usually), mutable connective tissue, a water vascular system, deuterostome development, an exclusively marine existence, and (usually) dioecious reproduction with external fertilization. The pentamerous radial symmetry as typified by the classic representation of starfish is secondarily derived both phylogenetically and ontogenetically from bilaterally symmetrical ancestors and larvae, respectively. Free-swimming ciliated planktonic larvae with a complete digestive tract are found in 40%–50% of echinoderms, with the remainder having lecithotrophic larvae or direct development. Early echinoderms first appear in the fossil record in the early Cambrian period, with typical crinoids, asteroids, and echinoids appearing in the Ordovician, and ophiuroids in the Mississippian; holothuroids are poorly represented as fossils, as would be expected from their soft bodies (Ruppert and Barnes, 1994).

Echinoderms are of restricted economic interest. Sea urchin gonads and sea cucumbers (trepang) are used as food in some regions, and sea stars are considered pest species for mussel and oyster aquaculture (Coteur et al., 2002). They serve as important determinants of community structure in some ecosystems, for example, sea urchins in kelp forests (Steneck et al., 2002), and ophiuroid beds of the deep sea and certain shallow-water communities (Aronson and Harms, 1985).

Anatomy and Physiology

Anatomy and physiology of echinoderms are thoroughly described by Ruppert and Barnes (1994). Major points are summarized here, beginning with features common to all echinoderm classes and then features of each class. Figures 17.1–17.4 illustrate the important anatomical features of the asteroids, echinoids, and holothuroids.

The main surface orientation terms for echinoderms are *oral* and *aboral*. For asteroids, ophiuroids, and echinoids, oral typically means the lower side; for crinoids, the oral surface is up; and, for holothuroids, which have an elongated polar (oral to aboral) axis, the oral surface is at one end, sometimes angled up. The dermis contains calcite ossicles that vary from sparse in holothuroids to tightly interconnected in echinoids.

The water vascular system is unique to echinoderms and functions variously in locomotion, gripping, and feeding. It consists of canals lined with ciliated epithelium and connects with the exterior surface through a cluster of pores called the *madreporite*. From the madreporite, the plumbing extends through pore canals to a vertical stone canal (with calcareous walls), a ring canal that circles the mouth, folded pouches called *Tiedmann's bodies* situated interradially on the inner side of the ring canal, (sometimes) muscular sacs also interradially along the ring canal called *polian vesicles*, radial canals extending into the arms (asteroids, ophiuroids, and crinoids) or along the sides nearly to the aboral pole (echinoids and holothuroids), valved lateral canals alternating sides along the radial canals, a muscular ampulla, and finally a podium (*tube foot*). Fluid in the water vascular system is similar to seawater except for the addition of coelomocytes, some protein, and a higher potassium concentration. Ampullar contraction closes the valve to the lateral canal, and water pressure elongates the podium. Adhesion of podia to substrate is chemically mediated. Contraction of longitudinal muscles of the podium retracts the podium and refills the ampulla. Cilia in the stone canal drive a primarily inward flow of water, while cilia in the madreporite pores filter out larger particles and phagocytes in the Tiedmann's bodies clear the fluid of bacteria and other foreign matter. Lines of podia further define

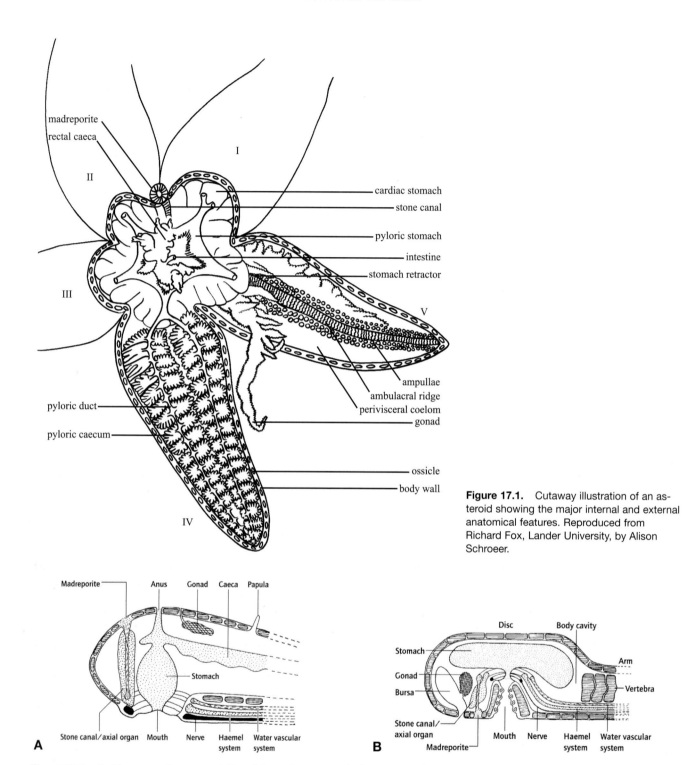

Figure 17.1. Cutaway illustration of an asteroid showing the major internal and external anatomical features. Reproduced from Richard Fox, Lander University, by Alison Schroeer.

Figure 17.2. **A:** Diagrammatic representation of the various anatomical structures of an asteroid body and arm. **B:** Diagrammatic representation of the various anatomical structures of an ophuroid body and arm. Both diagrams are from Barnes et al. (2001), after Nichols (1962).

regions of the echinoderm body surface, with podia (Figure 17.5) lining the ambulacral groove of asteroids, ophiuroids, and crinoids, or ambulacral regions of holothuroids and echinoids, with interambulacral regions intervening.

The hemal system for circulating coelomic fluids is rudimentary in asteroids, ophiuroids, and crinoids; more complex in echinoids; and most complex in holothuroids. In the basic plan, there are four coelomic circulatory systems: the water vascular system, perivisceral coelom supplying the viscera, hyponeural sinus system supplying the nerves, and genital coelom supplying the gonads. All are lined with cilia that help circulate fluid, and all contribute blood vessels that unite at a simple heart lo-

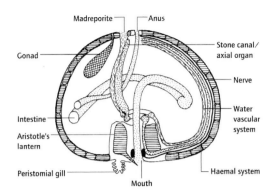

Figure 17.3. Cross-sectional illustration of an echinoid. From Barnes et al. (2001).

cated in the vicinity of the madreporite. In the starfish *Asterias forbesi*, the heart beats approximately 6 times per minute. Sea cucumbers lack a systemic heart but have a dorsal vessel and ventral vessel along the intestine, with numerous single-chambered hearts pumping blood from the dorsal vessel through intestinal lamellae, and also have a vascular plexus surrounding the respiratory tree. Sea cucumbers have a coelomocyte called a *hemocyte* that contains hemoglobin.

Mutable connective tissue, or *catch*, is another feature unique to echinoderms. Catch can vary rapidly between rigid and flexible based on nervous control and ion (particularly calcium) concentrations, though the precise mechanisms of control are not understood. Among other applications, the unique properties of mutable connective tissue are used in predator defense by brittle stars to cast off arm tips, by sea cucumbers to enable evisceration, and by sea urchins to lock spines to wedge into crevices.

Pathogen defense in echinoderms is mediated by the coelomocytes (or variously termed *amebocytes*, *mesodermic phagocytes*, or *immunocytes*) and is best described in asteroids. Coelomocytes accumulate around foreign bodies and sites of injury, phagocytosing small particles, walling off large objects, and forming clots (Sparks, 1985). Spent coelomocytes migrate to distal ends of papules and podia, or other epithelial sites, where they are pinched off and extruded (Ruppert and Barnes, 1994). Sea star coelomocytes produce reactive oxygen species and nitric oxide as part of the innate immune response (Beck et al., 2001;

Coteur et al., 2002). It was Elie Metchnikoff's observations in the late 1800s of sea star bipinnaria larvae coelomocytes' response to puncture by rose thorns that led to the development of the field of comparative and cellular immunology, for which he received the 1908 Nobel Prize in medicine (Beck and Habicht, 1996). Echinoderm coelomic fluid also contains hemolysins, hemagglutinins, and antimicrobial substances (Jangoux, 1990).

The nervous system of echinoderms is minimally ganglionated. A circumoral nerve ring lies in the peristomial epidermis, and a radial nerve extends from the nerve ring along the radial canal of the water vascular system. Tactile, photosensory, and chemosensory cells are dispersed within the epidermis.

Crinoids include the attached stalked forms called *sea lilies* and free-living forms called *feather stars* (order Comatula). Sea lilies are restricted to deep water, whereas feather stars are found in both shallow and deep water. The stalk of sea lilies may reach a length of 1 m, whereas it is lost in postlarval development of feather stars. The pentamerous body is called the *crown*. The *stalk* is composed of jointed skeletal ossicles and bear slender cirri, which are retained at the base of feather stars and used for grasping the substrate when at rest. The crown attaches to the stalk aborally at the cuplike *calyx*. The oral wall of the calyx is called the *tegmen*, with the mouth in the center and ambulacral grooves extending up each arm from the mouth. The anus is located in a prominence called the *anal cone* on the oral surface in one of the interambulacral areas. The arms are jointed like the stalk, and in most species they branch immediately after leaving the crown to form 10 arms, or more with further branching in some species. Arms are lined with small jointed pinnules, which are the source of the name feather star. Movable flaps called *lappets* can expose or cover the ambulacral grooves. Three podia united at the base underlie each lappet. Feather stars can crawl, or swim by alternating arm movements. Crinoids are suspension feeders, using the podia to capture suspended particles and transfer them to the mouth. The mouth leads to a short esophagus, an intestine that makes a complete turn around the calyx, and a terminal portion that extends upward to the anus at the anal cone. Five coelomic canals extend through the stalk and along the oral side of the arms. Gas exchange takes place at the podia. Instead of a madreporite, crinoids have numerous separate surface pores and pore canals in the tegmen that open into the coelom near the stone canals. Several stone canals join the

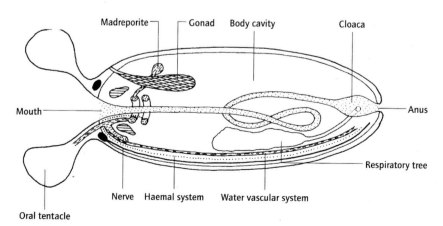

Figure 17.4. **A:** Longitudinal drawing of a typical holothuroid. From Barnes et al. (2001).

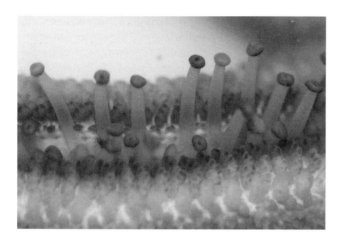

Figure 17.5. Magnified tube feet or podia from an asteroid. Courtesy of Kelly Krell.

ring canal, there are no ampullae, and each lateral canal supplies a trio of podia. All crinoids are dioecious. There are no distinct gonads; rather, germinal epithelium located in the proximal portion of the arms, in an extension of the coelom within pinnules or arms, give rise to gametes. Gametes are spawned by rupture of the pinnule walls. Some cold-water species brood eggs and juveniles.

Asteroids, the sea stars, typically have five arms, but sun stars may have 7–40 or more. Arms are not distinctly set off from the disc. Ambulacral groove extend radially on the oral surface and contain 2–4 rows of podia. On the aboral surface, the madreporite is located eccentrically, whereas the inconspicuous anus, if present, is located centrally. Small jawlike pedicellariae provide protection against settling larvae in two orders of asteroids, and small evaginations of the body wall called *papules* on the aboral surface are involved with gas exchange. The digestive system consists of a muscular peristomial membrane encircling the mouth, a short esophagus, a two-chambered (cardiac and pyloric) stomach filling the disc, pyloric cecae extending into the arms, and a short tubular intestine from the aboral surface of the pyloric stomach extending to the centrally located aboral anus. Many asteroids feed by everting the cardiac stomach through the mouth to engulf the prey or by inserting the everted stomach through a narrow gap in a bivalve's gape to digest the animal within its valves. Asteroids include scavengers, carnivores, and suspension feeders. Gas exchange and nitrogenous waste elimination take place by diffusion across thin areas of the body surface, such as tube feet and papules. Some asteroids reproduce asexually by disc division, each part regenerating a new whole. Gonads are contained within the arms, two per arm, and, when reproductively active, swell to fill most of the available space in the arms. Some cold-water species brood eggs.

Ophiuroids, the brittle stars and basket stars, like asteroids also have arms, but the arms are sharply demarcated from the central disc, lack an ambulacral groove, are more solidly constructed, and locomotion is primarily from direct arm movement rather than by podia. Surface features of the disc and arms include shields and spines. There are typically five arms, but in basket stars the arms branch repeatedly. The arms appear

jointed and are constructed of four longitudinal rows of shields (one aboral, two lateral, and one oral) surrounding internal vertebral ossicles. The vertebral articulations of the arms of most species enable ample lateral movement but restricted vertical movement. The ambulacrum is closed, with podia extending between the oral and lateral shields, one pair per joint. The mouth is surrounded by five interradial jaws, and one oral shield is modified to form the madreporite (in contrast to the aboral madreporite of asteroids). The madreporite has a single pore and canal, the stone canal ascends rather than descends to the ring canal, and ampullae are lacking. Ophiuroids include carnivores, scavengers, deposit feeders, and filter feeders. The digestive tract is simple, consisting of a prebuccal cavity, peristomial membrane with mouth, a short esophagus, and a large stomach filling most of the disc, with 10 marginal pouches. Undigested material is regurgitated; there is no intestine or anus. Bursal slits lie on either side of the arms on the oral side of the disc, and gonads are located on the coelomic side of the bursae within the disc. Dioecious species with external fertilization and development are most common. Some species brood eggs and juveniles in the bursae. Some ophiuroids are hermaphroditic, either simultaneous or protandric, and some reproduce by asexual division.

The regular echinoids, sea urchins, and the irregular echinoids—heart urchins (spatangoids) and sand dollars (clypeasteroids)—have surface spines and no arms, and the ossicles are flattened and tightly bound together to form a solid case called the *test*. Regular echinoids are radially symmetrical, roughly spherical, and have relatively long spines. The peristomial membrane surrounds the mouth, along with five buccal podia and five pairs of gills. The anal region, called the *periproct*, is at the aboral pole. The body surface is divided into five ambulacral areas, with podia and five interambulacral areas lacking podia. The madreporite is one of the five large genital plates surrounding the periproct, modified with multiple pores. Each genital plate has a gonopore. Spines are movable and sit in a ball-and-socket–type joint. Spines may be used for defense, locomotion (along with podia), or wedging into crevices. Spines of some species contain irritants and barbs. Three-jawed, sometimes poisonous, pedicellariae cover the test surface and function in defense and cleaning the body surface. Irregular echinoids are moderately to considerably flat in the oral–aboral axis, with elongation into an anterior–posterior axis, have small spines and no peristomial gills, and burrow in the substrate. The peristome is located anteriorly and the periproct posteriorly. Podia are degenerate or absent from the equator of the body surface. Aboral ambulacra are arranged in petaloids. Symmetrical notches or fenestrations in the test of sand dollars are called *lunules*. *Aristotle's lantern* is a complex five-jawed feeding apparatus of sea urchins that can be protruded and retracted. The buccal cavity and pharynx ascend within Aristotle's lantern into an esophagus that descends laterally to a tubular stomach. A cecum is usually located at the junction of the esophagus and stomach. The stomach takes one turn around the inside of the test wall and joins the thinner-walled aboral intestine, which makes a complete turn in the opposite direction and ascends to the rectum and anus. A narrow tube called a *siphon* parallels the stomach and empties into the intestine, functioning to remove excess water. Most regular urchins are grazers, whereas irregular urchins are selective deposit feeders. Gas exchange takes place at the peristomial gills as well as the podia. All echinoids are dioecious. A few species brood eggs on the peristome or around the periproct. Regular echinoids have five gonads suspended along the interambulacra, whereas most irregular echinoids lack the posterior gonad.

Holothuroids, the sea cucumbers, have mouth and anus at opposite poles, with meridional ambulacral and interambulacral areas, a greatly elongated polar axis, reduced microscopic dermal ossicles, and a row of 10–30 tentacles (modified podia) around the mouth. Holothuroids lie on one side, and the ventral surface, composed of three ambulacral areas, is called the *sole*. Dorsal podia are reduced or absent, and some burrowing species lack podia. Most species are epibenthic, some burrow, and a few deep-sea species are pelagic. Sea cucumbers are deposit or suspension feeders. The mouth and tentacles can be retracted within the adjacent body wall when disturbed. The mouth opens into a muscular pharynx surrounded by a calcareous ring. Many holothuroids lack a stomach, but when present it is muscular and gizzardlike. The intestine is long and convoluted, terminating in a cloaca. In most species, gas exchange takes place in the two respiratory trees, which are located to the right and left of the digestive tract and emerge at the cloaca. Water fills the respiratory trees by pumping action of the cloaca and is expelled by contraction of the respiratory trees. Filling requires 6–10 cloacal contractions, whereas water is expelled in a single action. The madreporite has no connection with the body surface but rather is unattached in the coelom. Fluid enters instead via ciliated cloacal perforations. Holothuroids have a single gonad, located anteriorly beneath the middorsal interambulacrum, with a gonopore middorsally between two tentacles or behind the tentacular collar. Most are dioecious, and a few, mostly cold-water species brood eggs and juveniles.

Environmental Disorders and Preventive Medicine

Like other aquatic invertebrates, echinoderms are susceptible to toxic effects of heavy metals. Copper toxicity occurs in sea stars at concentrations of 0.15 ppm maintained over several days, resulting in weakness, loss of righting reflex, stomach eversion, arm sloughing, and death (Sparks, 1985). In sea urchins, concentrations of 0.15 ppm resulted in death within 15 days, whereas concentrations of 0.10 ppm for 2 weeks resulted in delayed mortality by 70 days after exposure (Gore et al., 2003).

Infectious Diseases

Infectious diseases of echinoderms have been comprehensively reviewed (Jangoux, 1990). Agents associated with echinoderms as pathogens or symbionts with uncertain effects include bacteria, fungi, cyanophytes, flagellates, amoebae, apicomplexans, haplosporidians, ciliates, algae, sponges, cnidarians, turbellari-

ans, trematodes, nematodes, a nemertean (Berg and Gibson, 1996), gastropods, bivalves, entoproctans, polychaetes, myzostomid annelids, tardigrades, copepods, barnacles, amphipods, an arachnid, pycnogonids, an insect, bryozoans, and pearlfish. A selection of prominent or better-characterized conditions will be included here.

Bacterial Infections

Bacteremia

Healthy echinoderm coelomic fluid is normally sterile (Bang and Lemma, 1962; Jangoux, 1990). Experimental inoculations in healthy starfish or sea urchins are rapidly cleared by phagocytic coelomocytes when water quality is good. Physical trauma or autotomy can lead to bacterial colonization of the coelomic fluid, as can keeping starfish in stagnant water heavily contaminated with bacteria. Bacteremic starfish lose weight, move sluggishly, and become edematous, as demonstrated by swollen papules and paxillae (Bang and Lemma, 1962).

Bald Sea Urchin Disease

This graphically named disease is believed to have a bacterial etiology and can be transmitted by applying pieces of affected tissue to experimentally traumatized tissue of healthy sea urchins (Jangoux, 1990). Although numerous opportunistic bacteria may be cultured from lesions, of 14 such isolates the disease was reproduced experimentally in the purple sea urchin, *Strongylocentrotus purpuratus*, only with *Vibrio anguillarum* and *Aeromonas salmonicida* (Gilles and Pearse, 1986). Physical injury facilitates disease development. Lesions occur predominantly on the lateral and oral surfaces of the test and typically have a central necrotic region devoid of spines and tube feet surrounded by a ring of swollen and sometimes discolored tissue (Bower et al., 1994). Phagocytes and red spherule cells infiltrate affected tissues (Jangoux, 1990). Death reportedly occurs if the affected surface area exceeds 30% or the lesion extends deep to the test into the coelomic cavity, but recovery from lesser lesions is possible with sloughing and regeneration of affected tissue (Jangoux, 1990). Reported primarily in *Paracentrotus lividus* from France and *Strongylocentrotus franciscanus* from California, the condition is not species specific and has occurred naturally and experimentally in several other sea urchin species. Paramoebiasis (see the section *Paramoeba invadens* Infestation of Sea Urchins) can cause similar surface lesions.

A localized mortality event in the sea biscuit *Meoma ventricosa* in Curaçao, Netherlands Antilles, was attributed to bacterial infection (Nagelkerken et al., 1999). Affected animals lost spines progressively prior to death. Gram-negative bacteria were observed microscopically in the catch connective tissue of the spines. Inoculation of an uncharacterized bacteria isolated from affected sea biscuits into the sea urchin *Lytechinus variegatus* produced similar effects. The area affected was limited to 3.5 km of coastline down-current from the Curaçao main harbor, with significant decreases in the sea biscuit population, and greater mortality closer to the harbor.

Black Sea Urchin (Diadema antillarum) *Mass Mortality (Black Sea Urchin Plague)*

This sweeping die-off was first recognized in Panama in 1983, spread in a manner consistent with surface currents throughout the Caribbean and as far as Bermuda by 1984, subsided, and had a brief, less virulent resurgence in late 1985 (Lessios, 1988). Although the species specificity and pattern of dispersal indicated an infectious disease, the cause was never definitively identified. There was a possible association with *Clostridium perfringens* or *Cl. sordelli*, based on isolation of these anaerobes from affected laboratory urchins, and death of healthy individuals following injection of the bacteria isolated from mortalities (Bauer and Agerter, 1987). Mortality rates were high, with 85%–100% reduction in populations. Affected urchins had increased mucus production, began to lose spines, became lethargic and less cryptic, and died or succumbed to predation. Deaths began within 10 days of disease emergence in an area. No other urchin species were affected. The mass mortality contributed to dramatic shifts in community structure, with increased algae coverage of reefs. Interestingly, the ecological effects seem to have been better studied than disease etiology or the pathogenic effects on the urchins (e.g., see Liddell and Ohlhorst, 1986). Population recovery following the mass mortality has been limited, but the markedly lower population densities following the mass mortality have been associated with larger average size of existing black sea urchins (Hughes, 1994).

Parasitic Infections

Apicomplexan

Apicomplexan parasites have been reported from sea cucumbers and heart urchins, including 22 gregarines and one coccidian parasite (Jangoux, 1990). The primary genera of gregarine parasites are *Cytobia*, *Lithocystis*, and *Urospora*. Infestation is believed to occur by ingestion, with deposit-feeding echinoderms being most susceptible. Parasites occur primarily within the hemal system for at least part of the life cycle, with coelomic cavity, respiratory trees, and gonads also affected by some. Local host coelomocyte reaction can be observed microscopically, and intracoelomic free stages are presumed to compete for host energy supply, but pathological effects are otherwise not described.

Paramoeba invadens *Infestation of Sea Urchins*

Paramoebiasis occurs in the green sea urchin *Strongylocentrotus droebachiensis*, on the Atlantic Coast of Nova Scotia (Jones and Scheibling, 1985; Jellett et al., 1988; Jangoux, 1990; Bower et al., 1994). The amoeba causes muscle necrosis, leading to dysfunction of tube feet, spines, and mouth. Coelomocytes infiltrate tissues generally, coelomocyte cell count is reduced, coelomic fluid protein concentration increases, and coelomic fluid clotting is impaired. Affected urchins become immobile, stop feeding, lose attachment, and die. Disease can be reproduced by either injection or water-borne exposure with cultured *P. invadens* (Jones and Scheibling, 1985). The disease appears to be species spe-

cific, since other echinoderm species in the same areas as the green sea urchin mortalities are not affected. Natural disease and growth of *P. invadens* in culture are maximal from 15° to 20°C, with outbreaks ceasing below 10°C. Mass mortalities occurred from 1980 to 1983 and from 1992 to 1995, and have been linked to increased tropical storm activity, which drives warmer water to the coasts and may help disseminate the disease agent (Schiebling and Hennigar, 1997). Population declines of *S. droebachiensis* have resulted in increased algal coverage and marked ecological shifts, similar to the situation with the black sea urchin mass mortality (see the section Black Sea Urchin [*Diadema antillarum*] Mass Mortality [Black Sea Urchin Plague]).

Orchitophyra stellarum, *Ciliate Disease of Sea Stars*

This holotrichous ciliate parasite has a circumboreal distribution, infesting *Asterias* spp. and other sea stars of the family Asteriidae (Jangoux, 1990; Bower et al., 1994). *Orchitophyra stellarum* is not considered to be host specific, and although morphometric investigations suggest that more than one species may be involved in different regions, molecular analysis of rRNA internal transcribed spacers of widely distributed isolates revealed no sequence differences (Goggin and Murphy, 2000). The parasite invades the host gonad (primarily males) and causes gonadal atrophy, partial or complete castration, and autotomization of arms. Grossly the gonad may appear smaller and discolored, and numerous elongated ciliates may be observed on wet mounts of coelomic fluid or gonads. Infested tissues are invaded by host phagocytic cells apparently responding to damaged tissue rather than the ciliates, and phagocyte adhesion properties are altered in infested individuals (Jangoux, 1990). Because of its predilection for males (up to 28% prevalence in male and 1% prevalence in female *Asterias rubens* [Sparks, 1985], and 38%–100% in male and 0% in female *A. amurensis* [Byrne et al., 1997]), it can reduce the proportion of males and the reproductive potential in a population. Because of this property, it has attracted interest for potential use as a biological control agent for invasive sea stars and sea star predators on mussel and oyster beds, but its lack of host specificity should be a cautionary consideration against its wide dissemination (Byrne et al., 1997), and early experimental attempts were unsuccessful (Jangoux, 1990).

Algae

An algal parasite, *Coccomyxa ophiura*, has been reported from ophiuroids *Ophiura texturata*, *Ophiura albida*, and *Ophiura sarsi*, and *Coccomyxa astericola* has been reported from starfish *Hippasteria phryngiana* and *Solaster endeca* (Jangoux, 1990). Algae form small, green, subepidermal foci on the aboral surface of disc and arms, where they progressively dissolve skeletal plates and form irregular defects filled with algal cells. Lesions coalesce, the epidermis disintegrates, arms autotomize, and the coelomic cavity may be perforated, with subsequent fatality.

Mesozoans

Mesozoans comprise a small group of minute structurally simple animals of uncertain taxonomic affinity specialized as parasites of marine invertebrates (Ruppert and Barnes, 1994). Asexual parasitic forms alternate with free-living sexual forms. As a group, it is slightly better known for parasitizing cephalopod bladders, but one species, *Rhopalura ophiocomae*, parasitizes ophiuroids, primarily *Amphipholis squamata* (Jangoux, 1990). Ciliated larvae penetrate the bursal slits, attach to the bursal epithelium, and form plasmodia that penetrate to the coelomic side of the bursa. When mature, adults are emitted through the bursal slits. Pathogenicity derives from induced regression of the ovaries, but not testes, of the hermaphroditic host.

Helminths

Turbellarian flatworms as a group are primarily free living, but several species occur as symbionts and parasites of echinoderms. Despite over 65 species documented to live in the digestive tract or (possibly an artifact of dissection) coelomic cavity of echinoderms, reports on pathogenic effects are lacking, but nutrient competition with the host presumably occurs and some species feed on sloughed host intestinal epithelium (Jangoux, 1990). The family Umagillidae represents the most numerous of turbellarian parasites of echinoderms, with 52 species (Jangoux, 1990). One polyclad turbellarian, *Euplana takewakii*, feeds on ophiuroid gonads, castrating the infested bursae (Jangoux, 1990).

As hosts of trematodes and nematodes, echinoderms serve mainly as intermediate hosts for parasites of fish (Jangoux, 1990). Parasitic cysts may form in various tissues. Heavy infestations by metacercariae in ophiuroid arms can promote autotomization and may impair feeding in the Aristotle's lantern of sea urchins. The sea urchin *Strongylocentrotus droebachiensis* serves as definitive host for the nematode *Echinomermella matsi*, which is responsible for epidemic disease in Norway (Hagen, 1996). The nematode infests the perivisceral coelom and effectively castrates juveniles, and may cause death during synchronized internal release of massive numbers of larvae.

Spotted gonad disease of sea urchins in Japan has been loosely associated with trematode cysts (*Proctoeces maculatus*) in *Strongylocentrotus intermedius*, but the dark spots are apparently a host reaction not always directly associated with the trematode (Shimizu, 1994). The disease may reduce reproductive capacity slightly, but is mainly of some commercial concern in sea urchin gonads marketed for food, due to the aesthetic effect.

Gastropods

The gastropod family Eulimidae is composed of about 800 species almost exclusively associated with all major groups of echinoderms (Jangoux, 1990). Eulimids include both ectoparasites and endoparasites. Many attached ectoparasitic eulimids penetrate the echinoderm with their proboscis to reach the coelomic cavity, water vascular system, or hemal system, presumably feeding on host fluids, coelomocytes, or internal tissue. Some feed on echinoderm dermis. Endoparasitic eulimids occur in the digestive tract or coelomic cavity. In addition to their feeding activities, eulimids impact the host by causing attachment lesions and gall formation in asteroids, ophiuroids, and crinoids.

Annelids

Myzostomid annelids are related to polychaetes, and all (about 110 described species) are ectocommensal or parasitic on echinoderms, primarily crinoids, but also a few on asteroids and ophiuroids (Jangoux, 1990). Because most parasitic myzostomids infest bathyal echinoderms, their characterization is sparse. Gallicole species of the genus *Myzostomum* form galls under skeletal ossicles of crinoid arms or pinnules. Cysticole species of the genus *Cystimyzostomum* build stalked or unstalked subcutaneous cysts. A few species infest gonads of crinoids or ophiuroids, causing at least partial castration.

Crustaceans

Many species of copepods are reported associated with echinoderms, but host effects are poorly documented (Jangoux, 1990). Some species form galls on or in echinoids, and *Amphiurophilus amphiurae* inhibits development of host embryos in the genital bursae of the brooding ophiuroid *Amphipholis squamata*.

Some species of ascothoracid barnacles (naked barnacles) parasitize nonholothuroid echinoderms (Jangoux, 1990). They include ectoparasites of crinoids and ophiuroids, endoparasites in the coelomic cavity of sea stars and heart urchins, and genital bursa parasites of ophiuroids. Ascothoracids may castrate their hosts.

Pearlfishes

Pearlfishes of the genera *Carapus*, *Jordanicus*, and *Encheliophis* have an unusual association with holothuroids and some asteroids, using the body of the invertebrate host for shelter and, in some cases (particularly *Encheliophis* spp.), food (Jangoux, 1990). *Carapus* spp. and *Jordanicus* spp. pearlfishes usually enter the anus of a holothuroid tail first and reside in the respiratory tree or coelomic cavity during the day, coming out at night to forage. At low infestation rates damage is probably minimal and readily repaired, but at higher rates damage to the intestinal tract may ensue from repeated passages into and out of the coelomic cavity. *Encheliophis* spp., however, are true parasites, residing permanently within the echinoderm coelomic cavity and feeding on host viscera.

Neoplasia

Tumorlike epidermal lesions have been described in European brittle stars (*Ophiocomina nigra*), and a polypoid growth has been found on a sea cucumber (*Holothuria leucospilata*) (Sparks, 1985).

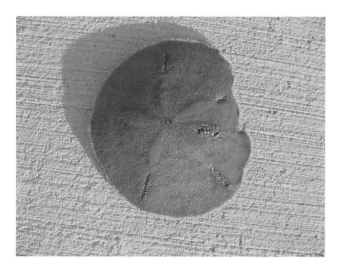

Figure 17.6. An apparently healthy wild keyhole urchin (*Mellita quinquiesperforata*) with a large healed area of its posterior surface (note the small size of the right rear hole). Trauma was the most likely cause of the defect in this animal.

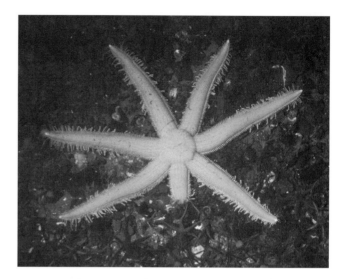

Figure 17.8. Limb breakage with initial regeneration in the sea star *Luidia ciliaris*, surrounded by brittle stars, Clyde Sea, Scotland. Courtesy of Richard Aronson.

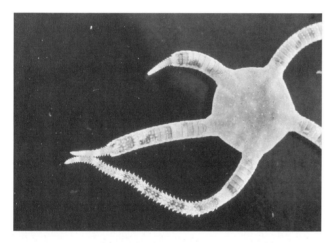

Figure 17.7. Three limbs at different stages of regeneration in the ophiuroid *Ophioderma appressum*. Courtesy of Richard Aronson.

Miscellaneous Conditions

General Trauma

Some echinoderms have remarkable regenerative abilities following trauma and the loss of tissue (see the following section). Animals that survive a traumatic event can heal and survive, although sometimes with a noticeable deformity (Figure 17.6).

Limb Breakage

Ophiuroids are known for their propensity to autotomize arms in response to predation or mishandling (akin to tail loss of some lizard species); hence their common name of brittle stars (Ruppert and Barnes, 1994). The disjoined arm typically

writhes vigorously for a time after separation. The ophiuroid *Ophiothrix oerstedi* can regenerate a missing arm completely in about 4 months (Aronson, 1987). A regenerating arm emerges from the severed arm tip at a smaller diameter and initially more brightly colored than the original base (Figure 17.7). Ophiuroid arm breakage and regeneration has been used as an index of predation pressure in both recent and fossil marine ecosystems (Aronson, 1987). Regenerative abilities of sea stars are also well known, as they can regenerate severed arms (Figure 17.8, Color Plate 17.8), and some species can even grow an entire organism from just an arm and one-fifth of the disc (less, if the madreporite is included in the disc portion) (Ruppert and Barnes, 1994). Related to this regenerative ability is normal asexual reproduction in some species in which the central disc divides and each part regenerates a new whole.

Evisceration and Tubules of Cuvier

Many holothuroids sometimes expel portions of the gastrointestinal tract and adnexa (Ruppert and Barnes, 1994). This is considered a normal seasonal phenomenon as a possible mechanism for reducing metabolic activity during periods of reduced food supply or eliminating waste. Regeneration follows evisceration. Certain *Holothuria* spp. and *Actinopyga* spp. holothuroids can forcibly expel adhesive or toxic tubules of Curvier from the base of the respiratory tree through a rupture in the cloaca and out the anus in a defense response (Ruppert and Barnes, 1994). These tubules are also regenerated following discharge.

Idiopathic Ulcers

Captive sun stars (*Solaster* sp.) can develop mild to severe multifocal ulcers in captivity. In some cases, these result in a full-

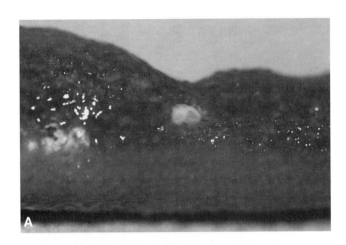

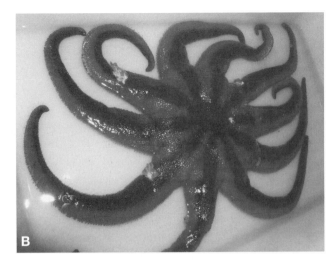

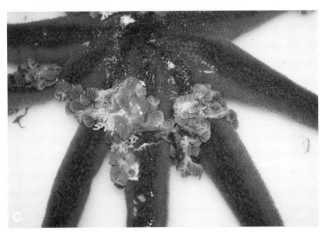

Figure 17.9.   A: Mild ulcer of a sun star. **B:** Moderate ulcers. **C:** Severe ulcers resulting in multifocal evisceration in a sun star. Both the pyloric cecae (ruffled tissue) and gonad (finer, branching tissue) are clearly evident. Courtesy of Kelly Krell.

thickness breach of the body wall and evisceration (Figure 17.9, Color Plate 17.9). Although a number of etiologies have been pursued (bacterial infection, poor water quality, and toxin from a neighboring sea star), the cause (or causes) of this condition remains unknown (K. Krell, personal communication, 2004).

Clinical Procedures

Most parasitic diseases of echinoderms are diagnosed based on wet-mount macroscopy or microscopy, or histopathology from postmortem specimens. Coelomic fluid can be collected nondestructively to harvest amebocytes for counts or functional studies, to assess bacteremia, and to measure coelomic fluid constituents such as total protein (Bang and Lemma, 1962; Jellett et al., 1988; Coteur et al., 2002). In sea urchins, coelomic fluid may be accessed by using needle and syringe via the peristomial membrane (Jellett et al., 1988). In starfish, coelomic fluid may be collected directly from a severed distal arm tip (Coteur et al., 2002), which regenerates, or by needle and syringe percutaneously through the arm tip (Bang and Lemma, 1962; K. Krell, personal communication, 2004) into the oral or aboral hemal

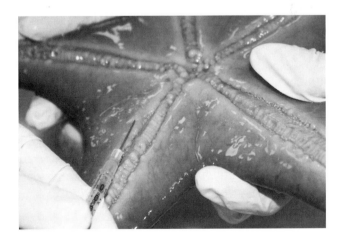

Figure 17.10.   Drawing hemolymph from the oral hemal ring of a sea star. Courtesy of Kelly Krell.

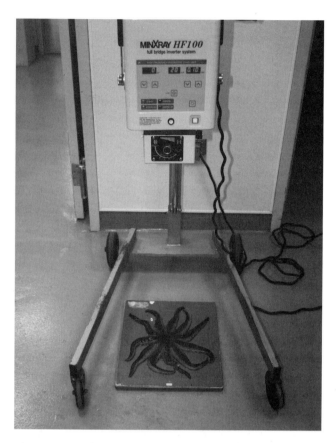

Figure 17.11.   A portable unit being used to radiograph a sun star (*Solaster* sp.). Courtesy of Kelly Krell.

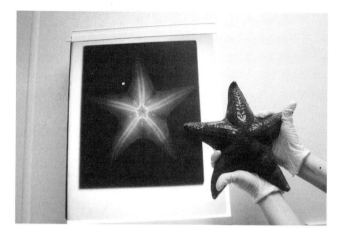

Figure 17.12.   A helpful orientation technique used by the Shedd Aquarium is to position the animal so the madreporite is in the *top left* corner (note location of the *M* marker). Courtesy of Kelly Krell.

cumbers, gradual dilution of sea water with freshwater for large sea stars, and 10 min. in calcium-free sea water followed by 10 min. in lg/L MS-222 for feather stars.

Some work has been done with imaging echinoderms (Figures 17.11 and 17.12, Color Plate 17.12). Radiographs can be used to evaluate the status of the ossicles and identify subclinical lesions of the skeleton (Figure 17.13).

Treatment Protocols

Published treatment protocols are lacking for echinoderms. Presumably principles of treating other marine invertebrates would apply, with many antibiotics being safe, whereas many parasiticides designed to kill pathogenic invertebrates are likely to be similarly toxic to the host invertebrate. Antibiotics could be delivered by injection into the coelom or by bath treatment, although basic parameters such as clearance rate or absorption from the water column have not been determined. One class of parasiticide that should be safe for echinoderms and effective against crustacean and other chitin-bearing parasites are the chitin synthesis inhibitors, such as lufenuron or diflubenzuron.

Human Health Hazards

The most common human health hazard associated with echinoderms is sea urchin spinal injury. Effects can be immediate, from physical injury and in some cases a painful toxin, secondary from seeding a bacterial infection, or chronic with granuloma formation occurring up to several months following initial injury (Sparks, 1985; Ruppert and Barnes, 1994; De la Torre and Toribio, 2001). Toxins from the pedicellariae of some species may also produce a painful reaction (Ruppert and Barnes, 1994).

ring (Figure 17.10). Anticoagulants used successfully include EGTA and EDTA. Workers at the Shedd Aquarium in Chicago have used sodium heparin with success (K. Krell, personal communication, 2004). Although anesthesia has not been routinely considered in echinoderm research, as with many other marine invertebrates they have been immobilized/anesthetized with magnesium chloride (MgCl$_2$, 8% solution in tap water for the sea star *Asterias forbesi* [Anderson, 1965]; and MgCl$_2$ · 6H$_2$O, 7.5% solution mixed with an equal volume of seawater for the sea stars *Luidia clathrata* and *Astropecten articulatus* [McCurley and Kier, 1995]). The fish anesthetic tricaine methanesulfonate (MS-222, 3-aminobenzoic acid ethyl ester) has been used in a concentrated form (10 g/L in seawater, versus approximately 100 mg/L for teleost fish) for the sea star *Coscinasterias calamaria* (O'Neill, 1994). Other anesthetic/immobilizing agents reported to be used in echinoderms include menthol (2.5%–5.0% in sterile seawater for the brittle star *Amphipholis squamata* [= *Axiognahus squamatus*] [Costello and Henley, 1971]) and propylene phenoxetol (propylenphenoxythol, 1-phenoxy-2-propanol, 1-phenoxypropan-2-ol; 2 mL/L saturated solution in seawater for the sea cucumbers *Holothuria forskali* [Van den Spiegel and Jangoux, 1987] and *Stichopus badionotus* [Hill and Reinschmidt, 1976]). For relaxation prior to preservation of specimens Hendler et al. (1995) recommend magnesium salts for general use, propylene phenoxytol for refractory sea cu-

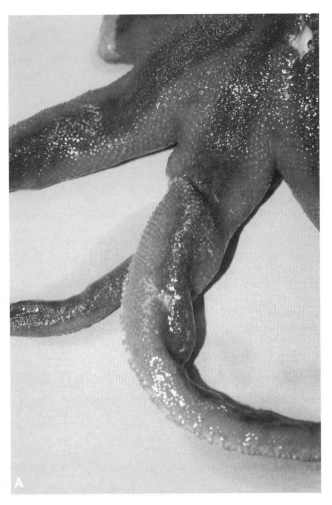
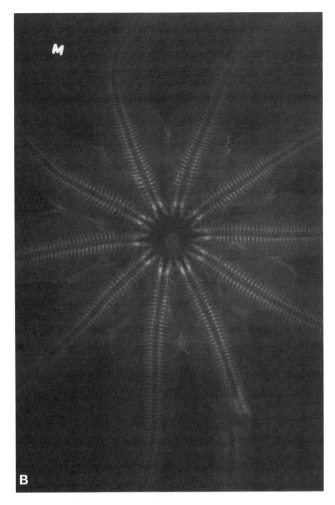

Figure 17.13.   A: Grossly visible osteolytic arm in a sun star. **B:** Radiographic view of an arm fracture. The osteolytic area can be seen at the *lower right*. *M*, madreporite. Courtesy of Kelly Krell.

References

Anderson JM (1965). Studies on visceral regeneration in sea-stars. III. Regeneration of the cardiac stomach in *Asterias forbesi* (Desor). Biol Bull 129:454–470.

Aronson RB (1987). Predation on fossil and recent ophiuroids. Paleobiology 13:187–192.

Aronson RB and Harms CA (1985). Ophiuroids in a Bahamian saltwater lake: The ecology of a Paleozoic-like community. Ecology 66:1472–1483.

Bang FB and Lemma A (1962). Bacterial infection and reaction to injury in some echinoderms. J Insect Pathol 4:401–414.

Barnes RSK, Calow P, Olive PJW, Golding DW, and Spicer JI (2001). The Invertebrates: A Synthesis, 3rd edition. Blackwell Science, Oxford, 497 pp.

Bauer JC and Agerter CJ (1987). Isolation of bacteria pathogenic for the sea urchin *Diadema antillarum* (Echinodermata: Echinoidea). Bull Mar Sci 40:161–165.

Beck G and Habicht GS (1996). Immunity and the invertebrates. Sci Am 275:60–66.

Beck G, Ellis T, Azhang HY, Lin WY, Beauregard K, Habicht GS, and Truong N (2001). Nitric oxide production by coelomocytes of *Asterias forbesi*. Dev Comp Immunol 25:1–10.

Berg G and Gibson R (1996). A redescription of *Nemertoscolex parasiticus* Greeff, 1879, an apparently endoparasitic heteronemertean from the coelomic fluid of the echiuroid *Echiurus echiurus* (Pallas). J Nat Hist 30:163–173.

Bower SM, McGladdery SE, and Price IM (1994). Synopsis of infectious diseases and parasites of commercially exploited shellfish. Annu Rev Fish Dis 4:1–199.

Byrne M, Cerra A, Nishigaki T, and Hoshi M (1997). Infestation of the Japanese sea star *Asterias amurensis* by the ciliate *Orchitophyra stellarum*: A caution against the use of this ciliate for biological control. Dis Aquat Org 28:235–239.

Costello DP and Henley C (1971). Methods for Obtaining and Handling Marine Eggs and Embryos, 2nd edition. Marine Biological Laboratory, Woods Hole, MA, 247 pp.

Coteur G, Corriere N, and Dubois P (2002). Environmental factors influencing the immune responses of the common European starfish (*Asterias rubens*). Fish Shellfish Immunol 12:187–200.

De la Torre C and Toribio J (2001). Sea-urchin granuloma: Histologic profile. A pathologic study of 50 biopsies. J Cutaneous Pathol 28:223–228.

Gilles KW and Pearse JS (1986). Disease in sea urchins *Strongylocentrotus purpuratus*: Experimental infection and bacterial virulence. Dis Aquat Org 1:105–114.

Goggin CL and Murphy NE (2000). Conservation of sequence in the internal transcribed spacers and 5.8S ribosomal RNA among geographically separated isolates of parasitic scutocociliates (Ciliophora, Orchitophryidae). Dis Aquat Org 40:79–83.

Gore SR, Lewbart GA, Christian L, and Law JM (2003). The effects of copper sulfate on the purple sea urchin *Arbacia punctulata*. Proc Int Assoc Aquat Anim Med 34:111–112.

Hagen NT (1996). Parasitic castration of the green echinoid *Strongylocentrotus droebachiensis* by the nematode endoparasite *Echinomermella matsi*: Reduced reproductive potential and reproductive death. Dis Aquat Org 24:215–226.

Hendler G, Miller JE, Pawson DL, and Kier PM 1995). Sea Stars, Sea Urchins and Allies: Echinoderms of Florida and the Caribbean. Smithsonian Institution Press, Washington, DC, pp. 21–27.

Hill RB and Reinschmidt D (1976). Relative importance of the antioxidant and anesthetic properties of propylene phenoxetol in its action as a "preservative" for living holothurians. J Invertebr Pathol 28:131–135.

Hughes TP (1994). Catastrophes, phase shifts, and large-scale degradation of a Caribbean coral reef. Science 265:1547–1551.

Jangoux M (1990). Diseases of Echinodermata. In: Kinne O, ed. Diseases of Marine Animals, volume 3. Biologische Anstalt Helgoland, Hamburg, pp 439–567.

Jellett JF, Wardlaw AC, and Scheibling RE (1988). Experimental infection of the echinoid *Strongylocentrotus droebachiensis* with *Paramoeba invadens*: Quantitative changes in the coelomic fluid. Dis Aquat Org 4:149–157.

Jones GM and Scheibling RE (1985). *Paramoeba* sp. (Amoebida, Paramoebidae) as the possible causative agent of sea urchin mass mortality in Nova Scotia. J Parasitol 71:559–565.

Lessios HA (1988). Mass mortality of *Diadema antillarum* in the Caribbean: What have we learned? Annu Rev Ecol Syst 19:371–393.

Liddell WD and Ohlhorst SL (1986). Changes in benthic community composition following the mass mortality of *Diadema* at Jamaica. J Exp Mar Biol Ecol 95:271–278.

McCurley RS and Kier WM (1995). The functional morphology of starfish tube feet: The role of a crossed-fiber helical array in movement. Biol Bull 188:197–209.

Nagelkerken I, Smith GW, Snelders E, Karel M, and James S (1999). Sea urchin *Meoma ventricosa* die-off in Curaçao (Netherlands Antilles) associated with a pathogenic bacterium. Dis Aquat Org 38:71–74.

Nichols D (1962). Echinoderms. Hutchinson University Library, London, 192 pp.

O'Neill PL (1994). The effect of anesthesia on spontaneous contraction of the body wall musculature in the asteroid *Coscinasterias calamaria*. Mar Behav Physiol 24:137–150.

Ruppert EE and Barnes RD (1994). Invertebrate Zoology, 6th edition. Saunders, Philadelphia, pp 920–995.

Schiebling RE and Hennigar AW (1997). Recurrent outbreaks of disease in sea urchins *Strongylocentrotus droebachiensis* in Nova Scotia: Evidence for a link with large-scale meteorologic and oceanographic events. Mar Ecol Prog Ser 152:155–165.

Shimizu M (1994). Histopathological investigation of the spotted gonad disease in the sea urchin, *Strongylocentrotus intermedius*. J Invertebr Pathol 63:182–187.

Sparks AK (1985). Synopsis of Invertebrate Pathology Exclusive of Insects. Elsevier, Amsterdam, 423 pp.

Steneck RS, Graham MH, Bourque BJ, Corbett D, Erlandson JM, Estes JA, and Tegner MJ (2002). Kelp forest ecosystems: Biodiversity, stability, resilience and future. Environ Conserv 29:436–459.

Van den Spiegel D and Jangoux M (1987). Cuverian tubules of the holothuroid *Holothuria forskali* (Echinodermata): A morphofunctional study. Mar Biol 96:263–275.

Chapter 18

UROCHORDATES

Robert S. Bakal

Introduction

The urochordates, or tunicates as they are often referred to, are an evolutionarily important group of animals. They represent a bridge between the invertebrates and the vertebrates. This has made them extremely interesting and valuable to researchers in a variety of disciplines. As a result many facilities currently maintain cultures of urochordates or cell lines derived from animals in this group. In addition to their value as research specimens, there is also some demand for these animals as human food items or for display in commercial or home aquaria. Currently these are very small markets, which are easily satisfied by collection of animals from the wild, but could expand in the future. Although there is relatively little information available on the diseases or treatments of these animals, their evolutionary and research importance, coupled with their potential future uses, make their inclusion in this book essential.

Natural History and Taxonomy

Complete body fossils of urochordates are rarely encountered due to the soft structure of their bodies. The oldest fossils of urochordates are believed to have come from the Early Cambrian period of the Paleozoic Era and are approximately 525 million years old. There is some debate over the actual classification of these fossils, as some researchers have reclassified these animals as cephalochordates (Chen et al., 1995). There have also been reports of fossil urochordates from the Precambrian period, but these have been met with skepticism. Despite the soft nature of their bodies, urochordate spicules have been found as microfossils; some paleontologists are unfamiliar with these structures and therefore may misidentify them as being of sponge origin.

There are approximately 1600 identified species of urochordates. They are exclusively marine and can be found in all the world's oceans.

The subphylum Urochordata, once referred to as Tunicata, exists within the phylum Chordata. The urochordates are subdivided into three classes: Ascidiacea, Thaliacea, and Larvacea. All chordates, including the urochordates, possess three unique characteristics at some point during their life cycle: a notochord, a dorsal hollow nerve cord, and pharyngeal gill slits. In addition, the urochordates and vertebrates all have blood contained in vessels, a ventrally located heart, and a post-anal tail. The tail is an extension of the notochord or backbone and musculature, beyond the anus, and contains no internal organs. In addition, all chordates exhibit bilateral symmetry.

Ascidians, commonly called sea squirts, are sessile organisms found in a wide variety of marine habitats. They exist as solitary animals or in colonies or groups fixed to some type of substrate (Barnes, 1987). Ascidians represent over 90% of all currently identified urochordates. They possess all three of the previously mentioned characteristics of chordates in the free-swimming larval stage. The larval stage is similar in appearance to a tadpole (larval amphibian) but loses the dorsal hollow nerve cord and notochord, as well as the tail, during metamorphosis into the sessile adult form. The pharyngeal gill slits are retained, enlarged, and function in particle capture for feeding by the animal.

The thaliacians, which include the salps and doliolids, are pelagic marine organisms. The class contains about 100 species in six genera. They are found in all the world's oceans but are more numerous in warmer climates (Barnes, 1987). Like the ascidians, they possess the three main characteristics of the chordates early in their life cycle but lose the dorsal hollow nerve cord and notochord during metamorphosis into the planktonic adult form. During metamorphosis, they lose their tails and use water currents generated by cilia or muscle contractions to propel them through the water column.

The larvacians, also called appendicularians, are so named because they are neotenic and retain their basic larval form. Even as adults the Larvacea have a dorsal hollow nerve cord and a notochord. They retain their tail, which is used for propulsion. These creatures inhabit the surface waters of all the world's oceans. There are approximately 70 species of Larvacea currently identified, and they are the most specialized of all the urochordates (Barnes, 1987).

Anatomy and Physiology

This section deals exclusively with the anatomy of the adult forms. There is extreme variability in the development and differentiation of the larvae of various species, making it nearly impossible to present a generalized anatomical plan. There is also extreme variability within the adult forms, but many characteristics are shared within the three classes.

The ascidians are spherical to cylindrical, range in size from 1 to 200 mm, and come in a variety of colors, with gray and green being the most common (Barnes, 1987). Their outermost surface is called the *tunic*. Its role is to support and protect the internal structures. The tunic itself is made up of protein, carbohydrates, and water. One of the primary structural elements of the tunic is *tunicin*, a cellulose-like compound. Some species also have spicules composed of calcium salts within their tunic, adding to the structure and texture of the tunic (Barnes, 1987). Additionally, amoeboid cells and blood cells are found within the tunic, and it is often directly supplied by blood vessels. In colonial species the tunic usually surrounds the entire colony (Barnes, 1987). Figure 18.1 illustrates the major anatomical features of a tunicate.

The body wall of the ascidian is covered by a single layer of epithelial cells and contains striated longitudinal and circular muscle bands within the mesenchyme. The circular muscle bands are very well developed in the siphon walls and function to close off the siphon while the remaining muscles can, to a small extent, contract the entire body. This process depends on the rigidity of the tunic (Barnes, 1987). It is the ability of these animals to constrict these muscles and force water out the siphons that has earned them the name sea squirts.

Ascidians possess two siphons through which water moves into and out of the animals: the incoming or *buccal siphon* and the outgoing or *atrial siphon*. Water flows through the buccal siphon, where a ring of tentacles prevents large items from getting past the siphon (Barnes, 1987). Once past the tentacles, the water enters the pharynx, which lies within a chamber called the *atrium* and is attached to the body wall along the ventral midline. The walls of the pharynx contain numerous slits that enable water to pass through into the atrium. Strands of tissue transverse the atrium, providing structural support and preventing overexpansion of the body due to the massive amounts of water filtered by the animal (Barnes, 1987). The pharyngeal slits are arranged in rows with transverse bars of tissue called *stigmata* between the rows. In many species there are also longitudinal bars or stigmata present. Cilia on the lateral aspects of

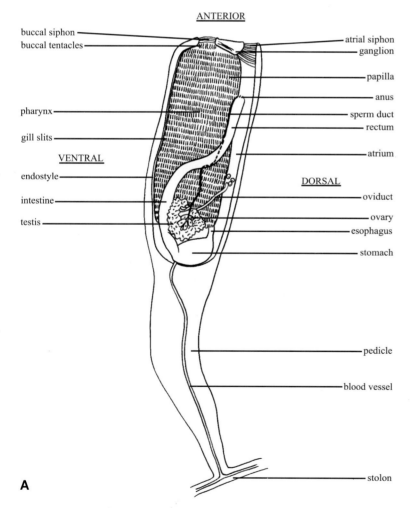

Figure 18.1.   A: Diagrammatic representation of a typical zoid from a colonial tunicate (*Ecteinascidia* sp.). Left-side view with a portion of the pharyngeal wall removed. Reproduced from Richard Fox, Lander University, by Alison Schroeer. Fox.

the stigmata move water through the pharyngeal slits and into the atrium while cilia on the internal surface of the bars move mucus perpendicular to the flow of the water (Barnes, 1987). The mucus is produced by the *endostyle*, which is a deep groove that extends the entire length of the pharyngeal wall and lies on the ventral side of the pharynx. The mucus produced by the endostyle, which is believed to be the origin of the vertebrate thyroid, is comprised of a mucoprotein that contains iodine-bound tyrosine. Flagella at the bottom of the endostyle force the mucus out and onto the bars, where the cilia move it in both directions toward the dorsal side of the animal. This mucus traps food particles as the water flows over it (Barnes, 1987). Opposite the endostyle is the *dorsal lamina*, a large ridge of tongue-like projections that guide the mucus posteriorly to the esophageal opening located on the dorsal side at the base of the pharynx (Barnes, 1987). The remainder of the digestive tract is U shaped. The esophagus forms the descending arm of the U. Closely associated and connected to this portion of the digestive system are numerous vesicles and tubules known as the *gastric* or *digestive glands*, which are secretory in nature, but the function of these secretions is currently unknown. The stomach, enlarged and located at the bend in the U, is responsible for extracellular digestion and lined with secretory cells. The intestine, or ascending arm of the U, opens distally into the atrium. The distal end of the intestine is modified to form a rectum. Waste products can then be expelled from the atrium through the atrial siphon (Barnes, 1987).

The circulatory system of the ascidian is characterized by the presence of a heart and a series of circulatory canals. Despite

their function and organization, these canals cannot be called vessels, because they lack true walls. The heart of the ascidian is a short, curved muscular tube that lies within a pericardial cavity located at the base of the digestive tract. The heart contains no valves. Rhythmic contractions are produced by excitation centers located at either end of the heart. The heart is aligned dorsoventrally with openings at either end (Barnes, 1987). Blood typically flows in a dorsal to ventral direction. From the ventral end of the heart the blood runs through the subendostylar sinus beneath the endostyle and through the branchial channels, which supply the bars of the pharynx. From here the blood is delivered, via canals, to the other visceral organs, including the digestive tract, and then back to the dorsal side of the heart (Barnes, 1987). Periodically these animals exhibit a reversal of blood flow. This is facilitated by the lack of heart valves and the presence of the excitation center at the dorsal end of the heart. This reversal is transient, and normal flow is resumed after 2–3 min. It is believed that since many of the major internal organs are in series (not in parallel), the periodic reversal of flow enables organs at the end of the line to have regular access to freshly oxygenated and nutrient-rich blood (Ruppert et al., 2004).

The cerebral ganglion, or brain, of the ascidian is a cylindrical or spherical structure found within the body wall connective tissue between the siphons (Rupert et al., 2004). Nerves emanating from this ganglion innervate all the major structures of the body. Urochordates do not possess any specialized sense organs but do have numerous sensory cells that are found on the buccal tentacles, within the atrium, and on the internal and external aspects of both siphons. These cells probably enable the animal to monitor, and therefore regulate, water flow. Immediately ventral to the cerebral ganglion lies the neural gland (which is a misleading name, since it lacks nerves and may not be glandular at all). A ciliated duct from the gland empties into the pharynx. The neural gland and ciliated duct help regulate the blood's fluid volume (Ruppert et al., 2004).

The vast majority of ascidians are hermaphroditic, possessing a single ovary and a single testis, which are generally located adjacent to the digestive tract, with the oviduct and spermatic duct coursing alongside the digestive tract and opening into the atrium (Barnes, 1987). Solitary animals generally release their eggs into the environment, where they are fertilized. The eggs of these animals are very small and surrounded by membranes that enhance their buoyancy. In contrast the eggs of the colonial species may be held within the atrium. In some species, the atrium develops special pouches to hold the developing eggs. Once hatched, the larvae may leave the parent or complete development may take place within the atrium. The larval form of the ascidians has a very short free-living period and does not exceed 36 h (Barnes, 1987).

In addition to sexual reproduction, many ascidians may undergo asexual reproduction, or *budding*. The process and tissue origins of budding are so complex and variable they preclude inclusion in this text.

The general anatomy of the thaliacians is similar to that of the ascidians, with some notable exceptions. Because the thaliacians are planktonic, their buccal and atrial siphons are located at opposite ends of their body. This enables them not only to

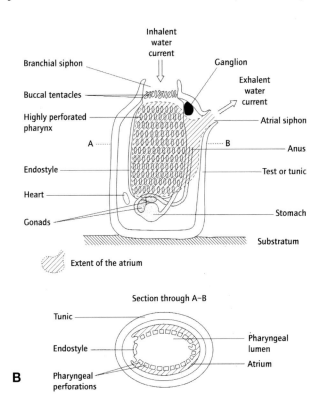

Figure 18.1.   B: Diagrammatic representation of a generalized solitary ascidian. From Barnes et al. (2001), Figure 7.32.

use the water currents developed by ciliary movements and muscle contractions for feeding and gas exchange but as a means of propulsion, as well. In addition, the animals of this class are all transparent, as are many planktonic creatures (Barnes, 1987).

The larvacians are quite a bit different from either the adult ascidians or the adult thaliacians and are the most specialized of all urochordates (Barnes, 1987). As previously described the larvacians are neotinic and retain many of their larval characteristics throughout life. They retain their tails (used for locomotion) and resemble the tadpole larvae of the other two classes of urochordates. The larvacians do not have siphons. The mouth is located on the anterior end of the body, and the distal digestive tract opens directly to the environment on the ventral body surface. The pharynx has only two pharyngeal clefts, which both open to the outside as opposed to opening into an atrium (Barnes, 1987). These animals do not have a tunic. Instead the surface epithelium secretes a gelatinous structure called a *house*, which surrounds the animal. The house has an incurrent orifice and an excurrent orifice (Barnes, 1987). The animal's tail movements cause currents to be produced that draw water into the house through the incurrent orifice, which is covered by a mesh of fine fibers that keeps large particles out. The water then passes through a second mesh filter, which serves to capture any nannoplankton in the water. The plankton is delivered to the mouth through a mucus tube (Barnes, 1987). The house itself is shed and replaced continuously. The house is produced in a compact mass and is expanded to full size by the animal's movements and water flow in a matter of seconds (Barnes, 1987). Studies of larvacians in the family Oikopleuridae have shown they retain their houses for a maximum of 4 h; a single animal can produce as many as 16 houses in a day. During spawning, house production ceases, and only sexual reproduction occurs in these species (Fennaux, 1985).

Infectious Diseases

Although their large body cavities with extensive water circulation make them exceedingly good parasitic and commensal hosts, there are no reports of any primary pathogen-induced mortality in this subphylum (Monniot, 1980). Secondary invasion of bacteria can and does occur as a result of injury to the animal or the decomposition of dead epibiota. The latter seems to be more common among aquarium animals and is a function of the deteriorating tissue remaining on the host as opposed to being removed by scavengers as in nature (Monniot, 1980). Besides these pathogenic bacterial conditions, some species of urochordates have commensal bacterial organisms. In many instances this commensal relationship is extremely specialized and may even be an obligate relationship. The commensal bacteria are often confined to specific organs and have special properties, such as luminescence. The commensal bacteria may be passed from parent to offspring in the egg, ensuring the continuation of the relationship (Julin, 1912; Pierantoni, 1921). At present there are no reports of any treatment for the pathogenic bacteria affecting these animals.

The line between parasitic and commensal organisms is often not clear in the literature. There is a vast array of protist organisms, including flagellates, apicomplexans, haplosporidians, ciliates, nephromyces, and even some algal organisms that are considered parasitic of or commensal with urochordates. In most cases the protist parasite or commensal appears to be species specific. These organisms are extremely common and in many cases animals may bear very heavy infestations (Monniot, 1980). In the case of haplosporidians, infestations may become so heavy that aggregations of the brown-pigmented spores can be seen by the naked eye, with little or no apparent affect on the host (Monniot, 1980).

Metazoan commensals and parasites of urochordates are numerous and varied. Cnidarians, ctenarians, turbellarians, annelids, bryozoans, nemerteans, gastropods, bivalves, cephalopods, copepods, amphipods, isopods, cirripedians, decapods, and fish have also been widely identified (Monniot, 1980). Although the metazoan parasites and commensals may be species specific, this host specificity seems less common for protists. In some instances the relationship between the host urochordate and the commensal or parasite is very simple, as in certain fish commensals. In this relationship the fish uses the urochordate as shelter and in return the urochordate receives food either from the fish's waste or from bits of uneaten food (Madin and Harbison, 1977; Janssen and Harbison, 1981). In other instances the relationship between the host and parasite or commensal can be extremely complex. In the case of certain copepod parasites the sexual development of the copepod is determined by the age of the host. If the copepod develops in a very young animal, the copepod will develop into a male. If the copepod develops in an adult animal, it will develop into a female, unless there is already a female present, in which case it will develop into a male (Hipeau-Jacquotte, 1982). This shows the extreme complexity of not only the relationship between this host and parasite but between two parasites within the same host.

No treatments are currently available or recommended for any of these parasitic organisms. Regimens that are used to treat these types of organisms in other hosts (e.g., vertebrates) are at risk of being as lethal to the urochordates as they are to the parasites themselves. The limited culture of these animals, coupled with the apparent minimal impact of the parasites on their hosts, make development of treatments for these parasites unlikely in the near future.

References

Barnes RD. 1987. Invertebrate Zoology, 5th edition. Saunders College, Philadelphia, pp 851–865.

Barnes RSK, Calow P, Olive PJW, Golding DW, and Spicer JI. 2001. The Invertebrates: A Synthesis, 3rd edition. Blackwell Science, Oxford, 497 pp.

Chen JY, Dzik J, Edgecombe GD, Ramskold L, and Zhouu GQ. 1995. A possible Early Cambrian chordate. Nature 377:720–722.

Fennaux R. 1985. Rhythm of secretion of oikopleurids' houses. Bull Mar Sci 37:498–503.

Hipeau-Jacquotte R. 1982. Host influence on the sex differentiation of its parasite. In: Parasites—Their World and Ours: Abstracts of the

Fifth International Congress of Parasitology, Toronto, Canada, 7–14 August 1982. Mol Biochem Parasitol (Suppl), p 586.

Jannsen J and Harbison GR. 1981. Fish in salps: The association of squaretails (*Tetragonursus* spp.) with pelagic tunicates. J Mar Biol Assoc UK 61:917–927.

Julin C. 1912. Reserches sur le developpement embryonnaire de *Pyrosoma giganteum*. Zool Jb 15(Suppl):775–863.

Madin LP and Harbison GR. 1977. The association of Amphipoda Hyperiidea with gelatinous zooplankton. I. Association with Salpidae. Deep Sea Res 24:449–463.

Monniot C. 1980. Diseases of Urochordata. In: Kinne O, ed. Diseases of Marine Animals, volume 3. John Wiley and Sons, New York, pp 569–636.

Pierantoni M. 1921. Gli organi luminosi simbiotici ed il loro ciclo ereditario in *Pyrosoma giganteum*. Pubbl Stn Zool Napoli, volume 4.

Ruppert EE, Fox RS, and Barnes RD. 2004. Invertebrate Zoology: A Functional Evolutionary Approach, 7th edition. Brooks/Cole—Thomson Learning, Belmont, CA, 963 pp.

Chapter 19

DIAGNOSTIC TECHNIQUES AND SAMPLE HANDLING

Ilze K. Berzins and Roxanna Smolowitz*

Introduction

Taking a clinical approach to invertebrate health is a relatively new, emerging field in veterinary medicine (Cooper, 1980, 1988, 2001; Frye, 1986; Cooper et al., 1992; Williams, 1999, 2001, 2003). Historically, detection of invertebrate diseases has been largely confined to the agricultural and aquaculture industries, with treatment, if any, based on a herd health approach. More recently, the evaluation and treatment of invertebrate disease are being focused on smaller groups of animals or the actual individual animal. The culture and use of invertebrates are steadily growing: as models for human and animal diseases in biomedical research expands (for invertebrate lab animal care, refer to www.nal.usda.gov/awic/pubs/invertebrates.htm); as pets and home aquarium systems in the private client sector; as display and educational animals in zoos and public aquariums; and finally, in the wild, as indicators of environmental health (Yevich and Yevich, 1994). Understanding the health and husbandry of this group of animals is becoming increasingly important to veterinary clinicians and, as part of this process, appropriate handling of specimens to aid in disease diagnosis is critical. Although specialized diagnostic techniques are used in detailed research studies (e.g., DNA probes [Stokes and Burreson, 2001; Stokes et al., 2001], in situ hybridization [Wang et al., 1998], freeze preparations for immunohistochemical studies [Strandberg et al., 1998], and scanning electron micrography [Hsu and Smolowitz, 2003]), the following discussion focuses on more practical methods for veterinary clinicians. It offers an overview of handling of samples from "mega"–invertebrates such as tarantulas, octopus, *nautilus*, or smaller specimens that can be found in aquarium and terrarium collections. Groups commonly encountered by practitioners include coelenterates (e.g., jellyfish, sea anemones, and corals); echinoderms (sea stars and sea urchins); arthropods, i.e., insects (e.g., butterflies, moths, stick insects, and grasshoppers); scorpions and tarantulas; crustaceans (e.g., crabs, lobster, and shrimp); and mollusks, i.e., bivalves (e.g., clams and oysters), gastropods (snails), and cephalopods (nautilus, octopus, cuttlefish, and squid). Other less commonly encountered groups include Porifera (sponges) and annelids, (oligochaetes, polychaetes, and leeches). Invertebrate parasites (e.g., nematodes, cestodes, and trematodes) are not covered. Excellent coverage of recommended methods of preservation for these organisms can be found in Noga (1996).

Data Collection from Living Specimens

Obtaining a History

Once a client has contacted you, an on-site evaluation of the situation is ideal. If this is not possible, the client should provide appropriate samples and a clinical history. For terrestrial animals, it is advisable that the client provide samples of the soil or bedding material. Evaluate the material for moisture content, uncharacteristic odors, mold or fungal growth, and coarseness or roughness of the substrate. For aquatic animals, the client should provide a recent sample of the water and submit it in a clean container such as a plastic or glass jar. Any water submitted must be separate from animal-transport water. Water samples should be evaluated immediately, but if this is not possible, they should be refrigerated and tested within 24 h. Prior to testing, the water sample should be allowed to return to the temperature of the exhibit system (if the client knows this). Key water parameters to evaluate include oxygen levels and temperature (more accurate if sampled on site), pH, ammonia, nitrite, nitrate, and salinity if dealing with marine or estuarine species. Other parameters such as alkalinity, hardness, and chloride can be tested for and often are more critical in freshwater systems. A variety of water-quality test kits are available. Basic kits offer semiquantitative results that will provide a general assessment of common problems encountered, whereas sophisticated equipment will be much more accurate, but more expensive, and may not be necessary for general clinical needs. Prices of kits and equipment do vary with accuracy and will range from

Acknowledgments. Dr. Susan Bower, Fisheries and Oceans Canada, Pacific Biological Station, Nanaimo, BC, Canada; Dr. Salvatore Frasca Jr., Department of Pathobiology and Veterinary Science, University of Connecticut; Dr. Michael Garner, Northwest ZooPath; Dr. Michael Kinsel, Zoological Pathology Program, University of Illinois; Ms. Carol McCollough, Diagnostics and Histology Laboratory, Maryland Department of Natural Resources, Cooperative Oxford Laboratory; Dr. Ester Peters from Tetra Tech, Inc.; Dr. Joseph Scimeca, Oak Ridge National Laboratory, Tennessee; and Ms. Peggy Reed, All Florida Veterinary Labs, Archer, Florida.

tens to thousands of dollars. An overview of kit selection, as well as testing for more specialized parameters (e.g., heavy metals and pesticides), is reviewed by Noga (1996).

Some of the animals that will be brought in for evaluation can be removed relatively easily from their home systems. However, when dealing with attached species (some echinoderms, anemones, and coral) advise clients to keep physical damage to a minimum when they are removing an animal from a tank. Also, animals that can bite, sting, or produce toxins that can result in skin irritation should be handled using powder-free latex gloves or rubber gloves.

During transport, animals should be housed in appropriately sized and shaped containers. For aquatic species, use the same general rule of thumb as is used for fish [for every 1 inch of fish (or invertebrate] use a half-gallon of water). For transport of terrestrial invertebrates, useful containers include the commercially available Critter Cages, which come in a variety of sizes and are fitted with a secure lid that provides adequate air exchange. If faced with extreme weather conditions outside, advise the client to place the animal container in an insulated cooler, with freezer packs if appropriate, before transporting the animal to the clinic.

Before physical examination of the animal, obtain a complete and accurate clinical history. Housing conditions (size, lighting, heat, humidity, and water parameters), source of the animal, presence of other animals, shipping conditions, supplier credentials if available, recent additions, food type and source, cleaning regimen, degree of water changes, and equipment type and maintenance (pumps, air stones, filters, lighting, ultraviolet light sterilizers, etc.) should be determined.

Physical Evaluation

When evaluating invertebrates, signs of stress and disease can be difficult to delineate. What is normal behavior? What is abnormal behavior? What are clinical signs to be aware of? A recent guide for assessing stress and disease in aquatic** invertebrates has been outlined by Miller-Morgan (2003) and is summarized here:

Cnidarians
Anorexia
Closed for long periods of time
Failure to display tentacles
Excess mucus production
Eversion of gastrodermis (GI tract lining, "stomach") for long periods
"Cannon ball" (overly rounded, margins of bell tucked under) appearance in jellyfish (normal though for the cannonball jellyfish, *Stomolophus meleagris*)
Erosions of the epidermis (Steers et al., 2003)

**Note that many of these clinical signs can also be applied to evaluating terrestrial invertebrates (which in most cases will be arthropods). Some specific signs for ill arachnids include anorexia, lethargy, damaged limb or body, loss of hairs (setae), retained slough (shed), presence of mites, abnormal discharge of fluids from external orifices, and twitching/incoordination (Cooper et al., 1992).

Mollusks
Anorexia
Lethargy
Gaping of shells
Excess mucus production
Sloughing of skin layers
Lowered threshold for inking
Pale color for extended periods
Self-mutilation
Abnormal swimming behavior (in cephalopods)

Arthropods
Anorexia
Lethargy
Erosions and darkening of the shell
Failure to right themselves
Leg or claw loss (may be a result of aggression, as well)
Incomplete molting

Echinoderms
Anorexia
Drooping of spines
Poor display of tube feet
Poor attachment to surfaces
Body whitening
Epithelial loss
Color loss
Failure to right themselves

Please refer to the individual chapters in this text for more taxa-specific details.

Sample Collection

Equipment for sample collection is relatively standard: needles and syringes of various sizes (tuberculin syringes with attached needles are ideal for smaller specimens), culturettes, glass slides and coverslips, capillary tubes, microcontainers, powder-free latex gloves, microscope, dissecting scope, forceps and scissors of various sizes, 70% ethanol (for quick sterilization of instruments or cleaning of collection sites if needed), and sterile water (not distilled) or seawater. Cutting shears, rongeurs, knives, a Dremel tool with small drill bits, and a hammer may also be required to gain access to internal spaces. When handling all specimens, be aware of the zoonotic disease potential (especially atypical mycobacterial infections) and remember that many of these animals can bite, sting, or produce toxins and irritants. Ensure you are properly protected when working with the specimens.

It is often necessary to sedate the organism for adequate sampling. Sedation as a means to provide analgesia is uncertain, because the capability of invertebrates to perceive pain is poorly understood (Williams, 1999) and much work is needed in this area. However, the animals can often be difficult to restrain properly, necessitating effective sedation. Ethanol (5%–10% solution), chlorobutanol (0.05%–0.5%), chloral hydrate (0.2%

solution in seawater), chloroform, urethane (1%), and Nembutal (sodium pentobarbital) (a barbiturate, 80–350 mg/L) are some of the compounds shown to be effective in mollusks (Ross and Ross, 1999). Two of the older, more commonly used agents are magnesium chloride or magnesium sulfate (magnesium competes with calcium for synaptic transmission). A general method is to add iso-osmotic 7.5% wt/vol magnesium chloride ($MgCl_2 \cdot 6H_2O$) slowly to the water containing the animal and monitor an appropriate dose level by noting when the animal does not respond to prodding. In addition to the immersion method, a 10% solution of magnesium chloride can be injected near the cerebral ganglia for a much faster effect. Tricaine methane sulfonate (MS-222) starting at a 0.3% solution and eugenol (the active ingredient in clove oil) are also noted to be effective, but concentrations used are variable depending on the animal group. In developing methods for euthanasia for green crabs, it was noted that 4.5 mL of eugenol (dissolved 1:10 in ethanol first) in a 1 L of water/seawater took 4h to death at about 18°C and that lesser times may be used for noninvasive procedures or gill clips (A. Hancock, unpublished data). Gaseous anesthetics (halothane, enflurane, and isoflurane) and carbon dioxide are also being used. For aquatic species, these anesthetics, usually administered with oxygen, can be added directly to the water or bubbled into the water. Carbon dioxide should be bubbled directly into the water. For terrestrial species, place the animal in a small induction chamber (for special designs, see Cooper [2001]) or, if small enough, a well-sealed jar. In all cases, take care to prevent release to the air. Although crustaceans may respond differently to some of the drugs listed for mollusks, presumably due to the difference in the chemicals involved at their synaptic receptor sites (Ross and Ross, 1999), many of the agents used are similar. Personal experiences with MS-222 in crustaceans have been unsuccessful but eugenol (clove oil) has been effective (R.S., unpublished data). Injectable agents being evaluated, procaine (25 mg/µg) and Saffan (alphaxolone–alphadolone, 30 mg/kg) have been shown to be effective in decapods (crabs) (Ross and Ross, 1999). Injection sites (as well as sampling sites) are the flexible arthrodial membranes between either the cephalothoracic and abdominal body segments, ventrally in the arthrodial membrane of the abdominal segments, or at the base of an appendage (Ross and Ross, 1999). Less information is available on echinoderms and cnidarians, but the magnesium-based solutions have been effective with most invertebrates and are known to be effective in these groups in particular. A more detailed discussion of appropriate anesthetic and monitoring techniques can be found in each speci-fic invertebrate-group chapter of this book, as well as in numerous papers, texts, and Web sites (Araujo et al., 1995; Ross and Ross, 1999; Biological Bulletin Compendia Web site www.hermes.mbl.edu/BiologicalBulletin/ANESCOMP/AnesComp-Tab1.html). It is also important to note that the concentrations of the various substances listed are for maintaining an anesthetic level. For euthanasia, it is advisable to increase the dose and/or time of exposure. Although an obvious choice for euthanasia would be pentobarbital, personal experience (R.S.) has shown that it was poorly effective and destroyed tissue at the injection site (in decapods [crabs]).

What actually can be collected? Surface tissue (skin scrapes), hemolymph and hemocytes (blood), and biopsy samples from easily accessible organs are some of the more commonly sampled specimens. However, clinicians will initially have to develop their own set of reference values because very little information is available for standard use. A general introduction to taking biological samples from invertebrates can be found in the work by Williams (1999). If one becomes involved with international health certification of invertebrates, more detailed information on internationally important diseases is found in the *Manual of Diagnostic Tests for Aquatic Animals* (OIE, 2003a), prepared by the Office International des Epizooties (OIE). The manual outlines accepted methods to use in the diagnosis of internationally important diseases and the *Aquatic Animal Health Code* (OIE, 2003b), provides health certification outlines. The aim is to ensure health safety of international trade in aquatic animals and products.

Prior to collecting samples, a thorough understanding of the anatomy is important in determining approach sites. A general invertebrate text will provide the basics (Brusca and Brusca, 1990), and more detailed information can be found in the 15-volume collection on general and microscopic invertebrate anatomy compiled by Harrison and Kohn (1991), as well as in the various chapters of this text.

Surface scrapes or swabs can be obtained from most invertebrates. The specimens are smeared or placed on glass slides, several drops of sterile saline or water (depending on the animal's environment) are added, and then a coverslip is added. The sample can be evaluated for parasites, mats of bacteria, and fungal elements. The samples can then be allowed to dry and subsequently stained with a variety of commercially available benchtop stains (such as Diff-Quik [Difco Laboratories, Sparks, MD]), Gram stains, and acid-fast stains (the cold-method stain, Kinyon's, is preferable for acid-fast evaluation). It is recommended that slides of interest be saved for future reference. Permanent slides can be made by adding several drops of mounting material (such as Permount) to the stained slide, applying a coverslip, and allowing the slide to dry for several days.

The *blood* of invertebrates is composed of hemolymph. Blood cells are named *hemocytes* or *amebocytes*. The oxygen-carrying pigment in most groups is *hemocyanin*, which will turn blue when exposed to air and circulate freely as proteinaceous crystals in the hemolymph. Invertebrates do not have adaptive immune capacity, but their innate immune system has been identified. The hemocyte types and some associated functions in some invertebrates have been identified, including bivalve mollusks, lobsters, sea urchins, horseshoe crabs, tarantulas, and others (e.g., see Carballal et al. [1997] and Schartau and Leiderscher [1983]). Not all studies agree on the types of hemocytes in the hemolymph of a species or the functions of each (Cheng, 1981; Cheng et al., 1984; Martin and Hose, 1997). More work needs to be done in this area. In general, hemocytes of bivalve mollusks and crustaceans are divided into hyalinocytes and granulocytes (Martin and Hose, 1997; Cheng, 1996; Carballal et al., 1997). Starfish, cephalopods, and horseshoe crabs (*Limulus polyphemus*) contain only one cell type, the amebocyte (Budelmann et al., 1997), whereas sea urchins are thought to contain several different hemocyte types (depending on the author and the species of urchin) (Cavey and Märkel, 1997). Functions attributed to hemocytes and amebocytes are pseudopodial movement and phagocytosis. Hemocyte encapsulation of parasites (nematodes) has been observed. Studies have begun to further characterize innate immune functions of hemocytes in oysters and American lobsters (Goedken and DeGuise, 2003; Hégaret et al., 2003a, 2003b; Morsey and DeGuise, 2003). Cell numbers and types appear to change significantly with seasons, size, gender, food availability, molt status, and gonadal development (Stolen et al., 1995; Carballal et al., 1998; Nollens et al., 2003). There have also been studies on hemolymph characteristics such as total protein, glucose, agglutinins, pH, lactic acid, and ion content (Cheng, 1981, 1996; Cheng et al., 1984; Santarém et al., 1994). Stolen et al. (1995) provide a variety of methods for collection and evaluation of defense mechanisms in bivalves. However, many of these tests require microtechniques that are not practical for the clinician, yet they do provide information on techniques used at a research level. With adequate sample size, some of the more basic parameters such as pH, glucose, hemocyte count, ion composition, and protein content, however, could be evaluated in the clinic.

When examining the hemocytes or hemolymph of any invertebrate, first review the types of cells, associated functions, and other known basic parameters for that animal.

Hemolymph collection sites are varied, and knowledge of the anatomy of the individual species is needed. Most invertebrates do not have closed circulatory systems, and much of the internal spaces are part of a hemocoelomic system. Collection sites include hemocoelomic spaces themselves, pericardial sacs, and pumping organs or hearts. In crustaceans, aspirates may be taken by inserting needles through the softer cuticle (arthrodial membrane) found between hard cuticle plates (at suture lines) and at the base of legs. Actual leg amputation will also provide samples of hemolymph from the wound site. In bivalves, the posterior adductor muscle sinus/pericardial sac is a common sampling site (Howard and Smith, 1983; Smolowitz and Reinisch, 1986; Ross and Ross, 1999). Samples can be obtained from the pericardial sac in oysters through a hole drilled in the ligament holding the shells together (Howard and Smith, 1983) or by inserting the needle through the ligament area in clams. At any collection site, it is advisable to clean the area first with 70%–80% ethyl alcohol.

The information available on the use of anticoagulants is minimal. EDTA has been used, but its efficacy is relatively unknown. R.S. dilutes hemolymph 1/10 into sterile seawater upon drawing out hemolymph (unpublished data).

Hemolymph smears can be made by placing several drops onto a glass slide coated with poly-L-lysine and allowing them to settle for several minutes (Smolowitz and Reinisch, 1986). Cells may be evaluated unstained, or standard benchtop stains may be used to delineate parasites and fungal or bacterial infections (Clauss et al., 2003).

Cell counts may also be attempted, but, as discussed previously, the results may be highly variable. Because of the mobility of the hemocytes, cells should be fixed prior to evaluation of their number. In a method described by Santarém et al. (1994), an aliquot of hemolymph/hemocytes is fixed in a solution of 1% formalin in TBS (0.05 M Tris–buffered saline, pH 8.4). Counts are then made using standard hemocytometer methods.

Evaluation of excretal products is another relative unknown, but if such substances can be obtained they should be examined. In arachnids (spiders), guanine, uric acid, adenine, and hypoxanthine are several of the products that have been identified (Williams, 1999).

Biopsies can also be attempted. Use of a swab of 70% ethyl alcohol to cleanse the site for internal biopsies may be appropriate in situations when dealing with relatively hard exteriors (arthropods) but is too harsh for softer invertebrate tissue. A thorough flushing of the sampling site with sterile water or saline (depending on aquatic habitat of the host) is more appropriate for sampling softer tissues. Wet mounts of gills (as used in fish evaluations) often reveal parasites and fungi even without a stain, but a stained smear is recommended. Pieces of shell (Sherrill et al., 2002) or exoskeleton can also be evaluated once fixed and prepared properly.

When sampling for bacterial and fungal diseases, it is important to learn pathogen from normal flora. Nonpathogenic species are often ubiquitous in water (both fresh and salt) and in soil. If possible, take samples from normal individuals or from unaffected sites on a diseased individual to aid in delineating pathogenic species. Selecting an appropriate diagnostic laboratory is also critical. Ideally, select a lab with experience in aquatic organisms. If this is not possible, select a diagnostic facility willing to work with unusual specimens. Much of the initial work will be experimental for all involved, which should not be viewed as a disadvantage but rather a challenge, because results will contribute to the field of invertebrate medicine. The best type of culture media for microbiological sampling is unclear in many cases, but plating on both a rich medium and a poor medium (both adapted to saltwater) is useful. Marine brain–heart infusion broth and agar (see the formulas at the end of this chapter) are examples of rich media (Difco, 1998). Blood and MacConkey's agar have been used with some success (Williams, 1999; P. Reed, personal communication). Special sea-salt agars for marine species can be obtained from commercial suppliers. Sauboraud's dextrose agar can be used for fungal cultures, but, again, the challenge to clinicians is to determine normal from abnormal, and some infections may be detectable only on histological examination. Finally, ideal incubation temperatures for both bacterial and fungal agents in general have not been well established. Culturing at room temperature and at the species preferred temperature in addition to routine settings used for warm-blooded species is recommended.

Surface lesions in aquatic animals can be very hard to culture because of the microbial mat that will cover any external surfaces. Samples from affected and unaffected sites can be used for comparison to determine whether different flora are isolated from diseased sites. General methods for culturing surface bacteria on invertebrates involve flushing the site with sterile seawater (or, if possible, heat-sear the surface) and then proceeding as usual with sampling by using a sterile loop or culturette. For juvenile oyster disease (*Roseimarina crassostreae* [Boettcher et al., 2000]), culture the mantle edge where the lesions most often occur (R.S., unpublished method).

Standard viral detection is difficult because appropriate cell lines have not been developed or are not readily available. Special techniques (Hasson et al., 1997; Rodríquez et al., 2003) usually are required to detect viral infections. Insect disease diagnostics are more developed, and clinicians can try to contact appropriate research facilities for assistance.

Invertebrates themselves can serve as hosts to parasitic invertebrate species. Larger specimens may be discovered upon dissection of the host, but more commonly they will be noted in fixed specimens on histological evaluation. These parasites may be difficult to categorize because life cycles are often inadequately described. Specialized techniques do exist for characterizing parasites (Mullen et al., 2003) but may not be practical for clinicians. An exception to the sparsity of detection techniques is the technique developed using thioglycolate media to detect the protozoal infection, *Perkinsus marinus*, in oysters (Ray, 1954; Mackin, 1962).

Necropsy Procedures

One of the most difficult questions when approaching an invertebrate necropsy is determining whether the animal is actually dead. Ideally, moribund individuals will be available for euthanasia (see Appendix 2 in this book). Many anesthetic agents (see the previous discussion and Chapters 9–14 on arthropods) can be used for euthanasia simply by overdosing the animal and/or increasing the exposure period. Examining more than one individual is ideal but often not possible. In addition to having difficulty in determining death, the condition of a certain tissue may vary because different organs/tissues deteriorate at different rates, even while the animal is still alive, and many of the invertebrate tissues tend to deteriorate at a faster rate than vertebrate equivalents. Processing the animal as rapidly as possible is recommended.

Routine dissecting equipment will be appropriate for most specimens: compound microscope, dissecting scope, slides, coverslips, surgical blades, scissors, forceps, sampling materials for microbiological pathogens (discussed in the preceding section) and sample containers with fixative of choice.

A thorough understanding of anatomical structures is critical, as is knowledge of normal versus abnormal. If adequate information is unavailable on anatomical features, it is recommended that serial photographs be taken while the specimen is being dissected. Line drawings can then be created from these photographs that can aid in future dissections (Berzins et al., 1990).

Evaluate external and internal structures carefully. In mollusks, first examine the shell. Look for mantle recession, parasites (boring sponges and worm tunnels), blisters, pustules, and calcareous malformations (Howard and Smith, 1983). During an internal examination, look for firmness of tissue, changes in color, and cyst or tumor formation. In cephalopods, examine for erosions or ulceration of skin, swelling of mantle edges (edema), and increased mucus around the tentacles (as in the chambered *nautilus*). In echinoderms, evaluate for discolorations (black/red indicate areas of inflammation), loss of spines, activity of feet, and spines in the water. In crustaceans, look for shell erosions (note location and severity), blackening of gills (possibly indicative of a fungal infection), and hemolymph color—red for gaffkemia (a Gram-positive bacterium, *Aerococcus viridans* var. *homari*), and paramoeba (Russell et al., 2000), and orange for mineral disease (A. Dove, personal communication). Sometimes one will be able to see the color of hemolymph through the soft cuticle on the ventral surface of lobsters. Hemolymph will be whitish in crabs with *Hematodinium* sp. (a dinoflagellate).

Wet mounts or squash preparations are recommended on all identifiable organs.

There is very little information on baseline parameters, so begin to evaluate as many specimens as possible to develop a catalog of normal and diseased conditions.

When handling any type of animal tissue, be aware of potential zoonotic diseases. Routine hygienic practices will be adequate for most of the necropsy procedures.

Fixation Procedures

Many proper fixation techniques rely on adequate sedation of the specimen if it still is alive. Most of these animals have a propensity to contract or pull in tentacles. Careful anesthetizing or narcotizing should precede fixation. Ideally, as with other animal tissues, 0.5–1.0 cm samples and proper volume ratios are recommended (1:10 parts tissue to fixative). Entire specimens can be fixed, if not too large, by injecting fixative solutions into internal spaces prior to immersing the entire animal. In bivalves, the shell ligament holding the two halves together may need to be cut to expose internal tissues properly to the fixative. To prevent tearing of the mantle, use a sweeping motion of a knife to loosen mantle and muscle, cutting the adductor muscle(s) (the muscles holding the valves together) from the shell. If the animal has been feeding on a hard substrate (e.g., coral or sand) and is still alive, one may want to hold it in a container without substrate for a few days to allow the gut to clear to facilitate cutting into tissues for histology. Shells of gastropods may need to be chipped back to extract the animal.

Choice of a particular fixative may be based on select research criteria, but, for general usage, several standard fixatives have proven to be effective (see the next section). Avoid using compounds, such as phenolics and strong acids or bases, that may damage tissue during fixation (Sparks, 1985). As with all tissues specimens, do not freeze tissue because that will create a variety of artifacts.

Common Fixatives

Formulas are provided at the end of this chapter.

Neutral 10% Buffered Formalin

This is the most common, general fixative employed for all animals (Davidson's fixative is the most common alternative for invertebrates, and Dietrich's fixative is often used when sampling abundant numbers of small animals such as amphipods, copepods, and other zooplankton). Ten percent formalin in seawater is recommended if working with marine organisms. Concerns with shrinkage, loss of cellular detail, and poor staining qualities may be unfounded and be more the result of an improper use of the fixative as opposed to the fixative itself. Ensure that fixatives are properly prepared and buffered prior to use. Concerns with staining qualities may also reflect familiarization with the use of a specific fixative.

Bouin's Fixative (Bouin, 1897)

This is selectively used with more gelatinous, amorphous specimens such as jellyfish (M. Kinsel, personal communication). Avoid long-term storage in this fixative, because it can cause severe hardening of the tissues.

Davidson's Fixative (Shaw and Battle, 1957)

This is the most common alternative fixative to formalin, especially with mollusks, crustaceans, and echinoderms (S. Bower, personal communication).

Dietrich's (Kahle's) Fixative (Thompson and Hunt, 1966)

This is often used when sampling abundant numbers of small animals such as amphipods and copepods (zooplankton) from the water column.

Helly's Fixative (with modifications [Barszcz and Yevich, 1975])

This is thought to provide superior cellular detail, including granules of secretory cells with little shrinkage or distortion of cells. Modifications were made to the formula to remove a toxic component.

Ethyl Alcohol, 70%–80%

Alcohol is not often used as a primary fixative but can be used for shipment of fixed specimens or their storage fixed in other media (although there is a concern of hardening of tissue with long-term storage).

Special Handling

Useful tips on special handling of specimens are provided in *Humason's Animal Tissue Techniques* (Presnell and Schreibman, 1997), and the *Animal Processing Manual* by Callis and Sterchi (2002), which are summarized here:

- Porifera (sponges): Most sponges are marine. They contain calcium-based and silica-based spicules. For marine species, suggested fixatives are Helly's, Bouin's, or 10% formalin in seawater and Bouin's or 10% buffered formalin in freshwater. Sponges containing calcium spicules need to be decalcified. Those with silica spicules can be desilicified in 80% alcohol plus 5% hydrofluoric acid added gradually in a glass dish coated with paraffin. After a few hours, the specimen should be transferred to 80% alcohol.
- Coelenterates
  - Hydrae: Place the animal in a shallow dish with a few drops of water and then slowly pipette fixative onto the specimen, adding the fixative first to the base of the animal

and then up toward the tentacles (this prevents the tentacles from withdrawing).
  - Sea anemones: First anesthetize the animal (a 30% magnesium chloride solution is recommended), leaving it in the solution until there is no contraction of tentacles. Pour off the solution and add the fixative (Bouin's or 10% formalin seawater) slowly down the side of the container. Pipette some through the oral cavity.
  - Jellyfish: First anesthetize the animal (magnesium solution). While the animal is in seawater, add fixative (10% buffered formalin) down the side of the container (10–100 mL seawater rough proportion). Stir. After 2–3 h, transfer to fresh 10% formalin seawater in solution.
  - Medusae: First anesthetize the animal (magnesium solutions). When the bell no longer contracts, slowly add fixative (10% buffered formalin in seawater), stirring gently.
  - Corals with extended polyps: First narcotize with magnesium solutions and then slowly add fixative (10% buffered formalin in seawater). The stony corals will need to be decalcified before trimming. Horny corals contain a compound known as gorgonin and do not need to be decalcified but may be difficult to trim. Soft corals can be processed for histology without decalcification, because they do not have a calcium base.
- Echinoderms
  - Narcotize first using a magnesium chloride or magnesium sulfate solution. When tube feet and pedicellaria are no longer moving, inject fixative into tips of the sea star and then drop the entire animal (if not excessively large) in a fixative solution such as 10% buffered formalin in seawater. Larger animals may need sectioning prior to fixation. Many in this group (sea stars, brittle stars, sea urchins, and sand dollars) have calcareous plates and spines. Helly's, Bouin's, or 10% formalin in seawater are recommended fixatives. Decalcification will be necessary for most specimens and may take longer for some of the structures, for example, the mouthpiece (Aristotle's lantern). Also, some of the animals feed by scraping algae from calcareous surfaces, so they may have calcareous material in the gastrointestinal tract. Either remove the tract or be sure to decalcify the tissue.
- Arthropods
  - Terrestrial: Anesthetize animals with a gaseous anesthetic (chloroform or ether can also be used) by adding the compound to an appropriately sized container with a sealed lid (see Chapters 9–14 on arthropods). If the animal's legs need to be spread prior to fixation, separate the appendages by pinning them down on a moderately pliable surface and then pipette fixative around them. If the entire animal is small enough, place it on a slide that is within a shallow container (e.g., a Petri dish) and, after positioning, slowly add a fixative of choice.
  - Aquatic: Anesthetize the animals prior to fixation. Hermit crabs need to be removed from their shells prior to fixation. One may need to inject fixative through arthrodial membranes (the soft cuticle at the suture lines and the base of the legs) to penetrate the internal organs ade-

quately if preserving whole organisms. Dietrich's or Davidson's fixative is recommended.

— Remember that the carapace contains chitin and calcium. Decalcification may be effective in most cases, but in thicker tissues may need dechitinization as well.

— For whole mounts, one may need to clear the exoskeleton.

  ▪ Lactophenol: This is actually a mounting medium, useful for clearing smaller specimens. Formula:
    – Melted phenol (carbolic acid), 3 parts
    – Lactic acid, 1 part
    – Glycerin, 2 parts
    – Distilled water, 1 part

  ▪ One can also bleach whole mounts in hydrogen peroxide for 12 h or longer, if needed.

• Annelids
— One may need to clear the gut first of sand, grit, and hard particles. Let the animals feed on soft food (e.g., cornmeal or gel) for about 3 days.

— A terrestrial or freshwater species should be placed in freshwater and 50% ethyl alcohol slowly added until the concentration of the mix reaches about 10% alcohol. One may also dip the animal in the fixative and then hang it from its posterior element into the solution. Alternatively, one may place the animal in short lengths of glass tubing to keep it straight during fixation.

— For saltwater forms, first anesthetize the animal and then fix it with a fast-penetrating fixative (e.g., Bouin's).

• Mollusks
— Marine species: Helly's solution or 10% formalin in seawater. For freshwater species, neutral buffered 10% formalin or Bouin's fixative is recommended.

— Gastropods (snails) and bivalves
  ▪ To open the operculum or shells for proper tissue fixation, the animal must be well anesthetized.
  ▪ Cut ligament and muscle by inserting a knife into the gap and cutting in sweeping motion, trying not to damage the mantle.
  ▪ Gastropods and cephalopods can be gently pulled from their shells when they are adequately anesthetized.

— Nudibranchs
  ▪ Use 10% buffered formalin in seawater for deeply anesthetized or freshly dead animals.

Decalcification

Most corals and echinoderms will need to be decalcified prior to sectioning of tissue for histological slide preparation. Most mollusks will be removed from their shells and do not need to be decalcified, except for beaks in some cephalopod species or if one wants to retain the shell, such as in very small bivalves (McCafferty and Smolowitz, 1995), or evaluate the interaction of specific lesions between the shell and tissue, such as in juvenile oyster disease (R.S., personal application). Arthropods with thinner exoskeletons can also be placed in decalcifying solutions, because calcium is deposited in the cuticle for strength (Bullis and McCafferty, 1995). Several commercial preparations

are available through the major scientific supply companies. A solution of formic acid and sodium citrate can be prepared, as well (the formula is at the end of this chapter). To help maintain specimen orientation during histological preparation, while there is still a little form left to the tissues, cut the tissue sections (or use the entire specimen) and position them in histology cassettes between sponges to hold the tissue in place. Then, finish the decalcification process. This is highly recommended for coral and urchins. To determine the point of decalcification, attempt to trim tissue. It is not advisable to leave tissue in decalcification solutions for excessive periods, because there is some indication of adverse effects on the staining reaction of tissues (i.e., a lack of uptake or a need to increase the time required for staining) (Yevich and Barszcz, 1981). Once the tissue is decalcified, wash the tissue with tap water before returning it to a clean container of fixative.

Dechitinization

For arthropods with thicker exoskeletons, removal of calcium deposits may not be sufficient to cut through the tissue. Chitin is another component of exoskeletons and may need to be removed in addition to calcium deposits. Once a tissue is dechitinized, it should be treated much as was described for decalcified tissue.

Preparation of Tissue Samples for Histology

If not evaluating the tissues, send the fixed tissues to pathologists who, ideally, have experience in examining invertebrate tissue or have a dedicated interest in learning. Properly seal and label sample containers. Do not send tissues in glass containers. Many of the commercial pathology laboratories specializing in exotic animal pathology will often provide shipping labels, information sheets, and containers filled with 10% buffered formalin. However, it is recommended that one cut and cassette tissues, identifying each cassette, so that the pathologist will have a good idea of what tissues will be evaluated. Also, request an extra set of slides for oneself. If one plans to work extensively with a species, developing a study set of normal anatomy and histology is recommended (Berzins et al., 1990).

When cutting into tissues, the necessary equipment includes a fume hood, tissue cassettes, pathology cutting blades and a handle, a cutting tray (often partially filled with paraffin to aid in the cutting process), a sieve, a funnel for draining fixatives from tissue, and plastic containers for used fixatives (arrange special disposal).

Label cassettes with a lead pencil or special histology markers, as the processing steps will remove ink, and transfer the tissue cassettes to a container with fresh fixative, usually 10% buffered formalin or 70%—80% ethyl alcohol (see what the laboratory prefers) prior delivery to the processing laboratory. (Note: When shipping formalin, due to its hazardous chemical status, special mailing precautions must be followed. Contact the shipping agent to ensure proper packaging.)

Embedding, Sectioning, Mounting, and Staining of Tissue Samples

These steps will most likely be outsourced. With a duplicate set of slides, a clinician can learn to evaluate the histology of specimens. Numerous texts and articles on invertebrate diseases and histology are available (Johnson, 1980; Bell and Lightner, 1988; Bullis, 1989; Perkins and Cheng, 1990; Messick and Sindermann, 1992; Smolowitz et al., 1992; Couch and Fournie, 1993; Yevich and Yevich, 1994; Stolen et al., 1995; Elston, 1999).

Once properly fixed, routine paraffin infiltration and standard stains for human tissues can be used (Luna, 1992). Harris's hematoxylin–eosin (H&E) is the basic stain for routine evaluation (hematoxylin stains the nucleus and some mucus cells, and the eosin stains the cytoplasm). Inform the processing laboratory if using fixatives other than 10% buffered formalin and if tissues were decalcified or dechitinized. There is concern that some of these methods may reduce stain uptake. The amount of time slides need to spend in stains may be influenced by type of fixative and whether tissues have been decalcified. If possible, submit soft tissue from the area of interest separate from decalcified or dechitinized tissue. Also, different processing schedules can be implemented for different groups of animals if results are not satisfactory with standard methods (such as when processing very fatty tissues) (Yevich and Barszcz, 1981; Howard and Smith, 1983; Callis and Sterchi, 2002; C. McCollough, personal communication).

Summary

Clinical invertebrate medicine is an exciting new and developing field. There are a lot of unknowns and much to be learned. However, this should not be viewed as a disadvantage but as a challenge and an opportunity to contribute to this emerging field. Remember, "The world is your oyster!"

Resources

Web Sites

1. Information on anesthesia: www.hermes.mbl.edu/BiologicalBulletin/ANESCOMP/AnesComp-Lit.html
2. Information on care and use of invertebrates in biomedical research: www.nal.usda.gov/awic/pubs/invertebrates.htm
3. Information on diagnostics of internationally important invertebrate diseases: www.oie.int
4. Registry of Tumors in Lower Animals: www.pathology-registry.org
5. Information from the Canadian Fisheries and Oceans Department on diseases and pathology of shellfish: www.pac.dfo-mpo.gc.ca/sci/shellfish
6. Information and services available for shrimp and bivalve histology: www.aquatichealth.org/services

Contacts

All Florida Veterinary Laboratory
6406 SW 170th Street
Archer, FL 32618

Maryland Department of Natural Resources
Cooperative Oxford Laboratory
904 South Morris Street
Oxford, MD 21654

Registry of Tumors in Lower Animals
22900 Shaw Road, Suite 107
Sterling, VA 20166
E-mail: administrator@pathology-registry.org

Journals

Diseases of Aquatic Organisms
Invertebrate Biology
Journal of Aquatic Animal Health
Journal of Crustacean Biology
Journal of Invertebrate Pathology
Journal of Shellfish Research
Malacologia

Organizations

International Association for Aquatic Animal Medicine
National Shellfish Association
Society for Invertebrate Pathology

Fixatives and Solutions

Bouin's Fixative (Bouin, 1897)

Formula taken from *Humason's Animal Tissue Techniques* (Presnell and Schreibman, 1997).

75 mL picric acid, saturated aqueous (be careful for the chemical to remain aqueous; dry picric acid is highly explosive)
25 mL 37% formaldehyde
5 mL glacial acetic acid

Wash tissue sections in 70%–80% alcohol until the yellow no longer leaches out. The yellow should disappear before sections are stained. If it doesn't, treat the slides with 70% alcohol plus a few drops of saturated lithium carbonate until the yellow disappears.

Davidson's (Hartmann's) Fixative (Shaw and Battle, 1957)

Formula provided by S. Bowers (personal communication).

100 mL glycerin (modification added by S. Bowers)
200 mL 37%–40% formaldehyde

300 mL 95% ethyl alcohol (ethanol)
300 mL water (or seawater, but that will cloud with seawater)

Add 100 mL glacial acetic acid per 900 mL of the above mixture just prior to use.

It is important to add these materials in the order given.

Dechitinizing Solution

Formula provided by the Johns Hopkins Comparative Medicine and Pathology histology laboratory. Extreme care must be taken in handling, as some ingredients are toxic:

4 g mercuric chloride
0.5 g chromic acid (chromic trichloride)
10 mL concentrated nictric acid
50 mL 95% alcohol
200 mL distilled water

Add in this order: water, alcohol, nitric acid, and powders. Fix the tissue first in formalin and then add tissues to fresh dechitinizing solution every 2 days or so. Periodically test to determine whether tissues are ready to cut. When ready, rinse samples several hours in running tap water prior to cutting.

Dietrich's (Kahle's) Fixative (Thompson and Hunt, 1966)

Formula taken from Callis and Sterchi (2002).

750 mL distilled water
375 mL 95% ethyl alcohol
125 mL 37% formaldehyde
25 mL glacial acetic acid

Combine ingredients in sequence listed, starting with water. Used primarily for small invertebrates such as copepods and other zooplankton. Rinse fixed tissue well with running water for 24 hours to prevent the formation of acid hematin (a brown/black precipitate) during processing.

Formalin in Seawater

Formula taken from Howard and Smith (1983) and modified by R.S.

100 mL 37% formaldehyde solution
900 mL seawater
6–8 marble chips for additional buffering (not necessary if unavailable)

If natural seawater is not available, commercial products such as Instant Ocean (Aquarium Systems, Mentor, OH) can be used. Individual formulas exist to make one's own (Howard and Smith, 1983), but it is easier to purchase commercial brands.

Formic Acid–Sodium Citrate (for Decalcification)

Formula taken from Luna (1992).

Solution A
    50 g sodium citrate
    250 mL distilled water
Solution B
    125 mL formic acid, 99%
    125 mL distilled water

1. Mix volumes of A and B 1:1 at the time of use.
2. Place a stir bar in the beaker and cover it with a plastic drain strainer. Place the fixed and rinsed samples/cassettes in the beaker. Add enough decalcification solution to cover the samples. Place the beaker on the stir plate. Stir constantly, changing the decalcification solution once each day. Most decalcification will be completed in 3 days.
3. Wash afterward for 1 h in running tap water.

Modified Helly's Fixative (Barszcz and Yevich, 1975)

Formula taken from Yevich and Barszcz (1981).

1 L deionized water
50 g zinc chloride ($ZnCl_2$)
25 g potassium dichromate ($K_2Cr_2O_7$)

Combine the ingredients in sequence and stir until dissolved. Add 5 mL of 37% formaldehyde per 100 mL of fixative at the time of use. Zinc chloride is used instead of the original mercuric chloride because zinc chloride is less toxic. Amount of time spent in fixatives depends on size and density of tissue, with a maximum of 24 h. Prolonged fixation will result in excessively hard and brittle tissue.

10% Neutral Buffered Formalin

This solution is also commercially available.

100 mL 37% formaldehyde
900 mL water
4 g sodium phosphate, monobasic, monohydrate (NaH_2PO_4)
6 g sodium phosphate, dibasic, anhydrous (Na_2HPO_4)

Combine the ingredients in the sequence listed, starting with water.

Marine Brain–Heart Infusion Broth (MBHI)

Formula provided by Robert Bullis (personal communication). In general, add 13.5 g NaCl for every 100 g of media:

g Media[a]	g NaCl	mL H$_2$O
4.625	0.625	1.875
9.250	1.250	3.750
18.500	2.500	7.500
37.000	5.000	15.000

[a]Difco Brain–Heart Infusion (237500 [0037-17]) (Difco Laboratories, Sparks, MD). The bottle label has information on making the media.

Marine Brain–Heart Infusion Agar (MBHIA)

Formula provided by Robert Bullis.

g Media[a]	g NaCl	g Agar[b]	mL H$_2$O	Approx. no. plates[c]
4.625	0.625	1.875	125	5
9.250	1.250	3.750	250	10
18.500	2.500	7.500	500	20
37.000	5.000	15.000	1000	40

1. Dissolve the desired quantity of media in the appropriate volume of deionized water and heat to boiling.
2. Sterilize the mixture by autoclaving at 121°C for 15 min.
3. Pour heated liquid agar into plates and allow to cool at room temperature until condensation disappears from lid. Refrigerate until needed.

[a]Difco Brain–Heart Infusion (237500 [0037 17]). The bottle label has information on making the media.
[b]BD Bacto Agar (214010) (Difco Laboratories, Sparks, MD).
[c]100 × 15-mm sterile Petri dishes.

References

Araujo R, Remón JM, Moreno D, and Ramos MA (1995). Relaxing techniques for freshwater molluscs: Trials for evaluation of different methods. Malacologia 36:29–41.

Barszcz CA and Yevich PP (1975). The use of Helly's fixative for marine invertebrate histopathology. Comp Pathol Bull 12:4.

Bell TA and Lightner DV (1988). A Handbook of Normal Penaeid Shrimp Histology. World Aquaculture Society, Baton Rouge, LA, 114 pp.

Berzins IK, Maslanka PL, Montali RJ, Davis KJ, and Pletcher JM (1990). Anatomy and histology of the common cuttlefish *Sepia officinalis*. Registry of Veterinary Pathology, Armed Forces Institute of Pathology, Washington, DC.

Boettcher KJ, Barber BJ, and Singer JT (2000). Additional evidence that juvenile oyster disease is caused by a member of the *Roseobacter* group, and colonization of non-affected animals by *Stappia stellulata*-like strains. Appl Environ Microbiol 66:3924–3930.

Bouin P (1897). Etudes sur l'evolution normale et l'involution du tube seminifere. Arch Anat Microsc 1:225–339.

Brusca RC and Brusca GJ (1990). Invertebrates. Sinauer Associates, Sunderland, MA, 880 pp.

Budelmann BU, Schipp R, and von Boltzky S (1997). Cephalopoda. In: Harrison FW and Kohn AJ, eds. Microscopic Anatomy of Invertebrates, volume 6A: Mollusca II. Wiley-Liss, New York. pp 117–146.

Bullis RA (1989). Etiology and pathology of shell disease [abstr]. J Shellfish Res 8:460.

Bullis RA and McCafferty M (1995). A method for the histological processing of crustacean exoskeleton: Techniques in fish immunology 4. In: Stolen JS, Fletcher TC, Smith SA, Zelikoff JT, Kaattari SL, Anderson RS, Söderhall K, and Weeks-Perkins BA, eds. Immunology and Pathology of Aquatic Invertebrates. SOS, Fair Haven, NJ, pp 215–222.

Callis G and Sterchi D (2002). Animal Processing Manual, 1st edition. National Society for Histotechnology: Veterinary, Industry and Research Committee, Bowie, MD.

Carballal MF, Lopez MC, Azevedo C, and Villalba A (1997). Hemolymph cell types of the mussel *Mytilus galloprovincialis*. Dis Aquat Org 29:127–135.

Carballal MJ, Villalba A, and Carmen L (1998). Seasonal variation and effects of age, food, availability, size, gonadal development and parasitism on the hemogram of *Mytilus galloprovincialis*. J Invertebr Pathol 72:304–312.

Cavey MJ and Märkel K (1997). Echinoidea. In: Harrison FW and Kohn AJ, eds. Microscopic Anatomy of Invertebrates, volume 14: Mollusca II. Wiley-Liss, New York, pp 345–400.

Cheng TC (1981). Bivalves. In: Ratcliffe NA and Rowley AF, eds. Invertebrate Blood Cells, volume 1. Academic, New York, pp 233–300.

Cheng TC (1996). Hemocytes: Form and functions. In: Kennedy VS, Newell RIE, and Eble AF, eds. The Eastern Oyster, *Crassostrea virginica*. Maryland Sea Grant College, College Park, MD, pp 299–333

Cheng TC, Marchalonis JJ, and Vasta GR (1984). Role of molluscan lectins in recognition processes. In: Cohen E, ed. Recognition Proteins, Receptors, and Probes: Invertebrates. Alan R Liss, New York, pp 1–15.

Clauss T, Taylor D, and Berzins IK (2003). Mycobacteriosis in a chambered nautilus, *Nautilus pompilius*. In: Proceedings of the 34th Annual Conference of the International Association for Aquatic Animal Medicine, pp 170–171.

Cooper JE (1980). Invertebrates and invertebrate disease: An introduction for the veterinary surgeon. J Small Anim Pract 21:495–507.

Cooper JE (1988). Emergency care of invertebrates. Vet Clin North Am Exotic Anim Pract 1:251–264.

Cooper JE (2001). Invertebrate anesthesia. Vet Clin North Am Exotic Anim Pract 4:57–67.

Cooper JE, Pearce-Kelly P, and Williams DL, eds (1992). Arachnids: The Proceedings of a Symposium on Spiders and Their Allies. Chiron, London, 207 pp.

Couch JA and Fournie JW (1993). Pathobiology of Marine and Estuarine Organisms. CRC, Boca Raton, FL, 552 pp.

Difco (1998). Difco Manual, 11th edition. Difco Laboratories, Sparks, MD, 862 pp.

Elston RA (1999). Health Management, Development and Histology of Seed Oyster. World Aquaculture Society, Baton Rouge, LA, 110 pp.

Frye FL (1986). Care and feeding of invertebrates kept as pets or study animals. In: Fowler ME, ed. Zoo and Wild Animal Practice. Philadelphia, WB Saunders, pp 1039–1054.

Goedken M and DeGuise S (2003). Flow cytometry as a tool to quantify oyster phagocytosis, respiratory burst and apoptosis. In: Proceedings of the 34th Annual Conference of the International Association for Aquatic Animal Medicine, p 124.

Gray P (1954). The Microtomist's Formulary and Guide. Blakiston, New York, 794 pp.

Harrison FW and Kohn AJ, eds (1991). Microscopic Anatomy of Invertebrates, volumes 1–15. Wiley-Liss, New York.

Hasson KW, Hasson J, Aubert H, Redman RM, and Lightner DV (1997). A new RNA-friendly fixative for the preservation of penaeid shrimp samples for virological detection using cDNA genomic probes. J Virol Methods 66:227–236.

Hégaret H, Wikfors GH, and Soudant P (2003a). Flow-cytometric analysis of haemocytes from eastern oysters, *Crassostrea virginica*, subjected to a sudden, high-temperature stress. I. Haemocyte types and morphology. J Exp Mar Biol Ecol 293:237–248.

Hégaret H, Wikfors GH, and Soudant P (2003b). Flow-cytometric analysis of haemocytes from eastern oysters, *Crassostrea virginica*, subjected to a sudden, high-temperature stress. II. Haemocyte functions: Aggregation, viability, phagocytosis and respiratory burst. J Exp Mar Biol Ecol 293:249–265.

Howard DW and Smith CS (1983). Histological Techniques for Marine Bivalve Mollusks. NOAA Technical Memorandum NMFS-F/NEC-25. National Marine Fisheries Service, Northeast Fisheries Center, Woods Hole, MA.

Hsu AC and Smolowitz RM (2003). Scanning electron microscopy investigation of epizootic lobster disease in *Homarus americanus*. Biol Bull 205:228–230.

Johnson PT (1980). Histology of the Blue Crab, *Callinectes sapidus*: A Model for the Decapoda. Praeger, New York, 440 pp.

Luna LG (1992). Histopathologic Methods and Color Atlas of Special Stains and Tissue Artifacts. American Histolabs, Gaithersburg, MD, 767 pp.

Mackin JG (1962). Oyster disease caused by *Dermocystidium marinum* and other micro-organisms in Louisiana. Publ Inst Mar Sci Univ Tex 7:132–229.

Martin GG and Hose JE (1997). Vascular elements and blood (hemolymph). In: Harrison FW and Kohn AJ, eds. Microscopic anatomy of invertebrates, volume 9: Mollusca II. Wiley-Liss, New York, pp 119–414.

McCafferty M and Smolowitz R (1995). A method for histological processing of larval bivalves: Techniques in Fish Immunology 4. In: Stolen JS, Fletcher TC, Smith SA, Zelikoff JT, Kaattari SL, Anderson RS, Söderhall K, and Weeks-Perkins BA, eds. Immunology and Pathology of Aquatic Invertebrates. SOS, Fair Haven, NJ, pp 215–222.

Messick GA and Sindermann CJ (1992). Synopsis of principal diseases of the blue crab, *Callinectes sapidus*. NOAA Technical Memorandum NMFS-F/NEC-88, 24 pp.

Miller-Morgan T (2003). Signs of stress and disease in aquarium animals. Ornamental Fish Health News 2:1.

Morsey BM and DeGuise S (2003). Natural killer cell activity in the eastern oyster and American lobster. In: Proceedings of the 34th Annual Conference of the International Association for Aquatic Animal Medicine, p 123.

Mullen TE, Nevis KR, Frasca S Jr, Gast RJ, Peglar MT, Gillevet PM, and O'Kelly CJ (2003). Characterization of the amoeba associated with paramoebiasis in the American lobster (*Homarus americanus*) by small subunit ribosomal gene analysis. In: Proceedings of the 34th Annual Conference of the International Association for Aquatic Animal Medicine, pp 105–106.

Noga EJ (1996). Fish Disease: Diagnosis and Treatment. Iowa State University Press, Ames.

Nollens HH, Keogh JA, and Probert PK (2003). Effect of shell lesions on survival, growth, condition, reproductive capacity and hematology of the New Zealand blackfoot abalone, *Haliotis iris*. In: Proceedings of the 34th Annual Conference of the International Association for Aquatic Animal Medicine, p 104.

OIE (Office International des Epizooties) (2003a). Manual of Diagnostic Tests for Aquatic Animals, 4th edition. OIE, Paris, 358 pp. Also available at http://www.oie.int/eng/normes/fmanual/A_summry.htm.

OIE (Office International des Epizooties) (2003b). Aquatic Animal Health Code, 6th edition. OIE, Paris, 165 pp. Also available at http://www.oie.int/eng/normes/fcode/A_summry.htm.

Perkins FO and Cheng TC (1990). Pathology in Marine Science. Academic, San Diego, 538 pp.

Presnell JK and Schreibman MP (1997). Humason's Animal Tissue Techniques, 5th edition. Johns Hopkins University Press, Baltimore, 572 pp.

Ray S (1954). Biological studies of *Dermocystidium marinum*, a fungus parasite of oysters. Rice Institute Pamphlet Special Issue, Houston, 114 pp.

Rodríquez J, Bayot B, Amano Y, Panchana F, de Blas I, Adlay V, and Calderón J (2003). White spot syndrome virus infection in cultured *Penaeus vanna* (Boone) in Ecuador with emphasis on histopathology and ultrastructure. J Fish Dis 26:439–450.

Ross LG and Ross B (1999). Anaesthetic and Sedative Techniques for Aquatic Animals. Blackwell Sciences, Cornwall, UK.

Russell S, Hobbie K, Burrage T, Koerting C, De Guise S, Frasca S, and French RA (2000). Identification of a protozoan parasite in the American lobster, *Homarus americanus*, from Long Island Sound [abstr]. J Shellfish Res 19:581.

Santarém MM, Robledo JAF, and Figueras A (1994). Seasonal changes in hemocytes and serum defense factors in the blue mussel *Mytilus galloprovincialis*. Dis Aquat Org 18:217–222.

Schartau W and Leiderscher T (1983). Composition of the hemolymph of the tarantula *Eurypelma californicum*. J Comp Physiol [A] 152:73–77.

Shaw BL and Battle HI (1957). The gross and microscopic anatomy of the digestive tract of the oyster *Crassostrea virginica* (Gmelin). Can J Zool 35:325–347.

Sherrill J, Reidel C, Raymond J, Holland M, Landman N, and Montali R (2002). Characterization of "black shell syndrome" in captive chambered nautilus (*Nautilus pompilius*) at the Smithsonian National Zoological Park. In: Proceedings of the American Association of Zoological Veterinarians, pp 337–338.

Smolowitz RM, Bullis RA, and Abt DA (1992). Pathologic cuticular changes of winter impoundment shell disease preceding and during intermolt in the American lobster, *Homarus americanus*. Biol Bull 183:99–112.

Smolowitz RM and Reinisch CL (1986). Indirect peroxidase staining using monoclonal antibodies specific for *Mya arenaria* neoplastic cells. J Invertebr Pathol 48:139–145.

Sparks AK (1985). Synopsis of Invertebrate Pathology (Exclusive of Insects). Elsevier Science, Amsterdam, 423 pp.

Steers JE, Sherrill J, Raymond J, and Garner M (2003). Characterization and treatment of necrotic dermatitis ("bell rot") in a collection of jellies. In: Proceedings of the 34th Annual Conference of the International Association for Aquatic Animal Medicine, pp 107–109.

Stokes NA and Burreson EM (2001). Differential diagnosis of mixed *Haplosporidium costale* and *Haplosporidium nelsoni* infections in the eastern oyster, *Crassostrea virginica* using DNA probes. J Shellfish Res 20:207–213.

Stokes NA, Calvo LMR, Apakupakul K, Burreson EM, Sunila I, and Smolowitz R (2001). Validation of DNA-based molecular diagnostics for the hard clam parasite QPX (Quahog Parasite Unknown) and the oyster parasite SSO (*Haplosporidium costale*). In: Aquaculture 2001: Book of Abstracts. World Aquaculture Society, Baton Rouge, LA, 599 pp.

Stolen JS, Fletcher TC, Smith SA, Zelikoff JT, Kaatari SL, Anderson RS, Soderhall K, and Weeks-Perkins BA, eds (1995). Immunology and Pathology of Aquatic Invertebrates. SOS, Fair Haven, NJ, 258 pp.

Strandberg JD, Rosenfield J, Berzins IK, and Reinish C (1998). Specific localization of polychlorinated biphenyls in clams (*Mya arenaria*) from environmentally impacted sites. Aquat Toxicol 41:343–354.

Thompson SW and Hunt RD (1966). Selected Histochemical and Histopathological Methods. Charles C Thomas, Springfield, IL, 1639 pp.

Wang CS, Tsai YJ, and Chen SN (1998). Detection of white spot disease virus (WSDV) infection in shrimp using in situ hybridization. J Invertebr Pathol 72:170–173.

Williams DL (1999). Sample taking in invertebrate veterinary medicine. Vet Clin North Am Exotic Anim Pract 2:777–801.

Williams DL (2001). Skin diseases of invertebrates. Vet Clin North Am Exotic Anim Pract 4:309–320.

Williams DL (2003). Oral biology and disease in invertebrates. Vet Clin North Am Exotic Anim Pract 6:459–65.

Yevich PP and Barszcz CA (1981). Preparation of Aquatic Animals for Histopathological Examination. In: Biological Field and Laboratory Methods for Measuring the Quality of Surface Waters and Wastes, 2nd edition. Cincinnati, OH, US Environmental Protection Agency, 38 pp.

Yevich PP and Yevich CA (1994). Use of histopathology in biomonitoring marine invertebrates. In: Kramer KJM, ed. Biomonitoring of Coastal Water and Estuaries. CRC, Boca Raton, FL, pp 179–204.

Chapter 20

LAWS, RULES, AND REGULATING AGENCIES FOR INVERTEBRATES

Daniel S. Dombrowski

Introduction

This chapter provides a summary of the current major international and United States (U.S.) regulations that apply to invertebrates in captivity. This information is to be used as a guide in the process of acquiring permits to import, export, transport, house, and display invertebrates. State and local laws vary considerably, and a comprehensive summary of these laws is beyond the scope of this review. However, references and contact information for each state are provided, and readers are encouraged to contact local government agencies when appropriate. A summary of current contact information for the authoritative agencies of foreign countries is also provided.

There are many and regulations to consider before obtaining and keeping invertebrates. Unfortunately, many people are unaware of these rules, and violations commonly occur. The Convention on International Trade in Endangered Species of Wild Fauna and Flora (CITES), the Endangered Species Act (ESA), and the Magnuson Fishery Conservation and Management Act (MFCMA) all have specific references to invertebrate species. As with vertebrates, the Lacy Act (LA) is a major tool for enforcement of international, national, and local wildlife laws that apply to invertebrates. The primary federal agencies with jurisdiction over invertebrate species in the United States include the U.S. Department of Agriculture: Animal and Plant Health Inspection Service (USDA: APHIS), the U.S. Fish and Wildlife Service (USFWS), and the National Oceanic and Atmospheric Administration: National Marine Fisheries Service (NOAA-NMFS). All U.S. states have their own agricultural protection and wildlife departments to enforce local regulations pertaining to invertebrates. The U.S. Animal Welfare Act and Animal Welfare Regulations specifically address vertebrate species, but for the most part exclude invertebrates. However, it is my opinion that invertebrate animals should be equally considered and proposals for research using live invertebrates be submitted for Institutional Animal Care and Use Committee (IACUC) approval.

As with familiar vertebrate species, there are several internationally recognized reportable diseases of invertebrates. The Office International des Epizooties (OIE) is an intergovernmental organization that disseminates current information on animal disease issues worldwide. They maintain a list of reportable diseases, including several that affect invertebrates. A list of these diseases (Table 20.1) and contact information for reporting them are provided.

Convention on International Trade in Endangered Species of Wild Fauna and Flora

CITES is an agreement between nations drafted to recognize those wildlife species whose survival is, or may become, threatened by international trade. Plants and animals are recognized by the convention. All endangered or threatened species of the participating countries are not necessarily listed by CITES—only those species that are actually threatened by trade. There are three major categories for species listed by CITES: Appendix I, Appendix II, and Appendix III. Species listed in Appendix I are the most highly regulated. These are threatened with extinction and are not available for commercial trade. Species listed in Appendices II and III are also regulated but are available for commercial trade with special permits. Species listed in Appendices II and III are not currently threatened with extinction but may become so if trade is not managed. There are currently 160 countries participating in CITES; approximately 60 invertebrate species are included in Appendix I, 2000 in Appendix II, and 16 in Appendix III. For a complete and current listing of all CITES species, refer to http://www.cites.org. The invertebrate species in CITES Appendices I and II are listed in Table 20.2.

CITES is only an agreement between governments. It has no enforcement body of its own. Each of the participating countries must recognize and enforce trade laws and provide or require permits for the importation and/or exportation of species listed by CITES. In the United States, agencies that enforce laws for the protection of CITES species and provide import and export permits are the USDA (plants), the USFWS (wildlife), and the NMFS (marine organisms). Permit requests and general inquiries about terrestrial and freshwater invertebrates listed by CITES should be directed to the USFWS:

U.S. Fish & Wildlife Service
Division of Management Authority
4401 North Fairfax Drive, Room 700
Arlington, VA 22203
(703) 358-2104
http://www.fws.gov

Table 20.1. Office International des Epizooties (OIE) Reportable Diseases of Invertebrates

Taxa	Diseases
Bees	Acarapisosis
	American foulbrood
	European foulbrood
	Tropilaelaps
	Varroosis
Mollusks	*Bonamia ostreae*
	Bonamia exitiosus
	Mikrocytos roughleyi
	Haplosporidium nelsoni
	Marteilia refringens
	Marteilia sydneyi
	Mikrocytos mackini
	Perkinsus marinus
	Perkinsus olseni/atlanticus
	Haplosporidium costale
	Withering syndrome of abalones *Candidatus Xenohaliotis californiensis*
Crustaceans	Taura syndrome
	White spot disease
	Yellowhead disease
	Tetrahedral baculovirosis (*Baculovirus penaei*)
	Spherical baculovirosis (*Penaeus monodon*-type baculovirus)
	Infectious hypodermal and hematopoietic necrosis
	Crayfish plague (*Aphanomyces astaci*)
	Spawner-isolated mortality virus disease

Permit requests and inquiries regarding marine invertebrates (including the corals, giant clams, and queen conch) listed by CITES should be directed to the NMFS:

NOAA Fisheries
1315 East West Highway
SSMC3, Silver Spring, MD 20910
http://www.nmfs.noaa.gov

For more information on wildlife issues, including laws and regulations pertaining to a specific country, visit the CITES Web site. CITES maintains a directory of contact information for wildlife management agencies of all nations (including non-CITES governments):

http://www.cites.org/common/directy/e_directy.html

Endangered Species Act

The ESA is designed to prevent the extinction of animal and plant species through conservation and protection of critical habitat. This act, which was passed in 1973, lists species that are in peril according to their current population status. In general, species are listed as endangered if they are faced with extinction in the near future throughout all or most of their range. Species that are likely to become endangered in the foreseeable future are listed by the ESA as threatened. Some species are protected by the ESA due to "similarity of appearance" to other species listed. Native U.S. species and some species native to other parts of the world are listed in the ESA. The ESA protects species through regulations on trade, limiting human impact, and conservation of critical habitats. It prohibits trade, import, export, transport, and possession of listed species except by special permit. The ESA states that no person may "take" an endangered or threatened species. *Take* is defined within the document as "harass, harm, pursue, hunt, shoot, wound, kill, trap, capture, collect, attempt to engage in any such conduct intentionally or unintentionally." There are currently over 1200 species listed as threatened or endangered, and about 200 of those are invertebrates, including the species of mollusks, crustaceans, arachnids, and insects listed in Table 20.3.

The U.S. agencies that regulate interstate trade, enforce the ESA, and issue permits to work with ESA species are the USDA (plants), the USFWS (wildlife), and the NMFS (marine organisms). Endangered species permits are granted only for scientific research, captive propagation, and incidental take. Threatened species permits may also be granted for educational exhibits. Permit requests and general inquiries about terrestrial and freshwater invertebrates listed by the ESA should be directed to the appropriate regional or main USFWS office (Table 20.4).

Magnuson–Stevens Fishery Conservation and Management Act

The MSFCMA is the primary legislation behind the activities of the NMFS. It calls for eight Regional Fishery Management Councils to be established to work with the NMFS to prepare fishery management plans for marine resources. These plans set regulations for taking fish, identify essential fish habitat, and recognize Marine Protected Areas. Essentially, marine fishery resources consist of all of the offshore living components that contribute to U.S. economy through food or recreation.

Within the MSFCMA, *fish* are defined as "finfish, mollusks, crustaceans, and all other forms of marine animal and plant life other than marine mammals and birds." *Fishing* is defined as (A) the catching, taking, or harvesting of fish; (B) the attempted catching, taking, or harvesting of fish; (C) any other activity which can reasonably be expected to result in the catching, taking, or harvesting of fish; or (D) any operations at sea in support of, or in preparation for, any activity described in subparagraphs A through C.

Several species of invertebrates are specifically addressed in this document as "Continental Shelf Fishery Resources" (Table 20.5). The NMFS should be contacted for information on all pertaining regulations.

In general, this act is designed to protect U.S. ocean resources, including fish and any other species that live on or around the U.S. Continental Shelf. For more information on the collection, import, or export of these organisms, contact

Table 20.2. Current Convention on International Trade in Endangered Species of Wild Fauna and Flora (CITES) Appendix I and Appendix II listed invertebrate species (June 2005)

Cnidaria: Hydrozoa
Fire corals (Milleporina: Milleporidae)
  Appendix II:
    All species of the family Milleporidae
Lace corals (Stylasterina: Stylasteridae)
  Appendix II:
    All species of the family Stylasteridae
Cnidaria: Anthozoa
Blue corals (Helioporacea: Helioporidae)
  Appendix II:
    Heliopora coerulea
Organ pipe corals (Stolonifera: Tubiporidae)
  Appendix II:
    All species of the family Tubiporidae
Black corals (Antipatharia)
  Appendix II:
    All species of the order Antipatharia
Marine mussels (Mytiloidas Mytilidae)
  Appendix II
    Lithophaga lithophaga
Stony corals (Scleractinia)
  Appendix II:
    All species of the order Scleractinia
Mollusca: Gastropoda
Agate snails and Oahu tree snails (Stylommatophora: Achatinellidae)
  Appendix I:
    Achatinella spp.
Green tree snails (Stylommatophora: Camaenidae)
  Appendix II:
    Papustyla pulcherrima
Queen conchs (Mesogastropoda: Strombidae)
  Appendix II:
    Strombus gigas
Mollusca: Bivalvia
Giant clams (Venerida: Tridacnidae)
  Appendix II: All species of the family Tridacnidae
Freshwater mussels and pearly mussels (Unionida: Unionidae)
  Appendix I:
    Conradilla caelata
    Dromus dromas
    Epioblasma curtisi
    Epioblasma florentina
    Epioblasma sampsoni
    Epioblasma sulcata perobliqua
    Epioblasma torulosa gubernaculum
    Epioblasma torulosa torulosa
    Epioblasma turgidula
    Epioblasma walkeri
    Fusconaia cuneolus
    Fusconaia edgariana

    Lampsilis higginsii
    Lampsilis orbiculata orbiculata
    Lampsilis satur
    Lampsilis virescens
    Plethobasus cicatricosus
    Plethobasus cooperianus
    Pleurobema plenum
    Potamilus capax
    Quadrula intermedia
    Quadrula sparsa
    Toxolasma cylindrella
    Unio nickliniana
    Unio tampicoensis tecomatensis
    Villosa trabalis
  Appendix II:
    Cyprogenia aberti
    Epioblasma torulosa rangiana
    Pleurobema clava
Annelida: Hirudinoidea
Leeches (Arhynchobdellida: Hirudinidae)
  Appendix II: *Hirudo medicinalis*
Arthropoda: Insecta
Butterflies (Lepidoptera: Papilionidae)
  Appendix I:
    Ornithoptera alexandrae
    Papilio chikae
    Papilio homerus
    Papilio hospiton
  Appendix II:
    Atrophaneura jophon
    Atrophaneura pandiyana
    Bhutanitis spp.
    Ornithoptera spp. (sensu D'Abrera) (all except species in
      Appendix I)
    Parnassius apollo
    Teinopalpus spp.
    Trogonoptera spp. (sensu D'Abrera)
    Troides spp. (sensu D'Abrera)
Arthropoda: Arachnida
Scorpions (Scorpiones: Scorpionidae)
  Appendix II:
    Pandinus dictator
    Pandinus gambiensis
    Pandinus imperator
Tarantulas (Araneae: Theraphosidae)
  Appendix II:
    Aphonopelma albiceps
    Aphonopelma pallidum
    Brachypelma spp.
    Brachypelmides klaasi

NOAA Fisheries
1315 East West Highway
SSMC3, Silver Spring, MD 20910
http://www.nmfs.noaa.gov

The Lacey Act

This is the major enforcement tool for U.S. agencies regarding wildlife protection. The Lacey Act makes it illegal to participate in the trade of animals or plants taken in violation of any local, state, federal or international law, including violations of foreign law.

Table 20.3. Invertebrate species listed by the U.S. Endangered Species Act as endangered or threatened (For the current list see http://llecos.fws.gov/tess.public.)

Species (common name)	Native country/state	Species (common name)	Native country/state
Gastropoda: Endangered		*Cyprogenia stegaria* (fan shell)	USA: AL, IL, IN, KY, OH, PA, TN, VA, WV
Achatinella spp. (Oahu tree snails)	USA: HI		
Antrobia culveri (Tumbling Creek cave snail)	USA: MO		
Athearnia anthonyi (Anthony's river snail)	USA: AL, GA, TN	*Cyrtonaias tampicoensis tecomatensis* (Tampico pearly mussel)	Mexico
Campeloma decampi (slender campeloma)	USA: AL		
Discus macclintocki (Iowa Pleistocene snail)	USA: IA, IL	*Dromus dromas* (dromedary pearly mussel)	USA: AL, KY, TN, VA
Fontelicella idahoensis (Idaho spring snail)	USA: ID	*Elliptio steinstansana* (Tar River spiny mussel)	USA: NC
Helminthoglypta walkeriana (Morro shoulderband snail)	USA: CA	*Epioblasma brevidens* (Cumberlandian combshell)	USA: AL, KY, MS, TN, VA
Lanx spp. (Banbury Springs limpet)	USA: ID	*Epioblasma capsaeformis* (oyster mussel)	USA: AL, GA, KY, NC, TN, VA
Leptoxis plicata (plicate rock snail)	USA: AL		
Lepyrium showalteri (flat pebble snail)	USA: AL	*Epioblasma florentina curtisii* (Curtis pearly mussel)	USA: AR, MO
Lioplax cyclostomaformis (cylindrical lioplax)	USA: AL, GA		
Oxyloma haydeni kanabensis (Kanab amber snail)	USA: AZ, UT	*Epioblasma florentina florentina* (yellow blossom)	USA: AL, TN
Papustyla pulcherrima (Manus Island tree snail)	Admiralty Island	*Epioblasma florentina walkeri* (Tan riffle shell)	USA: AL, KY, NC, TN, VA
Physa natricina (Snake River physa snail)	USA: ID	*Epioblasma metastriata* (upland combshell)	USA: AL, GA, TN
Polygyriscus virginianus (Virginia fringed mountain snail)	USA: VA	*Epioblasma obliquata obliquata* (catspaw)	USA: AL, IL, IN, KY, OH, TN
Pyrgulopsis pachyta (armored snail)	USA: AL	*Epioblasma obliquata perobliqua* (white cat's paw)	USA: IN, MI, OH
Pyrgulopsis bruneauensis (Bruneau hot spring snail)	USA: ID		
Pyrgulopsis neomexicana (Socorro spring snail)	USA: NM	*Epioblasma othcaloogensis* (southern acorn shell)	USA: AL, GA, TN
Pyrgulopsis ogmorhaphe (Royal Marstonia)	USA: TN	*Epioblasma penita* (southern combshell)	USA: AL, MS
Tryonia alamosae (Alamosa spring snail)	USA: NM	*Epioblasma torulosa gubernaculums* (Green blossom)	USA: TN, VA
Tulotoma magnifica (Tulotoma snail)	USA: AL		
Valvata utahensis (Utah valvata snail)	USA: ID	*Epioblasma torulosa rangiana* (northern riffle shell)	USA: IL, IN, KY, MI, OH, PA, WV Canada: Ont
Gastropoda: Threatened		*Epioblasma torulosa torulosa* (Tubercled blossom)	USA: AL, IL, IN, KY, TN, WV
Anguispira picta (painted snake coiled forest snail)	USA: TN		
Elimia crenatella (Lacy Elimia)	USA: AL	*Epioblasma turgidula* (turgid blossom)	USA: AL, TN
Erinna newcombi (Newcomb's snail)	USA: HI	*Fusconaia cor* (shiny pigtoe)	USA: AL, TN, VA
Leptoxis ampla (round rock snail)	USA: AL	*Fusconaia cuneolus* (finerayed pigtoe)	USA: AL, TN, VA
Leptoxis taeniata (painted rock snail)	USA: AL	*Hemistena lata* (cracking pearly mussel)	USA: AL, IL, IN, KY, OH, TN, VA
Mesodon clarki nantahala (noonday snail)	USA: NC		
Mesodon magazinensis (Magazine Mountain shagreen)	USA: AR	*Lampsilis abrupta* (pink mucket)	USA: AL, AR, IL, IN, KY, LA, MO, OH, PA, TN, VA, WV
Orthalicus reses (Stock Island tree snail)	USA: FL		
Succinea chittenangoensis (Chittenango ovate amber snail)	USA: NY		
Taylorconcha serpenticola (Bliss Rapids snail)	USA: D	*Lampsilis higginsii* (Higgins eye)	USA: IA, IL, MN, MO, NE, WI
Triodopsis platysayoides (flat-spired three-toothed snail)	USA: WV	*Lampsilis streckeri* (speckled pocketbook)	USA: AR
		Lampsilis subangulata (shinyrayed pocketbook)	USA: AL, FL, GA
Bivalvia: Endangered		*Lampsilis virescens* (Alabama lamp mussel)	USA: AL, TN
Alasmidonta atropurpurea (Cumberland elktoe)	USA: KY, TN	*Lasmigona decorata* (Carolina heel splitter)	USA: NC, SC
Alasmidonta heterodon (dwarf wedge mussel)	USA: CT, DC, DE, MA, MD, NC, NH, NJ, NY, PA, VA, VT Canada: NB	*Leptodea leptodon* (scaleshell mussel)	USA: AL, AR, IL, IN, IA, KY, MN, MO, OH, OK, SD, TN, WI
Alasmidonta raveneliana (Appalachian elktoe)	USA: NC, TN	*Medionidus parvulus* (Coosa moccasin shell)	USA: AL, GA, TN
Amblema neislerii (fat three-ridge)	USA: FL, GA	*Medionidus penicillatus* (Gulf moccasin shell)	USA: AL, FL, GA
Arkansia wheeleri (Ouachita rock pocketbook)	USA: AR, OK	*Medionidus simpsonianus* (Ochlockonee moccasin shell)	USA: FL, GA
Conradilla caelata (birdwing pearly mussel)	USA: TN, VA	*Megalonaias nicklineana* (Nicklin's pearly mussel)	Mexico

(continued)

Table 20.3. *(continued)*

Species (common name)	Native country/state	Species (common name)	Native country/state
Obovaria retusa (ring pink)	USA: AL, IL, IN, KY, OH, PA, TN, WV	*Cambarus zophonastes* (cave crayfish)	USA: AR
		Gammarus acherondytes (Illinois cave amphipod)	USA: IL
Pegias fibula (littlewing pearly mussel)	USA: AL, KY, NC, TN, VA	*Lirceus usdagalun* (Lee County cave isopod)	USA: VA
		Orconectes shoupi (Nashville crayfish)	USA: TN
Plethobasus cicatricosus (white warty back)	USA: AL, IL, IN, KY, TN	*Pacifastacus fortis* (Shasta crayfish)	USA: CA
		Palaemonias alabamae (Alabama cave shrimp)	USA: AL
Plethobasus cooperianus (orangefoot pimple back)	USA: AL, IA, IL, IN, KY, OH, PA, TN	*Palaemonias ganteri* (Kentucky cave shrimp)	USA: KY
		Spelaeorchestia koloana (Kauai cave amphipod)	USA: HI
Pleurobema clava (clubshell)	USA: AL, IL, IN, KY, MI, OH, PA, TN, WV		
		Streptocephalus woottoni (riverside fairy shrimp)	USA: CA
Pleurobema collina (James spiny mussel)	USA: VA, WV	*Stygobromus pecki* (Peck's cave amphipod)	USA: TX
Pleurobema curtum (black clubshell)	USA: AL, MS	*Stygobromus hayi* (Hay's Spring amphipod)	USA: DC
Pleurobema decisum (southern clubshell)	USA: AL, GA, MS, TN	*Syncaris pacifica* (California freshwater shrimp)	USA: CA
		Thermosphaeroma thermophilus (Socorro isopod)	USA: NM
Pleurobema furvum (dark pigtoe)	USA: AL		
Pleurobema georgianum (southern pigtoe)	USA: AL, GA, TN		
Pleurobema gibberum (Cumberland pigtoe)	USA: TN	**Crustacea: Threatened**	
Pleurobema marshalli (flat pig toe)	USA: AL, MS	*Antrolana lira* (Madison Cave isopod)	USA: VA
Pleurobema perovatum (ovate clubshell)	USA: AL, GA, MS, TN	*Branchinecta lynchi* (vernal pool fairy shrimp)	USA: CA, OR
		Palaemonetes cummingi (Squirrel Chimney Cave shrimp)	USA: FL
Pleurobema plenum (rough pigtoe)	USA: AL, IN, KY, PA, TN, VA	*Lepidurus packardi* (vernal pool tadpole shrimp)	USA: CA
Pleurobema pyriforme (oval pigtoe)	USA: AL, FL, GA		
Pleurobema taitianum (heavy pigtoe)	USA: AL, MS		
Potamilus capax (fat pocketbook)	USA: AR, IA, IL, IN, KY, MO, MS, OH	**Arachnida: Endangered**	
		Adelocosa anops (Kauai Cave wolf spider)	USA: HI
Ptychobranchus greeni (triangular kidney shell)	USA: AL, GA, TN	*Cicurina baronia* (Robber Barron Cave mesh weaver)	USA: TX
Quadrula cylindrica strigillata (rough rabbit's foot)	USA: TN, VA	*Cicurina madla* (Madla's Cave mesh weaver)	USA: TX
		Cicurina venii (Braken Bat Cave mesh weaver)	USA: TX
Quadrula fragosa (winged maple leaf)	USA: AL, IA, IL, IN, KY, MN, MO, NE, OH, OK, TN, WI	*Cicurina vespera* (Government Canyon Bat Cave mesh weaver)	USA: TX
		Microhexura montivaga (spruce-fir moss spider)	USA: NC, TN
Quadrula intermedia (Cumberland monkey face)	USA: AL, TN, VA	*Neoleptoneta microps* (Government Canyon bat cave spider)	USA: TX
Quadrula sparsa (Appalachian monkey face)	USA: TN, VA		
Quadrula stapes (stirrup shell)	USA: AL, MS	*Neoleptoneta myopica* (Tooth Cave spider)	USA: TX
Toxolasma cylindrellus (pale lilliput)	USA: AL, TN	*Tartarocreagris texana* (Tooth Cave pseudo-scorpion)	USA: TX
Villosa perpurpurea (purple bean)	USA: TN, VA		
Villosa trabalis (Cumberland bean)	USA: AL, KY, TN, VA	*Texella cokendolpheri* (Cokendolpher Cave harvestman)	USA: TX
		Texella reddelli (Bee Creek Cave harvestman)	USA: TX
Bivalvia: Threatened		*Texella reyesi* (Bone Cave harvestman)	USA: TX
Elliptio chipolaensis (Cipola slabshell)	USA: AL, FL		
Elliptoideus sloatianus (purple bank climber)	USA: AL, GA, FL	**Insecta: Endangered**	
Lampsilis altilis (finelined pocketbook)	USA: AL, GA	*Apodemia mormo langei* (Lange's metalmark butterfly)	USA: CA
Lampsilis perovalis (orangenacre mucket)	USA: AL, MS	*Batrisodes texanus* (Coffin Cave mold beetle)	USA: TX
Lampsilis powelli (Arkansas fat mucket)	USA: AR	*Batrisodes venyivi* (Helotes mold beetle)	USA: TX
Margaritifera hembeli (Louisiana pearl shell)	USA: LA	*Boloria acrocnema* (Uncompahgre fritillary butterfly)	USA: CO
Medionidus acutissimus (Alabama moccasin shell)	USA: AL, GA, MS	*Brychius hungerfordi* (Hungerford's crawling water beetle)	USA: MI Canada
Potamilus inflatus (Alabama heel splitter)	USA: AL, LA, MS	*Callophrys mossii bayensis* (San Bruno elfin butterfly)	USA: CA
Crustacea: Endangered		*Cicindela ohlone* (Ohlone tiger beetle)	USA: CA
Branchinecta conservatio (Conservancy fairy shrimp)	USA: CA	*Euphilotes battoides allyni* (El Segundo blue butterfly)	USA: CA
Branchinecta longiantenna (longhorn fairy shrimp)	USA: CA		
Branchinecta sandiegonensis (San Diego fairy shrimp)	USA: CA		
Cambarus aculabrum (cave crayfish)	USA: AR		

(continued)

Table 20.3. *(continued)*

Species (common name)	Native country/state	Species (common name)	Native country/state
Euphilotes enoptes smithi (Smith's blue butterfly)	USA: CA	*Rhadine infernalis* (ground beetle)	USA: TX
Euphydryas editha quino (Quino checkerspot butterfly)	USA: CA Mexico	*Rhadine persephone* (Tooth Cave ground beetle)	USA: TX
Glaucopsyche lygdamus palosverdesensis (Palos Verdes blue butterfly)	USA: CA	*Rhaphiomidas terminatus abdominalis* (Delhi Sands flower-loving fly)	USA: CA
Heraclides aristodemus ponceanus (Schaus swallowtail butterfly)	USA: FL	*Somatochlora hineana* (Hine's emerald dragonfly)	USA: IL, IN, OH, WI
Heterelmis comalensis (Comal Springs riffle beetle)	USA: TX	*Speyeria callippe callippe* (Callippe silverspot butterfly)	USA: CA
Icaricia icarioides fenderi (Fender's blue butterfly)	USA: OR	*Speyeria zerene behrensii* (Behren's silverspot butterfly)	USA: CA
Icaricia icarioides missionensis (Mission blue butterfly)	USA: CA	*Speyeria zerene myrtleae* (Myrtle's silverspot butterfly)	USA: CA
Lycaeides argyrognomon lotis (lotis blue butterfly)	USA: CA	*Stygoparnus comalensis* (Comal Springs dryopid beetle)	USA: TX
Lycaeides melissa samuelis (Karner blue butterfly)	USA: IL, IN, MA, MI, MN, NH, NY, OH, PA, WI Canada: Ont	*Texamaurops reddelli* (Kretschmarr Cave mold beetle)	USA: TX
Manduca blackburni (Blackburn's sphinx moth)	USA: HI	*Trimerotropis infantilis* (Zayante band-winged grasshopper)	USA: CA
Neonympha mitchellii francisci (Saint Francis' satyr butterfly)	USA: NC	*Troides alexandrae* (Queen Alexandra's birdwing butterfly)	Papua New Guinea
Neonympha mitchellii mitchellii (Mitchell's satyr butterfly)	USA: IN, MI, NJ, OH	**Insecta: Threatened**	
Nicrophorus americanus (American burying beetle)	USA: eastern states south to FL, west to SD and TX Eastern Canada	*Ambrysus amargosus* (Ash Meadows naucorid)	USA: NV
		Cicindela dorsalis dorsalis (Northeastern beach tiger beetle)	USA: CT, MA, MD, NJ, NY, PA, RI, VA
Papilio chikae (Luzon peacock swallowtail butterfly)	Philippines	*Cicindela puritana* (Puritan tiger beetle)	USA: CT, MA, MD, NH, VT
Papilio homerus (Homerus swallowtail butterfly)	Jamaica, entire	*Desmocerus californicus dimorphus* (valley elderberry longhorn beetle)	USA: CA
Papilio hospiton (Corsican swallowtail butterfly)	Corsica, Sardinia	*Elaphrus viridis* (Delta green ground beetle)	USA: CA
Polyphylla barbata (Mount Hermon June beetle)	USA: CA	*Euphydryas editha bayensis* (bay checkerspot butterfly)	USA: CA
Pseudocopaeodes eunus obscurus (Carson wandering skipper)	USA: CA, NV	*Euproserpinus euterpe* (Kern primrose sphinx moth)	USA: CA
Pyrgus ruralis lagunae (Laguna Mountains skipper)	USA: CA	*Hesperia leonardus montana* (Pawnee montane skipper)	USA: CO
Rhadine exilis (ground beetle)	USA: TX	*Speyeria zerene hippolyta* (Oregon silverspot butterfly)	USA: CA, OR, WA

U.S. Department of Agriculture

The Animal and Plant Health Inspection Service (APHIS) is a regulatory program of the U.S. Department of Agriculture (USDA). They are charged with the protection and promotion of U.S. agriculture and administration of the Animal Welfare Act. The USDA-APHIS is concerned with the international and interstate transport of organisms that could pose potential health or environmental risk to U.S. animal and plant crops and native fauna and flora. The service also responds to issues concerning human safety, wildlife health, wildlife damage management, and introduced pest species. APHIS directs many programs, including Veterinary Services, Animal Care, and Wildlife Services that administer animal health, safety, welfare, and wildlife control regulations. Plant Protection and Quarantine

(PPQ) is the USDA-APHIS program that focuses on safeguarding U.S. and international agricultural and natural resources through animal and plant pest control. It specifically regulates and provides permits for the import, export, transport, possession, and display of many invertebrate species. Bees, butterflies and moths, earthworms, snails, and slugs are directly addressed. Any arthropod species perceived to be a potential plant pest is under PPQ jurisdiction. Federal and accompanying state permits are required for all of these organisms.

Potential Vectors of Disease

Any arthropod that lives in dung during any of its life stages or is a potential vector for nonhuman disease is regulated by APHIS Veterinary Services. For information on international

Table 20.4.   Contact information for U.S. Fish and Wildlife Service regional offices

http://www.fws.gov/r9irmtsb/regional.html

Region 1 (California, Hawaii, Idaho, Nevada, Oregon, Washington)
911 NE 11th Avenue
Portland, Oregon 97232-4181
(503) 231-6118

Region 2 (Arizona, New Mexico, Oklahoma, Texas)
PO Box 1306
Albuquerque, New Mexico 87103
(505) 248-6282

Region 3 (Illinois, Indiana, Iowa, Michigan, Minnesota, Missouri, Ohio, Wisconsin)
Federal Building, Fort Snelling
Twin Cities, Minnesota 55111
(612) 713-5301

Region 4 (Alabama, Arkansas, Florida, Georgia, Kentucky, Louisiana, Mississippi, North Carolina, Puerto Rico, South Carolina, Tennessee, Virgin Islands)
1875 Century Boulevard
Atlanta, Georgia 30345
(404) 679-4000

Region 5 (Connecticut, Delaware, Maine, Maryland, Massachusetts, New Hampshire, New Jersey, New York, Pennsylvania, Rhode Island, Vermont, Virginia, West Virginia)
300 Westgate Center Drive
Hadley, Massachusetts 01035
(413) 253-8300

Region 6 (Colorado, Kansas, Montana, Nebraska, North Dakota, South Dakota, Utah, Wyoming)
PO Box 25486
Denver, Colorado 80025
(303) 236-7920

Region 7 (Alaska)
1011 East Tudor Road
Anchorage, Alaska 99503
(907) 786-3542

Main Office
U.S. Fish & Wildlife Service
Division of Management Authority
4401 N. Fairfax Drive, Room 700
Arlington, VA 22203
(703) 358-2104
http://www.fws.gov

NMFS currently has only one species of invertebrate listed as endangered under the ESA, the white abalone (*Haliotis sorenseni*). The black abalone (*Haliotis cracherodii*), the elkhorn coral (*Acropora palmata*), and the staghorn coral (*Acropora cervicornis*) are all currently candidates for listing. Permit requests and inquiries regarding these marine invertebrates should go to NMFS at

NOAA Fisheries
1315 East West Highway
SSMC3, Silver Spring, MD 20910
http://www.nmfs.noaa.gov

Table 20.5.   Invertebrate species specifically named in the Magnuson–Stevens Fishery Conservation and Management Act (MSFCMA)

Cnidaria: corals
Acanella spp. (bamboo coral)
Antipathes spp. (black coral)
Callogorgia spp. (gold coral)
Corallium spp. (precious red coral)
Keratoisis spp. (bamboo coral)
Parazoanthus spp. (gold coral)
Crustacea: crabs and lobsters
Cancer magister (Dungeness crab)
Chaceon quinquedens (deep-sea red crab)
Chionoecetes tanneri (tanner crab)
Chionoecetes opilio (tanner crab)
Chionoecetes angulatus (tanner crab)
Chionoecetes bairdi (tanner crab)
Homarus americanus (lobster)
Lithodes aequispinus (golden king crab)
Lithodes maja (northern stone crab)
Menippe mercenaria (stone crab)
Paralithodes brevipes (king crab)
Paralithodes californiensis (California king crab)
Paralithodes camtschatica (king crab)
Paralithodes platypus (king crab)
Paralithodes rathbuni (California king crab)
Mollusca: abalones, conchs, and clams
Arctica islandica (ocean quahog)
Haliotis corrugata (pink abalone)
Haliotis kamtschatkana (Japanese abalone)
Haliotis rufescens (red abalone)
Spisula solidissima (surf clam)
Strombus gigas (queen conch)
Porifera: sponges
Hippiospongia lachne (sheepswool sponge)
Spongia barbera (yellow sponge)
Spongia cheiris (glove sponge)
Spongia graminea (grass sponge)

trade, refer to the National Center for Import and Export (NCIE) by visiting their Web site:

http://www.aphis.usda.gov/vs/ncie/

One can otherwise contact them at

USDA-APHIS-VS-NCIE
4700 River Road, Unit 133
Riverdale, MD 20737
(301) 734-3277

Potential hosts and vectors of human disease, including species of snails and bloodsucking arthropods, are regulated by the Centers for Disease Control and Prevention (CDC). A permit is required from the CDC for the importation of any organism that may cause human disease. For more details or to download a copy of the required permit application and instructions, visit the CDC import–permit Web site:

http://www.cdc.gov/od/ohs/biosfty/imprtper.htm

One can otherwise contact them at

Centers for Disease Control and Prevention
Import Permit Program
1600 Clifton Road NE
Mailstop E-79
Atlanta, GA 30333
(404) 498-2260

Slugs and Snails

Slugs and snails are regulated by the APHIS-PPQ as potential plant pests. Several species are known to be pests and are banned from importation into the United States. Banned species include *Achatina fulica* (giant African snail), *Pomacea canaliculata* (channeled or golden apple snail), and *Rumina decollata* (decollate snail). Permits are required for importation, interstate transport, and possession of all other species. Permit (PPQ Form 526 [Section A]) applications may be obtained from the Web site:

http://www.aphis.usda.gov/ppq/permits/plantpest/snails_slugs.
    html

One can otherwise contact them at

PPQ Permit Staff
USDA, APHIS, PPQ
4700 River Road, Unit 133
Riverdale, MD 20737
(301) 734-8758

Earthworms

Due to the potential risk of plant pathogen introduction via contaminated soil in their guts, earthworms are regulated by the APHIS-PPQ. A permit (PPQ Form 526 [Section A]) and a detailed plan of containment and waste disposal are required prior to importation. For a copy of the permit application and for more details, visit the Web site:

http://www.aphis.usda.gov/ppq/permits/plantpest/earth-
    worm.html

One can otherwise contact them at

PPQ Permit Staff
USDA, APHIS, PPQ
4700 River Road, Unit 133
Riverdale, MD 20737
(301) 734-8758

Bees

The APHIS-PPQ regulates the bee trade in the United States. Currently, the interstate transport of bees within the United States does not require a permit. However, importation of bees (live or dead), honeybee semen (genus *Apis*), and beekeeping equipment including, but not limited to, used hives, boards, nests, and nonliquefied beeswax does require a permit (PPQ

Form 526). To download a copy of the permit application and instructions, visit the Web site:

http://www.aphis.usda.gov/ppq/permits/bees/index.html

Questions about bee regulations should be directed to

Dr. Wayne Wehling
Entomologist
USDA, APHIS, PPQ
4700 River Road, Unit 133
Riverdale, MD 20737
(301) 734-8700

Herbivorous Arthropods (Including Arthropod Pests, Butterflies and Moths, and Arthropods for Education and Display)

Several separate categories of plant-eating arthropods are regulated by the APHIS-PPQ and require different permits for import, interstate transport, and containment. General permit categories include Butterflies and Moths, Arthropod Pests, and Arthropods for Display or Educational Purposes. A few of the more common pet-trade species of invertebrates that pose a relatively low risk of introduction (for example, Madagascar hissing roaches [Figure 20.1] and giant African millipedes) may eventually be exempt from the permit requirements, although they, along with all other phytophagus arthropods, are currently considered possible plant pests and do require permits. Essentially, any arthropod that may directly or indirectly impact native flora or crop plants should be considered a potential risk. If the organism feeds on plants at any stage in its life, it is subject to regulation by the PPQ. A current list of specially regulated arthropods that have been determined by the USDA-APHIS to be plant pests (Table 20.6) is available on the Web site:

http://www.aphis.usda.gov/ppq/regpestlist/

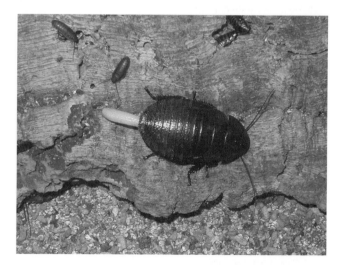

Figure 20.1. A Madagascar hissing cockroach (*Gromphadorhina portentosa*) with a developing and protruding egg case. Although common as pets, these animals currently require a USDA-APHIS permit. Photo courtesy Shane Boylan.

Table 20.6. Arthropod species specifically recognized and regulated by USDA-APHIS as plant pests (organized by family)

Insecta

Acrolepiidae
    Acrolepiopsis assectella
Aleyrodidae
    Aleurocanthus spiniferus
    Neomaskellia bergii
Alydidae
    Leptocorisa acuta
Apidae
    Apis mellifera capensis
    Apis mellifera scuttellata
Carposinidae
    Carposina niponensis
Cerambycidae
    Anoplophora glabripennis
Chrysididae
    Chrysis spp.
Chrysomelidae
    Exosoma lusitanica
Coccidae
    Coccus viridis
Coreidae
    Leptoglossus chilensis
Cossidae
    Dyspessa ulula
Crambidae
    Maruca vitrata
Curculionidae
    Brachycerus spp.
    Conotrachelus aguacatae
    Conotrachelus spp.
    Copturus aguacatae
    Cryptorhynchus mangiferae
    Curculio elephas
    Curculio nucum
    Elytroteinus subtruncatus
    Euscepes postfasciatus
    Heilipus lauri
    Listroderes subcinctus
    Megalometis chilensis
    Metamasius spp.
    Naupactus xanthographus
    Rhabdoscelus obscurus
    Sternochetus mangiferae
Cynipidae
    Dryocosmus kuriphilus
Dermestidae
    Trogoderma granarium
Diaspididae
    Furcaspis oceanica
Elachistidae
    Stenoma catenifer
Elateridae
    Conoderus rufangulus
Formicidae
    Solenopsis invicta
    Solenopsis richteri
    Solenopsis richteri X *Solenopsis invicta* hybrid
Gelechiidae
    Pectinophora gossypiella
    Pectinophora scutigera
    Conopomorpha cramerella

Hieroxestidae
    Opogona sacchari
Lycaenidae
    Lampides boeticus
Lymantriidae
    Lymantria dispar
Lyonetiidae
    Leucoptera malifoliella
Margarodidae
    Icerya aegyptiaca
Megachilidae
    Coelioxys spp.
Noctuidae
    Earias fabia
Phlaeothripidae
    Haplothrips chinensis
Plutellidae
    Prays endocarpa
Pseudococcidae
    Phenococcus manihoti
Pyralidae
    Chilo suppressalis
    Conogethes punctiferalis
    Omphisa anastomosalis
Scarabaeidae
    Adoretus sinicus
    Adoretus spp.
    Anomala sulcatula
    Holotrichia mindanaona
    Phyllophaga spp.
    Popillia japonica
Scolytidae
    Hypothenemus hampei
    Tomicus piniperda
    Xyleborus spp.
Sminthuridae
    Sminthurus viridis
Tephritidae
    Anastrepha fraterculus
    Anastrepha grandis
    Anastrepha ludens
    Anastrepha obliqua
    Anastrepha serpentina
    Anastrepha striata
    Anastrepha suspensa
    Bactrocera cucurbitae
    Bactrocera dorsalis
    Bactrocera tryoni
    Ceratitis capitata
    Ceratitis spp.
    Pterandrus spp.
    Toxotrypana curvicauda
Tortricidae
    Adoxophyes orana
    Argyrotaenia pulchellana
    Capua tortrix
    Cryptophlebia leucotreta
    Cydia funebrana
    Cydia splendana
    Epiphyas postvittana

(continued)

Table 20.6. *(continued)*

Hemimene juliana	Tenuipalpidae
Laspeyresia spp.	*Brevipalpus chilensis*
Lobesia botrana	Tetranychidae
Pammene fasciana	*Amphitetranychus viennensis*
Proeulia spp.	*Mononychellus tanajoa*
Arachnida (mites)	Varroidae
Eriophytidae	*Euvarroa sinhai*
Eriophyes gossypii	Varroidae
Eriophyes litchii	*Varroa jacobsoni*
Laelapidae	**Nematoda**
Tropilaelaps clareae	Heteroderidae
Tarsonemidae	*Globodera pallida*
Acarapis woodi	*Globodera rostochiensis*

Several specific permits may be issued with varying conditions, depending on the status of the organism and its potential or known risk as a pest species. Applications for permits should be submitted separately for known plant pests, arthropods for display and education, butterflies and moths for butterfly houses, and general possession. Specified levels of security and containment may vary depending on the potential risk of each organism in question. Facilities that plan to import arthropods from outside the United States must follow strict guidelines in the construction and maintenance of a receiving facility. These guidelines are intended to direct the creation of a facility that is *escape proof* to ensure that unwanted pest species do not escape and become established in the United States. A permit is required for transport (including interstate and international importation), possession, and display. A state permit must accompany this federal permit. A permit application (PPQ Form 526) may be downloaded from the agricultural permits page linked to the PPQ main Web page:

http://www.aphis.usda.gov/ppq/

Questions about plant pest permits can be directed to

PPQ Permit Staff
USDA, APHIS, PPQ
4700 River Road, Unit 133
Riverdale, MD 20737
(301) 734-5302

Table 20.7 lists all U.S. state agencies that belong to the National Plant Board (NPB) and are involved in plant protection and plant pest regulation within their state. For more information, visit the Web site:

http://www.aphis.usda.gov/npb/npbmemb.html

Invertebrate Predators and Nonherbivorous Arthropods

The APHIS-PPQ currently has no jurisdiction over spiders, centipedes, scorpions, and other predatory arthropods that are not considered potential pest species (unless they are meant for release as biological control agents). These species do not require permits from the USDA. If predators or parasitoid arthropods such as mites, lady beetles, wasps, or mantids are intended for release as biological control agents, Section A of PPQ Form 526 should be submitted as an application for the permit. For information, review the Web site:

http://www.aphis.usda.gov/ppq/permits/

One can otherwise contact them at

USDA, APHIS, PPQ
4700 River Road, Unit 133
Riverdale, MD 20737
(301) 734-8700

U.S. Fish and Wildlife Service (USFWS)

The USFWS is a branch of the U.S. Department of the Interior (DOI). It is the major U.S. agency focused on wildlife conservation and habitat preservation. The Lacey Act (LA) grants USFWS the authority to enforce state, federal, international, and foreign wildlife laws. They have many national and international departments and programs. The International Affairs (IA) department promotes Wildlife Without Borders and assists other nations through global partnerships and support of wildlife and habitat conservation. The USFWS Division of Law Enforcement watches over wildlife importation, exportation, trade, and sale. Their jurisdiction covers both live and dead animals and plants, including any parts or pieces. Permits for terrestrial invertebrate species listed by CITES, terrestrial invertebrate species listed by the ESA, and wildlife importation or exportation should be obtained through the USFWS. Applications can be obtained by downloading from the internet at the Web site:

http://permits.fws.gov/applicationmain.shtml

Table 20.7. Contact information for U.S. State Plant Protection and Regulation Offices

Alabama
Division of Plant Industry
Alabama Department of Agriculture & Industries
PO Box 3336
Montgomery, AL 36109-0336
(334) 240-7225
http://www.agi.state.al.us/pppm.htm

Alaska
Plant Industry Section
Alaska Department of Natural Resources Division of Agriculture
1800 Glenn Highway, Suite 12
Palmer, AK 99645-0949
(907) 745-7200
http://www.dnr.state.ak.us/ag

Arizona
Plant Services Division
Arizona Department of Agriculture
1688 West Adams
Phoenix, AZ 85007
(602) 542-0996
http://www.azda.gov/PSD/psd.htm

Arkansas
Division of Plant Industry
Arkansas State Plant Board
PO Box 1069
Little Rock, AR 72203
(501) 225-1598
http://www.plantboard.org

California
Plant Health & Pest Prevention Services
California Department of Food & Agriculture
1220 N Street
Sacramento, CA 95814
(916) 654-1022
http://www.cdfa.ca.gov/phpps

Colorado
Division of Plant Industry
Colorado Department of Agriculture
700 Kipling Street, Suite 4000
Lakewood, CO 80215-5894
(303) 239-4140
http://www.ag.state.co.us/DPI/

Connecticut
The Connecticut Agricultural Exp. Station
123 Huntington Street, PO Box 1106
New Haven, CT 06504-1106
(203) 974-8474
http://www.caes.state.ct.us

Delaware
Plant Industries Section
Delaware Department of Agriculture
2320 South DuPont Highway
Dover, DE 19901-5515
(302) 698-4587
http://www.state.de.us/deptagri/plantind/

Florida
Division of Plant Industry
Florida Department of Agriculture and Conservation Services
PO Box 147100
Gainesville, FL 32614-7100
(352) 372-3505
http://www.doacs.state.fl.us/~pi/

Georgia
Plant Protection Division
Georgia Department of Agriculture
19 Martin Luther King Drive, Room 243
Atlanta, GA 30334-4201
(404) 651-9486
http://www.agr.georgia.gov

Hawaii
Plant Industry Division
Hawaii Department of Agriculture
1428 South King Street
Honolulu, HI 96814
(808) 973-9535
http://www.hawaiiag.org/hdoa/pi.htm

Idaho
Division of Plant Industry
Idaho Department of Agriculture
PO Box 790
Boise, ID 83701-0790
(208) 332-8620
http://www.agri.state.id.us/plants/plant_industriesTOC.htm

Illinois
Bureau of Environmental Programs
Illinois Department of Agriculture
P.O. Box 19281, State Fairgrounds
Springfield, IL 62794-9281
(217) 782-2172
http://www.agr.state.il.us/Environment/

Indiana
Division of Entomology & Plant Pathology
Indiana Department of Natural Resources
Indiana Government Center South 402 West Washington,
  Room W290
Indianapolis, IN 46204-2748
(317) 232-4120
http://www.in.gov/dnr/entomolo/

Iowa
Iowa Department of Agriculture and Land Stewardship
Wallace State Office Building
502 East 9th Street
Des Moines, IA 50319-0051
(515) 281-6323
http://www.agriculture.state.ia.us/entomology.htm

(continued)

Table 20.7. *(continued)*

Kansas
Plant Protection and Weed Control Program
Kansas Department of Agriculture
PO Box 19282
Topeka, KS 66619-0282
(785) 862-2180
http://www.accesskansas.org/kda/Plantpest/plant-main.htm

Kentucky
Department of Entomology University of Kentucky
S-225 Agriculture Science Center North
Lexington, KY 40546-0091
(859) 257-5838
http://www.uky.edu/Agriculture/NurseryInspection/

Louisiana
Department Agriculture & Forestry
5825 Florida Boulevard, Suite 1023
Baton Rouge, LA 70806
(225) 952-8100
http://www.ldaf.state.la.us/horticulture&quarantine-programs.asp

Maine
Division of Plant Industry
Maine Department of Agriculture
28 State House Station
Augusta, ME 04333-0028
(207) 287-3891
http://www.state.me.us/agriculture/pi/

Maryland
Plant Protection Section
Maryland Department of Agriculture
50 Harry S. Truman Parkway
Annapolis, MD 21401
(410) 841-5920
http://www.mda.state.md.us

Massachusetts
Division of Regulatory Services
Massachusetts Department of Agricultural Resources
251 Causeway Street, Suite 500
Boston, MA 02114
(617) 626-1771
http://www.state.ma.us/dfa/farmproducts/

Michigan
Pesticide & Plant Pest Management Division
Michigan Department of Agriculture
PO Box 30017
Lansing, MI 48909
(517) 373-4087
http://www.michigan.gov/mda/

Minnesota
Division Agronomy and Plant Protection
Minnesota Department of Agriculture
90 West Plato Boulevard
St. Paul, MN 55107-2094
(651) 297-7174
http://www.mda.state.mn.us/appd

Mississippi
Bureau of Plant Industry
Mississippi Department of Agriculture and Commerce
PO Box 5207
Mississippi, MS 39762
(662) 325-7765
http://www.mdac.state.ms.us/Library/BBC/PlantIndustry/
    PlantIndustry.html

Missouri
Plant Industries Division
Missouri Department of Agriculture
PO Box 630
Jefferson City, MO 65102-0630
(573) 751-2462
http://www.mda.state.mo.us/d.html

Montana
Agricultural Sciences Division
Montana Department of Agriculture
PO Box 200201
Helena, MT 59620-0201
(406) 444-3730
http://www.agr.state.mt.us

Nebraska
Bureau of Plant Industry
Nebraska Department of Agriculture
PO Box 94756
Lincoln, NE 68509-4756
(402) 471-2394
http://www.agr.state.ne.us/division/bpi/bpi.htm

Nevada
Bureau of Plant Industry
Nevada Division of Agriculture
350 Capitol Hill Avenue
Reno, NV 89502-2992
(775) 688-1180
http://www.agri.state.nv.us/pl_ind2.htm

New Hampshire
Division of Plant Industry
New Hampshire Department of Agriculture Markets & Food
State Laboratory Building 6, Hazen Drive
Concord, NH 03301
(603) 271-2561
http://www.agriculture.nh.gov/about/plant_industry.htm

New Jersey
Division of Plant Industry
New Jersey Department of Agriculture
PO Box 330
Trenton, NJ 08625-0330
(609) 292-5441
http://www.state.nj.us/agriculture/plant

New Mexico
Bureau of Entomology & Nursery Industries
New Mexico Department of Agriculture, MSC 3BA
PO Box 30005
Las Cruces, NM 88003-0005
(505) 646-3207
http://www.nmdaweb.nmsu.edu/DIVISIONS/AESlent.html

Table 20.7. *(continued)*

New York
Division of Plant Industry
New York Department of Agriculture and Markets
1 Winners Circle Capitol Plaza
Albany, NY 12235-0001
(518) 457-2087
http://www.agmkt.state.ny.us/PI/PIHome.html

North Carolina
Plant Industry Division
North Carolina Department of Agriculture and Consumer Services
216 West Jones Street
Raleigh, NC 27603
(919) 733-3933
http://www.agr.state.nc.us/plantind

North Dakota
North Dakota Department of Agriculture
600 East Boulevard Ave.
Bismarck, ND 58505-0020
(701) 328-4765
http://www.agdepartment.com/Programs/Plant/PlantInd.html

Ohio
Plant Pest Control Section
Ohio Department of Agriculture Division of Plant Industry
8995 East Main Street
Reynoldsburg, OH 43068
(614) 728-6400
http://www.state.oh.us/agr/PlantIndustryDiv.html

Oklahoma
Plant Industry & Consumer Services Division
Oklahoma Department of Agriculture, Food, & Forestry
PO Box 528804
Oklahoma City, OK 73152-8804
(405) 521-3864
http://www.oda.state.ok.us/pics.htm

Oregon
Plant Division
Oregon Department of Agriculture
635 Capitol Street NE
Salem, OR 97301-2532
(503) 986-4663
http://www.egov.oregon.gov/ODA/PLANT/

Pennsylvania
Plant Protection Division
Bureau of Plant Industry
Pennsylvania Department of Agriculture
2301 North Cameron Street
Harrisburg, PA 17110-9408
(717) 772-5222
http://www.agriculture.state.pa.us

Puerto Rico
State Plant Quarantine Program
Puerto Rico Department of Agriculture
PO Box 10163
Santurce, PR 00908-1163
(787) 724-4627

Rhode Island
Department of Environmental Management
Rhode Island Division of Agriculture & Resource Marketing
235 Promenade Street, Room 370
Providence, RI 02908
(401) 222-2781
http://www.state.ri.us/dem/programs/bnatres/agricult

South Carolina
Department of Plant Industry
511 Westinghouse Road
Pendleton, SC 29670
(864) 646-2140
http://www.dpi.clemson.edu

South Dakota
South Dakota Department of Agriculture
Division of Agricultural Services
Office of Plant Protection
523 East Capitol Avenue, Foss Building
Pierre, SD 57501-3182
(605) 773-3796
http://www.state.sd.us/doa/das/hp-w&p.htm

Tennessee
Division of Plant Certification
Tennessee Department of Agriculture
PO Box 40627 Melrose Station
Nashville, TN 37204
(615) 837-5338
http://www.state.tn.us/agriculture/regulate/plants

Texas
Agri-Systems
Texas Department of Agriculture
PO Box 12847 Capitol Station
Austin, TX 78711
(512) 463-1145
http://www.agr.state.tx.us

Utah
Division of Plant Industry
Utah Department of Agriculture & Food
PO Box 146500
Salt Lake City, UT 84114-6500
(801) 538-7180
http://www.ag.utah.gov/plantind/plant_ind.html

Vermont
Plant Industry Section
Vermont Agency of Agricultural Food & Markets
116 State Street
Montpelier, VT 05620-2901
(802) 828-2431
http://www.state.vt.us/agric/pid.htm

Virginia
Office of Plant and Pest Services
Virginia Department of Agriculture & Consumer Services
PO Box 1163
Richmond, VA 23218
(804) 786-3515
http://www.vdacs.state.va.us/plant&pest

(continued)

Table 20.7. *(continued)*

Washington Plants and Insects Washington State Department of Agriculture PO Box 42560 Olympia, WA 98504-2560 (360) 902-2071 http://www.agr.wa.gov/PlantsInsects	**Wisconsin** Plant Industry Bureau Wisconsin Department of Agriculture, Trade & Consumer Protection PO Box 8911 Madison, WI 53708-8911 (608) 224-4590 http://www.datcp.state.wi.us
West Virginia Plant Industries Division West Virginia Department of Agriculture 1900 Kanawha Boulevard East Charleston, WV 25305-0191 (304) 558-2212 http://www.state.wv.us/agriculture/divisions/plant_industries.html	**Wyoming** Consumer & Compliance Division Wyoming Department of Agriculture 2219 Carey Avenue Cheyenne, WY 82002 (307) 777-6590 http://www.wyagric.state.wy.us/

One can otherwise contact the local regional USFWS office (Table 20.4). Wildlife importation and exportation in the United States must be declared to the USFWS. In most cases, these shipments must go through designated ports. The definition of *wildlife* for this purpose includes live or dead (parts or products) of vertebrates and invertebrates in any life stage whether they were bred in captivity or collected in the wild. For more information on U.S. importation and exportation, visit the Web page:

http://www.le.fws.gov/Contact_Info_Ports.html

One can otherwise contact the USFWS Office of Law enforcement:

Office of Law Enforcement
U.S. Fish and Wildlife Service
4401 North Fairfax Drive
MS-LE-3000
Arlington, VA 22203
(703) 358-2271

National Marine Fisheries Service (NMFS)

The NMFS is the U.S. federal agency responsible for the protection and preservation of living marine resources. This agency should be contacted for information regarding the collection, transport, importation, or exportation of marine invertebrates that occur outside of U.S. state waters. The NMFS jurisdiction extends from state coastal waters (3 miles off shore) to 200 miles off shore. The NMFS is located within the National Oceanic and Atmospheric Administration (NOAA) of the Department of Commerce. It operates primarily to implement and enforce U.S. federal laws, including the Endangered Species Act (ESA), the Lacey Act (LA), and the Magnuson–Stevens Fishery Conservation and Management Act (MSFCMA).

Details of the ESA, LA, and MSFCMA have been addressed previously in this chapter.

State and Local Regulations

Many state and local laws must be observed when collecting, transporting, or maintaining invertebrates in captivity. Contact information for state plant protection agencies that will regulate plant pest species is provided in Table 20.7. A list and contact information for all U.S. state wildlife protection offices are provided in Table 20.8. These state agencies maintain separate lists of recognized plant pests and state protected species. Each state also has its own laws, regulations, and requirements for permits. Unfortunately, it is beyond the scope of this chapter to try to address all of the states individually. When looking into the particular rules and regulations for a species, first contact the appropriate federal agencies. They will provide additional recommendations for state and local contacts.

Animal Welfare Act and Animal Welfare Regulations: Licenses and the Institutional Animal Care and Use Committees

In both the Animal Welfare Act and Animal Welfare Regulations, the legal definition of *animal* is limited to select warm-blooded vertebrates. Invertebrates appear to be excluded and not considered in any of the regulations referring to animals. However, depending on the interpretation of the definition of *exotic animal* and of *wild animal* in the Animal Welfare Regulations, invertebrates may be considered in either of these categories. In many cases, the interpretation is primarily left to the USDA official in charge.

The U.S. Animal Welfare Act as found in the U.S. code (Title 7—Agriculture; Chapter 54—Transportation, Sale, and Handling of Certain Animals) is a Congressional document

Table 20.8. Contact information for U.S. state, territorial, and tribal wildlife regulatory agencies

Alabama Department of Conservation and Natural Resources
Division of Wildlife and Freshwater Fisheries
64 North Union Street
Montgomery, AL 36130
(334) 242-3465
http://www.dcnr.state.al.us

Alaska Department of Fish and Game
PO Box 25526
Juneau, AK 99802-5526
(907) 465-4100
http://www.state.ak.us/local/akpages/FISH.GAME/adfghome.htm

Arizona Game and Fish Department
2221 West Greenway Road
Phoenix, AZ 85023-4399
(602) 942-3000
http://www.gf.state.az.us

Arkansas Game and Fish Commission
2 Natural Resources Drive
Little Rock, AR 72205
(800) 364-4263
http://www.agfc.state.ar.us

California Department of Fish and Game
1416 Ninth Street
Sacramento, CA 95814
(916) 445-0411
http://www.dfg.ca.gov

Colorado Division of Wildlife
6060 Broadway
Denver, CO, 80216
(303) 297-1192
http://www.wildlife.state.co.us

Connecticut Department of Environmental Protection
Bureau of Natural Resources: Wildlife Division
79 Elm Street
Hartford, CT 06106-5127
(860) 424-3011
http://www.dep.state.ct.us/

Delaware Department of Natural Resources and Environmental
  Control
Division of Fish and Wildlife: Wildlife Section
89 Kings Highway
Dover, DE 19901
(302) 739-5297
http://www.dnrec.state.de.us/fw/

District of Columbia Department of Health
Environmental Health Administration: Fisheries and Wildlife Division
51 N Street, NE
Washington, DC 20002
(202) 535-2500
http://dchealth.dc.gov/services/administration_offices/
  environmental/services2/fisheries_wildlife/

Florida Fish and Wildlife Conservation Commission
Division of Wildlife
620 South Meridian Street
Tallahassee, FL 32399-1600
(850) 488-3831
http://floridaconservation.org/

Georgia Department of Natural Resources
Wildlife Resources Division
2070 U.S. Highway 278, SE
Social Circle, GA 30025
(770) 761-3035
http://georgiawildlife.dnr.state.ga.us/

Guam Division of Aquatic and Wildlife Resources
192 Dairy Road
Mangilao, GU 96923
(671) 735-3986

Hawaii Department of Land and Natural Resources
1151 Punchbowl Street, Room 130
Honolulu, Hawaii 96813
(808) 587-0405
http://www.hawaii.gov/dlnr/Welcome.html

Idaho Department of Fish and Game
600 South Walnut, PO Box 25
Boise, ID 83707
(208) 334-3700
http://www.fishandgame.idaho.gov

Illinois Department of Natural Resources
Resource Conservation
1 Natural Resources Way
Springfield, IL 62702
(217) 785-8547
http://dnr.state.il.us/orc/index.htm

Indiana Department of Natural Resources
Division of Fish and Wildlife
402 West Washington Street, Room W273
Indianapolis, IN 46204
(317) 232-4080.
http://www.in.gov/dnr/fishwild/about/

Iowa Department of Natural Resources
Wildlife Bureau
502 East 9th Street
Des Moines, IA 50319-0034
(515) 281-5918
http://www.iowadnr.com/wildlife/index.html

Kansas Department of Wildlife and Parks
Wildlife Diversity Coordinator
512 SE 25th Avenue
Pratt, KS 67124-8174
(620) 672-5911
http://www.kdwp.state.ks.us/

Kentucky Department of Fish and Wildlife
1 Game Farm Road
Frankfort, KY 40601
(800) 858-1549
http://www.kdfwr.state.ky.us

(continued)

289

Table 20.8.   (continued)

Louisiana Department of Wildlife and Fisheries
Non-Game Animals: General Information
2000 Quail Drive
Baton Rouge, LA 70808
(225) 765-2976
http://www.wlf.state.la.us/

Maine Department of Inland Fisheries and Wildlife
284 State Street
41 State House Station
Augusta, ME 04333-0041
(207) 287-8000
http://www.state.me.us/ifw/

Maryland Department of Natural Resources
Wildlife & Heritage Services
580 Taylor Avenue, E-1
Annapolis, MD 21401
(401) 260-8540
http://www.dnr.state.md.us/wildlife

Massachusetts Division of Fisheries and Wildlife
251 Causeway Street, Suite 400
Boston, MA 02114-2152
(617) 626-1590
http://www.state.ma.us/dfwele/dfw

Michigan Department of Natural Resources
Mason Building
PO Box 30028
Lansing, MI 48909
(517) 373-2329
http://www.dnr.state.mi.us

Minnesota Department of Natural Resources
500 Lafayette Road
St. Paul, MN 55155-4040
(651) 296-6157
http://www.dnr.state.mn.us

Mississippi Department of Wildlife, Fisheries and Parks
1505 Eastover Drive
Jackson, MS 39211-6374
(601) 432-2400
http://www.mdwfp.com

Missouri Department of Conservation
2901 West Truman Boulevard
Jefferson City, MO 65109
(573) 751-4115
http://www.conservation.state.mo.us

Montana Fish, Wildlife, and Parks
1420 East Sixth Avenue
PO Box 200701
Helena, MT 59620-0701
(406) 444-2535
http://www.fwp.state.mt.us

Nebraska Game and Parks Commission
2200 North 33rd Street
Lincoln, NE 68503
(402) 471-0641
http://www.ngpc.state.ne.us

Nevada Department of Wildlife
1100 Valley Road
Reno, NV 89512
(775) 688-1500
http://www.nevadadivisionofwildlife.org

New Hampshire Fish and Game Department
11 Hazen Drive
Concord, NH 03301
(603) 271-3511
http://www.wildlife.state.nh.us

New Jersey Department of Environmental Protection
Division of Fish and Wildlife
501 East State Street
PO Box 400
Trenton, NJ 08625-0400
(609) 292-2965
http://www.state.nj.us/dep/fgw

New Mexico Department of Game and Fish
PO Box 25112
Santa Fe, NM 87507
(800) 862-9310
http://www.wildlife.state.nm.us

New York State Department of Environmental Conservation
Division of Fish, Wildlife & Marine Resources
625 Broadway
Albany, NY 12233-4750
(518) 402-8924
http://www.dec.state.ny.us/website/dfwmr

North Carolina Wildlife Resources Commission
Division of Wildlife Management
512 North Salisbury Street
Raleigh, NC 27604-1188
(919) 733-3391
http://www.ncwildlife.org

North Dakota Game and Fish Department
100 North Bismarck Expressway
Bismarck, ND 58501-5095
(701) 328-6300
http://www.state.nd.us/gnf

Ohio Department of Natural Resources
Division of Wildlife
1840 Belcher Drive
Columbus, OH 43224-1300
(614) 265-6300
http://www.dnr.state.oh.us/wildlife

Oklahoma Department of Wildlife Conservation
Wildlife Division
1801 North Lincoln Boulevard
Oklahoma City, OK 73105
(405) 521-2739
http://www.wildlifedepartment.com

Table 20.8.   *(continued)*

Oregon Department of Fish and Wildlife
2501 SW First Avenue
PO Box 59
Portland, OR 97207
(503) 872-5310
http://www.dfw.state.or.us

Pennsylvania Department of Conservation and Natural Resources
7th Floor Rachel Carson State Office Building
PO Box 8767
Harrisburg, PA 17105-8767
(717) 787-2869
http://www.dcnr.state.pa.us

Puerto Rico Department of Natural Resources and the Environment
Pda. 3_, Avenida Muñoz Rivera
Puerta de Tierra, Puerto Rico 00906-6600
(787) 724-8774 Ext. 2267
http://www.gobierno.pr/drna

Rhode Island Department of Environmental Management
Division of Fish and Wildlife
235 Promenade Street
Providence, RI 02908-5767
(401) 222-6800
http://www.dem.ri.gov/

Samoa
American Samoa Office of Marine Wildlife Resources
American Samoa Government
Pago Pago, American Samoa 96799
(684) 633-4456
http://www.samoanet.com/asg/asgomwr97.html

South Carolina Department of Natural Resources
Rembert C. Dennis Building
1000 Assembly Street
Columbia, SC 29201
http://www.dnr.state.sc.us

South Dakota Department of Game, Fish & Parks
523 East Capitol Avenue
Pierre, SD 57501-3182
(605) 773-3381
http://www.sdgfp.info

Tennessee Wildlife Resources Agency
Ellington Agricultural Center
PO Box 40747
Nashville, TN 37204
(615) 781-6552
http://www.state.tn.us/twra

Texas Parks and Wildlife
4200 Smith School Road
Austin, TX 78744
(800) 792-1112
http://www.tpwd.state.tx.us

Utah Division of Wildlife Resources
1594 W. North Temple
PO Box 146301
Salt Lake City, UT 84114-6301
(801) 538-4700
http://www.wildlife.utah.gov/

Vermont Fish and Wildlife Department
Law Enforcement Division
103 South Main Street
Waterbury, VT 05671-0501
(802) 241-3700
http://www.vtfishandwildlife.com

Virgin Islands (US) Department of Planning & Natural Resources
Division of Environmental Protection
Cyril E. King Airport, 2nd Floor
St. Thomas, US Virgin Islands 00802
(340) 774-3320
http://www.viczmp.com/DPNR%20Divisions.htm

Virginia Department of Game and Inland Fisheries
4010 West Broad Street
Richmond, VA 23230
(804) 367-1000
http://www.dgif.state.va.us

Washington Department of Fish and Wildlife
600 Capitol Way North
Olympia, WA 98501-1091
(360) 902-2200
http://www.wdfw.wa.gov

West Virginia Division of Natural Resources
Wildlife Resources Section
State Capitol Building 3, Room 812
Charleston WV 25305
(304) 558-2771
http://www.dnr.state.wv.us

Wisconsin Department of Natural Resources
101 South Webster Street
PO Box 7921
Madison, WI 53707-7921
(608) 266-2621
http://www.dnr.state.wi.us

Wyoming Game and Fish Department
5400 Bishop Boulevard
Cheyenne, WY 82006
(307) 777-4600
http://gf.state.wy.us/

written primarily to assure that animals intended for use in research, exhibits, and as pets are provided humane care and treatment. It applies to both housing and transport. It is also intended to prevent the use or sale of stolen pets. The document states that it is essential for Congress to regulate the transport, purchase, sale, housing, care, handling, and treatment of animals. Research facilities are required by this act to establish committees to oversee all activities with animals. All animal dealers and exhibitors are required to obtain a valid license.

The Animal Welfare Regulations are found in the Code of Federal Regulations (Title 9—Animals and Animal Products; Chapter 1—Animal and Plant Health Inspection Service; Department of Agriculture; Subchapter A—Animal Welfare; Parts 1-4). These regulations are intended to set forth the rules and procedures that must be followed by animal dealers, exhibitors, and animal research facilities. The details of the required license and the process by which animal dealers and exhibitors must obtain them are set forth. The registration requirements for animal research facilities are presented. Also included is a description of the Institutional Animal Care and Use Committee (IACUC), which is required to be appointed by the Chief Executive Officer of a research facility to assess animal programs, facilities, and procedures.

I recommend that animal dealers, exhibitors, and animal research facilities consider the proper care, husbandry, and transport of invertebrates as they would with any vertebrate species. Inquiries should be made to local USDA-APHIS officials about dealer licenses. Although currently individual IACUCs may not require prior approval for research projects using live invertebrates, I believe that research and use proposals should be submitted as they would for vertebrate species. Some invertebrate taxa in the United Kingdom require an IACUC protocol.

Office International des Epizooties

This is an international organization of member country governments that disseminates information on the worldwide status of current animal diseases. There are 164 member countries that each report on the diseases within their own territories. Information is made available through weekly, bimonthly, and annual publications. They publish a scientific journal, *Scientific*

and Technical Review, three times per year. The Office International des Epizooties (OIE) offers expertise to member countries on animal disease control and prevention to help stop the spread of disease to other countries. They maintain guidelines on important socioeconomic and public health-related animal diseases that impact international trade of animals and animal products. Both the International Animal Health Code, which addresses terrestrial animals, and the Aquatic Animal Health Code specifically note invertebrate diseases. There are five reportable diseases of bees listed in the former and 19 reportable diseases of various aquatic invertebrates in the latter (Table 20.1). For more information on the OIE, visit its Web site:

http://www.oie.int/eng/en_index.htm, or contact

The Central Bureau
12, rue de Prony
75017, Paris, France
Tel: 33-(0) 1 44 15 1888
Fax: 33-(0) 1 42 67 0987
http://www.oie.int

If any of these diseases are discovered or suspected in animals within the United States, immediately contact your local USDA-APHIS Veterinary Services (VS) office (Table 20.9).

Summary

There are many laws and regulations to be considered before obtaining and keeping invertebrates. Different activities such as collection, importation, exportation, interstate transportation, and containment may in some cases be addressed by different or multiple regulating agencies. With their high potential to become established plant pests, USDA-APHIS-PPQ regulations will probably become more stringent in the future. Prior to obtaining a species that is a potential pest, always contact the appropriate USDA and state agencies. Scientific studies involving live invertebrates should be designed with the same diligence as studies using vertebrate species. Proper permits, quality care, and secure containment should be the hallmarks of any activities with animals, backbone or not.

Table 20.9. Contact information for local state offices of USDA-APHIS-VS veterinarians (including Puerto Rico)

Alabama	Arizona
USDA, APHIS, VS	USDA, APHIS, VS
PO Box 70429	1400 East Southern Avenue, Suite 245
Montgomery, AL 36107	Tempe, AZ 85282
(334) 223-7141	(480) 491-1002
Alaska	**Arkansas**
USDA, APHIS, VS	USDA, APHIS, VS
2604 12th Court, SW, Suite B	1200 Cherry Brook Drive, Suite 300
Olympia, WA 98502	Little Rock, AR 72211
(360) 753-9430	(501) 224-9515

Table 20.9. (*continued*)

California
USDA, APHIS, VS
9580 Micron Avenue, Suite E
Sacramento, CA 95827
(916) 857-6170

Colorado
USDA, APHIS, VS
755 Parfet Street, Suite 136
Lakewood, CO 80215
(303) 231-5385

Connecticut
USDA, APHIS, VS
160 Worcester-Providence Road
Sutton Square Plaza, Suite 20
Sutton, MA 01590-9998
(508) 865-1421, 22

Delaware
USDA, APHIS, VS
1598 Whitehall Road, Suite A
Annapolis, MD 21401
(410) 349-9708

District of Columbia
USDA, APHIS, VS
1598 Whitehall Road, Suite A
Annapolis, MD 21401
(410) 349-9708

Florida
USDA, APHIS, VS
7022 NW 10th Place
Gainesville, FL 32605-3147
(352) 333-3120

Georgia
USDA, APHIS, VS
1498 Klondike Road, Suite 200
Conyers, GA 30094
(770) 922-7860

Hawaii
USDA, APHIS, VS
2604 12th Court, SW, Suite B
Olympia, WA 98502
(360) 753-9430

Idaho
USDA, APHIS, VS
9158 West Black Eagle Drive
Boise, ID 83709
(208) 378-5631

Illinois
USDA, APHIS, VS
2815 Old Jacksonville Road, Suite 104
Springfield, IL 62704
(217) 241-6689

Indiana
USDA, APHIS, VS
6960 Corporate Drive
Indianapolis, IN 46278-1928
(317) 290-3300

Iowa
USDA, APHIS, VS
Federal Building, Room 891
210 Walnut Street
Des Moines, IA 50309
(515) 284-4140

Kansas
USDA, APHIS, VS
1947 NW Topeka Boulevard, Suite F
Topeka, KS 66608
(785) 235-2365

Kentucky
USDA, APHIS, VS
PO Box 399
Frankfort, KY 40602
(502) 227-9651

Louisiana
USDA, APHIS, VS
5825 Florida Boulevard, Room 1140
Baton Rouge, LA 70806-9985
(225) 389-0436

Maine
USDA, APHIS, VS
160 Worcester-Providence Road
Sutton Square Plaza, Suite 20
Sutton, MA 01590-9998
(508) 865-1421, 22

Maryland
USDA, APHIS, VS
1598 Whitehall Road, Suite A
Annapolis, MD 21401
(410) 349-9708

Massachusetts
USDA, APHIS, VS
160 Worcester-Providence Road
Sutton Square Plaza, Suite 20
Sutton, MA 01590-9998
(508) 865-1421, 22

Michigan
USDA, APHIS, VS
3001 Coolidge Road, Suite 325
East Lansing, MI 48823
(517) 324-5290

Minnesota
USDA, APHIS, VS
251 Starkey Street
Bolander Building, Suite 229
St. Paul, MN 55107
(651) 290-3691

(*continued*)

Table 20.9. *(continued)*

Mississippi
USDA, APHIS, VS
345 Keyway Street
Flowood, MS 39232
(601) 965-4307

Missouri
USDA, APHIS, VS
PO Box 104418
Jefferson City, MO 65110-4418
(573) 636-3116

Montana
USDA, APHIS, VS
208 North Montana Avenue, Suite 101
Helena, MT 59601-3837
(406) 449-5407

New Hampshire
USDA, APHIS, VS
160 Worcester-Providence Road
Sutton Square Plaza, Suite 20
Sutton, MA 01590-9998
(508) 865-1421, 22

Nebraska
USDA, APHIS, VS
PO Box 81866
Lincoln, NE 68501
(402) 434-2300

Nevada
USDA, APHIS, VS
9580 Micron Avenue, Suite E
Sacramento, CA 95827
(916) 857-6170

New Jersey
USDA, APHIS, VS
Mercer Corporate Park
320 Corporate Boulevard
Robbinsville, NJ 08691-1598
(609) 259-8387

New Mexico
USDA, APHIS, VS
6200 Jefferson Street, NE, Suite 117
Albuquerque, NM 87109
(505) 761-3160

New York
USDA, APHIS, VS
One Winners Circle, Suite 100
Export/Area Office
Albany, NY 12205
(518) 453-0187

North Carolina
USDA, APHIS, VS
930 Main Campus Drive, Suite 200
Raleigh, NC 27606
(919) 716-5955

North Dakota
USDA, APHIS, VS
3509 Miriam Avenue, Suite B
Bismarck, ND 58501
(701) 250-4210

Ohio
USDA, APHIS, VS
12927 Stonecreek Drive
Pickerington, OH 43147
(614) 469-5602

Oklahoma
USDA, APHIS, VS
4020 North Lincoln Boulevard, Suite 101
Oklahoma City, OK 73105
(405) 427-9413

Oregon
USDA, APHIS, VS
530 Center Street, NE, Suite 335
Salem, OR 97301
(503) 399-5871

Pennsylvania
USDA, APHIS, VS
2301 North Cameron Street, Room 412
Harrisburg, PA 17110
(717) 782-3442

Puerto Rico
USDA, APHIS, VS
IBM Building
654 Munoz Rivera Avenue, Suite 700
Hato Rey, PR 00918
(787) 766-6050

Rhode Island
USDA, APHIS, VS
160 Worcester-Providence Road
Sutton Square Plaza, Suite 20
Sutton, MA 01590-9998
(508) 865-1421, 22

South Carolina
USDA, APHIS, VS
9600 Two Notch Road, Suite 10
Columbia, SC 29229
(803) 788-1919

South Dakota
USDA, APHIS, VS
314 South Henry, Suite 100
Pierre, SD 57501-0640
(605) 224-6186

Tennessee
USDA, APHIS, VS
PO Box 110950
Nashville, TN 37222
(615) 781-5310

Table 20.9. *(continued)*

Texas
USDA, APHIS, VS
Thornberry Building, Room 220
903 San Jacinto Boulevard
Austin, TX 78701
(512) 916-5551

Utah
USDA, APHIS, VS
176 North 2200 West, Suite 230
Airport Park, Building #4
Salt Lake City, UT 84116
(801) 524-5010

Vermont
USDA, APHIS, VS
160 Worcester-Providence Road
Sutton Square Plaza, Suite 20
Sutton, MA 01590-9998
(508) 865-1421, 22

Virginia
USDA, APHIS, VS
Washington Building, 6th Floor
1100 Bank Street
Richmond, VA 23219
(804) 771-2774

Washington
USDA, APHIS, VS
2604 12th Court, SW, Suite B
Olympia, WA 98502
(360) 753-9430

West Virginia
USDA, APHIS, VS
12927 Stonecreek Drive
Pickerington, OH 43147
(614) 469-5602

Wisconsin
USDA, APHIS, VS
6510 Schroeder Road, Suite 2
Madison, WI 53711
(608) 270-4000

Wyoming
USDA, APHIS, VS
5353 Yellowstone Road, Room 209
Cheyenne, WY 82009
(307) 772-2186

Appendix 1

INVERTEBRATE NEOPLASMS

Esther C. Peters

Examples of neoplastic lesions of invertebrates are archived in the Registry of Tumors in Lower Animals (RTLA), Sterling, Virginia, U.S.A. The RTLA is a collection of more than 7500 pathological specimens and associated literature pertaining to cold-blooded vertebrate and invertebrate animals. In Table A1.1, the number of cases archived in the RTLA is in parentheses after each type of neoplasm, and a semicolon separates different types of neoplasms in a single animal. This information is based on diagnoses made by the RTLA pathologists from 1965 through 2004.

From 1965 to 2001, the sites for many of the neoplastic lesions were not specified in the RTLA database. The registry staff is reviewing and updating the diagnoses to "Lesion: Site" format.

Reports of other types of neoplasms and other affected species appear in the published literature, but examples have not been contributed to the RTLA collection. Diagnostic terminology for neoplasia in invertebrates is, in many cases, under debate and requires discussion and reinterpretation (for example, the calicoblastic epithelioma of corals is being reexamined). Taxa spellings and relationships also change with time; the most recent listings from the Integrated Taxonomic Information System (ITIS) are provided in Table A1.1. For more information, contact the RTLA at administrator@pathology-registry.org.

Table A1. Invertebrate neoplasms in the RTLA collection

Phylum Class Order	Family	Species	Common name	Neoplasm (number of cases in RTLA)
Annelida Oligochaeta Haplotaxida	Lumbricidae	*Lumbricus terrestris*	Earthworm	Myoblastoma: ventral coelom (1)
Arthropoda Insecta Blattodea	Blattidae	*Leucophaea maderae*	Madeira cockroach	Neoplasm: salivary reservoir (1)
Diptera	Drosophilidae	*Drosophila melanogaster*	Fruit fly	Cystocyte neoplasm: ovary (3) Ganglioneuroblastoma: brain (1) Lethal (1) malignant blood neoplasm, l(1)mbn: systemic (1) Lethal (2) malignant blood neoplasm, 1(2)mbn: systemic (1) Lethal (3) malignant blood neoplasm, 1(3)mbn: systemic (1) Neoplasm: imaginal disk (3)
Malacostraca Decapoda	Lithodidae	*Paralithodes platypus*	Blue king crab	Carcinoma: antennal gland (1)
		Paralithodes camtschatica	Red king crab	Carcinoma: hindgut (1)
	Palaemonidae	*Exopalaemon* (formerly *Palaemon) orientis*	Oriental prawn or grass shrimp	Carcinoma: embryo (2)
	Penaeidae	*Farfantepenaeus* (formerly *Penaeus) aztecus*	Brown shrimp	Papilloma: epidermis (1)
		Farfantepenaeus (formerly *Penaeus) californiensis*	California brown shrimp	Papilloma: epidermis (1)
		Litopenaeus (formerly *Penaeus) vannamei*	Mexican white shrimp	Hemopoietic sarcoma: multicentric (1)

(continued)

Table A1.   (*continued*)

Phylum
  Class
    Order
	Family	Species	Common name	Neoplasm (number of cases in RTLA)

Cnidaria				
Anthozoa				
Scleractinia	Acroporidae	*Acropora cervicornis*	Staghorn coral	Epithelioma: calicoblastic epidermis (conjectured) (5)
		Acropora formosa	Formosan staghorn coral	Epithelioma: calicoblastic epidermis (4)
		Acropora palmata	Elkhorn coral	Epithelioma: calicoblastic epidermis (10)
		Acropora valenciennesi	Coral	Epithelioma: calicoblastic epidermis (4)
		Montipora sp.	Coral	Epithelioma: calicoblastic epidermis (conjectured) (1)
Mollusca				
Bivalvia				
Myoida	Myidae	*Mya arenaria*	Softshell	Adenoma: kidney (4)
				Disseminated neoplasia: systemic (27)
				Germinoma: gonad (114)
				Germinoma: gonad; carcinoma: stomach (1)
				Germinoma: gonad; papilloma: epidermis (1)
				Germinoma: multicentric (15)
				Papilloma: gill (1)
		Mya truncata	Truncate softshell	Disseminated neoplasia: systemic (1)
				Fibrosarcoma: multicentric (1)
Mytiloida	Mytilidae	*Geukensia demissa*	Ribbed mussel	Teratoma: gonad (1)
		Modiolus modiolus	Northern horse mussel	Vesicular cell sarcoma: visceral mass (1)
		Mytilus edulis	Blue mussel	Carcinoma: gill (1)
				Disseminated neoplasia: systemic (8)
				Germinoma: gonad (1)
		Mytilus galloprovincialis	Mediterranean mussel	Disseminated neoplasia: systemic (2)
				Fibroma: gonad (1)
				Germinoma: gonad (1)
		Mytilus sp.	Mussel	Vesicular cell sarcoma: gonad (1)
		Mytilus trossulus	Foolish mussel	Disseminated neoplasia: systemic (4)
		Mytilus trossulus(?)	Foolish mussel(?)	Disseminated neoplasia: systemic (2)
		Mytilus trossulus/ galloprovincialis	Mussel	Myxoma: multicentric (1)
Ostreoida	Ostreidae	*Crassostrea gigas*	Pacific oyster	Disseminated neoplasia: systemic (2)
				Epithelioma: mantle (1)
				Ganglioneuroma: visceral mass (1)
				Gonadoblastoma: gonad (1)
		Crassostrea virginica	Eastern oyster	Adenocarcinoma in situ: intestine (3)
				Adenoma: intestine (1)
				Adenoma: kidney (1)
				Adenoma: rectum (1)
				Adenopapilloma: gill (1)
				Disseminated neoplasia: systemic (69)
				Fibroma: blood vessel wall (1)
				Fibroma: gonad (1)
				Germinoma: gonad (3)
				Gonadoblastoma: gonad (2)
				Neuroblastoma: visceral ganglion (1)
				Papilloma: gill (1)
				Sarcoma: visceral mass (1)
		Ostrea conchaphila	Olympia oyster	Disseminated neoplasia: systemic (6)
		Ostrea edulis	Edible oyster	Disseminated neoplasia: systemic (14)
		Ostrea sandvicensis	Sandwich Island oyster	Disseminated neoplasia: systemic (1)
		Saccostrea glomerata (formerly *commercialis*)	Sydney rock oyster	Disseminated neoplasia: systemic (4)
				Papilloma: mantle (33)
				Germinoma: gonad (21)
		Tiostrea chilensis	Bluff oyster	Disseminated neoplasia: systemic (1)
	Pectinidae	*Argopecten irradians*	Bay scallop	Germinoma: gonad (1)

Table A1. (continued)

Phylum Class Order	Family	Species	Common name	Neoplasm (number of cases in RTLA)
		Pecten sp.	Scallop	Disseminated neoplasia: systemic (1)
Veneroida	Cardiidae	*Cerastoderma* (formerly *Cardium*) *edule*	Edible dwarf cockle	Adenoma: digestive gland (1) Disseminated neoplasia: systemic (2) Disseminated neoplasia: systemic; germinoma: gonad (1) Germinoma: gonad (1)
		Cerastoderma (formerly *Cardium*) *glaucum*	Cockle	Disseminated neoplasia: systemic (1)
	Dreissenidae	*Arctica islandica*	Ocean quahog	Disseminated neoplasia: systemic (1) Germinoma: gonad (1)
	Mactridae	*Spisula solidissima*	Atlantic surf clam	Myoma: foot (1) Neurofibroma: foot (1) Mesothelioma: heart (1)
	Tellinidae	*Macoma balthica*	Baltic macoma	Carcinoma: gill (2) Carcinoma: gill v. disseminated neoplasia: systemic (4)
		Macoma calcarea	Chalky macoma	Germinoma: gonad; disseminated neoplasia: systemic (1)
		Macoma inquinata	Stained macoma	Disseminated neoplasia: systemic (1)
		Macoma nasuta	Bent-nose macoma	Disseminated neoplasia: systemic (1)
	Veneridae	*Mercenaria mercenaria*	Northern quahog	Germinoma: gonad (13)
		Mercenaria mercenaria/ campechiensis	Northern × southern quahog (hybrid)	Germinoma: gonad (5)
		Tapes (= *Ruditapes*) *decussata*	Carpet shell clam	Disseminated neoplasia: systemic (5)
Cephalopoda				
Decabrachia	Sepiidae	*Sepia officinalis*	Common cuttlefish	Iridophoroma: dermis (1)
Octopoda	Octopodidae	*Octopus vulgaris*	Atlantic octopus	Fibropapilloma: mantle (1)
Gastropoda				
Archaeogas-tropoda	Haliotididae	*Haliotis* (formerly *Nordotis*) *discus*	Japanese abalone	Glioma: pleuropedal nerve cord (1)
Architaenio-glossa (formerly Mesogas-tropoda)	Ampullariidae	*Ampullarius australis*	Applesnail	Papilloma: epidermis; adenoma: digestive gland (1)
Polyplacophora				
Neoloricata	Chitonidae	*Chiton tuberculatus*	West Indian green chiton	Papilloma: gastrointestinal tract (1)
Platyhelminthes				
Trematoda				
Azygiida (formerly Digenea)	Azygiidae	*Otodistomum plunketi*	Trematode	Ganglioneuroblastoma: nerve cord, parenchyma (1)
Turbellaria				
Tricladida	Dugesiidae; Planariidae	*Dugesia; Crenobia* spp.	Planarians	Papilloma: epidermis (7)

RTLA, Registry of Tumors in Lower Animals.

Appendix 2

DISEASES OF INVERTEBRATES NOTIFIABLE TO THE WORLD ORGANIZATION FOR ANIMAL HEALTH (OIE)*

Mollusk Diseases

Infection with

Bonamia ostreae
Bonamia exitiosus
Mikrocytos roughleyi
Haplosporidium nelsoni
Marteilia refringens
Marteilia sydneyi
Mikrocytos mackini
Perkinsus marinus
Perkinsus olseni/atlanticus
Haplosporidium costale
Candidatus ✕*enohaliotis californiensis*

Crustacean Diseases

Taura syndrome
White spot disease
Yellowhead disease
Tetrahedral baculovirosis (*Baculovirus penaei*)
Spherical baculovirosis (*Penaeus monodon*-type baculovirus)
Infectious hypodermal and hematopoietic necrosis
Crayfish plague (*Aphanomyces astaci*)
Spawner-isolated mortality virus disease

Insect Diseases

Acarapisosis of honeybees
American foulbrood of honeybees
European foulbrood of honeybees
Varroosis of honeybees
Tropilaelap infestation of honeybees

*From the OIE (Office International des Epizooties) Web site: www.oie.int/eng/maladies/en_classification.htm (December, 2004).

Appendix 3

EUTHANASIA

Michael J. Murray

Little is written about euthanasia of invertebrates. One might suggest that euthanasia regarding these animals is a non sequitur, particularly in the more primitive groups (Porifera and Coelenterata), given the absence or limited development of a nervous system (Lewbart, 2005). This limited neural development raises the question as to whether invertebrates feel pain or experience distress. However, invertebrates can respond to stimuli that are regarded as noxious. Therefore, as an advocate for the well-being of animals, it is incumbent upon the veterinary profession to investigate and provide recommendations to the scientific community regarding the handling of this diverse group of creatures. At the very least, one should assure that invertebrates are not euthanized cavalierly; there should always be some consideration of the life of the animal.

In some invertebrate taxa, the method applied for euthanasia may be an extension of the standard techniques used to preserve the specimen for scientific study. In this case, the compounds employed tend to cause a relaxation of the animal, do not appear to destroy its architecture, and therefore may be interpreted as appropriate. In some instances, information concerning the anesthesia or immobilization of the animal group has been extrapolated and used as the technique for rendering the animal unconscious, and freezing or destruction of the brain or ganglia leads to death (Table A2.1 and specific chapters in this book).

The majority of the invertebrates described in Table A3.1 are aquatic. As a result, the use of immersion or bath-type compounds predominates. As actual death in many of these species may be difficult to confirm, it is recommended that an irreversible method for destruction of the animal follow anesthesia. In most cases, freezing, boiling, or immersion in alcohol or formalin is appropriate after the animal is determined to be nonresponsive after administration of other agents, such as magnesium chloride. However, freezing and boiling are not appropriate when tissues need to be submitted for histopathology.

In the terrestrial species, use of an inhalant, such as isoflurane, appears to produce adequate anesthesia. Again, death may be difficult to confirm, and methods such as freezing or alcohol/formalin immersion are recommended as second steps that ensure death. In either case (aquatic or terrestrial animal), the specific methodology applied must be consistent with the end use of the animal. For example, freezing would be inappropriate for specimens to be subjected to histological examination or formalin immersion inappropriate when microbiological sampling is anticipated.

As scientific endeavors are subjected to a justifiable increased scrutiny, it becomes incumbent upon the veterinary community to establish standards for the humane killing of animals, even those traditionally considered primitive, such as the invertebrates. It is hoped that further investigation into methodology will follow to assure that invertebrates are handled with the respect due any living creature.

References

Araujo R, Remon JM, Moreno D, Ramos MA. 1995. Relaxing techniques for freshwater mollusks: Trials for evaluation of different methods. Malacologia 36:29–41.

Battison A, MacMillan R, MacKenzie A, Rose P, Cawthorn R, Horney B. 2000. Use of injectable potassium chloride for euthanasia of American lobsters (*Homarus americanus*). Comp Med 50:545–550.

Boyle PR. 1991. The UFAW Handbook on the Care and Management of Cephalopods in the Laboratory. Universities Federation for Animal Welfare, Herts, UK.

Brusca RC. 1980. Common Intertidal Invertebrates of the Gulf of California, 2nd edition. University of Arizona Press, Tucson.

Cooper JE. 2001. Invertebrate anesthesia. Vet Clin North Am Exotic Anim Pract 4:57–67.

Lewbart GA. 2005. Aquatic invertebrate medicine. In: Proceeding of the North American Veterinary Conference, Orlando, FL, pp 1158–1162.

Messenger JB, Nixon M, Ryan KP. 1985. Magnesium chloride as an anesthetic for cephalopods. Comp Biochem Physiol [C] 82:203–205.

Reilly JS, ed. 2001. Euthanasia of Animals Used for Scientific Purposes, 2nd edition. Australian and New Zealand Council for the Care of Animals in Research and Teaching, Wellington, New Zealand, pp 85–86.

Roper CFE, Sweeney MJ. 1983. Technique for fixation and preservation of cephalopods. Mem Nat Mus Vic 44:28–47.

Scimeca JM, Oestmann DJ. 1995. Selected diseases of captive and laboratory reared cephalopods. Proc Int Assoc Aquat Anim Med 27:79–88.

Table A3.1. Acceptable methods of euthanatizing invertebrates

Taxon	Preferred method	Provisional method	References
Porifera (sponges)	10% buffered formalin	70% Ethanol	Brusca, 1980
Coelenterates: (comb jellies, coral, anemones)	Magnesium chloride	70% Ethanol 5% Formalin	Brusca, 1980
Gastropod mollusks (snails, slugs, sea hares)	Carbon dioxide in water Magnesium sulfate: 20%–30% added slowly	70% Alcohol added slowly 10% Formalin added slowly	Brusca, 1980 Brusca, 1980
Bivalve mollusks (clams, mussels, oysters)	Magnesium sulfate: 20%–30% added slowly	Submerge in boiling water after presedation with magnesium chloride	Brusca 1980; Araujo et al., 1995
Cephalopod mollusks (octopus, squid, cuttlefish)	Magnesium chloride MS-222	Gradually cool to 1.7°C and then freeze after presedation with magnesium chloride	Roper and Sweeney, 1983; Messenger et al., 1985; Boyle, 1991; Scimeca and Oestmann, 1995; Reilly, 2001; Lewbart, 2005
	Anesthesia followed by brain destruction	Brain destruction or decapitation	
Annelids (segmented worms)	Carbon dioxide in water MS-222 (0.5%)	Magnesium sulfate (7.3 g/100 mL water)	Brusca, 1980; Battison et al., 2000
Crustaceans (crabs, lobster, insects, spiders)	Isoflurane MS-222 Clove oil (0.125 mL/L) Cooling and then freezing: KCl, 100 mg/100 g into hemolymph	Immobilization followed by destruction of brain or ganglia	Battison et al., 2000; Cooper, 2001; Reilly, 2001
Echinoderms (sea stars, urchins, sea cucumbers)	Magnesium chloride	Add slowly to water: 50%–60% Ethanol 5% Formalin	Brusca, 1980

INDEX

A

AAS. *See* American Arachnological Society
(AAS)
Abalone, 65
black, 71, 74, 75, Color Plate 5.17
red, 67, 71
Withering syndome in, 71
Abdomen, spiders and, 166
Aber disease, 105, 106, Color Plate 7.12
Aboral orientation, echinoderms and, 245
Absorption anesthetics, insects and, 216
Acanthaster planci, 31
Acanthocephala, 4
Acaricides, 156, 159
Acarii mites, 159
Acaropsis woodi, 211
Accessory fertilization cells (AFCs), 237
Acclimation, postshipment, coelenterates
and, 48
Ace Quick Plug, corals and, 43–44
Acetic acid baths, horseshoe crabs and, 139
Achaeranea sp., 145
Achatina fulica, 282
Achetta domestica, 147
Acinarium, bees and, 210
Acinetobacter calcoaceticus, 176
Acoel flatworms, 53
Acoelomorpha, 53
Acoels, 53
Acroceridae spider flies, spiders and, 159
Acropora, 24, 25, 30, 33, 47
Acropora microphthalma, 32
Acropora palmata, 34, 36, 38
Acropora plana, 44
Acropora sp., 39, 42, 47, Color Plate 3.15
Acroporidae, coral bleaching and, 32–33
Acroporids, 34–35, 36
Actinaria, 24
Actinolaimus, 230
Actinopyga spp., 252
Actinula, 20
Adelea spp., 230
Adenophorea, 224
Adenovirus, *Hydra,* coelenterates and, 35
Adhesisagitta hispida, 237, 239
Adult male spiders, death of, 160

Advances in Insect Physiology, 206–207
Aebutina binotata, 145
Aeolosoma travancorense, 126
Aequipecten irradians concentricus, 96
Aerococcus viridans, 186
Aerococcus viridans var. *homari,* 185
Aeromonas hydrophila, 124, 229
Aeromonas salmonicida, 249
Aeromonas sp., 127–129
AFCs. *See* Accessory fertilization cells
(AFCs)
African baboon spiders, 143
African carpenter bees, 210
African emperor scorpions, 170
African funnel web spiders, 145
African millipedes, giant, 282
African snails, giant, 282
Agar, marine brain–heart infusion, 272
Agaricia agaricites, 37
Agaricia lamarcki, 37
Agariciidae, 33
Agelena consociata, 145
Agelenids, 145
Aggregata, 86
Aggregata sp., 86
Aggressiveness
of corals, 29
intraspecific, coelenterates and, 29
Agriculture, U.S. Department of, 277–284
Aiptasia anemones, 31
Aiptasia pallida, 23
AK1-S, corals and, 33
Alcohol, ethyl, as fixative, 268
Alcyonarians, 46
Algae
blue-green, 8, 31
brown, 30–31
brown hair, 31
bubble, 30
coralline, 31
green, 30
green hair, 30
nematodes and, 221
red, 31
red hair, 31
wire, 31

Algal competition, coelenterates and, 29–31
Algal overgrowth, corals and, 29–30
Algal scrubbing, 30
Allometric scaling and dosage selection,
spiders and, 164
Alonia macrophysa, 30
Alopecia, opisthosoma, 160
a-ecdysone, nematodes and, 223
Amazonian leech, 126
Amblypygi, 144
Amebocytes, 133, 247
American Arachnological Society (AAS),
144
American cockroaches, 215
American horseshoe crabs, 133, 134
American lobsters, 179, 185, 186, 187, 190
American oysters, 105
American Tarantula Society (ATS), 144
Ammonia
coelenterates and, 26
jellyfish sting and, 25
sponges and, 8
Amoco Cadiz supertanker wreck, 119
Amoebiasis, 40
Amoebic trophozoites, 40
Amoebocytes, 9, 265–266
Amphiopholis squamata, 250, 253
Amphipods, 15, 179
Amphiurophilus amphiurae, 251
Amphiurophilus squamata, 251
Ampullae, turbellarians and, 58
Amputation, limb autotomy as technique of,
spiders and, 161–162
Anadara trapezia, 93
Anadonta anatina, 95
Anal cone, crinoids and, 247
Analgesia
arrowworms and, 242
centipedes and, 202
cephalopods and, 86–87
chaetognaths and, 242
coelenterates and, 42–43
crustaceans and, 191–192
gastropods and, 74, 76–77
insects and, 215–216
millipedes and, 202